ANNUAL PROGRESS IN CHILD PSYCHIATRY AND CHILD DEVELOPMENT 1994

ANNUAL PROGRESS IN CHILD PSYCHIATRY AND CHILD DEVELOPMENT 1994

Edited by

MARGARET E. HERTZIG, M.D.

Associate Professor of Psychiatry
Cornell University Medical College

and

ELLEN A. FARBER, Ph.D.

Assistant Professor of Psychology in Psychiatry
Cornell University Medical College

BRUNNER/MAZEL *Publishers* ● New York

Library of Congress Card No. 68-23452
ISBN 0-87630-744-6
ISSN 0066-4030

Published by
BRUNNER/MAZEL, Inc.
19 Union Square West
New York, New York 10003

Manufactured in the United States of America
10   9   8   7   6   5   4   3   2   1

CONTENTS

v

ANNUAL PROGRESS IN CHILD PSYCHIATRY AND CHILD DEVELOPMENT 1994

Part I

DEVELOPMENTAL ISSUES

The papers in this section cover diverse topics including cognitive assessment in infancy, emotional development and peer acceptance in preschool and middle childhood, and self-esteem in adolescence and adulthood.

The predictability of childhood intelligence from infant assessments has long been of interest. In the last decade, it has been suggested that habituation or recognition memory paradigms with infants yield greater predictability of childhood IQ than traditional infant measures. In the first paper in this section, McCall and Carriger examine the evidence for predictability by conducting a meta-analysis using 31 samples from 23 studies. Habituation is defined as the decrement of attention or responsiveness to a repeatedly presented stimulus. It is assessed by the number of presentations of the standard stimulus that are necessary for the infant to look 50 percent as long as he looked on the first presentation of that stimulus. Recognition memory is assessed by presenting for five to 30 seconds a pair of identical stimuli for familiarization. Then two brief test trials (five to 20 seconds each) are presented. They consist of a simultaneous presentation of the familiar and a completely novel stimulus with the left-right positions reversed on the second trial. The ratio of looking time to the novel divided by the total looking time to both familiar plus novel stimuli during the two test trials is recorded.

Both habituation and recognition memory reflect the infant's ability to encode a stimulus into memory, to recognize that stimulus as familiar, and to cease looking at the familiar. Proponents of these paradigms suggest that speed and accuracy of encoding a stimulus into memory may be related more to capacities measured by childhood standardized intelligence tests than to the action and imitation skills measured on standardized infant tests.

The meta-analysis indicates that although predictions of childhood IQ based on habituation and recognition memory are consistently higher than for standardized infant tests, they are not consistently higher than predictions based on parental education and socioeconomic status. The average, weighted, normalized coefficient over all samples was .39. There was no significant difference in predictability between the two paradigms. Although predictions were higher for risk (low SES, preterm or disordered infants) than for nonrisk samples, prediction was not the product of a few extremely disordered infants. The level of prediction was remarkably consistent over the outcome ages of two to eight years. The authors conclude that it is not clear what process accounts for the significant associations. It may be skill at encoding, memory, or the disposition to inhibit responding to

1

familiar stimuli and stimuli of minor prominence. Future research is needed to determine how these early skills are important for, or a part of, later intelligence.

Social acceptance, particularly as defined by sociometric measurement, has been widely studied as an important predictor of later adaptation. The next two papers present new approaches to exploring correlates of sociometric status. Eisenberg and colleagues use concepts from the temperament and coping literature to examine social competence in preschoolers. The goal of the study was to determine the degree to which children's social competence could be predicted from emotionality (intensity and negative affect) and regulation (attentional regulation and mode of coping). Attentional regulation is a somewhat narrower construct than coping. Both involve controlling internal emotional arousal and the input of emotion-producing stimuli. These concepts are usually applied to problem behaviors and not to normative development. Multiple informants and multiple measures were used with a sample of 45 girls and 48 boys from five different classrooms. Ratings of temperament and social skills were provided by teachers, observers, and parents twice during the school year. Children completed a sociometric measure.

The authors hypothesized that the relationship between emotionality and social competence would be moderated by the ability to regulate emotion and behavior. Efforts to tease apart the influences of aspects of temperament in the development of social competence were hindered in part by the overlap between emotionality and regulation. However, there were differences among observers in the degree to which they responded to the temperament constructs. Teachers judged children's general social skills primarily based on their regulation, whereas peers' sociometric nominations gave an equal role to ratings of regulation and reactivity. There were also gender differences in the association of temperament with social skills. For boys more than for girls, emotionality, attentional control, and coping were all important correlates of social competence. Based on these preliminary results, the authors propose that variations in emotionality lead to differential acquisition of coping, which in turn affects social functioning and social acceptance.

The next paper also uses sociometric status as an indicator of adaptation. Parker and Asher extend the concept of group acceptance by focusing on friendship, an aspect of social development that has received little attention. In a sample of 881 third through fifth graders, they assessed dyadic friendships, revised a measure of friendship quality, compared friendships of accepted and low-accepted children, and examined the association of friendship quality with loneliness. High-accepted and average-accepted children were about twice as likely to have a best friend as low-accepted children. However, a third of the high-accepted children did not have a best friend; that is, the child they selected as a best friend did not name them among their list of three friends. Many low-accepted children did have friends. Measurement of children's self-reports of friendship quality revealed differences in friendship quality based on acceptance and gender. Both friendship adjustment and peer group acceptance had an association with loneliness. Results indicate that friendship is an area worthy of investigation that can enhance our understanding of peer acceptance and individual adaptation.

The final paper in this section tracks changes in self-esteem across the important transition from teenager to young adult and examines the personality correlates of high and low self-esteem. Block and Robins present a subset of data from the Berkeley Longitudinal study based on a sample of 47 girls and 44 boys assessed as high school freshmen and seniors and 5-years-post-high school graduates. Subjects completed Q-sorts for the real and ideal self. Congruence between perceived-self and ideal-self descriptions was considered indicative of high levels of self-esteem. They found gender differences in the development and levels of self-esteem. Males had higher self-esteem than females at every age, with males' self-esteem increasing over time and females' self-esteem decreasing over time. For females, self-esteem was reasonably well-established by adolescence, while for males, self-esteem was still evolving through adulthood. Examining the personality correlates of self-esteem indicated that changes in self-esteem were associated with an other orientation in females and a self orientation in males. Conclusions address the issue of consistency and change throughout the life course.

1

A Meta-Analysis of Infant Habituation and Recognition Memory Performance as Predictors of Later IQ

Robert B. McCall and Michael S. Carriger

University of Pittsburgh

A meta-analytic review of the literature on infant habituation and recognition memory performance as predictors of later IQ suggests several conclusions: (1) Habituation and recognition memory assessments made on a variety of risk and nonrisk samples in the first year of life predict later IQ assessed between 1 and 8 years of age with a weighted (for N) average of normalized correlations of .36 or a raw median correlation of .45 (2) The size of the predictive correlation is essentially the same for habituation and for recognition memory paradigms. (3) This prediction phenomenon is not obviously associated solely with one laboratory, one particular infant response measure, or a few extremely disordered infants. (4) The level of prediction to childhood IQ is substantial given the reliability of the infant measures. (5) Predictions are somewhat higher for risk than for nonrisk samples. (6) Predictions are consistently higher than for standardized infant tests of general development for nonrisk but not for risk samples, and they are not consistently higher than predicting from parental education and socioeconomic status or a few other infant behaviors for nonrisk samples. (8) Coefficients may be higher when the predicting assessments are made between 2 and 8 months of age than earlier or later, but prediction coefficients are remarkably consistent across the observed outcome age period of 2–8 years.

Reprinted with permission from *Child Development,* 1993, Vol. 64, 57–79. Copyright © 1993 by the Society for Research in Child Development, Inc.

The authors thank John Colombo, Jerome Kagan, and several psychology faculty and graduate students at the University of Pittsburgh for their detailed comments on an early draft of this paper; an unknown reviewer who suggested plotting the raw *r*'s; Cathy Kelley for preparing the manuscript endless times; and Trisha McCall for preparing some of the figures.

Prior to approximately 1960, intelligence, at least as reflected in scores within the normal range on standardized IQ tests, was considered stable, if not fixed, across the lifespan (Hunt, 1961). In 1961, Hunt questioned this assumption, suggesting that mentality was not fixed, at least not early in life. Subsequently, in the 1970s and early 1980s, several students of mental development emphasized the lack of stability in early mental test performance for normal samples (e.g., McCall, 1979; McCall, Hogarty, & Hurlburt, 1972) as well as for samples including at-risk and neurologically disordered infants (Kopp & McCall, 1982). This led to the conclusion that standardized tests of infant development did not predict later intelligence at useful levels until after 18 to 24 months of age for either nonrisk, at-risk, or some obviously disordered groups. This lack of stability, it was thought, was partly the result of profound qualitative changes in the nature of intelligence from infancy through childhood to adulthood (e.g., Kopp & McCall, 1982).

But the search for early predictors of later IQ continued (McCall, 1981), and recently habituation and recognition memory measured during the first year of life have been found to predict later IQ scores (e.g., Bornstein & Sigman, 1986). This finding suggests that while the sensorimotor capacities measured by standardized infant tests are not related conceptually or empirically to childhood intelligence, the encoding, storage, retrieval, discrimination, and recognition presumably measured by habituation and recognition memory tests may be related to the vocabulary, abstract reasoning, and memory skills assessed on childhood intelligence tests (e.g., Bornstein, 1985; Bornstein & Sigman, 1986; Colombo & Mitchell, 1988, 1991; Fagan, 1988; Fagan & Singer, 1983). The previous failure to predict, it was assumed, was simply a consequence of measuring the wrong attributes in infancy.

The Prediction Phenomenon

More specifically, *habituation* is defined as the decrement of attention or responsiveness to a repeatedly presented or continuously available stimulus (called the "standard" or "familiar" stimulus) that is not simply a consequence of sensory receptor fatigue. Currently, habituation is often measured by the number of presentations of the standard stimulus (presented for as long as an infant visually fixates it) that are necessary for the infant to look 50% as long as he or she looked on the first presentations(s) of that stimulus. However, the percent decrement in attention during familiarization, the total looking time during the familiarization period, or the response to a new stimulus presented after familiarization also have been used as the predicting measure (see Table 1). Presumably, rapid habituation reflects the infant's ability to quickly encode a stimulus into memory, to recognize the familiar stimulus when it is presented again, and to cease looking further at it.

TABLE 1

Studies and Sample Used in the Meta-Analyses

Authors (Lab Letter)	Sample Size	Included Preterm	Included Low SES	Included Disordered	Infant Age	Child Age	Predictor Measure	Outcome Measure	Correlation Coefficient
Habituation:									
Slater, Cooper, Rose, & Morrison, 1989 (S)	11 21	No No	⋮ ⋮	⋮ ⋮	6 mos. 3 mos.	8 yrs. 1 yr. 6 mos.	Mean length of fixation to novel stimulus (response recovery)	Wechsler Bayley	.61 .43
Sigman, Cohen, Beckwith, & Parmelee, 1986 (P)	91	Yes	Yes	Yes	Birth	8 yrs.	Total length of fixation to a redundant stimulus	Wechsler	.29
Bornstein, 1985 (B) ..	18	No	⋮	⋮	5 mos.	2 yrs.	Index-first fixation, total fixation, decrement in fixation to a redundant stimulus	Other	.55
O'Connor, Cohen, & Parmelee, 1984 (P) ...	28	Yes	Yes	Yes	4 mos.	5 yrs.	Change in heart rate to novel stimulus (response recovery)	Binet	.60
Bornstein, 1984 (B) ..	14	No	⋮	⋮	4 mos.	4 yrs.	Total length of fixation to a redundant stimulus	Wechsler	.54
Cohen & Parmelee, 1983 (P)	96	Yes	Yes	Yes	Birth	5 yrs.	Total length of fixation to a redundant stimulus	Binet	.29
Ruddy & Bornstein, 1982 (B)	20	No	No	No	4 mos.	1 yr.	Percent response decrement to a redundant stimulus	Bayley	.46

Continued

TABLE 1 (*cont.*)
Studies and Sample Used in the Meta-Analyses

Authors (Lab Letter)	Sample Size	Included Preterm	Included Low SES	Included Disordered	Infant Age	Child Age	Predictor Measure	Outcome Measure	Correlation Coefficient
Lewis & Brooks-Gunn, 1981 (L)	22	No	No	...	3 mos.	2 yrs.	Fixation to a novel stimulus (response recovery)	Bayley	.52
	57	No	Yes	...	3 mos.	2 yrs.		Bayley	.40
Miller et al., 1979 (M)	29	No	...	...	1,2,3 mos.	3 yrs. 3 mos.	Response decrement in first fixation	Language Comprehension	.39
Lewis, Goldberg, & Campbell, 1969 (L)	40	No	...	...	12 mos.	3 yrs. 8 mos.	Response decrement to a redundant stimulus	Binet	.39
Recognition memory: Rose, Feldman, Wallace, & McCarton, 1989 (R)	46	Yes	Yes	Yes	7 mos.	5 yrs.	Percentage of looking time to novel stimulus	Wechsler	.61
	45	No	Yes	No	7 mos.	5 yrs.		Wechsler	.54
Rose, Feldman, & Wallace, 1989 (R)	40	Yes	Yes	Yes	7 mos.	4 yrs.	Percentage of looking time to novel stimulus	Binet	.58
	42	No	Yes	No	7 mos.	4 yrs.		Binet	.45
Gottfried, Guerin, & Bathurst, 1989 (G)	130	No	No	No	6 mos.	8 yrs.	Percentage of looking time to novel stimulus	Wechsler	.25
DiLalla & Fulker, 1989 (D)	58	...	...	...	8 mos.	3 yrs.	Visual anticipation of the side a redundant stimulus would appear[a]	Binet	.23
Colombo, Mitchell, Dodd, Coldren, & Horowitz, 1989 (C)	23	No	...	No	4 mos.	1 yr. 4 mos.	Mean percentage of looking time to novel stimuli across five tasks	Binet Spatial Task	.53

Study	N					Age at test		Measure	Test	r
Rose, Feldman, & Wallace, 1988 (R)	84	Yes	Yes	Yes	Yes	6 mos.	3 yrs.	Percentage of looking time to novel stimulus	Binet	.46
Fulker et al., 1988 (D)	51	No	No	No	No	9 mos.	3 yrs.	Percentage of looking time to novel stimulus	Binet	.32
	143	No	No	No	No	9 mos.	2 yrs.		Bayley	.01
Rose & Wallace, 1985 (R)	35	Yes	Yes	Yes	Yes	6 mos.	6 yrs.	Mean proportion of looking time to novel stimuli across six tasks	Wechsler	.56
Fagan, 1984 (F)	36	No	No	No	. . .	7 mos.	5 yrs.	Mean percentage of looking time to novel stimuli across three tasks	PPVT	.42
Caron, Caron, & Glass, 1983 (A)	31	No	No	No	Yes	5 mos.	3 yrs.	Percentage recovery of fixation to a novel stimulus[b]	Binet	.42
Fagan & McGrath, 1981 (F)	19	No	No	No	No	5 mos.	4 yrs. 4 mos.	Percentage of looking time to novel stimulus	WISC Vocab	.33
	20	No	No	No	No	4 mos.	6 yrs. 6 mos.		WISC Vocab	.66
	19	No	No	No	No	5 mos.	7 yrs. 6 mos.		WISC Vocab	.46
O'Connor, 1980 (O)	17	Yes	No	No	No	4 mos.	1 yr. 6 mos.	Change in heart rate to novel stimulus[c]	Bayley	.61
	12	Yes	No	No	No	4 mos.	1 yr. 6 mos.		Bayley	.06
Yarrow, Klein, Lomonaco, & Morgan, 1975 (Y)	39	No	No	. . .	. . .	6 mos.	3 yrs. 7 mos.	Percentage of looking time to novel stimulus	Binet	.35

NOTE.— . . . signifies that this information could not be determined from the article.

[a] This was a procedure suggested by Marshall Haith. While it is neither traditional habituation (decrement in responding to a redundant signal is not measured) nor recognition memory (response to novel relative to familiar stimuli is not measured), it was included under recognition memory because presumably the infant was required to learn an alternating left-right position sequence which was displayed by choosing between two simultaneously available alternatives (i.e., left vs. right) which characterizes recognition memory paradigms.

[b] Caron, Caron, and Glass (1983) presented two familiar faces followed by two novel faces and measured fixation to the novel divided by the fixation to novel plus familiar.

[c] O'Connor (1980) presented alternating 400 and 1,000 Hz pure tones, replaced the first with a 200 Hz pure tone, and measured cardiac deceleration to the change in tone.

Typically, *recognition memory* is assessed by presenting for 5 to 30 sec a pair of identical stimuli (i.e., the "familiar" or "standard" stimulus) for familiarization, followed by two very brief test trials (e.g., 5 to 20 sec each) consisting of a simultaneous presentation of the familiar (i.e., standard) and a completely novel stimulus with the left-right positions reversed on the second trial. The predicting variable typically is the ratio of looking time to the novel divided by the total looking time to both familiar plus novel stimuli during the two test trials. Presumably, recognition memory reflects the infant's ability to encode a stimulus into memory, to recognize that stimulus as familiar or an alternative stimulus as not being familiar, and to cease looking at the familiar and/or to look longer at the novel stimulus.

The mental functions required by habituation and recognition memory collectively have been interpreted to reflect "information processing" capacities, such as the speed, accuracy, and completeness of encoding a stimulus into memory; the ability to recognize a familiar stimulus; and the propensity to avoid looking at the familiar and to study the novel stimulus (Bornstein & Sigman, 1986; Colombo & Mitchell, 1988, 1991; Fagan & McGrath, 1981; Lewis & Brooks-Gunn, 1981; McCall & Carriger, 1991; O'Connor, 1980; O'Connor, Cohen, & Parmelee, 1984; S. Rose, Feldman, & Wallace, 1988; D. Rose, Slater, & Perry, 1986; S. Rose & Wallace, 1985; Ruddy & Bornstein, 1982; Sigman, Cohen, Beckwith, & Parmelee, 1986). These skills would seem to be more obviously related to capacities measured by childhood standardized tests of intelligence (Bornstein & Sigman, 1986) than would the sensorimotor, action-consequence, and imitation skills represented on standardized infant tests (McCall, Eichorn, & Hogarty, 1977).

Regardless of the actual processes involved, individual differences in habituation and recognition memory do seem to predict later intelligence test scores better than those associated with standardized tests of general developmental level. Bornstein and Sigman (1986) reviewed the early prediction literature and found that habituation and recognition memory assessed between birth and 7 months of age correlated approximately .47 (median of raw r's) with childhood intelligence (usually IQ) assessed between 2 and 8 years of age, and the degree of relation was the same for each paradigm. In comparison, the average correlation between scores on standardized infant tests given between 1 and 6 months of age and childhood intelligence measured between 5 and 7 years of age for nondisordered samples is .09, although this correlation is somewhat higher when predicting from 7 to 12 months ($r = .20$) and at every infant age for risk ($r = .20$) and at every infant age for risk ($r = .54-.57$) and disordered (r $= .26-.51$) samples (Kopp & McCall, 1982). Presumably, habituation and recognition memory predict better because those measures reflect abilities that are more similar to those underlying intelligence test performance than do standardized infant tests.

Early Criticisms

However, while this newly found predictability has generated considerable excitement, some scholars have been more tempered, if not skeptical, in their response (e.g., McCall, 1981). Their concerns have taken three separate but related forms: (1) the underlying nature of habituation and recognition memory may not be what it appears, (2) the reliability and generality of infant measures are poor, and (3) the observed phenomenon may be artifactual.

The nature of habituation and recognition memory performance. Some researchers have disputed that habituation or recognition memory reflect any interesting "cognitive" process (Lecuyer, 1988, 1989; Malcuit, Pomerleau, & Lamarre, 1988). Malcuit et al. (1988), for example, argued that habituation procedures (and, by implication, recognition memory procedures) are nothing more than an operant paradigm involving a synchronous reinforcement schedule. Specifically, a particular behavior (an ocular movement or head turn) leads to a particular consequence (a stimulus enters the visual field), which reinforces the attending behavior. With repeated exposure, the consequence (i.e., the stimulus) loses its reinforcing properties, causing the behavior (i.e., looking) to stop. Therefore, habituation reflects nothing more than an operant behavior plus the well-known decline in the reinforcing potency of sensory/perceptual stimulation.

Lecuyer (1989) also suggested that individual differences in habituation may not index information processing. For example, he observed that infants can distinguish novel from familiar stimuli prior to having habituated to the familiar stimulus (Kagan, 1989; Lecuyer, 1989). Presumably, then, it is not necessary to habituate to a stimulus to process information about that stimulus, so the important information processing may not be reflected in habituation measures at all. Rather, habituation may simply reflect the ability to allocate attention to the various familiar and novel aspects of the environment. Although this ability may have importance in its own right, this argument potentially impugns the conceptual link between habituation and childhood measures of intelligence. Generally, researchers in the field have argued against these extreme conceptual criticisms (see Kuhn, 1989).

Reliability and generality problems. The short-term test-retest reliability of habituation and recognition memory behavior has been found to be quite low—approximately .30 to .45 (e.g., Bornstein, 1989; Bornstein & Sigman, 1986; Cohen, 1988; Fagan, 1984; Fagan & McGrath, 1981; Fagan & Singer, 1983; Lecuyer, 1989; McCall, 1989; Slater, 1988), varying with the individual measure (Colombo, Mitchell, & Horowitz, 1988; Colombo, Mitchell, O'Brien, & Horowitz, 1987). This level of reliability is no higher and often lower than the size of the predictive correlations. In addition, the generality of habituation and recognition memory performance across different stimuli and sensory modalities is similarly low (see Kagan, 1989; McCall, 1989). These observations, which are not disputed, raise questions about the nature of the endogenous thread that presumably ties together these different behaviors across the early years of life.

Prediction artifact. Some investigators have suggested that the relation between measures of habituation and recognition memory assessed during infancy and later childhood IQ scores may be an artifact of small sample sizes, the inclusion of a small number of organically damaged or at-risk infants with extreme values (Kagan, 1989; Lecuyer, 1989), or the presence of a subgroup of fast habituators who show high intelligence in childhood due to environmental enrichment (Kagan, 1989).

To demonstrate that this is at least possible, Gottfried (1988, personal communication) and Lecuyer (1989) computed the correlation between sample size and the predictive correlation between habituation/recognition memory and later childhood intelligence as reported in Bornstein and Sigman (1986). They found a correlation of −.60. This indicates that studies with a smaller sample showed higher predictive correlations, raising at least the possibility that the relation was produced or increased by one or two extreme infants who have a more substantial effect on the correlation in a small than in a large sample.

Other criticisms. Other students of infancy have voiced a variety of additional concerns when discussing this literature. For example, they worry that (1) the evidence for predictability for certain subgroups (e.g., at-risk or disordered infants assessed with the recognition memory paradigm) comes from one or two laboratories, (2) some samples contain infants having a great variety of syndromes known to be associated with retardation, (3) criteria for eliminating subjects from a sample are not always clear, (4) the variability of recognition memory scores is too high relative to the mean and the total exposure duration to permit much meaningful prediction, (5) the variability of infant performance is atypically large in the studies producing some of the best predictions, and (6) predictions do not occur for all measures of infant habituation and the best predicting measure is not consistent from one study to another.

Each of these criticisms is aptly leveled at some studies, and collectively they have fueled considerable skepticism about the validity of the prediction phenomenon. The question is whether the entire literature can be explained away by such concerns, and no one has seriously and publicly attempted to do so.

The Current Paper

The literature on the prediction of childhood IQ from habituation and recognition memory was reviewed by Bornstein and Sigman as recently at 1986, and numerous subsequent reviews have been published (e.g., Bornstein, 1989;

Colombo & Mitchell, 1991; Rose, 1989; Rose & Feldman, 1991). Why another review?

First, many of the recent reviews are selective, covering only habituation, only recognition memory, or mainly the work of one laboratory. A major purpose of the present paper was to compare habituation and recognition paradigms with respect to the level of prediction, as did Bornstein and Sigman (1986), and with respect to certain parameters of prediction (e.g., N, risk status, age), some of which have been given potential importance by the recent criticisms described above.

Second, the current literature is substantially larger. Early findings generated more research, and at least 77% more studies and 63% more samples are now available than when Bornstein and Sigman (1986) wrote their influential review. In addition to providing a larger database for review, the expanded literature now permits a more detailed meta-analysis of several parameters of this prediction phenomenon. Therefore, although only a few years have elapsed since Bornstein and Sigman's 1986 paper, this literature is worthy of being reviewed again.

Specifically, we asked several questions that could not be addressed previously because of the limited number of studies then available:

1. Do habituation and recognition memory tasks display similar patterns of correlation with childhood intelligence across several potential parameters?

2. What is the relation between the sample size and the predictive correlations for habituation and recognition memory tasks? Could this signal an artifactual effect based upon one or two extreme scores?

3. Is the risk status of the sample associated with the level of prediction for habituation and recognition memory?

4. What is the pattern of predictive correlations for habituation and recognition memory as a function of the age at assessment in infancy and the age at assessment in childhood?

META-ANALYTIC REVIEW

Sampling

Relevant articles on the predictive validity of habituation and recognition memory were generated by a computerized search of *Psychological Abstracts* for the years 1974 to 1989, a review of the bibliographies contained in this literature, and an examination of the personal files of the first author. The search produced a total of 23 studies (see Table 1), a substantial increase over the 13 studies reviewed by Bornstein and Sigman (1986).

A study was included in the review if (1) it was reported in full in a standard empirical report or with sufficient methodological detail in a chapter, (2) the sample did not contain frankly disordered infants having known syndromes associated with retardation, (3) it employed habituation, recognition memory, or both measures assessed between birth and 12 months, and (4) it measured childhood intelligence with some measure of general mental performance (usually IQ but sometimes vocabulary or memory) at least 1 year after the infant measure was taken (i.e., between 1 and 8 years of age).

These criteria meant that certain studies that appear relevant were not included in this analysis. For example, some unpublished studies and most data reported in book chapters were typically not included because they often lacked parametric details needed for the meta-analyses. Also, some studies of habituation or recognition memory used unique infant assessments or childhood mental behaviors (e.g., play) but not general IQ or a major component of it (e.g., vocabulary or memory subtests) as the outcome measure. These studies were not included because sufficient variability and numbers of studies employing these independent and dependent variables were not available on which to conduct meta-analyses and because they might introduce irrelevant variance if these procedural differences influenced the predictive correlations. Sometimes more than one predicting variable was available, and we tended to favor the most common variable first or, subsequently, that which produced the highest or most consistent predictive r. These several choices meant that our set of samples and r's were not always the same as those used by Bornstein and Sigman (1986). The potential bias that this could introduce did not seem to matter (see below).

Seven of the 23 studies that were included employed multiple (2 or 3) samples (e.g., preterm and full-term, younger and older infants), and these independent samples, not the studies, constituted the unit of analysis here. Although it might be argued that multiple samples within a study are not independent, we adopted the strategy of using sample as the unit of analysis, because it would increase the size of the meta-analytic sample and because Bornstein and Sigman (1986) also used sample, not study, as the unit of analysis. It must be acknowledged, however, that most meta-analytic strategies require independent samples, which assumption is violated to an unknown extent when more than one sample comes from the same study. We examined this possibility informally, feeling that the number of instances of multiple samples was too few for more formal statistical treatment.

Thirty-one samples from 23 studies were analyzed, 12 samples from 10 habituation studies and 19 samples from 13 recognition memory studies. This is a substantial increase over the previous review (Bornstein & Sigman, 1986) of 19 samples, 8 habituation and 11 recognition memory.

Variables

Once the samples were selected, several potential parameters of the subjects, procedures, outcome measures, and results were identified (see Table 1).

Independent variables. For each sample we recorded paradigm (habituation or recognition memory), birth status of the infants (i.e., the sample included some preterm infants or it included only full-term infants), socioeconomic status of the families (i.e., the sample included some low-SES families or the sample included only middle- to upper-SES families), health status of the infants (i.e., the sample included neurologically disordered infants or the sample included only neurologically healthy infants), the nature of the infant and childhood measures, sample size, age of infants at the initial assessment, and age of children at the outcome assessment.

Dependent variable. The dependent variable for the meta-analyses is the correlation coefficient (typically the z-transformed correlation coefficient, see below) between infant and outcome measures. We used one correlation from each sample. Data from a single sample were sometimes reported in more than one paper, in which case only one r from each sample was used, and, as a result, some reports are not cited. Unfortunately, the lack of details in reports about previous publications on the same sample or changes in a sample over time sometimes made these decisions uncertain.

In those cases in which more than one correlation was available, the correlation between the youngest infant age and the oldest childhood age was selected. This was done because it was possibly (see immediately below) the most conservative approach and because some interest focuses on the ability of the infant measures to predict "mature intelligence."

Ordinarily, as stated above, this approach would seem to bias the results toward lower predictions, because the longer the intertest interval the lower the correlation for standardized tests (Kopp & McCall, 1982; McCall, 1989). But this decreasing trend may not occur when predictions are made with habituation or recognition memory. For example, as indicated above, the test-retest reliabilities and short-term stabilities of these infant measures are often lower than their prediction coefficients, and predictions from these infant measures to intelligence tests given in the first 8 years of life may not show the typical decline in r with increasing childhood age (see below). So it is an empirical question whether this approach actually biases the size of the prediction and by how much.

Statistical considerations. Because the sample correlation is a biased estimator of the population correlation, all sample correlations were subjected to an r-to-z transformation (normalizing). The z-transformed coefficients were then weighted by the size of the sample minus 3, and this quantity was then divided by the sum of all sample sizes minus 3 for the set of samples included in the analysis (e.g., for the entire set of samples, for habituation samples only, and for recognition memory samples only). This has the effect of normalizing the sample correlations and rendering them unbiased estimators of the population correlation. This is the most common method of estimating the population correlation using independent samples (Hedges & Olkin, 1985).

This weighted normalized correlation coefficient, then, was the main dependent variable analyzed below. However, for comparison purposes, we also report in parentheses following the weighted normalized values the nonnormalized (i.e., untransformed) value corresponding to the weighted normalized average r. Note that this is merely transforming the weighted normalized average to a nonnormalized value (z_r to r transformation); it is *not* the mean unweighted nonnormalized value. We also report distributions and scatterplots of raw (i.e., untransformed, unweighted) prediction correlations as well as the median raw r of these distributions. Such plots help to depict graphically certain results, they demonstrate that the transformation and weighting procedures did not distort or produce the findings (except the central tendency of the predictions), and they provide a look at certain parameters that could not be analyzed statistically because of a limited number of cases.

The average transformed, weighted r and the median raw r each have certain advantages and limitations. The average transformed, weighted r is an unbiased estimator of the population average, and the weighting process roughly eliminates sample size as a potential contributor to estimates of central tendency. The median treats each sample as a unit and weights each sample equally, but it minimizes the influence of extreme results. While the weighted average r is a good estimate of the *population*, the median raw r is a good estimate of the typical *reported r*.

Using a single r per sample was an attempt to satisfy the statistical requirement that independent r's be used in a meta-analysis. However, dependencies could exist among r's derived from different samples but from the same laboratory, sometimes reported in the same article. While it is possible to deal with such potential dependencies in a statistical manner, the number of such samples was small. So we observed these possibilities more informally by examining scatterplots (see below).

Analytic strategy. Meta-analyses were conducted in two steps. First, the weighted normalized correlation coefficients were analyzed to determine their difference from zero and their homogeneity within a set of samples. Second, the weighted normalized coefficients were entered into separate correlational and difference-between-means analyses to determine if they varied as a function of subject and/or procedural variables. However, the *un*weighted normalized correlation coefficients were entered into correlational analyses with sample size (which otherwise is used to determine the weights). Then graphic displays of raw r's are presented to illustrate and extend the statistical results.

The Size and Significance of the Prediction of Later IQ from Infant Habituation and Recognition Memory

The first task was to test the size and significance of the relation between habituation and recognition memory assessed during infancy and childhood IQ. This was done for all samples regardless of paradigm and then separately for habituation and recognition memory samples. Further, tests of homogeneity were conducted to determine if the set of correlations could be viewed as being sampled from a single population or whether the correlations might derive from two or more populations, suggesting the influence of sampling or procedural parameters that varied within the set of samples (Hedges & Olkin, 1985).

All samples. The average weighted normalized correlation coefficient over all samples was .39 (comparable to a weighted but nonnormalized $r = .36$), which was significantly different from zero ($z = 13.82, p < .001$).

Across all samples, the hypothesis of homogeneity of the weighted normalized correlation coefficients was rejected, $Q(30) = 47.99, p < .001$. Therefore, one might infer that one or more sampling or procedure parameters that varied among samples in the total set influenced the size of the predictive relation.

Habituation versus recognition memory. The first potential parameter that might influence the predictive relation was type of infant assessment paradigm (i.e., habituation vs. recognition memory).

The separate average coefficients for the habituation and the recognition memory samples were each significantly different from zero. The average weighted normalized correlation coefficient for habituation was 0.41 ($r = 0.39; z = 8.40, p < .001$), and the average for recognition memory was 0.37 ($r = 0.35; z = 10.60, p < .001$). The weighted normalized correlation coefficient for the habituation samples was not significantly greater than the comparable coefficient for recognition memory samples. These and subsequent results are summarized in Table 2.

Although the weighted normalized correlation coefficients were not different for habituation and recognition memory paradigms, the significant heterogeneity result suggests that other parameters of the samples and procedures may influence the size of the predictions, perhaps interacting with paradigm. To evaluate this possibility in general, tests of homogeneity were conducted separately on the habituation and recognition memory samples. The coefficients for the habituation samples were homogeneous within sampling error, $Q(11) = 6.77, p < .10$, but the coefficients for the recognition memory samples were not homogeneous, $Q(18) = 40.68, p < .01$.

The above test is not equivalent to a test of the *difference* in homogeneity between paradigms, and the closeness to significance of the habituation test guards against the conclusion that the paradigms are different in this way. So, we

TABLE 2
Mean Weighted, Normalized Correlation Coefficients

Variable	Full Sample	Habituation	Recognition Memory
Paradigm:			
Habituation	.41 $(r = .39)$[a]		
Recognition memory	.37 $(r = .35)$		
Preterm infants:			
Included	.47 $(r = .43)$*	.35 $(r = .33)$[b]	.58 $(r = .52)$***
Not included	.35 $(r = .34)$	.48 $(r = .45)$	.30 $(r = .29)$
Low socioeconomic status:			
Included	.48 $(r = .45)$***	.35 $(r = .33)$[b]	.58 $(r = .52)$***
Not included	.27 $(r = .26)$	.54 $(r = .49)$	.24 $(r = .24)$
Disordered infants:			
Included	.45 $(r = .42)$*	.30 $(r = .29)$[b]	.58 $(r = .52)$***
Not included	.31 $(r = .30)$	.61 $(r = .55)$	.28 $(r = .28)$

[a] Values in parentheses represent the nonnormalized correlation corresponding to the weighted normalized r.
[b] Groups differ by sample size, and therefore differences in weighted, normalized correlation coefficients may be confounded by sample size. Groups did not differ by unweighted normalized correlation coefficients.
* $p < .05$.
** $p < .01$.
*** $p < .001$.

related the weighted normalized correlation coefficients to various potential parameters separately for both the habituation and recognition memory samples. *Raw data.* The use of transformed and weighted correlations is appropriate for the statistical meta-analysis, but some would argue that such procedures may distort results. Consequently, we present simple distributions and scatterplots of *untransformed, unweighted r's* as a complement to the formal meta-analyses. Specifically, Figure 1 presents the distribution of r's separately for the habituation and recognition memory paradigms taken from Table 1 in which the r's are represented by a Lab Code Letter corresponding to each laboratory (also given in Table 1). These distributions illustrate and amplify the statistical results reported above.

First, the median raw r is exactly .45 for each paradigm and for the combined sample. This value is higher than the average weighted transformed r of .39 (or its nonnormalized equivalent of .36) in part because of sample size. As reported below, r's were higher for small samples. The weighting process essentially combines subjects across samples, ignoring individual sample sizes, whereas the median allows sample size to operate. The former value (.36) is a better population estimate, but the latter (.45) is more typical of values reported in the literature.

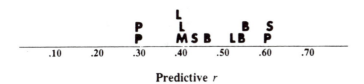

Habituation Paradigms

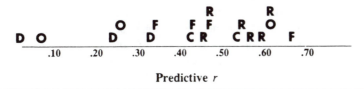

Recognition Memory Paradigms

Figure 1. The distribution of raw predictive *r*'s for habituation and recognition memory paradigms designated by the Lab Codes given in Table 1.

Second, the variability is only slightly greater for recognition memory than for habituation paradigms. This corresponds to the statistical results for homogeneity reported above.

Third, while in Figure 1 there appears to be greater similarity among *r*'s within than between laboratories, and some laboratories tend to report higher *r*'s than others, the general prediction phenomenon is not obviously and exclusively tied to one or even two laboratories.

While the predictive response measure for recognition memory paradigms is usually percent of looking time to the novel relative to the sum of looking to novel plus familiar stimuli (see footnotes to Table 1 for exceptions), a much greater variety of response measures has been used in habituation paradigms. These measures fall roughly into three types: *Habituation (H)*—response decrement over familiarization trials, *Fixation (F)*—the average or total looking at the standard stimulus during the familiarization phase, and *Recovery (R)*—the amount of response recovery to the novel stimulus relative to the last familiar stimulus.

Habituation Paradigms

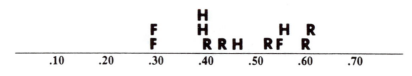

Predictive *r*

Figure 2. The distribution of raw predictive *r*'s for habituation paradigms designated by the type of predictor response: *H* = habituation or response decrement during familiarization, *F* = average or total fixation time during familiarization, and *R* = recovery of response to the presentation of a new stimulus following familiarization.

Figure 2 presents the same distribution of untransformed *r*'s for habituation paradigms as in Figure 1, but this time each *r* is represented by the type of infant predictive response measure (i.e., *H, F, R*). While the number of *r*'s is too small for formal statistical treatment, a few trends for future systematic study are apparent.

First, the prediction from habituation paradigms does not rest solely on any one of the three infant response measures. All three types of predictors can be found around the median *r* of .45, and no type of predictor measure always falls above or below the median. Second, and notwithstanding the first point, there is a slight tendency for the lowest predictive *r*'s to be based on average or total fixation times during familiarization (*F*) and the highest predictive *r*'s to be based on the recovery of response to a novel stimulus presented immediately after the familiarization phase. However, in addition to the small size of this trend, it should be observed that the two lowest *r*'s for Fixation both derived from the same laboratory, and two of the three highest *r*'s for Recovery come from the same (but another) laboratory. More tantalizing, though, is the observation that the same laboratory that reported the two lowest values for Fixation reported one of the highest values (*r* = .60) for Recovery. It should be noted, however, that sometimes studies assessed several predictor measures, only one of which is presented in the current review. Much more systematic study of the possible differential predictability of various response measures, especially from previously reported data, might help to focus interpretation on a particular mental process that mediates this predictive relationship (see McCall & Carriger, 1991).

Sampling and Procedural Parameters

The weighted normalized correlation coefficients were entered into a series of correlational analyses and *z* tests for the difference between average normalized correlation coefficients to determine their potential association with the inclusion of preterm infants, the inclusion of low socioeconomic status infants, the inclusion of disordered infants, sample size, and age of subject at infant and at outcome assessment.

Risk samples. Three series of *z* tests for the difference between weighted normalized correlation coefficients for the various sampling groups (i.e., risk factors of the presence of preterm, low SES, or disordered infants) were conducted, one for the entire set of samples and separately for samples employing a habituation and a recognition memory assessment (see Table 2 for details).

For *all samples,* the weighted normalized correlation coefficients were significantly *greater* for samples that included preterm infants, low socioeconomic status families, and neurologically damaged infants.

For the *habituation samples,* the weighted normalized correlation coefficients were not significantly related to any subject variable, but *r*'s tended to be *lower* in atypical samples.

For the *recognition memory samples,* however, the weighted normalized correlation coefficients were significantly *greater* for samples including preterm infants, low SES families, and neurologically damaged infants.

Therefore, it appears that atypical samples produce higher predictions to later IQ, especially for recognition memory paradigms (but see next section).

Figure 3 presents these data graphically, but for untransformed, unweighted *r*'s and for a single risk dimension. Specifically, the three indices of risk in Tables 1 and 2—the presence of preterm, low SES, or disordered infants—were not independent, because seven out of 13 samples that had one risk factor had all three. So samples were divided simply into No-Risk and Risk, the latter being any sample that had at least one of the three risk-factor groups included. Second, as one might expect, some laboratories concentrated on risk samples, and because only 13 risk samples are available from only five laboratories, confounds between laboratory and risk samples are likely at this early stage of the literature. So, distributions of predictive correlations represented by Lab Code Letters are graphed in Figure 3 separately for Risk and No-Risk samples within habituation (top) and recognition memory (bottom) paradigms.

For habituation paradigms, the four available *r*'s for risk samples span the entire range but include the two *lowest* *r*'s, both of which derive from the same laboratory (*P* = Parmelee), but one which also contributed the highest Risk *r*. For recognition memory paradigms, the nine risk samples also span the range of predictive *r*'s, but they predominate at the *high* end, again largely due to one laboratory (*R* = Rose). Therefore, there is a slight tendency for risk samples to produce higher predictive *r*'s, at least within recognition memory paradigms (but see next section).

Sample size. Three series of correlational analyses were conducted, one each for the entire set of samples, the habituation samples, and the recognition memory

Habituation Paradigms

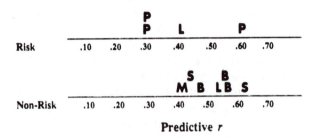

Predictive *r*

Recognition Memory Paradigms

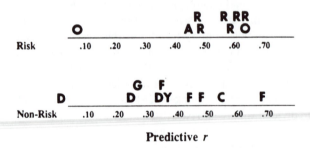

Predictive *r*

Figure 3. The distribution of raw predictive *r*'s for habituation and recognition memory paradigms as a function of Risk vs. Non-Risk samples designated by the Lab Codes given in Table 1.

samples. Sample size was the independent variable, and the *un*weighted but normalized predictive correlation coefficient was the dependent variable. The *un*weighted values were used only in the analyses on sample size, because *r*'s should not be weighted with the variable they are being correlated with (i.e., sample size).

For *all samples,* the unweighted normalized predictive correlation coefficients were significantly inversely related to the sizes of the samples ($r = -.56$, $p < .001$), a result similar to the $-.60$ observed by Gottfried (1988, personal communication) and Lecuyer (1989) for the samples reviewed by Bornstein and

Sigman (1986). Samples employing smaller numbers of subjects tended to show larger predictive relations.

This significant inverse relation between sample size and predictive coefficient was also present for both the *habituation* and *recognition memory* samples. Specifically, *r* equaled −.79, *p* < .01, for the habituation samples, and *r* was −.46, *p* < .05, for the recognition memory samples.

Figure 4 presents a slightly different view of this issue using the untransformed, unweighted *r*'s. Samples were divided as above into Risk (*R*) and Non-Risk (*O*), and then the predictive *r* was plotted as a function of *N* ignoring paradigm (since the relation occurred statistically in both paradigms).

Several points may be observed. First, two samples are clearly extreme, both recognition memory samples. O'Connor's (1980) risk sample of *N* = 12, *r* = .06 is very much off trend (i.e., an "outlier"; Belsley, Kuh, & Welsch, 1980), although the same study produced an on-trend *N* = 17, *r* = .61 (i.e., an "influential observation"). Fulker et al.'s (1988) nonrisk recognition memory sample of *N* = 143, *r* = .01 is extreme in both *N* and *r*, but it is basically an on-trend influential observation.

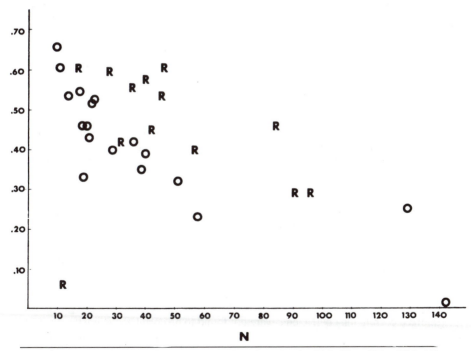

Figure 4. The scatterplot of predictive *r* as a function of *N* for Risk (*R*) and Non-Risk (*O*) samples ignoring paradigm.

Second, the weak general trend for Risk samples (*R*) to have higher predictive *r*'s than Non-Risk samples (*O*) is more clearly present when viewed conditional upon sample size. That is, collapsed across *N* onto the ordinate of Figure 4 (see also Fig. 3), only a slight tendency can be seen for risk samples to have higher *r*'s as reported above from the statistical analyses. But when viewed within samples of particular sizes (i.e., conditional distributions), the risk sample *r*'s are clearly above the regression line of *r* on *N*, and this is true for both paradigms (separate scatterplots were examined but not presented here). Therefore, the trend toward higher predictive *r*'s for risk samples *of comparable sizes* is general across paradigms, a theme consistent with the literature predicting later IQ from standardized infant tests (Kopp & McCall, 1982).

Third, even excluding the extreme values, a trend toward higher *r*'s for smaller samples exists for Risk (*R*) and Non-Risk (*O*) samples and for both paradigms (not separately shown graphically).

A major issue, however, is whether the inverse relation between *N* and *r* reflects a few extreme points *within individual samples* that produce the high predictive correlations, especially within small samples (e.g., Kagan, 1989). While it is impossible to determine the answer to this without examining scatterplots for individual samples, a case can be made that this potential artifact is unlikely to explain away the entire predictive phenomenon. If this hypothesis were true, one would expect risk samples to be more likely to contain extreme scores and therefore have higher *r*'s and, crucially, a larger inverse *r*-to-*N* relation. While the predictive correlations are higher for risk samples, the uniformity of this relation across all levels of *N* suggests it is not produced solely by extreme scores, which should have less influence in larger samples. Furthermore, the *r*-to-*N* relation exists equally in risk and nonrisk samples. More specifically, this relation occurred for samples having no preterm ($r = -.79$, $p < .001$), low SES ($r = -.61$, $p < .01$), no low SES ($r = -.64$, $p < .001$), disordered ($r = -.59$, $p < .01$), and no disordered ($r = -.62$, $p < .001$) infants. The relation was weakest for samples having preterm infants ($r = -.28$), opposite to what one would expect if developmentally persistent disordered subjects were producing these predictions.

In short, while higher predictive *r*'s are obtained for smaller samples, this does not appear to be simply produced by a few extreme scores, presumably from disordered infants (but no scatterplots for individual samples are presented in the literature).

Age of assessment in infancy and childhood. For all samples, the weighted normalized correlation coefficients were not found to be correlated significantly with either the age of the infants at the initial assessment or the age of the children at the outcome assessment. This also was true within both the habituation and recognition memory sets. However, infants responding to habituation tasks were younger (average of 3.83 months of age) than infants responding to recognition memory tasks (6.10 months of age), $F(1, 29) = 7.17$, $p = .01$.

While the meta-analyses did not reveal an effect of age at infant testing, this analysis is limited in two ways. First, in only three samples was the recognition memory assessment given at ages older than 7 months (i.e., at 8 and 9 months), and in only one sample was the habituation assessment administered at an age older than 6 months (i.e., at 12 months). Similarly, infants in only two samples in either paradigm were assessed before 2 months of age. Therefore, there is little power in our analyses to detect trends that might occur before 2 months or after 8 months. Furthermore, such analyses could not reveal any combined effect of age at infant and age at childhood assessments.

To look at the age data more closely, at least for heuristic purposes, Figure 5 presents the predictive correlations (ignoring paradigm and risk status) as a func-

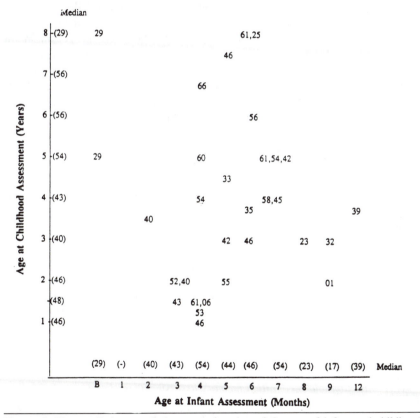

Figure 5. The predictive correlations as a function of the age of infant and childhood assessments. Marginal median *r*'s are given in parentheses along each axis.

tion of the age of infant and childhood assessments, with the marginal median correlations given within parentheses along each axis.

Notice first the marginal medians along the ordinate. They indicate a remarkably consistent level of prediction between $r = .40$ and $.56$ as a function of the
age of the childhood assessment between 1 and 8 years. The apparently lower
value of $.29$ at 8 years is fragile because of the great variability at that age (e.g.,
$.25$, $.29$, and $.61$) and because the $.48$ at 7 years, 6 months was arbitrarily
included in the calculation of the 7-year rather than the 8-year median. The level
prediction pattern between 1 and (at least) 8 years is remarkable, because most
longitudinal data display declining prediction coefficients with increases in outcome age and interest interval. It also means that selecting correlations that span
the longest intertest intervals did not bias the results toward lower values.

Now turn to the marginal values in parentheses along the abscissa. While the
number of samples is small at crucial points, a trend is suggested, namely, that
prediction is best from infant assessments made between approximately 2 and 8
months and poorer from assessments made earlier or later than this period. While
the data are very fragmentary, it would not be surprising to find low predictions
from the first month of life, since low correlations are typical from such ages in
other domains, reliability of measurement is likely poorer, state plays a greater
interfering role, etc. But the four relatively lower predictions from 8 months and
older are more notable. They represent three different paradigms and measures
($r = .01$ and $.32$ for recognition memory, Fulker et al., 1988; $r = .23$ for the
anticipation of left-right stimulus position, DiLalla & Fulker, 1989; $r = .39$ for
response decrement in habituation, Lewis, Goldbert, & Campbell, 1969). They
also constitute a prediction pattern that is opposite to the usual increase in correlations with increasing age at infant testing and shorter intertest intervals (note
that the intertest intervals for these r's are 2–3 years, whereas most r's for longer
intertest intervals are actually *higher*).

CONCLUSIONS AND ANALYSIS

The meta-analysis, coupled with other elements of the literature, lead to several
conclusions about the prediction phenomenon, its parameters, and the processes
that mediate the relation.

The Prediction Phenomenon

1. *Habituation and recognition memory assessments made on a variety of risk
and nonrisk samples of infants in the first year of life predict later IQ assessed
between 1 and 8 years of age with a weighted (for* N*) average of normalized correlations of .36 or a raw median correlation of .45. The literature now includes*

at least 31 samples representing a substantial diversity of ages, stimuli, subject characteristics, laboratories, and specific procedures, making it unlikely that the entire set of predictions is simply a collection of change phenomena or produced by a few procedural artifacts. While methodological issues may plague individual studies (e.g., McCall, 1981), it is becoming increasingly unlikely that extraneous factors can explain away the entire literature.

2. *The size of the predictive correlation is essentially the same for habituation and for recognition memory paradigms.* The average of the weighted normalized *r*'s was .39 for habituation and .35 for recognition memory studies, and the median raw correlation was .45 for both paradigms. While comparable prediction coefficients do not necessarily mean the same mechanism operates in each paradigm, this is the simplest and most parsimonious hypothesis. The median raw *r*'s are nearly identical to those reported in 1986 by Bornstein and Sigman.

3. *This prediction phenomenon is not obviously associated solely with one laboratory or one particular infant response measure.* While predictive *r*'s from single laboratories are often higher or lower than average, this is not consistently the case even within a laboratory, and the data from one laboratory are not solely responsible for the entire prediction phenomenon. Similarly, while predictions are slightly higher for some infant measures than others (especially within the habituation paradigm in which a greater variety of measures has been used), no one measure is solely responsible for the general prediction. At the same time, some measures may predict better than others, and more comparisons of different predicting measures within studies are needed.

4. *It seems unlikely that such predictions are simple products of extreme scores, presumably those of a few extremely disordered infants who remain low scoring or retarded in childhood.* Some scholars had raised this as a potential explanation, partly because a correlation of $-.60$ was found in Bornstein and Sigman's (1986) review between sample size and the size of the predictive correlation (Gottfried, 1988, personal communication; Lecuyer, 1989). Further, Kagan (1989) and Lecuyer (1989) speculated that it was possible that a few organically damaged or at-risk infants alone might produce these correlations, and one might expect this to be especially true in small samples in which one or two individuals would have a more substantial effect.

In the present meta-analysis, this inverse relation between sample size and the level of prediction was $-.56$ for all samples, $-.79$ for habituation samples, and $-.46$ for recognition memory samples. However, contrary to what might have been expected by the extreme-score hypothesis, the negative relation between sample size and predictive *r* was remarkably similar in subsamples containing or not containing at-risk infants. Of course, the only real way to evaluate the extreme-score hypothesis is for individual studies to publish scatterplots for their predictive correlations, which has not been done in the past.

It is crucial to point out, however, that it is still possible, perhaps likely, that *low-scoring infants, especially those from relatively unstimulating and unsupportive home environments, carry a disproportionate amount of the prediction load.* That is, the scatterplot may not reflect a uniformly linear relation or homogeneous oval; the predictive slope may be produced disproportionately by cases in the lower left quadrant. For example, standardized infant tests predict somewhat better for low-scoring than for high-scoring infants (McCall, 1979). Furthermore, infants with prenatal problems and depressed performance on standardized infant tests are more likely to remain low scoring on tests of mental performance during early childhood if they are reared in impoverished or other environments that are less likely to support mental development (Sameroff & Chandler, 1975). It is interesting to note in this regard that the heredity × environment reaction surface for IQ (Turkheimer & Gottesman, 1991) shows that extremely poor environments interrupt the otherwise consistent and fairly high genetic correlations with childhood IQ. Finally, although not always reported or systematically examined in this meta-analysis, the correlation between general measures of socioeconomic status is typically higher with childhood IQ (e.g., .50, McCall, 1979) than with the infant measures (e.g., r is approximately .40; Cohen & Parmelee, 1983; Fagan, 1984; Gottfried, Guerin, & Bathurst, 1989; O'Connor, Cohen, & Parmelee, 1984; Rose, Feldman, Wallace, & McCarton, 1989).

These observations collectively support a "Sameroff-Chandler lower-left quadrant prediction phenomenon." That is, while poorly scoring infants may be more likely to come from low SES homes, others score poorly because of temporary medical problems and, with extensive medical care and a rich environment, recover to have average or above IQs as children (top left quadrant of the prediction scatterplot). But those poor scoring infants reared in very mentally unstimulating circumstances may not recover, and it is their presence in the lower-left quadrant that produces much of the prediction correlation (but see Fagan & Knevel, 1989). They are not flukes, because there are more than one or two (especially in risk samples which do produce higher correlations) and because they could be meaningfully identified and explained.

Unfortunately, such a possibility has rarely been examined directly in research using either paradigm. When SES variables have been examined, they typically are combined with the infant assessment in a multiple regression, a statistical procedure that would not be as sensitive as other analyses to nonlinear relations and the specific combinations of circumstances hypothesized above to mediate this relation. Old data could be reexamined to test this hypothesis.

The fact remains, however, that a relation does exist between small samples and large predictive correlations in the total sample set ($r = -.56$), in recognition memory samples ($r = -.46$), and in habituation samples ($r = -.79$). What explains this consistent relation? The answer is not clear, but one possibility may lie in the interplay between statistical significance, *N*, and publishing practices. Specifically, correlations, like most other statistics, are more variable for smaller samples. Therefore, extremely high as well as extremely low correlations are more likely to be found in small than in large samples, but only extremely high correlations will be significant and therefore likely to get published. In contrast, smaller correlations are more likely to be significant in large samples and will be published. The total result is a negative relation between sample size and prediction level in the published literature. If this publishing bias has any explanatory power, it should apply to other behavioral domains as well, and its validity assumes that small data sets with nonsignificant *r*'s repose unpublished in the files of researchers.

5. *The level of predictions to childhood IQ is substantial given the reliability of the infant measures.* The short-term test-retest reliability of habituation and recognition memory scores has been found to be quite low (Bornstein, 1989; Bornstein & Sigman, 1986; Cohen, 1988; Fagan, 1984; Fagan & McGrath, 1981; Fagan & Singer, 1983; Lecuyer, 1989; McCall, 1989; Slater, 1988). Reliabilities typically are between .30 and .45, varying with the test-retest interval and with the particular measure (Colombo et al., 1987, 1988). Note that the reliabilities are approximately the same or lower than the predictive correlations. It is technically possible to have a predictive correlation that is higher than the reliability of the predictor if the reliability of the outcome variable is very high, because the maximum predictive *r* is the square root of the product of the two reliabilities (Ghiselli, 1964). The year-to-year reliability of the childhood IQ test is approximately .85 (McCall, 1989), sufficiently high to allow predictions to be higher than the much lower reliability of the infant assessment.

Many explanations for the poor reliability of the infant measures have been offered. Younger infants, for example, may process a different aspect of the stimuli presented in these tasks than they do when older (Cohen, 1988). Therefore, reliability measured across age may be low because the habituation (or recognition memory) procedures are actually measuring the processing of different elements of a single physical stimulus at the two ages. One may find higher test-retest reliabilities across two ages in infancy using different stimuli than across the same two ages using the same stimuli (Cohen, 1988), if the two different stimuli are similarly matched to the infants' abilities at each age.

Alternatively, poor short-term reliability may be due to the structure of the habituation and recognition memory assessments (McCall, 1989). In general, relatively few habituation or recognition memory tasks are given to the subjects in a session (Bornstein & Sigman, 1986; McCall, 1989). Therefore, only a brief sampling is taken of the infant's behavior, which is likely to be unreliable. A single memory task may be analogous to a single item on a paper and pencil test, and the reliability of .30–.45 for these infant measures is roughly similar to the correlation between single items on paper and pencil psychometric tests for older children and adults. Therefore, the reliability of the habituation and recognition memory scores may be adequate, but the number of "items" usually assessed is psychometrically insufficient (for a general discussion of this issue, see Rushton, Brainerd, & Pressley, 1983).

This explanation receives only partial empirical support. For example, Rose, Feldman, and Wallace (1988) found a median interitem correlation (i.e., "alternative forms" reliability) for 12 recognition memory tasks given at 6, 7, and 8 months of age to be −.10, with the range of average intertask correlations to be −.16 to .13. The mean test-retest correlation for single tasks across the 1-month interval was .18, with a range of −.16 to .47. However, combining the 12 tasks into summary scores at each age increased the age-to-age reliability to .30 to .49. Colombo et al. (1988) also raised the reliability of novelty preference scores to .50 from .24 by combining tasks. However, while reliability is increased by adding more tasks, even having 12 tasks, which is more than in most studies, does not produce a very reliable measure.

The lack of reliability, as well as the low generality of habituation and recognition memory measures across tasks using different stimuli (Kagan, 1989) or different stimulus modalities (McCall, 1989), suggests that whatever is being measured by these assessments may not be a single process and/or may not be solely or even largely an endogenous process. Instead, it may be influenced substantially by particular stimuli and other exogenous aspects of the total assessment situation.

Nevertheless, long-term predictions are obtained, and their level is substantial, especially when the low reliability of the predictor is considered. For example, with reliabilities ranging between .30 and .45 for the infant measures and a conservative .85 for the childhood IQ test, the maximum possible prediction is approximately .50−.62. Observed weighted predictions average .36, which means that the predictions account for 34%−52% of the "reliable" variance in this assessment system. This figure is higher (e.g., 53%−81%) if the median raw prediction of .45 is used. It is in this relative sense, more than the absolute level of prediction (see next section), that the infant measures potentially reflect a powerful predictor of later mental performance.

It should be noted that the calculations in this section are based on classical true-score test theory, which assumes that a "true score" remains constant over settings, occasions, and age. This assumption may not be valid (e.g., Lumsden, 1976), especially for developmental phenomena, and other approaches, such as Cronback's Generalizability Theory (Cronbach, Rajasatnam, & Glaser, 1963; Shavelson & Webb, 1981), may be more appropriate.

   6. *Predictions to childhood IQ from habituation and recognition memory are consistently higher than for standardized infant tests of general development for non-*

risk but not for risk samples, and they are not consistently higher than predicting from parental education and socioeconomic status or a few other infant behaviors for nonrisk samples. The average weighted correlation of .36 and certainly the median raw correlation of .45 for habituation and recognition memory is notably higher than correlations from standardized tests of general infant development, which display a median (raw) value of .09 for nondisordered samples for predicting 5–7-year IQ from the first 6 months of life (Kopp & McCall, 1982). On the other hand, the correlation for standardized infant tests to later IQ is .54 for risk samples (Kopp & McCall, 1982), and parental education and other measures of socioeconomic status tend to correlate approximately .40–.60 with children's IQ depending on age and the prediction interval (McCall et al., 1972). Also, while not often measured or reported, race and birth order have sometimes predicted almost as well as recognition memory in samples containing severely disordered infants (Fagan & Singer, 1983). Finally, and more startling as well as forgotten, the early onset of vocalization during the first year of life was observed to correlate .71 with IQ at age 26 years (Cameron, Livson, & Bayley, 1967), a result also found ($r = .50$) for similar behaviors by Moore (1967). Curiously, this result has only been reported for females. Therefore, while predictions from early habituation and recognition memory to later IQ are consistent, exist for both sexes (although sexes are not always reported separately; see O'Connor, 1980, for a very large sex difference), and are higher than from standardized tests of general infant development in nonrisk samples, they are not necessarily higher than for infant tests for risk samples, not the highest predictors ever found, and certainly not the easiest to obtain.

This observation has several implications. First, from the standpoint of sheer prediction accuracy, which may be of practical importance in screening, selection of infants for intervention programs, and counseling of parents, habituation and recognition memory are still of limited utility. Second, the field has become preoccupied with habituation and recognition memory, forgetting that other behaviors, such as early vocalization, may also predict later IQ. Third, this observation highlights the proposition that the importance of the habituation/recognition memory prediction phenomenon lies more in what it may reveal about the process of mental development than in the fact of the prediction per se or its size. Unfortunately, nearly all the empirical effort has been expended demonstrating the prediction, which is the first step; but very little research has been directed at discerning the nature of the processes or mechanisms responsible for the correlations (see below), which now should receive more emphasis.

Parameters

7. Predictions are somewhat higher for risk than for nonrisk samples. While this difference was observed statistically only for recognition memory samples (the averages of weighted r's were .52 vs. .27), the plot of prediction r's as a function of sample size (Fig. 4) clearly shows the correlations for risk samples to be uniformly higher within an N, and this is true for both paradigms. This result conforms to a similar finding for the prediction from standardized infant tests (Kopp & McCall, 1982). The presumption in both cases is that some low-scoring infants, likely those who are neurologically disordered *and* who are reared in intellectually unstimulating environments, score poorly as infants and as children, and such cases are more prevalent in risk samples and thus more likely to increase the size of the prediction for risk samples. This interpretation is consistent with the "Sameroff-Chandler lower-left quadrant hypothesis" described above as well as the notion that standardized infant tests predict better for poor-scoring than for average- or above-average-scoring infants (McCall, 1979).

8. *Predictions from habituation and recognition memory may be stronger when such assessments are made between 2 and 8 months of age than earlier or later.* The data for this proposition are fragmentary, involving only six of the 31 samples in Figure 5; and longitudinal data, while consistent with this theme, are also sparse (e.g., Cardon & Fulker, 1990; Rose et al., 1988). Nevertheless, the trend in Figure 5 is obvious, especially in contrast to the consistently high r's between 2 and 8 months, and is worthy of future study.

It is not unusual to find cross-age correlations to increase from birth to 2–3 months of age, as they do for standardized infant tests (McCall, 1979; McCall, Eichorn, & Hogarty, 1977). At the very least, the infant measures before 2 months may be less reliable than after 2 months. But the possible decline in predictability after 8 months, if substantiated by further study, would be more unusual and provocative. It would suggest, for example, that the simplest model of stability and continuity—that is, that the same behavior correlates consistently with itself across age—is not the case for this situation, and, indeed, two reports suggest that infant recognition memory predicts later IQ better than it predicts itself in childhood (Fagan, 1984; Slater, Cooper, Rose, & Morrison, 1989). This might imply that some qualitative transformation of the mediating mechanism occurs during development, in the manner theorized by Piaget and observed by McCall et al. (1977) for the same ages.

Alternatively, the mechanism may remain essentially the same, but the stimuli, behaviors, and measurement of it might change with development. For example, perhaps habituation and recognition memory to simple stimuli can be accomplished very quickly by the time the infant reaches approximately 8 months of age, and salient individual differences thereafter are not revealed unless the task is cognitively more difficult, presumably as in cross-modal transfer, which Gottfried et al. (1989) found to predict later IQ better than habituation at 12 months.

In any case, if these curious observations are supported by future research, something more complicated—and interesting—than simple stability in the same behavior may be involved in this prediction phenomenon.

9. *The level of prediction coefficients is remarkably consistent across the observed outcome age period of 2–8 years.* The marginal distribution along the ordinate of Figure 5 shows that the sizes of the *r*'s do not obviously vary with the age at which the childhood IQ test is given, and no statistically significant relation was found between weighted prediction *r*'s and age at outcome. What little longitudinal data are available (not reported here) also support the proposition of minimum effect for outcome age within studies (e.g., Fagan, 1984; Fagan & McGrath, 1981; Gottfried et al., 1989; Rose, Feldman, & Wallace, 1989; Slater et al., 1989), although some longitudinal studies (Colombo, Mitchell, Dodd, Coldern, & Horowitz, 1989; Thompson, Fagan, & Fulker, 1991) suggest that predictive *r*'s increase through the first 3 years.

The consistency of the predictive *r*'s between 2 and 8 years (and perhaps to age 12; Sigman, Cohen, Beckwith, Asarnow, & Parmelee, 1989) is unusual but not unprecedented in the longitudinal literature, and that exception is provocative. Specifically, the typical pattern is for longitudinal predictions to decline with increasing age at outcome, which is the case, for example, for predictions to later IQ from total scores on standardized infant tests (McCall, 1979). But this trend for total scores actually masks a pattern for subsets of items on these tests that mimics the persistent high predictions observed for habituation and recognition memory through the childhood years. Specifically, the first principal component at and following approximately 21 months of age predicts at very high levels IQ assessments given throughout childhood and adolescence (McCall et al., 1977).

The parallel observations that habituation and recognition memory in the first year of life and consensual vocabulary and symbolic thought in the second year both predict later IQ between 2 and 8 years and do so at the same, undecreasing level regardless of the age of the child at outcome assessment might be a homologous coincidence. But recent studies have suggested that habituation and recognition memory predict certain language and memory functions in young children (Bornstein & Sigman, 1986; Colombo et al., 1989; Fagan & Knevel, 1989; Rose, Feldman, Wallace, & McCarton, 1989), even when IQ is covaried from such skills (Thompson et al., 1991). Could habituation and recognition memory in the first year, consensual vocabulary and early symbolic functions in the second and third years, and IQ, verbal skill, and certain memory functions in childhood all be threads of the same developing mental fabric?

Conceptual Mechanism

The overt behaviors that correlate across development, such as those mentioned immediately above, are clues to the underlying mechanisms that mediate the predictions. While a few have wondered if habituation, at least, required any serious cognitive processes (e.g., Lecuyer, 1988, 1989; Malcuit et al., 1988), most students of the field (e.g., see Kuhn, 1989) have argued that performance in these paradigms reflects "information processing," that is, the ability to encode the familiar stimulus, remember it, compare a presented stimulus with the remembered engram, recognize the familiar stimulus when it is represented, discriminate a new stimulus from the familiar or its engram, and encode the new stimulus into memory (e.g., Bornstein, 1985; Bornstein & Sigman, 1986; Colombo & Mitchell, 1988, 1991; Fagan, 1988; Fagan & Singer, 1983; Lewis et al., 1969). Presumably, those infants who perform these tasks most rapidly turn out to have higher IQs, and that relative performance on these processes is stable from infancy to childhood.

Without question, accomplishing these tasks is required in the habituation or recognition memory paradigms, but it is not necessarily the case that such processes are sufficient to make the prediction or that the speed of their execution is the primary component of the predicting measures. McCall and Carriger (1991) make the case that they are not. While they acknowledge these information processing tasks must occur, they speculate that these processes are conducted very rapidly, and variance in the predicting measures reflects in substantial part another disposition—the disposition to *inhibit* responding to familiar stimuli and to stimuli of minor prominence (e.g., low energy, static, etc.). Similarly, Dempster (1991) recently argued that mature intelligence is typically discussed in terms of speed of information processing, the quality or quantity of information represented, executive processes, and processing capacity, but that it cannot be understood without reference to inhibitory processes, which have been largely ignored.

Whatever the mechanism, it seems clear that the prediction phenomenon has been established, and that much future research, including reanalyses of existing data, should be directed at crafting tasks and measures that differentiate these several skills during infancy and early childhood and discerning how they become woven into the fabric of mature intelligence.

REFERENCES

Belsley, D. A., Kuh, E., & Welsch, R. E. (1980). *Regression diagnostics: Identifying influential data and sources of collinearity.* New York: Wiley.

Bornstein, M. H. (1984, April). *Infant attention and care-giver stimulation: Two contributions to early cognitive development.* Paper presented at the International Conference on Infant Studies, New York.

Bornstein, M. H. (1985). Habituation of attention as a measure of visual information processing in human infants: Summary, systematization, and synthesis. In G. Gottlieb &

N. H. Krasnegor (Eds.), *Measurement of audition and vision in the first year of post-natal life: A methodological overview* (pp. 253–300). Norwood, NJ: Ablex.

Bornstein, M. H. (1989). Stability in early mental development: From attention and information processing in infancy to language and cognition in childhood. In M. H. Bornstein & N. A. Kresnegor (Eds.), *Stability and continuity in mental development* (pp. 197–170). Hillsdale, NJ: Erlbaum.

Bornstein, M. H., & Sigman, M. D. (1986). Continuity in mental development from infancy. *Child Development, 57,* 251–274.

Cameron, J., Livson, N., & Bayley, N. (1967). Infant vocalizations and their relationship to mature intelligence. *Science, 157,* 331–333.

Cardon, L. R., & Fulker, D. W. (1990). *Sources of continuity in infant predictors of later IQ.* Unpublished manuscript, authors.

Caron, A. J., Caron, R. F., & Glass, P. (1983). Responsiveness to relational information as a measure of cognitive functioning in non-suspect infants. In T. Field & A. Sostek (Eds.), *Infants born at-risk: Physiological, perceptual, and cognitive processes* (pp. 181–209). New York: Grune & Stratton.

Cohen, L. B. (1988). The relationship between infant habituation and infant information processing. *European Bulletin of Cognitive Psychology, 8,* 445–454.

Cohen, S. E., & Parmelee, A. H. (1983). Prediction of five-year Stanford-Binet scores in preterm infants. *Child Development, 54,* 1242–1253.

Colombo, J., & Mitchell, D. W. (1988). Infant visual habituation: In defense of an information-processing analysis. *European Bulletin of Cognitive Psychology, 8,* 455–461.

Colombo, J. C., & Mitchell, D. W. (1991). Individual differences in early visual attention: Fixation time and information processing. In J. Colombo & J. W. Fagen (Eds.), *Individual differences in infancy: Reliability, stability, and prediction* (pp. 193–227). Hillsdale, NJ: Erlbaum.

Colombo, J., & Mitchell, D. W., Dodd, J., Coldren, J. T., & Horowitz, F. D. (1989). Longitudinal correlates of infant attention in the paired-comparison paradigm. *Intelligence, 13,* 33–42.

Colombo, J., Mitchell, D. W., & Horowitz, F. D. (1988). Infant visual attention in the paired-comparison paradigm: Test-retest and attention-performance relations. *Child Development, 59,* 1198–1210.

Colombo, J., Mitchell, D. W., O'Brien, M., & Horowitz, F. D. (1987). The stability of visual habituation during the first year. *Child Development, 58,* 474–487.

Cronbach, L. J., Rajasatnam, N., & Glaser, B. (1963). Theory of generalizability: A liberalization of reliability theory. *British Journal of Statistical Psychology, 16,* 137–163.

Dempster, F. N. (1991). Inhibitory processes: A neglected dimension of intelligence. *Intelligence, 15,* 157–173.

DiLalla, D. L., & Fulker, D. W. (1989). Infant measures as predictors of later IQ: The Twin Infant Project (TIP). *Behavior Genetics, 19,* 753–754.

Fagan, J. F. (1984). The relationship of novelty preferences during infancy to later intelligence and later recognition memory. *Intelligence, 8,* 339–346.

Fagan, J. F. (1988). Evidence for the relationship between responsiveness to visual novelty during infancy and later intelligence. A summary. *European Bulletin of Cognitive Psychology,* **8,** 469–475.

Fagan, J. F., & Knevel, C. (1989, April). *The prediction of above-average intelligence from infancy.* Paper presented at the meeting of the Society for Research in Child Development, Kansas City.

Fagan, J. F., & McGrath, S. K. (1981). Infant recognition memory and later intelligence. *Intelligence,* **5,** 121–130.

Fagan, J. F., & Singer, L. T. (1983). Infant recognition memory as a measure of intelligence. In L. P. Lipsitt & C. K. Rovee-Collier (Eds.), *Advances in infancy research* (Vol. **2,** pp. 31–79). Norwood, NJ: Ablex.

Fulker, D. W., Plomin, R., Thompson, L. A., Phillips, K., DiLalla, L. F., Fagan, J. F., & Haith, M. M. (1988). *Rapid-screening of infant predictors of adult IQ: A study of infant twins and their parents.* Unpublished, authors.

Ghiselli, E. E. (1964). *Theory of psychological measurement.* New York: McGraw-Hill.

Gottfried, A. W., Guerin, D., & Bathurst, K. (1989). *Infant predictors of intelligence and achievement: A comparative analysis of sensorimotor, environmental, and recognition memory measures.* Unpublished, authors.

Hedges, L. L., & Oklin, I. (1985). *Statistical methods for meta-analysis.* Orlando, FL: Academic Press.

Hunt, J. McV. (1961). *Intelligence and experience.* New York: Ronald.

Kagan, J. (1989). Commentary: Does infant boredom reflect intelligence? *Human Development,* **32,** 172–176.

Kopp, C. B., & McCall, R. B. (1982). Predicting later mental performance for normal, at-risk, and handicapped infants. In P. B. Baltes & O. G. Brim, Jr. (eds.) *Life-span development and behavior* (Vol. **4,** pp. 33–61). New York: Academic Press.

Kuhn, D. (Ed.). (1989). Special issue. *Human Development,* **32,** 177–186.

Lecuyer, R. (1988). Please infant, can you tell me exactly what you are doing during a habituation experiment? *European Bulletin of Cognitive Psychology,* **8,** 476–480.

Lecuyer, R. (1989). Habituation and attention, novelty and cognition: Where is the continuity? *Human Development,* **32,** 148–157.

Lewis, M., & Brooks-Gunn, J. (1981). Visual attention at three months as a predictor of cognitive functioning at two years of age. *Intelligence,* **5,** 131–140.

Lewis, M., Goldberg, S., & Campbell, H. (1969). A developmental study of information processing within the first three years of life: Response decrement to a redundant signal. *Monograph of the Society for Research in Child Development,* **34**(9, Serial No. 133).

Lumsden, J. (1976). Test theory. In M. R. Rosenzweig & L. W. Porter (Eds.), *Annual review of psychology* (Vol. **27,** pp. 251–280). Palo Alto, CA: Annual Reviews.

Malcuit, G., Pomerleau, A., & Lamarre, G. (1988). Habituation, visual fixation, and cognitive activity in infants: A critical analysis and attempt at a new formulation. *European Bulletin of Cognitive Psychology,* **8,** 415–440.

McCall, R. B. (1979). The development of intellectual functioning in infancy and the prediction of later IQ. In J. D. Osofsky (Ed.), *Handbook of infant development* (pp. 707–740). New York: Wiley.

McCall, R. B. (1981). Early predictors of later IQ: The search continues. *Intelligence, 5,* 141–147.

McCall, R. B. (1989). Commentary: Issues in predicting later IQ from infant habituation rate and recognition memory performance. *Human Development, 32,* 177–186.

McCall, R. B., & Carriger, M. S. (1991). *Infant habituation and recognition memory performance as prediction of later IQ: A review and conceptual analysis.* Unpublished paper, authors.

McCall, R. B., Eichorn, D. H., & Hogarty, P. S. (1977). Transitions in early mental development. *Monographs of the Society for Research in Child Development, 42*(3, Serial No. 171).

McCall, R. B., Hogarty, P. S., & Hurlburt, N. (1972). Transitions in infant sensorimotor development and the prediction of childhood IQ. *American Psychologist, 27,* 728–748.

Miller, D. J., Ryan, E. B., Alberger, E., McGuire, M. D., Short, E. J., & Kenny, D. A. (1979). Relationships between assessments of habituation and cognitive performance in the early years of life. *International Journal of Behavioral Development, 2,* 159–170.

Moore, T. (1967). Language and intelligence: A longitudinal study of the first eight years: I. Patterns of development in boys and girls. *Human Development, 10,* 88–106.

O'Connor, M. J. (1980). A comparison of pre-term and full-term infants on auditory discrimination at four months and on Bayley Scales of Infant Development at eighteen months. *Child Development, 51,* 81–88.

O'Connor, M. J., Cohen, S. L., & Parmelee, A. H. (1984). Infant auditory discrimination in pre-term and full-term infants as a predictor of 5-year intelligence. *Developmental Psychology, 20,* 159–165.

Rose, D. H., Slater, A., & Perry. H. (1986). Prediction of childhood intelligence from habituation in early infancy. *Intelligence, 10,* 251–263.

Rose, S. A. (1989). Measuring infant intelligence: New Perspectives. In M. H. Bornstein & N. A. Krasnegor (Eds.), *Stability and continuity in mental development* (pp. 171–188). Hillsdale, NJ: Erlbaum.

Rose, S. A., & Feldman, J. F. (1991). Infant cognition: Individual differences and developmental continuities. In J. Colombo & J. W. Fagen (Eds.), *Individual differences in infancy: Reliability, stability, and prediction* (pp. 229–246). Hillsdale, NJ: Erlbaum.

Rose, S. A., Feldman, J. F., & Wallace, I. F. (1988). Individual differences in infants' information processing: Reliability, stability, and prediction. *Child Development, 59,* 1177–1197.

Rose, S. A., Feldman, J. F., & Wallace, I. F. (1989). *Language: A partial link between infant attention and later intelligence.* Unpublished manuscript, authors.

Rose, S. A., Feldman, J. F., Wallace, I. F., & McCarton, C. (1989). Infant visual attention: Relation to birth status and developmental outcome during the first five years. *Developmental Psychology, 25,* 560–576.

Rose, S. A., & Wallace, I. F. (1985). Visual recognition memory: A predictor of later cognitive functioning in pre-terms. *Child Development, 56,* 843–852.

Ruddy, M. G., & Bornstein, M. H. (1982). Cognitive correlates of infant attention and maternal stimulation over the first year of life. *Child Development, 53,* 183–188.

Rushton, J. P., Brainerd, C. J., & Pressley, M. (1983). Behavioral development and construct validity: The principle of aggregation. *Psychological Bulletin, 94,* 18–38.

Sameroff, A. J., & Chandler, M. J. (1975). Reproductive risk and the continuum of caretaking casualty. In F. D. Horowitz (Ed.), *Review of child development research* (Vol. **4,** pp. 187–244). Chicago: University of Chicago Press.

Shavelson, R. J., & Webb, N. M. (1981). Generalizability theory: 1973–1980. *British Journal of Mathematical and Statistical Psychology, 34,* 133–166.

Sigman, M., Cohen, S. E., Beckwith, L., Asarnow, R., & Parmelee, A. H. (1989, April). *Infant attention and sleep organization and cognitive skills in early adolescence.* Paper presented at the meeting of the Society for Research in Child Development, Kansas City.

Sigman, M., Cohen, S. E., Beckwith, L., & Parmelee, A. H. (1986). Infant attention in relation to intellectual abilities in childhood. *Developmental Psychology, 23,* 788–792.

Slater, A. (1988). Habituation and visual fixation in infants: Information processing, reinforcement, and what else? *European Bulletin of Cognitive Psychology, 8,* 517–523.

Slater, A., Cooper, R., Rose, D., & Morrison, V. (1989). Prediction of cognitive performance from infancy to early childhood. *Human Development, 32,* 137–147.

Thompson, L. A., Fagan, J. F., & Fulker, D. W. (1991). Longitudinal prediction of specific cognitive abilities from infant novelty preference. *Child Development, 62,* 530–538.

Turkheimer, E., & Gottesman, I. I. (1991). Individual differences and the canalization of human behavior. *Developmental Psychology, 27,* 18–22.

Yarrow, L. J., Klein, R. P., Lomonaco, S., & Morgan, G. A. (1975). Cognitive and motivational development in early childhood. In B. X. Friedlander, G. M. Sterritt, & G. E. Kirh (Eds.), *Exceptional infant* (Vol. **3,** pp. 491–502). New York: Brunner/Mazel.

2

The Relations of Emotionality and Regulation to Preschoolers' Social Skills and Sociometric Status

Nancy Eisenberg, Richard A. Fabes, Jane Bernzweig,
Mariss Karbon, Rick Poulin, and Laura Hanish
Arizona State University, Tempe

The purpose of this study was to examine the relations of emotionality (intensity and negative emotion) and regulation (coping and attentional regulation) to preschoolers' social skills (as rated by adults) and sociometric status. Teachers' ratings of children's constructive coping and attentional control were positively related to boys' social skills and peer status, whereas negative affect was negatively related. Acting out (vs. avoidant) coping and emotional intensity were negatively related to girls' and boys' social skills and boys' peer status. In addition, mothers' reports of boys' coping by seeking social support and low emotional intensity were associated with boys' positive social functioning, whereas avoidant coping was positively related to girls' rated social skills. The results are discussed in relation to research on emotion regulation and coping with emotion in interpersonal contexts.

In recent years, researchers and theorists have increasingly recognized the role of both regulatory and emotional components of temperament in the development of social competence. Indeed, in current conceptualizations of temperament, regulation and reactivity (including emotional reactivity) are viewed as interre-

Reprinted with permission from *Child Development,* 1993, Vol. 64, 1418–1438. Copyright © 1993 by the Society for Research in Child Development, Inc.

This research was supported by a grant from the National Science Foundation (DBS-9208375) to the first two authors and a Research Scientist Development Award from the National Institute of Mental Health (K02 MH00903-01) to Nancy Eisenberg. The authors wish to thank the parents, teachers, and children at the Child Development Laboratory and Child Study Laboratory, as well as the many students that assisted in this study.

lated and perhaps interacting (Fox, 1989; Rothbart & Derryberry, 1981), and the joint contributions of emotion and regulation are cited in recent models of social behavior and psychological disorder (Cummings & Cummings, 1988; Eisenberg & Fabes, 1992; Weinberger & Schwartz, 1990).

Information on the roles of emotionality and regulation in social competence frequently is embedded in the more global measures of temperament (e.g., of general reactivity or difficult temperament) or in the literature on stress and coping. Consider first the construct of regulation, which has been defined in many ways. Temperament theorists (e.g., Rothbart, 1989) tend to define regulation in terms of controlling impinging stimuli and internal states (i.e., regulating the input of emotion-producing stimuli as well as internal emotional arousal resulting from processing external stimuli). Regulation in current models of temperament frequently involves attentional processes (such as attention shifting and attention focusing) and the ability to activate or inhibit behavior (Rothbart, 1989; Windle & Lerner, 1986). However, as noted by Prior (1992) in a recent review, whereas attentional regulation is examined in many models of temperament, self-regulation of behavior has not been central in any documented temperament system.

Although not usually explicitly labeled as regulation, coping theorists also discuss the regulation of emotion and emotion-related behaviors. Lazarus and Folkman (1984) defined coping as changing cognitive and behavioral efforts to manage specific external or internal demands that are appraised as taxing or exceeding the resources of the individual. Two general modes of coping have been differentiated: problem-focused (efforts to modify the source of the problem) and emotion-focused (efforts to reduce emotional distress). Thus, coping behaviors include ways of modulating the degree of emotional arousal by altering the experience of emotion (emotion regulation, e.g., by switching one's attention to some different aspect of the situation, avoiding the situation, or by involving oneself in a distracting activity), as well as mechanisms for changing aspects of the emotion-laden situation (e.g., by enacting instrumental behaviors intended to alleviate the emotion-inducing problem). Although temperament and coping theorists discuss some identical or similar modes of regulation, temperament researchers tend not to study problem-focused coping (including self-regulation of behaviors; see, however, Derryberry & Rothbart, 1988), and the two groups of researchers discuss and operationalize attentional regulatory mechanisms in somewhat different ways.

Constructs of emotionality are also operationalized in a variety of ways in the developmental, personality, and clinical literature. Usually negative emotionality in children is assessed as part of measures of temperament (see Bates, 1989), and frequency and intensity of negative emotionality sometimes are combined into a single construct (Buss & Plomin, 1984). In other conceptualizations of temperament, such as those of Thomas and Chess (1977) and Strelau (1983), the more general dimension of reactivity includes intensity of emotional responding. In recent work in personality psychology, Larsen and his colleagues (Larsen & Diener, 1987) have studied a dimension of personality (viewed as an aspect of temperament) that reflects primarily affective intensity, that is, the intensity of positive and negative emotions when they are experienced (rather than merely the frequency of experiencing such emotions). Affective intensity, as assessed by Larsen, correlates positively with negative affectivity as well as with autonomic arousal and reports of distress in emotion-inducing contexts (Eisenberg et al., 1991; Larsen & Diener, 1987), but appears to reflect more than just frequency of negative emotionality (see Larsen & Diener, 1987).

What do we know about the role of regulatory processes in individual differences in social competence? Although coping has been intensely studied in recent years, there is relatively little research concerning *individual differences* in coping style and resultant social behavior. This is no doubt in part because effective coping is viewed as changing with contextual demands (Lazarus & Folkman, 1984). Nonetheless, many researchers who view coping as a process also assume that coping style influences the choice of a coping strategy in stressful contexts (e.g., Carver, Scheier, & Weintraub, 1989; Kliewer, 1991). Consistent with this view, individual differences in coping style have been associated with variables such as internalizing and externalizing behavior (Compas, Malcarne, & Fondacaro, 1988) and psychological distress (Glyshaw, Cohen, & Towbes, 1989).

Most studies of coping are focused on psychological dysfunction or coping with major life events (such as divorce). However, normative stressors may be more strongly associated with well-being than are major stressors (Compas, 1989; Kanner, Coyne, Schaefer, & Lazarus, 1981). In one of the few studies of the relation of coping to normal children's social competence, Kliewer (1991) found that children's social competence, as rated by teachers, was positively associated with avoidant modes of coping (i.e., avoidant actions and cognitive avoidance) and negatively related to displayed problem behaviors.

Although there is relatively little empirical work on the relation of attentional control (rather than on mere distractibility or soothability when individuals are distressed; see Bates, 1989) to children's social competence, Rothbart and her colleagues have found that the ability to control attention is associated with relatively low levels of negative emotion in adults (Derryberry & Rothbart, 1988) and infants (Rothbart, Ziaie, & O'Boyle, 1992). Moreover, deployment of attentional control and related strategies sometimes is useful in children's coping with stress and frustration (Miller & Green, 1985). Thus, based on the work of Kliewer and Rothbart, it would appear that the use of avoidant strategies (including psychological as well as behavioral avoidance or distraction), perhaps used to reduce aversive affective stimulation, sometimes is associated with positive outcomes (see

Roth & Cohen, 1986), particularly in uncontrollable situations (Altshuler & Ruble, 1989; Forsythe & Compas, 1987). In addition, however, instrumental problem-focused modes of coping also frequently have been associated with positive outcomes, especially when the stressful situation is viewed as controllable (e.g., Compas et al., 1988; Folkman, Lazarus, Dunkel-Schetter, DeLongis, & Gruen, 1986). Further, the availability of social support and the tendency to cope by seeking support or help often have been cited as reducing the negative effects of stress (Cohen & Wills, 1985; Nelson-Le Gall, 1981), although there is little research to directly support the contention that coping by seeking emotional support is associated with children's emotional functioning (see Kliewer, 1991).

In comparison to work on examining the relation of coping and regulation to children's social competence, there is considerable research on the relation of reactivity and negative emotionality to social and problem behaviors. In general, temperamental reactivity and negative affective tone have been associated with negative behaviors (e.g., aggression, angry outbursts) and behavioral problems in childhood (Barron & Earls, 1984; Bates, 1990; Billman & McDevitt, 1980; Brody, Stoneman, & Burke, 1988; Kyrios & Prior, 1990; Teglasi & MacMahon, 1990). However, in only a few studies have researchers examined emotional intensity rather than the broader construct of reactivity (e.g., Brody et al., 1988). Moreover, relatively few data are available on the relation of emotionality to peer relationships (Parker-Cohen & Bell, 1988), although there is some evidence that intense, moody, or emotionally negative children are less popular with peers (Stocker & Dunn, 1990), or are more reactively hostile (Olweus, 1980; Stevenson-Hinde, Hinde, & Simpson, 1986) than are other children. However, the pattern of findings for peer relationships is weak (see Parker-Cohen & Bell, 1988), and in most studies on temperament and social functioning both temperament and behavior/adjustment were assessed by means of adults' reports (with the same adults often reporting on both).

The purpose of the present paper was to examine the contributions of both regulation (including attentional control and various modes of coping) and emotionality (including both negative affectivity and intensity of emotion, particularly negative emotions) to normal children's social skills and sociometric status. As noted previously, the empirical research on the relations of emotionality and regulatory processes to social competence in normal populations of children is limited. Much of the available research has been conducted with clinical populations or has been focused on behavioral problems rather than general social competence. Further, in much of the relevant research, predictor variables (e.g., emotionality) and outcome measures were obtained from a single informant (usually the mother). In the present study, multiple informants were used to assess temperamental and coping variables, as well as sociometric status and social skills. Because measures of temperament often differ across informants and settings (Goldsmith, Rieser-Danner, & Briggs, 1991), we obtained measures of regulation and emotionality from both mothers and adults at school so that we could determine if prediction from the home and school differed. In addition, few researchers have considered both aspects of temperament and coping (including regulation and emotionality) in the same study (see Compas, 1987). This is true despite the fact that children's temperament may define a range of responsivity to stress and influence the child's coping style (Compas, 1987), and coping can mediate the valence of emotion experienced in stressful situations (Folkman & Lazarus, 1988). In the present study, we examined the joint and overlapping contributions of regulation and emotionality to the prediction of social competence.

Based on the prior literature and on current theory, we expected both emotional aspects of temperament (negative affectivity and emotional intensity) and aspects of regulation (coping/attentional control) to be associated with social competence (including social skills and sociometric status). Specifically, attentional control and modes of coping such as instrumental problem solving, seeking support (especially at home), cognitive restructuring, and perhaps distracting actions and thoughts were expected to be associated with positive social functioning, whereas negative affect and hostile modes of coping (e.g., aggression) and venting of emotion were expected to be negatively related. In addition, we expected emotional intensity in regard to general arousability and negative emotions, as well as the tendency to experience negative emotions, to be associated with negative social functioning. Hot-headed boys (Olweus, 1980) and children who report high intensity of anger (Klaczynski & Cummings, 1989) tend to be aggressive. Moreover, socially inappropriate ways of dealing with aggression tend to be associated with low sociometric status and adults' ratings of social competence (Coie, Dodge, & Kupersmidt, 1990; Fabes & Eisenberg, 1992a). High regulatory capacities also have been associated with socially competent behaviors such as low levels of aggression (e.g., Block & Block, 1980; Pulkkinen, 1982), as well as with delay of gratification, prosocial behaviors, the ability to deal with frustration, and low levels of jealousy and exploitive behavior (Block & Block, 1980).

Although we expected some correlation between emotionality and social competence, we also expected this relation to be at least partially moderated by the ability to regulate emotion and behavior. Specifically, we hypothesized that children who were high in emotional intensity and low in regulatory/coping capabilities would be lower in social competence and sociometric status than would other children (see Fig. 1 for a depiction of our view of the links among emotionality, regulation, and social competence). However, the degree to which it is possible to isolate children's regulatory processes from their emotional tendencies was unclear given that their observable behavior undoubtedly reflects both. Thus, we assessed the associations among measures of regulation and emotionality, as well as their additive and relative prediction of indexes of social competence.

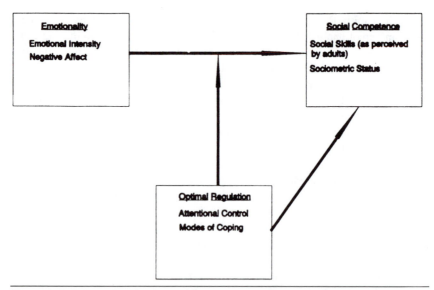

Figure 1. Relations of optimal regulation and emotionality to social competence

Finally, Prior (1992) recently argued that there is a need for research on gender differences in the association between temperament and outcome variables, and that the interaction effects between aspects of temperament and sex may be more important than main effects when examining psychosocial adjustment. She noted that there appear to be gender differences in some aspects of social functioning (including higher aggression and anger for boys) as well as in some modes of emotionality (including higher fear and anxiety in girls; also see Bates, 1989), and that socializers may respond differently to various temperamental characteristics when expressed by girls versus boys. Thus, in the present study we computed most of the major analyses separately by sex of child, although we did not have firm predictions regarding differences in the relations of regulation and emotionality to girls' and boys' social competence.

METHOD

Subjects

Participants were children in five classes at two preschools. In fall semester (henceforth labeled T1), 42 girls and 49 boys participated (no families declined participation in the aspects of the research described in this paper). All except one boy continued the second semester (henceforth labeled T2); in addition, three new girls participated at T2 for a total of 45 girls and 48 boys. Girls' and boys' mean ages were 61.4 and 62.1 months figured midway (i.e., 4 months) through the study (range = 52–76). The children were predominantly from Caucasian, non-Hispanic, middle-class families in suburbs of a large city; 3% were black, 4% were of Asian heritage, 1% was Hispanic, and 3% were of mixed origin. Mean numbers of years of maternal and paternal education were 16.40 (SD = 2.36; range = 12 [high school] to 20 [graduate school]) and 17.39 (SD = 2.18), respectively. Family income ranged from $15,000 to $200,000 (M = $66,000, SD = 31,755). Thus, the parents involved generally were well educated, and family income was relatively high.

Adult Report Measures

The study took place during two academic semesters (T1 and T2). Various measures were administered to teachers (N = 5) and teacher aides (N = 10), undergraduate observers (N = 15), mothers, and children. The children's teachers, but not aides, were the same at T1 and T2.

Social skills and popularity. At T1 and T2 the teachers and aides rated the children's social competence, including social skills and popularity. The measure of social competence was a 10-item adaptation of Harter's (1979) Perceived Competence Scale for Children (see Fabes & Eisenberg, 1992a). Seven items assessed general social skills (henceforth called SS); three explicitly assessed popularity. A typical item on the SS scale was "This child usually acts appropriately" versus "This child is often not well-behaved"; an item on the popularity subscale was "This child has a lot of friends" versus "This child doesn't have a lot of friends." Respondents used Harter's 4-point response scale (i.e., selected an option and then indicated if the item was "sort of" or "really" true, scored so a high score indicated high SS or popularity). Alphas for the scale for aides and teachers at the two administrations ranged from .89 to .91 for SS and from .94 to .95 for popularity. Alphas for the entire scale (including all 10 items) ranged from .87 to .88.

In addition, the same scale was completed at the end of T2 by undergraduate observers who observed the children for over 3 months each semester. These observers rotated around the classrooms and playgrounds in a systematic order obtaining information on anger reactions (the data on anger reactions are not reported in this paper; see Fabes & Eisenberg, 1992a, for a general description of the observation procedures). Because different numbers of observers viewed each child (with the minimum for each child being two observers and most being observed rated by three to five observers), observers' responses for each child were averaged for each item. The alphas for these averaged responses were .93 and .98, respectively, for SS and popularity (the alpha for the entire scale was

.89). Because of the drop in reliability when the items for general social skills and popularity were combined (see above for teacher/aide data), and because we wanted to differentiate between adults' conceptions of social skills and their perceptions of children's social status, the items assessing social skills and popularity were not combined.

Teachers' and aides' ratings of social skills were correlated with one another at both T1 and T2, r's(86 and 81) = .72 and .63, and across time, r's(88 and 78) = .75 and .66 for teachers and aides (although aides differed at T1 and T2), all p's < .001. As a result, their ratings were standardized and averaged both within time period and across time. In addition, the observers' ratings at T2 were significantly correlated with the composite measure of teachers'/aides' ratings at T2 only and combined across both T1 and T2, r's(90) = .72 and .75, p's < .001, respectively. Thus, a composite measure of rated social competence at T2 was obtained by standardizing and averaging teachers', aides', and observers' ratings, although observers' ratings also were used separately in analyses in which the predictor variables were teacher/aide measures (so that predictors and outcome variables were obtained from different sources). In addition, in some analyses we report findings within a given time period (T1 or T2).

Similarly, teachers' and aides' ratings of children's popularity were significantly correlated with each other, r's(86 and 81) = .48 and .62, p's < .001, at T1 and T2, respectively. Moreover, the undergraduate observers' ratings of the children's popularity at T2 were significantly correlated with the teachers' and aides' ratings of popularity at T2, r's(81 and 90) = .48 and .73, p's < .001. Also, teacher/aide combined ratings of popularity at T1 and T2 were associated with respective sociometric ratings, r's(89 and 91) = .40 and .46, p's < .001, as were observers' ratings at T2, r(91) = .58, p < .001. Because of the overlap in measures, and because sociometric status is a more direct measure of popularity, the latter was used in all subsequent analyses.

Coping. Children's preferred coping behaviors were assessed in two ways. First, teachers and aides (at T1 and T2) and mothers (at T1) rated on a 7-point scale the likelihood that the child would engage in each of 13 general types of coping responses. These ratings reflected the following types of responses used to study coping with stress (Ayers et al., 1990; Kliewer, 1991): (1) instrumental coping (takes some constructive action to improve a problem situation), (2) emotional intervention (cries to elicit assistance from others to help solve the problem), (3) instrumental aggression (resolves problems through physical or verbal aggression), (4) avoidance (leaves or avoids a problem situation), (5) distraction (keeps him- or herself busy so as not to think about the problem), (6) venting (cries to release pent-up feelings or elicit comfort from others), (7) emotional aggression (uses physical or verbal aggression to release pent-up feelings), (8) cognitive restructuring (tries to think about the situation in a positive way), (9) emotional support (talks about his or her problems with friends or a teacher in hope of getting support), (10) cognitive avoidance (avoids thinking about a problem or attempts to ignore it), (11) instrumental intervention (asks an adult or another child to help solve the problem), (12) instrumental support (talks with a friend or teacher about the problem to help find a solution), and (13) denial (denies that there really is a problem). The aforementioned definitions, sometimes accompanied by an example, were provided to raters.

In addition, at T1, prior to filling out the aforementioned ratings, teachers and aides were presented with three scenarios about everyday conflicts and asked to rate (on the same 1–7 scale) the likelihood of the children responding in each of nine ways (the first nine types of coping listed above), as well as "doing nothing." The scenarios concerned when the child was hurt or angry because a peer purposely knocked over the block tower he or she was building, or because he or she was excluded from peers' play or being made fun of by peers. Concrete examples of these coping behaviors were provided; for example, for the exclusion scenario, the option for avoidance was "Stays away from the children or leaves the scene," whereas the option for instrumental coping was "Asks the other children why they won't let him/her play." Alphas for each of the 10 ratings across the three scenarios ranged from .88 to .98 for teachers and from .88 to .96 for aides.

Thus, at T1, both the global coping ratings and the ratings for the three coping vignettes (which were averaged) were obtained from teachers and aides. Items for the same mode of coping generally were highly related across these two types of measures (alphas for the two-item scales ranged from .80 to .98 for teachers and .75 to .96 for aides). Moreover, denial (in global ratings only) and doing nothing (in story ratings only) were related (alphas = .78 for teacher, .92 for aides), as were the two ratings of instrumental support and instrumental intervention (in global ratings only; alphas = .86 and .68). In addition, based on correlational analyses, it was clear that many conceptually related modes of coping were empirically related. Thus, we combined a number of indexes of coping (after standardization) into the following composite scores (which reflect conceptual distinctions in the literature): (1) distraction/avoidance—distracting actions and avoidant behavior (measures from both story and global ratings), doing nothing (from vignettes), denying (from global ratings), and cognitive avoidance (global rating) (alphas for seven-item scale = .88 for teachers, .92 for aides); (2) aggression—global and story ratings for both emotional and instrumental aggression (alphas for this four-item scale = .88 and .97 for teachers and aides); (3) venting—global and story ratings of venting emotion and emotional intervention (alphas for four-item scale = .98 and .94); and (4) seeking support (global ratings for instrumental intervention and instrumental support, as well as story and global measures of emotional support; alphas for the 4-item scale = .90 and .84). In addition, as described previously, there were measures of instrumental coping and cognitive restructuring based solely on a single global rating and the mean score of the three vignette ratings (see above).

At T1 for mothers and at T2 for teachers and aides, global ratings but not story ratings were obtained. For teachers, aides, and mothers, composites similar to those from T1 were formed (in addition to single item measures of cognitive restructuring and instrumental coping). Mothers' coping composites at T1 were the same as for the teachers/aides at T2, except denial did not cluster with the other distracting/avoidant modes of coping. The composites were (1) denial, avoidance, distracting actions, cognitive avoidance (four-item alphas = .75 and .74 for teachers and aides; alpha for three-item composite for mothers = .61); (2) instrumental and reactive aggression (alphas = .88, .93, and .88 for teachers, aides, and mothers); (3) instrumental support, instrumental intervention, and emotional support (three-item alphas = .95, .96, and .56); and (4) venting and emotional intervention (two-item alphas = .93, .88, and .64). The items in the aforementioned groupings were standardized and averaged to form composites.

Test-retest correlations for the teachers' ratings taken approximately 5 months apart ranged from .52 to .74 (all except instrumental coping were .59 or higher), even though the stories were part of the composite measures at T1 and not at T2. Moreover, teachers' and aides' scores for each given coping composite were significantly interrelated at both time periods (r's ranged from .35 to .74 at T1 and from .39 to .58 at T2). Thus, teachers' and aides' scores were standardized and averaged at both T1 and T2. Correlations of the teacher/aide combined composites from T1 to T2 ranged from .51 for instrumental coping to .78 for aggression. Therefore, aggregate measures across T1 and T2 frequently were used in subsequent analyses.

Because a number of the coping aggregates were significantly interrelated, they were further reduced. Teachers'/aides' (combined) responses were factor analyzed, as were mothers'. For teachers/aides, there were two factors (using loadings of .70 or higher): (1) distraction/avoidance (.82), cognitive restructuring (.79), aggression (−.75), and venting (−.71), and (2) instrumental problem solving (.91) and seeking support (.90). No category scored higher than .46 on the other factor. Separate analyses for girls and boys resulted in very similar factors. Thus, two composite coping scores were computed by combining the standardized values of the aforementioned categories: acting out versus avoidance (with a high score indicating more aggression/venting and low levels of distraction/avoidance and cognitive restructuring) and constructive coping. These composite scores, including data from T1 and T2 (each of which was positively related over time; r's[90] = .61 and .83 for constructive and acting out coping), were used in subsequent analyses unless specified otherwise.

Similar factor analyses resulted in quite different factors for mothers' ratings of boys and girls. Thus the maternal data were not reduced further.[1]

Emotional intensity. Teachers, aides, and mothers rated children's emotional intensity (EI) both semesters. At T1, the scale consisted of five items (e.g., "This child responds very emotionally to things around him/her" and "This child tends to get nervous or distressed easily") adapted from Larsen's (Larsen & Diener, 1987) Affective Intensity Scale (1 = usually false; 5 = usually true). At T2, the EI scale included eight items (rated on a 7-point scale; 1 = extremely untrue, 7 = extremely true). Four of the items at the two times were virtually identical in wording; five pertained to negative emotions such as anger, upset, or anxiety. Alphas for teachers, aides, and mothers were .88, .87, and .79, respectively, at T1, and .84, .67, .62 at T2 (after dropping one item that lowered the alpha).

Teachers' and aides' ratings of EI were significantly related at T1 and T2, r's(84 and 83) = .59 and .43, p's < .001. Thus, their ratings were averaged at each time period (only the teacher's rating was used if the aide's was missing). Moreover, the two composites were correlated across T1 and T2, $r(89) = .64$, $p < .001$, and therefore were averaged. Similarly, mothers' ratings of EI were correlated across time, $r(71) = .54$, $p < .001$, and were averaged. The composite T1/T2 measures were used in all analyses unless specified otherwise.[2]

Attentional control. Attention shifting and attention focusing were assessed with items adapted from Derryberry and Rothbart's (1988) temperament scale. Both were assessed with three items (e.g., "When interrupted or distracted, my child often forgets what he/she was about to say" and "My child's attention is easily disrupted if there are people talking in the room around him/her" for attention shifting and focusing). Attention focusing and shifting were positively correlated,

---

[1]For 3 months at T2, four new and different observers conducted "scan" observations of the children in random order and coded their behaviors during free play into the following mutually exclusive categories (from Mize & Ladd, 1988): physical/verbal aggression, social conversations, cooperative play (with or without conversation), solitary play, onlooking, and teacher-oriented. Kappas for reliability codings (215 to 332 per observer) for each observer for each category ranged from .72 to 1.00 (except aggression was observed only three times during reliability coding; agreement was 67%). For teacher/aide ratings, constructive coping was positively related to cooperative interactions and negatively related to onlooker and solitary behavior, partial r's(89) = .32, −.24, and −.25, p's < .002, .024, and .015 (controlling sex and age). Acting out versus avoidance was positively related to observed aggression and negatively related to onlooker behavior, partial r's(89) = .32 and −.27, p's < .002 and .009. For mothers' ratings of coping, avoidance/distraction was negatively related to observed aggression and positively related to teacher-oriented behavior, partial r's(74) = −.31 and .23, p's < .007 and .049; venting was positively related to solitary play and negatively related to cooperation, partial r's(76) = .23 and −.24, p's < .041 and .034; and aggressive coping was negatively related to observed cooperation, partial $r(76) = −.23$, $p < .045$ (partialing age and sex). These data provide some validity of our indexes of coping behaviors.

[2]An observational measure of anger intensity when children were angered (a 3-point rating) was also obtained by the 15 undergraduate observers (interrater reliability = .79 at T2; see Fabes & Eisenberg, 1992b, for discussion of this measure in another study). This measure was positively related to teacher/aide ratings of EI, $r(73) = .53$, $p < .001$ (r = .09 for mothers).

$r(91) = .63, p < .001$ for averaged teachers/aides and $r(77) = .34, p < .002$ for mothers, as well as conceptually related; thus, a composite attention measure was computed using the items from both scales (alphas = .83, .80, and .71 for teachers, aides, and mothers with one item dropped).

Teachers' and aides' ratings of attentional control at T2 were positively related, $r(83) = .40, p < .001$. Thus, they were averaged across the two to form composite measures.

Negative affect. We created a negative affect scale with items adapted from Derryberry and Rothbart's (1988) fear (e.g., "This child often feels uneasy when he/she enters a darkened room"), sadness (e.g., "This child frequently misses friends and relatives"), and autonomic reactivity (e.g., "This child's palms usually sweat during an important event") subscales. Many of the items on these scales were intercorrelated, and alphas for sadness or fear alone sometimes were relatively low. Moreover, the sadness, fear, and autonomic reactivity scales grouped together in a factor analysis, whereas the two attention subscales grouped on another factor. Alphas for the 10-item scale for teachers, aides, and mothers were .86, .80, and .68, respectively. Because ratings of negative affect were positively correlated for aides and teachers, $r(83) = .25, p < .019$, they were aggregated to create a more reliable measure.

Sociometric Status

Each semester children's sociometric status was assessed using procedures similar to those of Asher, Singleton, Tinsley, and Hymel (1979). Children sorted pictures of the children in their classroom into three piles ("really like to play with," "like to play with some," and "like to play with *only* a little bit"). Pictures of faces varying in smiling (from a lot to virtually not at all) were used to mark each pile. Nearly all children in the classes rated all their classmates (a couple were unwilling to do so).

To compute a summary score for sociometric status, children were assigned a score of 3 for every time they were placed by peers in the "really like to play with" pile, a 2 for the middle pile, and a 1 for the least positive pile. These scores were summed and standardized within class and sex. Sociometric status was only moderately stable from T1 to T2, $r(88) = .45, p < .001$ (r's = .53 and .38, p's $< .001$ and .008, for girls and boys, respectively). Given the amount of change over time, most analyses pertaining to sociometric status were conducted separately for T1 and T2.[3]

---

[3]We also formed sociometric groups using Coie and Dodge's (1988) formula for popular and rejected children (all other children were in an average group). The only modification was that we used .5 SD rather than I SD in the formula so that our three groups would be approximately equal in size. Multivariate and discriminant analyses using these three groups resulted in findings quite similar to those reported for our primary index of sociometric status.

Procedure

At T1 and T2, teachers and aides completed the measures of EI, coping, SS, and popularity for each child near the end of the semester (at least 12 weeks into the school term, and often later). Mothers completed the measures of coping (only the global rating scale) and EI at T1. At T2, teachers, aides, and mothers were administered the measures of children's attentional control and negative affect. Maternal data were obtained (sometimes with missing data) from 81 mothers at T1 and 80 at T2 (89 had EI ratings at one time or the other). At T1 and T2, the children's behaviors on the playground and in classrooms were observed by undergraduate observers who rated the children's social competence and popularity (only for those children that they felt they knew fairly well). Sociometric ratings were collected near the end of each semester, starting about 11 weeks into the children's school semester (the two evaluations were about 5 months apart).

RESULTS

Overview of the Analyses

The primary goal of the analyses was to examine the degree to which indexes of children's social competence could be predicted from school and maternal measures of their regulation and emotionality. In preliminary analyses, we examined the relations of analogous ratings of the major constructs across settings, as well as interrelations among the various predictor variables (i.e., measures of regulation and emotionality) and between the two major dependent variables (sociometric status and adult-rated social skills). Then the relations of the predictor variables to our measures of social competence were examined with correlational and regression analyses.

Our original intent was to examine the interaction between indexes of emotionality and regulation in predicting social competence (i.e., the moderating role of regulation on emotionality). However, the ability to interpret interaction terms is severely limited if the two predictor variables are highly correlated (see Baron & Kenny, 1986). As is discussed in the results, our measures of emotionality and regulation generally were moderately to highly correlated, probably due to the fact that adults' ratings of children's regulation and emotionality were based on observations of children's behaviors—behaviors that already reflect both regulatory processes and the expression of emotion. Thus, in the analyses we focused primarily on the cumulative and relative contributions of our indexes of emotionality and regulation to prediction of social competence.

   In the analyses, measures usually were aggregated across reporters and time (when possible and when the same reporter was not used for both the assessment of predictors and dependent variables); our primary purpose was not to examine influences across time (in part because the time gap between measures was relatively short and because the aggregate measures appeared to be more reliable; see Rushton, Brainerd, & Pressley, 1983). Nonetheless, limited information regarding correlations within a given time period or from the first to the second assessment is provided. Moreover, because of the number of analyses, we try to emphasize patterns of findings rather than isolated findings.

Preliminary Analyses

Interrelations of analogous measures in the home and school contexts. To examine the relations between measures of regulation and emotionality in the home and school, analogous measures for teacher/aides (henceforth called school ratings) and mothers were correlated. Home and school ratings of coping generally were positively correlated. Correlations between the two at T1 (when maternal ratings were obtained and prior to reducing the school data further) for instrumental problem solving, distraction/avoidance, aggression, seeking support, venting, and cognitive restructuring were .28, .28, .29, .26, .33, and .06, p's < .001, .013, .008, .017, .002, and N.S. Mothers' ratings of EI were not significantly related to school ratings at T1 (r = .09) and were only marginally related at T2, $r(79) = .21, p < .055$. Moreover, consistent with prior findings on temperament ratings at home and at school (e.g., Goldsmith, Riesser-Danner, & Briggs, 1991), home and school ratings of negative affect and attentional control were not significantly related to the analogous ratings for mothers at T2.

Interrelations of regulation and emotionality measures. To examine the correlations between the regulation measures (the composite coping indexes, combined across time and rater and attentional control at T2) and those of emotionality (including rated EI, averaged across time, and negative affect), partial correlations (controlling age) were computed (see Table 1 for means). The findings are presented separately by sex in Table 2.

   As can be seen in Table 2, the patterns of rated EI and negative affectivity (which were positively correlated) to indexes of regulation were similar. Both were positively related to girls' and boys' acting out versus avoidance and negatively related to boys' constructive coping. In addition, both were negatively correlated with attentional control. Correlations within T1 and T2 are not presented in Table 2. However, the relations between EI and aspects of regulation generally were similar using T1 and T2 measures of EI except, for girls, EI at T2 but not T1 was negatively related to attentional control, partial r's(42 and 39) = −.43, p < .001 and −.06, N.S., respectively (correlations were quite similar for boys

TABLE 1
Means and Standard Deviations for the Measures of Regulation, Emotionality,
and Social Competence

MEASURES	GIRLS		BOYS	
	M	SD	*M*	SD
oping:				
School constructive coping[a]	.18	.64	−.18	.71
School acting out vs. avoidant coping[a]	−.38	2.32	.43	2.37
School attentional control	4.54	.83	4.17	.94
Mother: cognitive restructuring	3.83	1.56	3.64	1.30
Mother: avoidance/distraction	3.46	1.12	3.51	1.09
Mother: aggression	2.97	1.7	3.77	1.63
Mother: support seeking	5.01	1.03	4.88	1.08
Mother: venting	4.50	1.45	3.48	1.33
Mother: instrumental coping	5.39	1.00	5.26	1.18
Mother: attentional control	4.82	1.03	4.86	1.05
motionality:				
School emotional intensity[a]	−.23	.69	.25	.82
School negative affect	3.63	.71	3.74	.72
Mother: emotional intensity[a]	.07	.84	−.01	.96
Mother: negative affect	4.20	.85	3.97	.74
Teacher/aide/observer composite[a]	.41	.69	−.38	1.00
Observers only (T2 only)	3.54	.55	3.35	.59
T1 sociometric status[b]	0	.95	0	.96
T2 sociometric status[b]	0	.95	0	.96
T1 and T2 sociometric status	−.03	.83	.00	.79

NOTE.—School measures indicate teacher and aide aggregate measures.
[a] Standardized and averaged across semesters.
[b] Standardized within sex.

for the T1 and T2 measures of EI). In addition, the correlations of attentional control to constructive coping and acting out versus avoidant coping both were significant for boys, whereas neither were significant for girls.

This pattern of findings was not due solely to coping and EI being rated by the same persons. Most of the intercorrelations were significant when the ratings of one person were correlated with those of the other (e.g., when teacher ratings were correlated with aides' ratings, or vice versa; see footnotes for Table 2). Thus, our measures of emotionality were often related to indexes of regulation in the school setting even when the raters were different, although constructive coping was unrelated to other indexes of emotionality or regulation for girls, and girls' attentional control was unrelated to both modes of coping.

We also examined the correlations of maternal reports of children's negative affect and emotional intensity to the indexes of maternal reported regulation (i.e., attentional control and the six coping categories). For girls, although emotional intensity and negative affect were positively correlated, partial $r(36) = .50$,

TABLE 2

Partial Correlations among School-based Measures of Emotionality and Regulation
(Controlling Age)

Coping and Emotionality Composites	Constructive Coping	Acting Out vs. Avoidant Coping	Attentional Control	Emotional Intensity	Negative Affect
Constructive coping	. . .	−.02	.01	.16	−.03
Acting out versus avoidance coping	−.25[+]	. . .	−.20	.82[***c,f]	.33[*a]
Attentional control	.39[**c]	−.50[***b]	. . .	−.27[*]	−.53[***a]
Emotional intensity	−.39[**d]	.82[***c,]	−.51[***a]	. . .	.52[***c]
Negative affect	−.34[*]	.47[***e]	−.58[***d]	.51[***a,d]	. . .

NOTE.—Correlations for girls are above the diagonal; those for boys are below.
[a] The correlation of teachers' ratings (on left) to aides' ratings (on top) was significant at $p < .05$.
[b] The correlation of teachers' ratings (on left) to aides' ratings (on top) was significant at $p < .01$.
[c] The correlation of teachers' ratings (on left) to aides' ratings (on top) was significant at $p < .001$.
[d] The correlation of aides' ratings (on left) to teachers' ratings (on top) was significant at $p < .05$.
[e] The correlation of aides' ratings (on left) to teachers' ratings (on top) was significant at $p < .01$.
[f] The correlation of aides' ratings (on left) to teachers' ratings (on top) was significant at $p < .001$.
[+] $p < .10$.
[*] $p < .05$.
[**] $p < .01$.
[***] $p < .001$.

$p < .001$, negative affect was unrelated to indexes of regulation, whereas emotional intensity was negatively related to instrumental coping and avoidance/distraction, partial r's(35 and 33) = −37 and −.35, p's < .026 and .04, and positively related to aggression and venting, partial r's(35 and 36) = .36 and .45, p's < .028 and .005. For boys, negative affect and emotional intensity also were positively related, partial $r(38)$ = .68, $p < .001$; negative affect was negatively related to positive cognitive restructuring, partial r's(33) = −.34, $p < .044$, and positively related to aggressive coping, partial r (34) = .45, $p < .006$. EI was negatively related to boys' positive cognitive restructuring and instrumental coping, partial r's(39 and 40) = −.52 and −.30, p's < .001 and .057, and positively related to boys' aggressive coping, partial $r(40)$ = .43, $p < .004$. Thus, for mothers as well as school personnel, there were often moderate associations between reports of regulation and of emotionality.

Interrelations of Measures of Indexes of Social Skills and Sociometric Status

The measures of social functioning used in the major analyses were ratings of children's social skills at school (as reported by adults) and their sociometric status. Correlations (partialing age and sex) were computed to examine their interrelations. Peer ratings at T1 were unrelated to teacher/aide ratings of social competence at T1 ($r = .09$), but the T2 ratings of sociometric status were related to school composite ratings of social competence at T2, partial $r(89) = .41$, $p < .001$, as well as to the ratings of the undergraduate observers, partial $r(88) = .46$, $p < .001$ (controlling sex and age). The pattern of correlations was similar for boys and girls.[4]

Prediction of Social Functioning from School Rated Temperament and Coping

In this section, we examine the relations of measures of emotional responding (EI, negative affect) and coping/regulation (constructive and acting out vs. avoidance, attentional control) to sociometric status and adults' reports of social skills. Prediction to T2 indexes of social functioning is emphasized (indeed, undergraduates rated social skills only at T2) because children knew each other better by T2 (which would affect ratings of sociometric status) and because their patterns of behavior at school would be expected to be better established later in the school year.

Sociometric status. As presented in Table 3, peer status at T2 was correlated primarily with boys' regulation and emotionality (age was partialed in all analyses); it was positively related to boys' attentional process and constructive coping, and negatively related to negative affect, rated EI, and acting out versus avoidant coping. Interestingly, at T1 (which is not in Table 3), acting out versus avoidant coping (measured at T1), EI (T1), and attentional control (assessed only at T2), were not significantly related to boys' sociometric status, although constructive coping at T1 and negative affect were still at least marginally positively and negatively correlated with status at T1, partial r's(46 and 45) $= .28$ and $-.31$, p's $< .055$ and .037. For girls, the pattern of correlations was very similar (and nonsignificant) at T1 and T2. Correlations between T1 measures of EI or the coping composites and T2 sociometric status were similar to those presented in Table 3.

[4]Teachers/aides rated boys as higher on aggressive coping and lower on coping by seeking support, p's $< .001$; lower on constructive coping (composite measure), $p < .01$; higher on acting out versus avoidant coping (composite), but only at T1, $p < .03$; lower on social competence and attentional control, $p < .001$ and .003; and marginally higher on EI, $p < .056$. Mothers rated boys higher on aggressive coping and lower on venting coping, p's $< .036$ and .001 (there were no findings for temperament); observers rated boys as lower on social competence, $p < .001$. With regard to correlations with age, older children were rated as lower on distraction/avoiding coping, cognitive restructuring, negative affect, and EI (the latter only at T1), and higher on instrumental problem-solving (all teacher/aide ratings), p's $< .001$, .028, .059, .046, and .039. There were no significant relations of age to ratings of social skills. Finally, verbal intelligence, as assessed with Ammons and Ammons' (1962) Quick IQ test for 80 children at T1 and 90 children at T2 (and averaged across T1 and T2 when possible), was positively related to mothers' assessments of aggressive coping and school ratings of instrumental coping, and negatively related to school assessments of avoidant coping, p's $< .029$, .026, and .003 (it was unrelated to any other indexes).

TABLE 3
Partial Correlations of Indexes of
Regulation and Emotionality with
Sociometric Status and Observers' Ratings
of Social Skills (Controlling Age)

	Rated Social Skills	Sociometric Status
Constructive coping:		
Girls	.04	.26$^+$
Boys	.36*	.30*
Acting out versus avoidance:		
Girls	−.65***	−.16
Boys	−.65***	−.39**
Attentional control:		
Girls	−.22	−.17
Boys	.64***	.41**
Negative affect:		
Girls	.13	−.01
Boys	−.39**	−.43**
Rated EI:		
Girls	−.45**	−.17
Boys	−.62***	−.32*

NOTE.—Both the sociometric ratings and the observers' ratings were from T2 (findings were similar when the
combined T1 and T2 sociometric ratings were used). The
coping measures were the combined T1 and T2 composites, although the findings generally were stronger when
only the T2 coping scores were used.
$^+$ $p < .10$.
* $p < .05$.
** $p < .01$.
*** $p < .001$.

In regression equations, we examined the joint contribution of the coping/
regulation and emotionality to sociometric ratings at T2 separately for boys and
girls. Due to the relatively small number of subjects and the fact that age did not
contribute significantly to prediction, age was not included in these regression
analyses. Thus, the two composite coping variables, negative affect, and composite EI were entered in a single step (see Table 4). When controlling for all other
variables, negative affect was marginally negatively related to peer status,
whereas constructive coping was marginally positively related. The contribution
of individual variables to prediction was undoubtedly limited because of the overlapping variance in predictors. In a similar regression analysis for girls, the multiple R was only marginally significant (see Table 4). In an additional regression
equation in which interactions with sex were entered on the third step (and sex on
the first step with age), the change in R^2 was not significant. Thus, although

TABLE 4
The Relations of Sociometric Status and Observers' Ratings of Social Skills to Teacher/Aide Skills of
Regulation and Emotionality: Regression Equations

| | CRITERION VARIABLES | | | |
| | Observers' Ratings of Social Skills | | Sociometric Status (T2) | |
PREDICTORS	Boys	Girls	Boys	Girls
Betas:				
Constructive coping	.09	.06	.25$^+$	.37*
Acting out versus avoidant coping	-.43*	-.72****	.00	.29
Rated emotional intensity	.19	-.10	.02	-.59*
Attentional control	.44**	-.24$^+$	.11	-.04
Negative affect	.14	.27$^+$	-.32$^+$	.20
F value	$F(5, 42) = 10.84$****	$F(5, 38) = 11.94$****	$F(5, 42) = 3.39$*	$F(5, 39) = 2.06^+$
Multiple R	.75	.78	.54	.46

$^+$ $p < .10$.
* $p < .05$.
** $p < .01$.
*** $p < .001$.
**** $p < .0001$.

prediction of sociometric status from regulation and emotionality was considerably better for boys and girls, there were not significant differences in the degree of prediction for the two sexes.

In another analysis, we compared children who were high in EI and low in regulation with other children. Specifically, we divided subjects into high versus low groups on attentional control, EI, and constructive coping (based on median splits within each sex; using the composite T1/T2 data when possible). Acting out versus avoidant coping was not used because it included items more directly indicative of unregulated behavior (Sanson, Prior, & Kyrios, 1990) and was highly correlated with EI (thus our analyses were conservative). Negative affect was not used to group children because of its high correlation with EI and the more central role of EI in regard to uncontrolled behavior. Then subjects who were high on EI and low on the two measures of regulation ($N = 18$; 3 girls, 15 boys) were compared with other subjects ($N = 75$). According to a two-level (regulation/EI group) analysis of covariance (covarying age and sex), children high in EI but low in regulation/constructive coping were significantly lower in sociometric status ($M = -.55$) than were other children ($M = .13$), $F(1, 89) = 8.68$, $p < .004$.

Finally, with regression analyses we examined the prediction of sociometric status from regulatory capacities and emotionality while controlling for one another. Thus, in one set of regression equations the three indexes of regulation (attentional control, constructive coping, and acting out vs. avoidant coping) were entered as a set on the first step and then the two indexes of emotionality (EI and negative affect) were entered on the second step; in a second set of equations, the order of entry for the two sets of variables was reversed. As can be seen in Table 5, for girls, neither set of variables predicted more clearly when the other set was controlled (recall, also, that prediction for girls was only marginally significant). For boys, whichever set of variables was entered first predicted relatively strongly, whereas those entered on the second step did not. Thus, regulatory and emotional characteristics of children overlapped in the variance they explained in predicting peer status, and neither was a clearly stronger predictor.

Observers' ratings of social skills. Because children's temperament and coping were rated by teachers and aides, we used the undergraduate observers' ratings of general social competence (obtained only at T2) in analyses of the relations between coping or temperament and social competence (so the raters were not the same).

As can be seen in Table 3, girls' rated social skills were negatively correlated with acting out versus avoidance coping and rated EI. Boys' social skills were negatively related to the same variables as well as negative affect, and were positively related to attentional control and constructive coping. In general, the pattern of findings using T2 measures of coping and EI was similar to the pattern of findings at T1 with two exceptions: (*a*) girls' rated social skills were significantly nega-

TABLE 5

Regression Equations Examining the Prediction of Social Skills and Sociometric Status from Regulation and Emotionality While Controlling for One Another

Girls:						
Step 1: Emotionality	.61	.38	12.34****	.25	.06	1.41
Step 2: Regulation	.78	.24	7.66***	.46	.15	2.40+
Step 1: Regulation	.76	.57	17.77****	.31	.10	1.48
Step 2: Emotionality	.78	.04	1.94	.46	.11	2.73+
Boys:						
Step 1: Emotionality	.59	.34	11.79****	.47	.22	6.40**
Step 2: Regulation	.75	.22	7.04***	.54	.07	1.30
Step 1: Regulation	.74	.55	18.01****	.48	.23	4.28**
Step 2: Emotionality	.75	.01	.59	.54	.06	1.83

NOTE.—Emotionality includes negative affect and emotional intensity; regulation includes attentional control, constructive coping, and acting out versus avoidant coping. The steps indicate order of entry in the regression analyses; for each sex, the results for two different orders of entry (emotionality, then regulation and vice versa) are presented for both rated social skills and sociometric status.

+ $p < .10$.
* $p < .05$.
** $p < .01$.
*** $p < .001$.
**** $p < .0001$.

tively related to EI at T1, partial $r(38) = -.54$, $p < .001$, but not at T2, partial $r(41) = -.18$, N.S., and (*b*) girls' social skills were positively, nonsignificantly related to constructive coping at T1, partial $r(38) = -.23$, but negatively, nonsignificantly related to T2, partial $r(41) = -.10$. Moreover, correlations between observed social skills at T2 and T1 measures of EI and coping were similar to the aggregate data presented in Table 3 (albeit often slightly weaker).

In regression analyses, we examined the joint prediction of teachers'/aides' ratings of EI, negative affect, attentional control, and coping on rated social skills (separately by sex). As can be seen in Table 4, prediction was significant for both sexes, p's $< .0001$. These variables accounted for 57% and 61% of the variance in predicting boys' and girls' social skills, respectively. When controlling for other variables in the equation, girls who were low on acting out coping were viewed as more socially competent, and attention control was marginally, negatively related to status. Because the zero-order correlations between attentional control and girls' social skills were not even marginally significant, the unexpected effect for attentional control may be due to a suppression effect (Cohen & Cohen, 1983) and should be interpreted with caution. Boys' acting out versus avoidant coping was negatively related to rated social skills, whereas attentional control was positively related.

In an additional regression equation, we entered five interaction terms (between sex and each of the measures of emotionality and regulation) on a third step (and sex was entered in the first step). The change in R^2 for the third step was significant, $F(5, 80) = 4.06$, $p < .002$, R^2 change $= .09$, multiple $r = .80$. As is evident in Table 4, the findings for attention control differed significantly for boys and girls, beta $= .31$, $p < .0004$.

In addition, as discussed above, children were divided into two groups: those high on EI and low on attentional control/ constructive coping and other children. Children high in EI and low in regulation were significantly lower ($M = 2.98$) than other children ($M = 3.68$) in rated social skills, $F(1, 88) = 25.16$, $p < .001$.

Finally, as for sociometric status, two sets of regression equations were computed to assess the relative contributions of regulatory and emotional variables to predicting social skills when controlling for the contributions of one another. As can be seen in Table 5, for both girls and boys, regulatory capacities predicted above and beyond the contribution of emotionality (although the degree of prediction was reduced), whereas the reverse was not true. Thus, whatever variance emotionality accounted for in social skills was mediated or subsumed by regulatory abilities, whereas regulatory skills contributed to predictor above and beyond emotionality.

Prediction of Social Functioning from Mothers' Ratings of
Temperament and Coping

Mothers' ratings of their children's coping, attentional control, and emotional intensity were less often related to indexes of children's social functioning than were teacher/aide ratings, particularly for sociometric status. Mothers' ratings were unrelated to girls' peer status at T1 or T2. Mothers' ratings of boys' EI were negatively correlated with sociometric status at T2, partial $r(43) = -.45$, $p < .002$ (as well as for sociometric status at T1 and T2 combined); none of the correlations was significant for boys at T1 (i.e., using T1 indexes), although mothers' reports of EI at T1 were marginally, negatively related to peer status at T2, partial $r(45) = -.30$, $p < .055$. In addition, the composite of teacher, aide, and observers' ratings of social skills at T2 was positively related to mothers' reports of girls' distraction/avoidant coping and negative affect, partial r's(32 and 35) $= .40$ and $.35$, p's $< .02$ and $.034$, and boys' seeking of support, partial $r(39) = .36$, $p < .022$, and negatively correlated with boys' EI, partial $r(39) = -.42$, $p < .004$.

Regression analyses were computed to determine the joint contribution of maternal reported regulation and emotionality to children's social skills (using the composite score of standardized scores for teacher, aide, and observers' reports of social skills at T2). The variables that were significantly related to social skills in the aforementioned correlations were included, as was age, in the analyses (the number of predictors had to be limited due to sample size). For girls, age did not significantly contribute to prediction on the first step (multiple $R = .29$), however, addition of avoidance/distraction coping (beta $= .40$, $p < .012$) and negative affect (beta $= .38$, $p < .023$) increased prediction significantly, F for change in r^2 $(1, 29) = 6.64$, $p < .005$; R^2 change $= .29$, multiple $R = .61$. Thus, girls who were viewed as using avoidant and distracting ways of coping and who were high in negative affectivity were reported as having higher social skills at school. For boys, age did not significantly predict social skills on the first step (multiple $R = .20$); however, adding mothers' report of EI (beta $= -.25$, $p < .09$) and seeking support (beta $= .35$, $p < .019$) significantly enhanced prediction, F for change in R^2 $= 5.83$, $p < .006$, R^2 change $= .22$, multiple $R = .51$. According to an additional regression equation in which interactions with sex were included, there were no significant sex differences in the pattern of relations (although the betas for the interactions with sex for seeking support and negative affect were marginally significant).

Finally, high EI/low regulation (uncontrolled) children were compared to other children on our indexes of social functioning. Groups were constructed in a manner analogous as for school ratings; children high on maternal ratings of EI and low on support seeking and instrumental coping (the two types of coping behaviors that were in the teacher/aide index of constructive coping; seven children of each sex) were compared with other children (31 girls, 35 boys; median splits within sex were used to form groups). Mothers' ratings of attentional control were not used in the construction of groups because they were not a good predictor of children's functioning, and the group of uncontrolled children was too small ($N = 7$ rather than 14) if low attentional control was necessary for placement in the uncontrolled group. Based on a 2 (sex) $\times$ 2 (EI/regulation group) ANCOVA (covarying age), uncontrolled but reactive children were lower in sociometric ratings ($M = -.46$) than were other children ($M = .15$), $F(1, 77) = 6.06, p < .016$. In a similar ANCOVA in which the dependent variable was observers/teacher/aide ratings of social competence, the main effects of sex and group and the interaction of group and sex were significant, F's$(1, 75) = 19.85, 5.52$, and 4.05, p's $< .001, .021$, and $.048$, respectively. Uncontrolled, reactive boys ($M = -.959$) were rated lower in social competence than other boys ($M = -.063$), $F(1, 39) = 7.30, p < .01$; uncontrolled and more controlled girls (M's $= .401$ and $.448$) did not differ.

DISCUSSION

The results of the present study are consistent with the view that the emotional aspects of temperament as well as regulatory and coping capabilities are associated with children's general social skills (as rated by adults) and sociometric status. In addition, the combination of high emotional intensity with low levels of constructive coping and attentional regulation (the latter for teacher/aide but not mothers' ratings) was associated with low social skills and sociometric status (although findings sometimes were obtained only for one sex). These findings highlight the importance of considering both children's emotional proclivities and the ways in which they regulate emotion arousal as influences on their social behavior.

Our findings are relatively compelling for several reasons: (*a*) some of the relations were relatively strong, and the percentages of variance accounted for tended to be high (especially in the regression equations for school data); (*b*) multiple informants were used to assess many of the central constructs, and social functioning was examined in three different ways; and (*c*) our measures of emotion and coping/regulation were obtained independently of our measures of social functioning (e.g., different raters/observers were involved in data collection). In addition, we have some evidence of the validity of our measures; for example, school-based measures of coping were associated with relevant observed behavior (e.g., cooperative behavior; see footnote no. 4). Further, our findings regarding emotional intensity and negative emotion, as well as coping and attentional control, generally are consistent with expectations and with the limited available data (e.g., Kliewer, 1991; Stocker & Dunn, 1990).

Interestingly, school ratings of high attentional control, low negative affect, and constructive coping were primarily related to boys' social functioning (and not girls'). Acting out versus avoidant coping and emotional intensity tended to negatively relate to social functioning for both sexes (although neither was related to girls' sociometric status). For boys, then, indexes reflecting both the positive and negative dimensions of regulation as well as emotionality were related to their social functioning. In contrast, for girls, indexes of positive modes of regulation (e.g., attentional control, constructive coping) generally were unrelated to social functioning, whereas indexes of EI and negative modes of coping (e.g., acting out vs. avoidance) were associated with low social skills. Although the difference in relations across the sexes usually was not significant in regression analyses (except for attentional control in regard to the prediction of social skills), certain variables obviously were predictors of social competence for one sex but not the other.

It is unclear why this difference in pattern of findings for boys and girls occurred. There were not ceiling or floor effects for relevant variables for girls, and the SDs for attentional control and constructive coping, albeit somewhat smaller for girls, were not greatly different from those for boys. However, girls did score higher on constructive coping and lower on emotional intensity; perhaps most girls were above a threshold of constructive coping needed for positive social functioning and/or were not as likely as boys to become overly emotionally aroused. Moreover, very few girls fell into the grouping of children who were high in EI *and* low in constructive modes of regulation, at least as rated by school personnel in the classroom setting. Indeed, for girls but not boys, there was little association between constructive coping and measures of emotionality or attentional control; girls' constructive coping seemed to be independent of the temperamental constructs assessed in this study. Perhaps most girls are socialized to display constructive modes of coping regardless of temperamental predispositions. Alternatively, perhaps girls are expected to be well regulated; consequently, maybe it is only the lack of regulation that affects observers' assessments of girls' social competence.

Another interesting finding is that regulatory capabilities appeared to be more important than emotionality in predicting adults' perceptions of children's social skills at school (although both were predictors), whereas the two sets of factors contributed approximately equally to the prediction of sociometric status and overlapped considerably in the variance they accounted for in peer status. Adults in the school setting seem to judge children's general social skills (excluding popularity) primarily on the way emotional arousal and behavior are regulated, whereas peers seem to view emotionality and regulation as one and the same in choosing playmates. This difference was not due primarily to the content of the criterion measures for peers (sociometric evaluations) and adults (evaluations of how socially skilled and well behaved children were). When undergraduate observers' ratings of popularity with peers were the criterion variable in regressions in which the order of entry of the two sets of variables (regulation vs. emotionality) was varied, prediction of popularity was high (the multiple R's were .68 and .56 for girls and boys), but emotionality did not account for a significant amount of additional variance once regulation was entered (whereas regulation was a significant predictor even when entered second). In fact, emotionality was not a significant predictor of adults' ratings of girls' popularity even when the emotionality variables were entered first in the equation. Thus, preschoolers probably focus primarily on peers' behaviors as enacted in social contexts and do not, or are not able to, consider the reasons why a peer acts in a given way; in contrast, adults may be more likely to focus on the degree to which a given behavior is well regulated. Alternatively, well-regulated children may be better liked by adults than less regulated children, and this may have led to a positive bias in adults' assessments of well-regulated children's social competence.

Mothers' reports of children's coping/temperament also were related to children's social competence, particularly children's social skills as perceived by adults in the school setting. Boys' sociometric status and social skills were associated with maternal reports of low EI; their social competence was correlated with reported support seeking as a mode of coping. In contrast, girls' social skills at school were positively correlated with mothers' reports of using distracting/ avoidant coping and with negative affect. For girls, avoiding a potential social conflict seemed to be associated with adults' perceptions of social competence, and this perception is consistent with gender role stereotypes. In addition, girls who are sad or fearful at home seem to be perceived as better behaved at school, perhaps because they are relatively unlikely to get into trouble. The limited association of maternal ratings of emotionality and regulation to children's sociometric status may be due to mothers' limited observation of their children with larger groups of peers (resulting in their assessments being based primarily on behavior in the home). In addition, characteristics deemed socially competent in the home often may not be those that facilitate peer acceptance.

The finding that girls' use of avoidant/distracting coping at home was associated with school personnel's perceptions of good behavior is consistent with Kliewer's (1991) data indicating that avoidant coping was positively related to teacher-rated social competence at school and negatively related to problem behaviors. In addition, in the present study, teacher/aide assessments of avoidance/ distraction were positively related to undergraduates' assessments of social competence for boys and girls when the acting out/avoidance composite score was broken into its component parts (i.e., aggression/venting versus behavioral and cognitive avoidance, distracting actions, and denying). Thus, at least among normal children in a preschool setting, avoiding social conflict with peers seems to be associated with adults' perceptions of children's social competence. In contrast, avoidant modes of coping generally were unrelated to children's peer status. Interestingly, boys' avoidant coping (as rated by school personnel) at T1 was not significantly correlated with peer status at T1 or T2, r's $= -18$ and .07, whereas low peer status at T1 was significantly correlated with avoidant coping at T2, $r(48) = -.31, p < .028$. This pattern of findings suggests that for boys, lack of acceptance by peers leads to avoidance in peer conflicts rather than vice versa. In considering these findings, it is important to keep in mind that avoidant coping in social conflicts is not the same as general social avoidance, the latter of which has been associated with low peer status, particularly for girls (Coie et al, 1990).

In the present study, regulatory and emotional tendencies predicted social skills for both sexes, but sociometric status primarily for boys (although the difference in prediction between the sexes was not significant). In addition, there were fewer findings for sociometric status at T1 than later in the school year. It is likely that children's choices of playmates increasingly are based on the characteristics of their peers as they become better acquainted with them. In fact, in the present study, the correlation between peer status in the fall and in the spring was relatively modest, a finding that is consistent with the view that children's peer preferences and relationships develop over time. Nonetheless, it is unclear why regulatory and emotional characteristics were relatively weak predictors of girls' peer status. Most girls may exhibit relatively controlled and competent social behavior (recall they were lower than boys in EI and higher in constructive coping, acting out vs. avoidant coping at T2, attentional control, and rated social skills), with the result that other characteristics of girls (such as similarity in toy choices, attractiveness, or familiarity) largely determine whether or not girls are preferred as playmates.

It appears that mothers and teacher or aides differed in their perspectives of children's emotional intensity. Similar to Stocker and Dunn's (1990) findings for negative emotionality, school personnel and mothers' ratings of EI were unrelated at T1 and only marginally, positively related at T2. Moreover, teacher/aide but not mothers' ratings of EI were positively correlated with observed intensity of anger (see footnote 2). In additional analyses using scan observations (see footnote 3), mothers who rated their children as high in EI had children who exhibited solitary and dependent (teacher-oriented) behavior, partial r's(84) $= .30$ and .24, p's $< .006$ and .026, and were low in sociability and cooperation, partial r's(84) $= -.32$ and $-.27, p$'s $< .003$ and .011. In contrast, children rated as high on EI at school exhibited relatively high levels of both aggression and sociability, partial r's(89) $= .35$ and .23, p's $< .001$ and .03, and low levels of onlooking behavior, partial $r(89) = -.21, p < .044$. It appears that mothers' perceptions of children's emotional intensity were generally based on children's sadness, fear, sulking, and anxiety, whereas teachers'/aides' perceptions appeared to be influenced by instances of anger reactivity as well as other negative emotions. Clearly this is a topic that merits more attention.

Consistent with current discussions of coping and regulation (e.g., Compas, 1987), regulatory skills generally were negatively correlated with negative affect and emotional intensity, particularly for boys (note that in this study EI pertained primarily to intensity of negative emotions). Indeed, the two sets of dispositional characteristics (regulation and emotionality) are probably so intertwined by childhood that it is somewhat difficult to examine either one independent of the other. Especially when observations or ratings made on the basis of daily observation are the measures of regulation and emotionality, the two are difficult to isolate. This is because social behavior is the outcome of both emotional arousal and regulation of that arousal and related desires, needs, or action tendencies. Moreover, when using measures other than self report, it is difficult to know if emotional responsivity occurs but is well regulated and/or masked. Thus, research with older children and adults who are capable of reporting on their internal emotions and attempts to regulate those emotions is needed.

Because of the correlational nature of our data, it is impossible to determine cause and effect relationships. However, given the evidence of a genetic basis for negative affect and emotional intensity (at least after infancy; Plomin & Stocker, 1989; Reynolds, Barker, & Sakai, 1991), it seems likely that these components of temperament affect social functioning more than vice versa. Moreover, it seems reasonable to assume that the acquisition of constructive coping behaviors enhances social functioning, although well-liked children may have more opportunities to learn constructive rather than disruptive modes of coping. The situation is further complicated by the fact that emotional intensity was associated with coping behaviors. Thus, differences in temperament may affect the probability of children learning and implementing various modes of coping in social conflicts. For example, emotional children, especially those prone to negative affect, may be likely to vent emotion or agress in stressful situations, whereas less emotional children, and/or those who can regulate their emotion (e.g., with attentional processes), may be better able to react in constructive ways. An important task in future research is to start to disentangle these complex relations.

REFERENCES

Altshuler, J. L., & Ruble, D. N. (1989). Developmental changes in children's awareness of strategies for coping with uncontrollable stress. *Child Development*. **60.** 1337–1349.

Ammons, R. B., & Ammons, C. H. (1962). *The Quick Test: Provisional manual*. Missoula, MT: Psychological Tests Specialists.

Asher, S. R., Singleton, L. C., Tinsley, B. R., & Hymel, S. (1979). A reliable sociometric measure for preschool children. *Developmental Psychology, 15,* 443–444.

Ayers, T., Sandler, I., Bernzweig, J., Harrison, R., Wampler, T., & Lustig, J. (1990). *Handbook for the content analysis of children's coping responses.* Unpublished manuscript, Arizona State University.

Baron, R. M., & Kenny, D. A. (1986). The moderator-mediator variable distinction in social psychological research: Conceptual, strategic, and statistical considerations. *Journal of Personality and Social Psychology, 51,* 1173–1182.

Barron, A. P., & Earls, F. (1984). The relation of temperament and social factors to behavior problems in three-year-old children. *Journal of Child Psychology and Psychiatry, 25,* 23–33.

Bates, J. E. (1989). Concepts of measures of temperament. In G. A. Kohnstamm, J. E. Bates, & M. K. Rothbart (Eds.), *Temperament in childhood* (pp. 3–73). New York: Wiley.

Bates J. E. (1990). Conceptual and empirical linkages between temperament and behavior problems: A commentary on the Sanson, Prior, and Kyrios study. *Merrill-Palmer Quarterly, 36,* 193–199.

Billman, J., & McDevitt, S. C. (1980). Convergence of parent and observer ratings of temperament with observations of peer interaction in nursery school. *Child Development, 51,*395–400.

Block, J. H., & Block, J. (1980). The role of ego-control and ego-resiliency in the organization of behavior. In W. A. Collins (Ed.), Development of cognition, affect, and social relations. *Minnesota symposium on child psychology* (Vol. **13,** pp. 39–101). Hillsdale, NJ: Erlbaum.

Brody, G. H., Stoneman, Z., & Burke, M. (1988). Child temperament and parental perceptions of individual child adjustment: An intrafamilial analysis. *American Journal of Orthopsychiatry, 58,* 532–542.

Buss, A. H., & Plomin, R (1984), *Temperament: Early developing personality traits.* Hillsdale, NJ: Erlbaum.

Carver, C. S., Scheier, M. F., & Weintraub, J. K. (1989). Assessing coping strategies: A theoretically based approach. *Journal of Personality and Social Psychology, 56,* 267–283.

Cohen, J., & Cohen, P. (1983). *Applied multiple regression/correlation analysis for the behavioral sciences.* Hillsdale, NJ: Erlbaum.

Cohen, S., & Wills, T. A. (1985). Stress, social support, and the buffering hypothesis. *Psychological Bulletin, 98,* 310–317.

Coie, J. D., & Dodge, K. A. (1988). Multiple sources of data on social behavior and social status in the school: A cross-age comparison. *Child Development, 59,* 815–829.

Coie, J. D., Dodge, K. A., & Kupersmidt, J. B. (1990). Peer group behavior and social status. In S. R. Asher & J. D. Coie (Eds.), *Peer rejection in childhood* (pp. 17–59). Cambridge: Cambridge University Press.

Compas, B. E. (1987). Coping with stress during childhood and adolescence. *Psychological Bulletin, 101,* 393–403.

Compas, B. E. (1989, April). *Vulnerability to stress in childhood and adolescence.* Paper presented at the biennial meeting of the Society for Research in Child Development, Kansas City, MO.

Compas, B. E., Malcarne, V. L., & Fondacaro, K. M. (1988). Coping with stressful events in older children and young adolescents. *Journal of Consulting and Clinical Psychology,* **56,** 405–411.

Cummings, E. M., & Cummings, J. L. (1988). A process-oriented approach to children's coping with adults' angry behavior. *Developmental Review,* **8,** 296–321.

Derryberry, D., & Rothbart, M. K. (1988). Arousal, affect, and attention as components of temperament. *Journal of Personality and Social Psychology,* **55,** 958–966.

Eisenberg, N., & Fabes, R. A. (1992). Emotion, regulation, and the development of social competence. In M. S. Clark (Ed.), *Emotion and social behavior: Vol. 14. Review of personality and social psychology* (pp. 119–150). Newbury Park, CA: Sage.

Eisenberg, N., Fabes, R. A., Schaller, M., Miller, P. A., Carlo, G., Poulin, R., Shea, C., & Schell, R. (1991). Personality and socialization correlates of vicarious emotional responding. *Journal of Personality and Social Psychology,* **61,** 459–471.

Fabes, R. A., & Eisenberg, N. (1992a). Young children's coping with interpersonal anger. *Child Development,* **63,** 116–128.

Fabes, R. A., & Eisenberg, N. (1992b). Young children's emotional arousal and anger/ aggressive behaviors. In A. Fraczek & H. Zumkley (Eds.), *Socialization and aggression* (pp. 85–102). Berlin: Springer-Verlag.

Folkman, S., & Lazarus, R. S. (1988). Coping as a mediator of emotion. *Journal of Personality and Social Psychology,* **54,** 466–475.

Folkman, S., Lazarus, R. S., Dunkel-Schetter, C., DeLongis, N., & Gruen, R. (1986). Dynamics of a stressful encounter: Cognitive appraisal, coping, and encounter outcomes. *Journal of Personality and Social Psychology,* 1986, **50,** 992–1003.

Forsythe, C. J., & Compas, B. E. (1987). Interaction of cognitive appraisals of stressful events and coping: Testing the goodness of fit hypothesis. *Cognitive Therapy and Research,* **11,** 473–485.

Fox, N. A. (1989). Psychophysiological correlates of emotional reactivity during the first year of life. *Developmental Psychology,* **25,** 364–372.

Glyshaw, K., Cohen, L. H., & Towbes, L. C. (1989). Coping strategies and psychological distress: Prospective analyses of early and middle adolescents. *American Journal of Community Psychology,* **17,** 607–623.

Goldsmith, H. H., Rieser-Danner, L. A., & Briggs, S. (1991). Evaluating convergent and discriminant validity of temperament questionnaires for preschoolers, toddlers, and infants. *Developmental Psychology,* **27,** 566–580.

Harter, S. (1979). *Perceived Competence Scale for Children: Manual.* Denver: University of Denver.

Kanner, A. D., Coyne, J. C., Schaefer, D., & Lazarus, R. S. (1981). Comparison of two modes of stress measurement: Daily hassles and uplifts versus major life events. *Journal of Behavioral Medicine,* **4,** 1–39.

Klaczynski, P. A., & Cummings, E. M. (1989). Responding to anger in aggressive and nonaggressive boys: A research note. *Journal of Child Psychology and Psychiatry,* **30,** 309–314.

Kliewer, W. (1991). Coping in middle childhood: Relations to competence, type A behavior, monitoring, blunting, and locus of control. *Developmental Psychology, 27*, 689–697.

Kyrios, M., & Prior, M. (1990). Temperament, stress and family factors in behavioural adjustment of 3–5-year-old children. *International Journal of Behavioral Development, 13*, 67–93.

Larsen, R. J., & Diener, E. (1987). Affect intensity as an individual difference characteristic: A review. *Journal of Research in Personality, 21*, 1–39.

Lazarus, R. S., & Folkman, S. (1984). *Stress, appraisal, and coping.* New York: Springer.

Miller, S. M., & Green, M. L. (1985). Coping with stress and frustration: Origins, nature and development. In M. Lewis & C. Saarni (Eds.), *The socialization of emotions* (pp. 263–314). New York: Plenum.

Mize, J., & Ladd, G. W. (1988). Predicting preschoolers' peer behavior and status from their interpersonal strategies: A comparison of verbal and enactive responses to hypothetical social dilemmas. *Developmental Psychology, 24*, 782–788.

Nelson-Le Gall, S. (1981). Help-seeking: An understudied problem-solving skill in children. *Developmental Review, 1*, 224–246.

Olweus, D. (1980). Familial and temperamental determinants of aggressive behavior in adolescent boys: A causal analysis. *Developmental Psychology, 16*, 644–666.

Parker-Cohen, N. Y., & Bell, R. Q. (1988). The relationship between temperament and social adjustment to peers. *Early Childhood Research Quarterly, 3*, 179–192.

Plomin, R., & Stocker, C. (1989). Behavioral genetics and emotionality. In J. S. Reznick (Ed.), *Perspectives on behavioral inhibition* (pp. 219–240). Chicago: University of Chicago Press.

Prior, M. (1992). Childhood temperament. *Journal of Child Psychology and Psychiatry, 33*, 249–279.

Pulkkinen, L. (1982). Self-control and continuity from childhood to late adolescence. In P. B. Baltes & O. Brim, Jr. (Eds.), *Life-span development and behavior* (Vol. 4). New York: Academic Press.

Reynolds, C. A., Baker, L. A., & Sakai, L. M. (1991, November). *The development of affect intensity: A cross-sectional biometrical approach.* Paper presented at the "Lives through Time" Conference, Palm Springs, CA.

Roth, S., & Cohen, L. J. (1986). Approach, avoidance, and coping with stress. *American Psychologist, 41*, 813–819.

Rothbart, M. K. (1989). Behavioral approach and inhibition. In J. S. Reznick (Ed.), *Perspectives on behavioral inhibition* (pp. 139–157). Chicago: University of Chicago Press.

Rothbart, M. K., & Derryberry, D. (1981). Development of individual differences in temperament. In M. E. Lamb & A. L. Brown (Eds.), *Advances in developmental psychology* (Vol. 1, pp. 37–86). Hillsdale, NJ: Erlbaum.

Rothbart, M. K., Ziaie, H., & O'Boyle, C. (1992). Self-regulation and emotion in infancy. In N. Eisenberg & R. A. Fabes (Eds.), *Emotion and self-regulation in early development: New Directions in Child Development* (pp. 7–24). San Francisco: Jossey-Bass.

Rushton, J. P., Brainerd, C. J., & Pressley, M. (1983). Behavioral development and construct validity: The principle of aggregation. *Psychological Bulletin,* **94,** 18–38.

Sanson, A., Prior, M., & Kyrios, M. (1990). Contamination of measures in temperament research. *Merrill-Palmer Quarterly,* **36,** 179–192.

Stevenson-Hinde, J., Hinde, R. A., & Simpson, A. E. (1986). Behavior at home and friendly or hostile behavior in preschool. In D. Olweus, J. Block, & M. Radke-Yarrow (Eds.), *Development of antisocial and prosocial behavior* (pp. 127–145). Orlando, FL: Academic Press.

Stocker, C., & Dunn, J. (1990). Sibling relationships in childhood: Links with friendships and peer relationships. *British Journal of Developmental Psychology,* **8,** 227–244.

Strelau, J. (1983). *Temperament, personality, and activity.* New York: Academic Press.

Teglasi, H., & MacMahon, B. H. (1990). Temperament and common problem behaviors of children. *Journal of Applied Developmental Psychology,* **11,** 331–349.

Thomas, A., & Chess, S. (1977). *Temperament and development.* New York: Brunner/Mazel.

Weinberger, D. A., & Schwartz, G. E. (1990). Distress and restraint as superordinate dimensions of self-reported adjustment: A typological perspective. *Journal of Personality,* **58,** 381–417.

Windle, M., & Lerner, R. M. (1986). Reassessing the dimensions of temperamental individuality across the life span: The revised dimensions of temperament survey (DOTS-R). *Journal of Adolescent Research,* **1,** 213–230.

Zuckerman, M., Kuhlman, D. M., & Camac, C. (1988). What lies beyond E and N? Factor analyses of scales believed to measure basic dimensions of personality. *Journal of Personality and Social Psychology,* **54,** 96–107.

3

Friendship and Friendship Quality in Middle Childhood: Links with Peer Group Acceptance and Feelings of Loneliness and Social Dissatisfaction

Jeffrey G. Parker and Steven R. Asher

University of Illinois at Urbana-Champaign

The distinction between friendship adjustment and acceptance by the peer group was examined. Third- through 5th-grade children (N = 881) completed sociometric measures of acceptance and friendship, a measure of loneliness, a questionnaire on the features of their very best friendships, and a measure of their friendship satisfaction. Results indicated that many low-accepted children had best friends and were satisfied with these friendships. However, these children's friendships were lower than those of other children on most dimensions of quality. Having a friend, friendship quality, and group acceptance made separate contributions to the prediction of loneliness. Results indicate the utility of the new friendship quality measure

Reprinted with permission from *Developmental Psychology,* 1993, Vol. 29, No. 4, 611–621. Copyright © 1993 by the American Psychological Association, Inc.

This article is based on a doctoral dissertation carried out by Jeffrey G. Parker in the Department of Psychology at the University of Illinois at Urbana-Champaign. Portions of this article were presented at the annual meeting of the American Educational Research Association, Boston, in April 1990.

The research reported in this article was supported by National Institute of Child Health and Human Development Training Grant HD07205, by an American Psychological Association Dissertation Fellowship to Jeffrey G. Parker, and by a research grant to Steven R. Asher from the W. T. Grant Foundation.

We express our deepest appreciation to the students, teachers, and principals of Bottenfield, Carrie Busey, Ben Franklin, Dr. Howard, Thomas Paine, and Robeson Elementary Schools. Without the considerable cooperation and support of everyone involved, this research would not have been possible. We also thank Carol Rockhill and Kathryn Zelis for their help with data collection and Ben Wallace for developing a program to calculate reciprocal sociometric nominations.

and the value of distinguishing children's friendship adjustment from their general peer acceptance.

Researchers have made considerable progress in understanding the emergence, maintenance, and consequences of acceptance versus rejection by the peer group (see Asher & Coie, 1990, for reviews). Although group acceptance is an important facet of children's successful adaptation to peers, greater attention is needed to children's ability to form and maintain satisfying and supportive specific dyadic friendships as distinct from their ability to gain acceptance in the classroom more generally. Indeed, several authors (e.g., Blyth, 1983; Bukowski & Hoza, 1989; Furman & Robbins, 1985) argued that problems in group acceptance do not necessarily preclude satisfactory friendship adjustment, and they pointed out that concerns about the emotional well-being of low-accepted children might be attenuated if it could be established that low-accepted children have satisfying one-to-one friendships. To date, however, children's friendship adjustment has been studied far less frequently and less systematically than children's group acceptance, and the links between these two forms of peer adjustment are poorly understood.

Although little consensus exists as yet regarding the most appropriate means of assessing friendship success or adjustment, several reviews (e.g., Berndt, 1984; Bukowski & Hoza, 1989) suggested that two different elements of friendship adjustment could be examined. The first is the extent of a child's participation in friendship, that is, whether or not the child has an acknowledged, mutual friendship with another child. The second is the quality of a child's best friendship, that is, the degree of companionship the relationship provides, its supportiveness, and its level of conflict.

One can gauge the first element—children's participation in friendship—in school settings by identifying reciprocal choices among the patterns of nominations children give in response to questions about who their best friends are (see Berndt, 1984). Studies of this type have documented differences in participation in friendship as a function of gender, classroom and school structure, age, and several other variables (see Epstein, 1986, for a review). Moreover, recent research has documented the existence of important behavioral and social–cognitive differences between children involved in mutual friendships and children without mutual friendships (Carlson-Jones & Bowling, 1988; Howes, 1988; Mannarino, 1976; McGuire & Weisz, 1982; Roopnarine & Field, 1984).

To date, however, it is unclear how participation in friendship varies as a function of group acceptance. In studying the relationship between friendship and acceptance, one must have clearly distinct measures of each dimension. As Bukowski and Hoza (1989) pointed out, certain commonly used sociometric measures of acceptance actually confound acceptance with friendship. This occurs

particularly when group acceptance is assessed with sociometric nomination procedures, which typically require children to indicate their best friends or children
they like most within a particular group (often only three choices are allowed).
The number of nominations children receive is then taken as their level of acceptance, or these positive nominations are used in combination with negative nominations to identify poorly-accepted children. Although nomination measures are
highly valid for certain research questions, when limited-choice positive nominations are used to assess peer acceptance, certain interpretative problems arise.
When friendship is the explicit criterion (e.g., "Name your three best friends"),
error is likely to be introduced, because children will fail to nominate other children whom they actually like or accept but do not view as a best friend. Even
when friendship is not the explicit criterion (e.g., "Name three children you like
most"), there is still a problem. Because children are restricted in the number of
choices they can make, they are likely to limit their choices to their best friends.
Moreover, by allowing only a limited number of choices, information is missing
about how children feel about most of the children in their classroom.

A conceptually clearer approach would be for one to use reciprocal friendship-
nomination sociometric measures to assess friendship and to use a "roster-and-
rating scale" sociometric measure of liking to assess children's overall acceptance
by their peers (for early steps in this direction, see Asher, Singleton, & Taylor,
1982; Oden & Asher, 1977). Reciprocal friendship nominations provide face-valid
indicators of friendship (see Bukowski & Hoza, 1989), and rating-scale measures
of acceptance provide complete information about how much each child likes
every other child in the group (Asher & Hymel, 1981). For rating-scale measures
to serve this purpose, it is important that children be asked to rate how much they
like or like to play with every other classmate, rather than be asked to rate how
much they view every other child as a friend.

One aim of the present research was to evaluate differences in the prevalence
of friendship among low-, average-, and high-accepted children. Of particular
interest was whether many low-accepted children, despite their low overall status,
nonetheless have best friends. Although several studies contain information about
this issue (Berghout-Austin, 1985; Bukowski, Hoza, & Newcomb, 1987;
Buzzelli, 1988; Drewry & Clark, 1984; Feltham, Doyle, Schwartzman, Serbin,
& Ledingham, 1985; Howes, 1988; Mannarino, 1976; Rizzo, 1988; Roopnarine
& Field, 1984), none of the research combines reciprocal nomination measures of
friendship with rating-scale measures of acceptance.

A second aim of the present research was to develop an instrument for assessing
children's perceptions of the qualitative features of their best friendships. A third,
related aim was to examine how the qualities of accepted children's friendships
differ from the qualities of low-accepted children's friendships. Several studies
have examined age and gender differences in the quality of children's friendships

by obtaining from children estimates of the extent to which their friendships meet certain relationship needs (Berndt & Perry, 1986; Buhrmester & Furman, 1987; Bukowski et al., 1987; Furman & Buhrmester, 1985; Sharabany, Gershoni, & Hofman, 1981). In this research, there is general consistency across studies concerning the qualitative aspects of friendship that are important to consider (see Asher & Parker, 1989). These include (a) the extent to which the relationship offers children opportunities for play, companionship, and recreation; (b) the degree of intimate disclosure and exchange that characterizes the relationship; (c) the extent to which the friends share, help, and guide one another; and (d) the extent to which children find the relationship validating and enhancing of self-worth.

In existing research on individual differences in friendship quality, researchers have sometimes also considered the types of stress as well as support present in children's friendships (e.g., Berndt & Perry, 1986; Bukowski et al., 1987). For example, Berndt and Perry found that conflict and disagreement are common in children's close friendships (see also Gottman, 1983) and, at least among older children, are independent of the level of positive, supportive aspects of friendship. A distinction needs to be made, however, between the level of conflict children experience and the ease and manner with which their conflicts are resolved. Several investigators have found that it is the ability to resolve conflicts quickly and amicably, not the ability to avoid conflict altogether, that distinguishes close peer relationships from other peer relationships in early childhood (Gottman & Parkhurst, 1980; Hartup & Laursen, 1989; Vespo & Caplan, 1988). Other authors (e.g., Carlson-Jones, 1985; Hartup & Laursen, 1989) have reported similar findings with respect to the friendships of older, school-age children. The amount of conflict children experience and the ease and readiness with which conflict is resolved represent, therefore, somewhat distinct dimensions.

The nature of the link between acceptance by the peer group and the quality of children's friendships is virtually unexplored. Scholars of personal relationships caution against being too ready to make inferences about the properties of dyadic relationships from measures of an individual's group functioning and behavior. Hinde (1979), Hartup (1986), Sroufe (e.g., Sroufe & Fleeson, 1986), Furman (1984a, 1984b), and others have noted that behavior in dyadic relationships is always the product of a complex, idiosyncratic interaction among the personal characteristics of an individual, the personal characteristics of his or her partner, and the relationship's history and circumstances. Furthermore, friendships, like all other personal relationships, have emergent properties, such as role expectations and obligations, that can mute, alter, or amplify an individual's personality characteristics or typical patterns of behavior.

On the other hand, a number of behavioral and social skills deficits have been shown to distinguish children who are rejected by their peer group from better-accepted children (see Asher & Coie, 1990); these deficits could be expected to contribute to problems in functioning between low-accepted children and their friends. Furthermore, several studies (e.g., Buzzelli, 1988; Gottman, Gonso, & Rasmussen, 1975; Kurdek & Krile, 1982) have shown that unpopular children reason in less sophisticated ways about friendship and friendship-related issues than other children (but see Bichard, Alden, Walker, & McMahon, 1988, for an exception).

In the present study, we compared high-, average-, and low-accepted children on the qualities of their best friendships. Specifically, we examined whether the friendships of poorly-accepted children differed from better-accepted children with respect to six qualitative aspects: *validation and caring* (i.e., the degree to which the relationship is characterized by caring, support, and interest); *conflict and betrayal* (i.e., the extent to which the relationship is typified by argument, disagreement, annoyance, and mistrust); *companionship and recreation* (i.e., the extent to which the friends spend enjoyable time together inside or outside of school); *help and guidance* (i.e., the extent of the friends' efforts to assist one another with routine or challenging tasks); *intimate exchange* (i.e., the extent to which the relationship is characterized by disclosure of personal information and feelings); and *conflict resolution* (i.e., the degree to which disagreements in the relationship are resolved efficiently and fairly). In addition, we compared high-, average-, and low-accepted children with respect to the level of satisfaction they expressed with their best friendship. We included a satisfaction measure, because children of different levels of acceptance might report similar amounts of satisfaction even though there are differences in the specific qualities they perceive in their friendships.[1]

A fourth aim of the present research was to examine children's friendship adjustment in relation to children's feelings of loneliness and social dissatisfaction. The link between friendship adjustment and loneliness has been the subject of considerable theorizing but little empirical inquiry. Sullivan (1953) drew specific attention to the putative links between friendship and loneliness, ascribing special significance to preadolescent friendship as a means of staving off feelings of loneliness and isolation. Over the past several years, considerable progress has been made in the reliable measurement of loneliness in children (see Asher, Parkhurst, Hymel, & Williams, 1990), and loneliness has been found to be correlated with low group acceptance or rejection as measured by sociometric ratings or a combination of positive and negative sociometric nominations (e.g., Asher, Hymel, & Renshaw, 1984; Asher & Wheeler, 1985; Cassidy & Asher, 1992; Crick & Ladd, 1993). Dyadic friendships were not assessed in these studies, however. Therefore,

---

[1] We are indebted to Carol Dweck for suggesting an independent assessment of children's friendship satisfaction.

it remains to be seen whether friendship bears a similarly strong relationship to loneliness or whether the apparent relation between loneliness and acceptance might be accounted for by differences in the friendship adjustment of accepted and unaccepted children. Furthermore, it is of theoretical and practical interest to learn whether having a friend has positive emotional benefits for low-accepted children who might otherwise report high levels of loneliness. Such a possibility is suggested by Bukowski et al. (1987), who focused on friendship adjustment, acceptance, and children's feelings of general self-worth and perceived cognitive and social competence.

In summary, the specific aims of the present research were (a) to examine the prevalence of mutual friendship among children in general and among low-accepted children in particular; (b) to develop a new measure of friendship quality; (c) to compare friendships of accepted and low-accepted children in terms of specific qualitative features and with respect to children's satisfaction with their friendships; and (d) to examine how acceptance, having a friend, and the quality of one's best friendship are related to the degree of loneliness and social dissatisfaction in middle childhood.

METHOD

Subjects

Eight hundred and eighty-one children were recruited from 36 third- through fifth-grade classrooms of five public elementary schools located in a mid-sized, midwestern community in the United States. The participants represented 98.5% of all children enrolled in these classrooms (13 children were excluded at parental request). Two hundred and ninety-six children (163 boys and 133 girls) were in the third grade, 251 children (135 boys and 116 girls) were in the fourth grade, and 334 children (174 boys and 160 girls) were in the fifth grade. The sample was 73.2% White, 23.4% Black, and 3.4% Asian or Hispanic.

All children completed all measures. However, for certain analyses (see the following sections) only children ($n = 484$) with at least one mutual, very best friend were of interest. The distribution of gender and grade for this subsample of friended children was as follows: 154 third graders (71 boys and 83 girls), 141 fourth graders (68 boys and 73 girls), and 189 fifth graders (95 boys and 94 girls).

Measures

Level of acceptance. We used a "roster-and-rating" sociometric procedure (Singleton & Asher, 1977) to assess children's level of classroom acceptance. Children were provided with rosters of all classmates and were asked to indicate on a 1-to-5 rating scale how much they liked to play with each of their classmates. A child's level of acceptance was determined from the average rating received from his or her classmates, standardized within gender within each classroom. Children were classified as *high-accepted* (n = 65 boys and 63 girls) if their received rating z score was greater than or equal to 1. Children were classified as *low-accepted* (n = 74 boys and 76 girls) if their z score was less than or equal to −1. The remaining children (n = 333 boys and 269 girls) were classified as *average-accepted*. The high-accepted and low-accepted groups represented the highest 14.5% and lowest 17% of the sample in terms of acceptance, respectively. *Friendship assessments.* Children's friendships were identified by using data from a two-step sociometric nomination procedure. In the first step, children were asked to indicate their three "best friends" from a roster of the names of all other children in their class. In the second step, children were then asked to review their three choices and to indicate which of the three choices represented their single, "very best friend." We then examined the choice matrix within each classroom to identify children who nominated each other.[2] Children were considered to have a very best friend if the classmate they designated as their very best friend in turn included them among his or her list of three best-friend choices. In other words, it was not necessary that the chosen classmate designate the choosing child as a very best friend (as opposed to a best friend) in order for the choosing child to be considered to have a very best friend, although this strict reciprocity held for 266 (55%) of the 484 cases of children who were identified as having a very best friend.[3]

---

[2]An issue that arises concerns the appropriateness of restricting friendship choices to within classrooms. It is possible that children who differ in acceptance also differ in their tendency to have a friend outside the classroom and that restricting friendship nominations to within the class could underestimate the friendship status of certain groups. In a previous study, we reported the results of a direct appraisal of this possibility using a sample of 278 elementary school-age children (Parker & Asher, 1989). In that study, before children completed any other sociometric measure, they were asked to write the names of their three very best friends. The children were told that these friends could live anywhere but should be other children and not adults. The number of friends listed who were not class members was tallied for each child. On average, children included just under one (M = 0.90) nonclassmate on this list of friends. A Gender × Level of Acceptance analysis of variance indicated no significant main effects or interaction. Thus, high-accepted, average-accepted, and low-accepted children did not differ in the number of nonclassmates they included. Because these nominations were of children outside the classroom, it was not possible to verify whether friendships were actually reciprocal relationships. But the important finding is that whatever underestimation of friendship does take place by restricting friendship assessment to the classroom seems to be limited and not particularly biased toward one acceptance group or another.

[3]A small minority of children (n = 3, or less than 1%) failed or refused to designate one or more friends at the initial step. These children were excluded from analyses. Another small minority (n = 4, also less than 1%) indicated one or more friendship choices but failed or refused at the second step to designate a "very best friend" among the friendship choices. These children could not be included in analyses requiring knowledge of their very best friendship. Their data could be used in other analyses, however, and their choices could be used to examine the reciprocity of other children's choices. In three additional cases, children ignored instructions and indicated more than one "very best friend-

In addition to this primary operationalization of friendship, a second, more inclusive criterion for friendship was established. For this second operationalization, children's "very best" designations were ignored. Thus, *best* (as opposed to *very best*) friendship was defined as a reciprocity across children for any of their three best-friend nominations. Unlike the more restrictive primary criterion, then, children could have more than one (but no more than three) best friendships by this criterion. We felt that this supplemental operationalization of friendship was essential to a comprehensive appraisal of children's participation in friendship. It also was of interest by virtue of being more directly comparable with operationalizations used in past studies.

Friendship quality. We examined the quality of children's very best friendship by using a questionnaire designed to assess children's perceptions of various qualitative aspects of their very best friendship. This questionnaire, the *Friendship Quality Questionnaire* (FQQ), contained 40 primary items and an initial "warm-up" item. The items asked children to indicate on a 5-point scale how true a particular quality is of their relationship with a specific friend (e.g., "Jamie and I loan each other things all the time"). The scale ranged from *not at all true* (0) to *a little true* (1) to *somewhat true* (2) to *pretty true* (3) to *really true* (4). The child completed the questionnaire with reference to a specific friend, whose name was inserted at the top of the questionnaire and embedded in each individual item by using a personal computer and word-processing software with data-merging capabilities. This reference to a specific friend was done to discourage children from completing the questionnaire on the basis of an internal representation of a stereotypic or idealized friendship or based on a mental composite of several different friendships. The target friend was the child's very best mutual friend as determined from the sociometric assessment described earlier.[4] The questionnaire was group administered in the child's classroom. We began administration by giving children instruction in using the scale. After this, children completed the questionnaire individually. Each item was read aloud to make as few demands as possible on children's reading ability.

The FQQ evolved over time through two administrations and appraisals before the present study. An initial pool of potential items was derived from a similar

---

ship" from among the three choices. In these cases, one choice was randomly designated the very best friendship, within the constraint that a nonmutual choice could not take precedence over a mutual choice (one case).

[4]For those children without a mutual very best friend, one of the child's mutual best friendship choices (top three) was substituted. For children without either type of friendship, the name of the child's unilateral (i.e., nonreciprocated) very best friend choice was substituted. These substitutions were necessary to avoid drawing undue attention during administration to children without mutual very best friends. Data from subjects without mutual very best friends were excluded from data analyses concerning the qualities of children's best friendships.

questionnaire developed by Bukowski et al. (1987).[5] We made some changes to the wording and response format of these initial items to clarify potential ambiguities in interpretation. In addition, the practice of customizing each questionnaire with the name of a specific friend was introduced. The FQQ was administered initially to 278 third- through sixth-grade children (see Parker & Asher, 1989) and subsequently to 153 third- through fifth-grade children. We used each evaluation to identify and replace weak or ambiguous items and to clarify the underlying factor structure. These evaluations resulted in the final pool of 40 items used in the present study and are shown in Table 1. The scoring and the derivation of subscales are described in the Results section.

Friendship satisfaction. Two questions were used to assess children's satisfaction with their friendship. These questions were administered separately from the FQQ. The first question asked, "How is this friendship going?" The second question asked, "How happy are you with this friendship?" For both questions, children indicated their satisfaction along a continuum anchored at the low end by a stylized line-drawing of a frowning, unhappy face and at the opposite, high end by a complementary stylized line-drawing of a smiling, happy face. Fifteen evenly spaced ticks were marked along the continuum to assist with measurement, and a child's score was based on which tick was circled, with higher scores indicating more satisfaction. To familiarize children with the use of the scale, we first guided the children through several examples involving school activities and hobbies. The two friendship satisfaction questions were then read aloud. The responses of children with very best friends to the two questions were highly related ($r = .85$), and ratings were therefore averaged into a single satisfaction score for each child.

Loneliness and social dissatisfaction. Children's feelings of loneliness and social dissatisfaction were assessed by using Asher and Wheeler's (1985) modification of a 24-item self-report questionnaire developed by Asher et al. (1984). This questionnaire contains 16 items focused on feelings of loneliness and social dissatisfaction in school and 8 filler items. The 16 primary items include four different kinds of items. These items assessed (a) children's feelings of loneliness (e.g., "I'm lonely at school"), (b) children's appraisal of their current peer relationships (e.g., "I don't have any friends in class"), (c) children's perceptions of the degree to which important relationship needs are being met (e.g., "There're no other kids I can go to when I need help at school"), and (d) children's perceptions of their social competence (e.g., "I'm good at working with other children in my class"). Children responded to each item on a 5-point scale, indicating the degree to which each statement is a true description of themselves. Total scores could range from 16 to 80, with greater scores indicating greater loneliness and social dissatisfac-

---

[5]We are indebted to William Bukowski and his colleagues for providing information about the reliability of their items.

TABLE 1
Items and Subscales of the Friendship Quality Questionnaire

Subscale/item[a]	Structure coefficient
Validation and Caring (α = .90)	
15. Makes me feel good about my ideas	.783
4. Tells me I am good at things	.780
6. Make each other feel important and special	.729
13. Tells me I am pretty smart	.703
8. Says "I'm sorry" if [he/she] hurts my feelings	.695
5. Sticks up for me if others talk behind my back	.662
10. Has good ideas about games to play	.644
41. Cares about my feelings	.635
12. Would like me even if others didn't	.595
30. Does not tell others my secrets	.547
Conflict Resolution (α = .73)	
26. Make up easily when we have a fight	.880
35. Get over our arguments really quickly	.840
11. Talk about how to get over being mad at each other	.573
Conflict and Betrayal (α = .84)	
20. Argue a lot	.844
27. Fight a lot	.822
3. Get mad a lot	.782
37. Doesn't listen to me	.696
31. Bug each other a lot	.652
9. Sometimes says mean things about me to other kids	.638
21. Can count on to keep promises	−.635
Help and Guidance (α = .90)	
34. Helps me so I can get done quicker	.823
39. Help each other with schoolwork a lot	.768
24. Gives advice with figuring things out	.757
36. Count on each other for good ideas on how to get things done	.744
32. Come up with good ideas on ways to do things	.702
33. Loan each other things all the time	.640
28. Share things with each other	.595
18. Do special favors for each other	.576
17. Help each other with chores a lot	.567
Companionship and Recreation (α = .75)	
2. Always sit together at lunch	.802
7. Always pick each other as partners for things	.728
23. Always play together at recess	.690
19. Do fun things together a lot	.660
22. Go to each others' houses	.571
Intimate Exchange (α = .86)	
14. Always tell each other our problems	.755
25. Talk about the things that make us sad	.740
16. Talk to her when I'm mad about something that happened to me	.709
40. Tell each other secrets	.690
38. Tell each other private things	.674
29. Talk about how to make ourselves feel better if we are mad at each other	.653

[a] Numbers are item numbers from the Friendship Quality Questionnaire.

tion. This questionnaire has been used in several studies with elementary school-age children and has proved to have excellent internal consistency (Cronback α $\geq$ .90; see Asher et al., 1990). The internal reliability in the present sample was comparable (α = .91).

One limitation of the Asher and Wheeler (1985) measure in the context of the present study is that a number of its items overlap in content with items that assess the quality of children's best friendships. This means that significant correlations could be found between this measure and items assessing the quality of children's friendships simply because of the partially overlapping content (see Nicholls, Licht, & Pearl, 1982, for a discussion of this issue). Accordingly, we constructed a secondary measure of children's loneliness using a subset of three of the Asher and Wheeler questionnaire items: "I feel alone at school," "I feel left out of things at school," and "I'm lonely at school." This secondary measure, then, represents a "pure" assessment of children's feelings of loneliness and social dissatisfaction, uncontaminated by their appraisals of the quality of their friendships, their perception of their social competence, or their estimate of the state of their current peer relationships. The internal consistency of this 3-item pure scale was α = .77. The correlation between the pure loneliness scale and the larger, 16-item scale was .84. Whenever loneliness and social dissatisfaction was analyzed in relation to measures of friendship quality, the 3-item pure loneliness scale was substituted for the 16-item measure, and this fact is noted accordingly. For the sake of continuity with other research, scores for the larger scale were used in analyses in which the possibility of overlapping content was not an issue (i.e., in analyses that did not involve friendship quality or friendship satisfaction).

Procedure

In the late fall, the parents of all children in the third through fifth grades of each participating school were mailed first-class letters describing the study. Parents were asked to contact either the principal or the experimenters if they did not want their child to participate or if they required more information about the study before deciding. Data collection took place in three sessions in the winter and spring of the school year. Each session lasted about 1 hr. The first session began with an introduction to the project and project staff. This introduction stressed that participation was voluntary and confidential. After this, we administered sociometric measures to assess peer acceptance and to identify best friendships. Other measures were also administered in this session that are not relevant to the present study. In the second session, approximately 1 month later, the loneliness and social dissatisfaction questionnaire was administered. In the third session, several weeks later, children's perception of the quality of their best friendship was assessed, as was their satisfaction with their friendship. All measures were group administered in class, and each session was conducted by a different investigator to minimize reactivity across sessions.

RESULTS

Preliminary Analyses

Preliminary analyses indicated that children's grade level was not significantly related to any of the independent and dependent variables under consideration. Furthermore, there were no instances in which it was necessary to qualify any of the findings on the basis of grade. However, including grade did adversely affect the size of some cells in several analyses. For this reason, the analyses reported here are derived after collapsing the data across grades.

Prevalence of Friendship

Using the criterion of reciprocated best friendship, 77.6% of the children in this sample had at least one friend. However, as noted earlier, 484, or 54.9%, of the 881 children in the sample had *very* best friends. Thus, the narrowing of the focus from best friendship to very best friendship had the impact of doubling the proportion of friendless children identified (45.1% vs. 22.4%).

Of primary interest was the prevalence of best friendship among groups of children differing in level of acceptance. We expected that the likelihood of friendship would increase as level of acceptance increased but that many low-accepted children would nevertheless have friends. Logit analysis was used to model the odds of having versus not having a mutual best friend as a function of children's gender and level of acceptance. We evaluated the significance of individual terms (main effects and their interaction) by comparing the goodness of fit of the model that included the term to the goodness of fit of the model without the term. A backward elimination procedure was used to arrive at a parsimonious model that fit the data. For cases in which significant effects were found, we examined adjusted residuals to assess the effects of membership in particular categories of the independent variables (i.e., low- vs. average- vs. high-acceptance). We ran separate analyses for the two distinct operationalizations of friendship to learn how estimates of the prevalence of friendship, particularly among low-accepted children, are affected by changes in the stringency of the criterion.

The first logit analysis, using the looser, best friendship criterion, found a significant effect for children's level of acceptance, likelihood ratio $\chi^2(2, N = 881) = 103.64$, $p < .001$. Membership in the low-accepted group significantly depressed the odds of having a friend, whereas membership in the high-accepted group significantly augmented these odds. Specifically, 45.3% of low-accepted, 82.3% of average-accepted, and 93.8% of high-accepted children had at least one friend. A main effect of gender was found, likelihood ratio $\chi^2(1, N = 881) = 7.09$, $p < .01$: Girls (81.6%) were more likely than boys (74.2%) to have a friend. The interaction of gender and level of acceptance did not significantly alter the odds of having versus not having a friend.

The second logit analysis, using the stringent, very best friendship criterion, revealed a highly significant effect for children's level of acceptance, likelihood ratio $\chi^2(2, N = 881) = 53.10$, $p < .001$, and a nearly significant Gender × Level of Acceptance interaction, likelihood ratio $\chi^2(2, N = 881) = 5.26$, $p < .07$. Membership in the low-accepted group significantly depressed the odds of having a very best friend, whereas membership in the high-accepted group significantly augmented these odds. Whereas 58.2% of average-accepted children and 69.5% of high-accepted children had very best friends, only 29.3% of low-accepted children had very best friends. Furthermore, whereas the proportion of boys with very best friends and the proportion of girls with very best friends were roughly equivalent in both the high- and average-accepted groups (72.3% vs. 66.7% and 56.2% vs. 60.7%, respectively), low-accepted girls (39.5%) were twice as likely as low-accepted boys (18.9%) to have a mutual very best friend. A comparison of these results with the corresponding results from the earlier analyses suggests that tightening the friendship criterion is particularly likely to affect the estimate of the number of low-accepted boys with friends.

Next, using the more inclusive definition, we examined whether there were differences in the number of best friends children had as a function of gender and level of acceptance. A 2 (gender) × 3 (level of acceptance) analysis of variance (ANOVA) yielded a highly significant effect for level of acceptance, $F(2,875) = 81.02$, $p < .0001$; a main effect for gender, $F(1,875) = 10.39$, $p < .001$; and no Gender × Level of Acceptance interaction, $F(2,875) = 0.79$, *ns*. Post hoc (Tukey) comparisons indicated that low-accepted children had significantly fewer friends ($M = 0.65$, $SD = 0.82$) than average-accepted children ($M = 1.50$, $SD = 0.98$), who in turn had significantly fewer friendships than high-accepted children ($M = 2.03$, $SD = 0.89$). Girls ($M = 1.54$, $SD = 1.01$) had significantly more friends than boys ($M = 1.35$, $SD = 1.02$).

Finally, we studied the relationship between the acceptance levels of very best friends. To accomplish this, we identified all dyads that met our sociometric criteria for very best friendship ($N = 351$). We then classified each dyad according to the level of acceptance of the partners. Of the 351 friendships, there were 9 dyads involving 2 low-accepted children, 36 dyads involving a low-accepted and an average-accepted child, 3 dyads involving a low-accepted and a high-accepted child, 179 dyads involving 2 average-accepted children, 104 dyads involving an average-accepted and a high-accepted child, and 20 dyads involving 2 high-accepted children. A one-sample chi-square test revealed that the observed distribution of configurations departed significantly from its expected distribution χ^2(5, $N = 351$) = 79.23, $p < .0001$, given random pairing and the relative frequency of children in the three acceptance groups. Inspection of the standardized residuals from this analysis indicated that the principal reason for this disparity rests with the pattern of low-accepted children's involvement in friendships. Whereas the number of low–low friendship dyads was consistent with expectations (9 observed vs. 10 expected), the number of dyads involving a low-accepted child with either an average-accepted or a high-accepted partner was markedly less than the number expected through random pairing (36 observed vs. 82 expected and 3 observed vs. 17 expected, respectively). Thus, low-accepted children's relative lack of involvement in friendships can be understood as a tendency for lower participation in friendships with better-accepted children, specifically, and not as an indiscriminant tendency toward less involvement in friendship. At the same time, it is important to note that low-accepted children's involvement in friendship is not restricted to involvement in dyads with other low-accepted partners. Indeed, the majority of dyads involving low-accepted children were dyads involving a low-accepted child and an average-accepted partner (36 out of 48 dyads, or 75%).

Friendship Quality

Identification of subscales. To identify subscales on the FQQ, we performed a principal-components analysis (oblique rotation) on the responses of the 484 children with very best friends to the 40 primary items in the FQQ. This analysis resulted in six factors with eigenvalues greater than 1. The six factors, which were in close agreement with the predicted underlying structure of the measure based on pilot testing, were labeled Intimate Exchange, Conflict Resolution, Companionship and Recreation, Help and Guidance, Validation and Caring, and Conflict and Betrayal. The rightmost column of Table 1 shows the structure coefficient from the principal-components analysis for each item in relation to the factor on which it showed the highest loading.

The principal-components analysis was used to guide the clustering of items into subscales. Specifically, we formed one subscale for each factor in the principal-components analysis by combining the items that loaded highly on each factor. Table 1 displays the Cronbach alpha for these six subscales. As is evident, the internal consistency of each subscale was satisfactory. A child's score for each subscale was the average of his or her ratings for the relevant items (unit weighting), after appropriate reverse scoring if necessary. The six subscales were moderately to highly intercorrelated, with *rs* ranging from .16 to .75 in absolute

TABLE 2

Comparisons of Boys and Girls on Friendship Quality Variables

	Girls			Boys				
Variable	*n*	*M*	*SD*	*n*	*M*	*SD*	*df*	*F*
Validation and caring	230	2.85	0.82	238	2.61	0.96	1, 462	10.40**
Conflict and betrayal	232	1.04	0.94	237	1.04	0.90	1, 463	0.15
Companionship and recreation	231	2.71	0.87	238	2.60	0.91	1, 463	2.50
Help and guidance	232	2.54	0.93	238	2.36	0.99	1, 464	5.84*
Intimate exchange	231	2.47	0.98	238	1.98	1.09	1, 463	31.65***
Conflict resolution	231	2.95	1.02	237	2.63	1.10	1, 467	13.91***

* $p < .05$. ** $p < .001$. *** $p < .0001$.

magnitude.[6] Conflict and Betrayal correlated negatively with all other subscales. All other subscales were positively intercorrelated.

Acceptance and friendship quality. The focus of this analysis was on whether low-accepted children who have mutual very best friendships have friendships that are of comparable quality to the friendships of other children. This issue was examined in a 2 (gender) $\times$ 3 (level of acceptance) multivariate analysis of variance, with the six subscale scores from the FQQ serving as dependent variables.[7]

The results of this analysis yielded a significant multivariate main effect for gender, $F(6, 454) = 4.87$, $p < .001$; a significant multivariate main effect for level of acceptance, $F(12, 910) = 3.17$, $p < .001$; and a nonsignificant multivariate Gender $\times$ Level of Acceptance interaction, $F(12, 910) = 1.32$. Follow-up univariate analyses revealed gender differences for four of the six friendship quality variables. Table 2 gives the mean, standard deviation, and sample size for each gender on each of the six friendship quality variables and the corresponding F value for the gender comparison. Boys and girls did not differ in their characterizations of their very best friendship with respect to either conflict and betrayal

---

[6]A table of these correlations is available on request from Jeffrey G. Parker.

[7]In these and subsequent analyses of friendship quality, all children's responses were included as long as the child was a participant in a very best friendship. We assume that the perceptions of the individual children, and not the dyad itself, are the appropriate unit of analysis in this context. Thus, ratings by 2 children of the same friendship are considered separate data points. As a precaution against violations of the independence of the data, however, we repeated all analyses in the present study involving friendship quality after eliminating any possibility of dependencies across subjects. Specifically, there were 133 friendships (involving 266 children) in which potential dependencies in the data existed (i.e., where both partners contributed data on friendship quality). For these pairs, the data of one member of the dyad were randomly dropped from statistical analyses, with the qualification that in mixed-acceptance group pairs involving an average-accepted child with either a high-accepted child or a low-accepted child, the high-accepted or low-accepted child was preferentially retained to maximize the sample sizes of these extreme groups. Analyses were then rerun on the new, reduced data set ($N = 484 - 133 = 351$). These reanalyses resulted in no qualifications concerning significant versus nonsignificant effects.

or companionship and recreation. However, boys did report less intimate exchange, more difficulty resolving conflict, less validation and caring, and less help and guidance in their friendships than did girls.

Follow-up univariate analyses indicated acceptance-level differences for five of the six friendship quality variables. Table 3 shows these results. The mean, standard deviation, and sample size for each acceptance group for each friendship quality variable are also shown in Table 3, along with the F statistic for each corresponding comparison and the results of post hoc pairwise comparisons of means (Tukey).

As shown in Table 3, children of differing levels of acceptance did not differ significantly with respect to how much companionship and recreation they saw their friendships as providing. However, by their reports, low-accepted children's friendships were less adequate than the friendships of other children in every other respect. Low-accepted children reported significantly less validation and caring, more difficulty resolving conflict, and less help and guidance than both high-accepted and average-accepted children, who did not differ from one another in these respects. Low-accepted children also reported significantly less intimate disclosure in their friendships than high-accepted children. Low-accepted children reported more conflict and betrayal in their friendships than did average-accepted children but not more conflict and betrayal than high-accepted children, although the means were in that direction. High-accepted children reported somewhat more conflict and betrayal than average-accepted children, but this difference was not significant. Finally, it is of interest that low-accepted children showed the greatest variability of any group on every friendship quality, except conflict and betrayal (see the standard deviations in Table 3).

Acceptance, Friendship Quality, and Friendship Satisfaction

In general, children with very best friends expressed relatively high satisfaction with these relationships. Low-accepted children ($M = 11.95$, $SD = 4.28$) reported slightly less friendship satisfaction than did either average-accepted ($M = 13.04$, $SD = 3.07$) or high-accepted ($M = 13.19$, $SD = 3.04$) children. However, these differences were not significant, $F(2,458) = 1.89$. Boys tended to express more satisfaction ($M = 13.28$, $SD = 2.82$) with their very best friendships than girls ($M = 12.65$, $SD = 3.52$), but this difference did not reach significance, $F(1,458) = 3.35$, $p < .07$. The Gender $\times$ Acceptance Level interaction was not significant, $F(2,458) = 2.04$.

Correlations computed between each of the friendship quality subscales and the satisfaction composite indicated that positive friendship qualities (i.e., validation and caring, companionship and recreation, help and guidance, and intimate exchange) were associated with higher satisfaction with the relationship, whereas

TABLE 3
Comparisons of Low-Accepted, Average-Accepted, and High-Accepted Children on Friendship Quality Variables

Variable	Low-accepted			Average-accepted			High-accepted			df	F
	n	M	SD	n	M	SD	n	M	SD		
Validation and caring	43	$2.36_{a,b}$	1.17	336	2.72_a	0.87	89	2.95_b	0.83	2, 465	6.52**
Conflict and betrayal	44	1.41_a	1.01	336	$.98_a$	0.82	89	1.07	1.19	2, 466	4.25*
Companionship and recreation	44	2.44	1.06	337	2.69_a	0.88	88	2.60	0.84	2, 466	1.36
Help and guidance	44	$1.99_{a,b}$	1.23	337	2.46_a	0.92	89	2.63_b	0.91	2, 467	6.58**
Intimate exchange	44	1.81_a	1.23	336	2.21	1.05	89	2.46_a	1.10	2, 466	5.41**
Conflict resolution	44	$2.33_{a,b}$	1.27	335	2.78_a	1.06	89	3.02_b	0.96	2, 465	6.22***

Note. Means with common subscripts differ from one another at $p < .05$.
* $p < .05$. ** $p < .01$.

perceptions of conflict and betrayal were associated with lower satisfaction. These correlations ranged in absolute magnitude from .35 to .52 and were highly similar across the three acceptance groups.[8] All correlations were statistically significant ($p < .01$). A multiple regression analysis with satisfaction regressed simultaneously on the six friendship quality subscales indicated that the six friendship quality variables accounted for 46% of the variance in satisfaction, $R = .68$, $F(6, 452) = 65.01$, $p < .0001$.[9]

Friendship Adjustment, Acceptance, and Loneliness

Sociometric ratings of acceptance were negatively correlated with loneliness, $r = -.39$, $p < .001$, for the entire sample. This correlation is consistent with past research (see Asher et al., 1990). We performed a Friendship Status (friended vs. friendless) × Level of Acceptance (high, average, low) × Gender ANOVA to examine differences between friended and friendless children with respect to loneliness and whether friendship and acceptance interacted concerning loneliness. This analysis yielded a significant main effect for acceptance level, $F(2, 848) = 65.29$, $p < .0001$, and a significant main effect for friendship status, $F(1, 848) = 14.58$, $p < .0001$, but no Friendship Status × Acceptance Level interaction, $F(2, 848) = 0.30$. There was no significant effect of gender, $F(1, 848) = 0.44$, nor did gender significantly interact with level of acceptance, $F(2, 848) = 2.56$, with friendship status, $F(1, 848) = 0.48$, or with acceptance level and friendship status, $F(2, 848) = 0.01$. Post hoc comparisons (Tukey) indicated that low-accepted children ($M = 42.11$, $SD = 16.10$) reported significantly higher loneliness than average-accepted children ($M = 30.56$, $SD = 10.69$), who in turn reported significantly higher loneliness than high-accepted children ($M = 25.46$, $SD = 8.99$). Likewise, the main effect for friendship status indicated that children without very best friends ($M = 34.74$, $SD = 13.88$) were significantly more lonely than children with very best friends ($M = 29.31$, $SD = 10.84$). The absence of a significant interaction of level of acceptance with friendship status is important, because it suggests that friendship offers low-accepted children the same kind of buffer against loneliness that it offers better-accepted children, but in the context of a greater degree of loneliness in general.

Next, for the subsample of 484 children with close friends, we conducted six parallel hierarchical multiple regression analyses on children's pure (i.e., three-item) loneliness scores to assess whether the quality of children's friendships

---

[8]A table of these correlations is available on request from Jeffrey G. Parker.

[9]Although the regression analysis provided information about the beta weights for each of the friendship quality variables, comparisons among these betas would be misleading because the existence of substantial correlations between these variables resulted in multicollinearity and mutual suppression among the predictors in the multivariate context.

added significantly to the prediction of loneliness after considering children's level of acceptance. Each of the six friendship quality variables served as a predictor in one of the regressions. In each regression, gender was entered first, followed in turn by the standardized sociometric acceptance ratings, the Gender × Acceptance interaction, the friendship quality variable, the Gender × Friendship Quality interaction term, the Acceptance × Friendship Quality interaction term, and finally, the three-way Gender × Acceptance by Peers × Friendship Quality interaction.

Consistent with past research, level of acceptance was a strong negative predictor of loneliness, $\beta = -.266$, $F(1, 455) = 34.66$, $p < .0001$. But importantly, each of the six FQQ variables also strongly predicted loneliness, even after controlling for level of acceptance, gender, and the Gender × Acceptance interaction. Table 4 summarizes the results for the six regressions. The columns of Table 4 present the simple correlation, beta, change in R^2, and the F statistic associated with this change for each friendship quality variable. Note that the conflict and betrayal variable was positively predictive of loneliness, whereas all other variables were negatively related. A comparison of the beta coefficients shown in Table 4 indicates that the six quality variables were roughly equally strong predictors of loneliness. Neither gender nor the interaction terms involving gender, acceptance by peers, or friendship quality significantly predicted loneliness in any regression.

We conducted a second set of six hierarchical regressions to examine whether level of acceptance by peers continued to predict loneliness after the effects of friendship quality were considered. These regressions were identical to the six previous regressions, except that the order in which variables entered the equation was reversed such that gender, friendship quality, and the interaction of gender and friendship quality were entered before sociometric acceptance ratings and interaction terms involving sociometric acceptance ratings. Not surprisingly, the

TABLE 4
Summary of Hierarchical Regressions of Friendship Qualities on "Pure" Loneliness

Quality	r	β^a	R^2_{change}	$F(1, 455)$
Validation and caring	−.29	−.262	.07	34.26**
Conflict and betrayal	.18	.160	.03	12.84*
Companionship and recreation	−.26	−.250	.06	32.57**
Help and guidance	−.26	−.229	.05	26.21**
Intimate exchange	−.19	−.175	.03	14.03*
Conflict resolution	−.29	−.276	.07	38.77**

^{a} Controlling for gender, sociometric rating, and Gender × Sociometric Rating interaction.
* $p < .001$.   ** $p < .0001$.

six friendship quality variables were each strong predictors of loneliness (absolute value of all betas $> .226$; all $ps < .0001$). More important, in each regression, level of acceptance by peers significantly negatively predicted loneliness even after controlling for friendship quality (all betas $> -.222$; all $ps < .0001$). Again, neither gender nor the interaction terms involving gender, acceptance by peers, or friendship quality significantly predicted loneliness in any regression.

DISCUSSION

The present data suggest that the distinction between acceptance and friendship adjustment is a meaningful one and should be preserved. With respect to the prevalence of friendships, for example, we found that not all highly accepted children had friends, even when the focus was on best as opposed to very best friendship. Indeed, just under a third of high-accepted children did not have the child they named as their very best friend include them among his or her list of three friends. Conversely, many, although certainly not most, low-accepted children did have friends. Relaxing the criteria for identifying a dyad as friends led to many more children at all levels of acceptance identified as having friends, especially low-accepted boys. Thus, it would be incorrect to characterize all low-accepted children as children without friends.

Similarly, the analyses involving children's reports of loneliness and social dissatisfaction indicated that children's friendship adjustment had an influence on children's feelings of loneliness above and beyond the influence of peer group acceptance, further supporting the distinction between friendship adjustment and group acceptance. Two different sets of findings support this point. First, children without best friends were more lonely than children with best friends, and this was true regardless of how well accepted they were. Thus, an additive relationship between acceptance and friendship obtained with respect to loneliness. Second, the regression analyses that focused on the qualities of children's best friendships indicated that friendship quality and acceptance contributed separately and about equally to the prediction of loneliness. Together, these findings suggest that children's feelings of loneliness can arise from several sources that, in combination, can seriously undermine children's feelings of well-being. Receiving poor acceptance by peers, lacking a friend, or having a friendship that fails to meet important relationship needs each contribute. (See Weiss, 1973, for a related discussion in the literature on loneliness in adulthood.)

Although results of the present study support the distinction between group acceptance and friendship, the extent of the connection between children's adjustment in the two domains should not be minimized. Better-accepted children were more likely to be involved in specific dyadic friendships than were less-accepted children. Indeed, high-accepted and average-accepted children were about twice as likely to have a very best friend as low-accepted children. This disparity was large for girls but was especially large for boys; fewer than 1 in 5 low-accepted boys had very best friends.

Likewise, analyses involving the new measure of friendship quality pointed to important differences between low-accepted, average-accepted, and high-accepted children's friendships with respect to validation and caring, help and guidance, conflict resolution, intimate exchange, and conflict and betrayal. Low-accepted children's very best friendships were more problematic in each of these respects than the friendships of other children.

The development of a self-report instrument for assessing children's perceptions is another contribution of this research. The friendship quality measure contains subscales with good internal consistency indicating that children can reliably describe features of their close peer relationships. In addition to the several differences noted for low-accepted versus better-accepted children, results from the friendship quality measure also yielded interesting information about gender in relation to friendship quality. Whereas two dimensions of friendship quality did not distinguish boys' and girls' friendships from one another (i.e., conflict and betrayal, companionship and recreation), girls reported higher levels than boys of validation and support, help and guidance, conflict resolution, and intimate exchange. These findings are consistent with the findings of most (e.g., Buhrmester & Furman, 1987; Furman & Buhrmester, 1985; Sharabany et al., 1981) but not all (e.g., Berndt & Perry, 1986) past studies that have compared boys' and girls' friendships. Research is needed on the factors that give rise to these gender differences. One suggestion has been that differences in the play preferences and group structures of boys and girls (e.g., the greater tendency for boys to play in large groups and for their groups to be hierarchically organized) give rise to differences in the qualities of their close personal relationships (see Maccoby, 1990). To date, however, this hypothesis has not received empirical scrutiny or support.

A further point about friendship quality concerns the heterogeneity within the low-accepted group. This group showed the largest within-group variability of all groups on five of the six qualities. An important task for future research will be to document and account for cases in which low-accepted children have friendships that are not dissimilar from those of other children. Recent research suggests the existence of aggressive versus withdrawn subgroups of low-accepted children, with the withdrawn subgroup reporting more loneliness and social dissatisfaction (Parkhurst & Asher, 1992; Williams & Asher, 1987). Attention to these subgroups might also reveal differences in the quality of their friendships.

Friendship quality was assessed in this research through the reports of the children themselves. There is much to recommend this way of assessing the properties of friendship (see Furman, 1984b). It is particularly useful when the qualities under study are infrequent and difficult to observe, as is the case for many of the qualities of friendship under study here (e.g., conflict and betrayal, intimacy), or when it is the subjective impact of behavior (such as a personal feeling of validation) that is of most interest. At the same time, relying on children's reports also poses certain important interpretative challenges to understanding children's friendship experiences. To begin with, because there are two parties to the relationship, friendships have two subjective realities rather than one (Furman, 1984b), and these may not always coincide. To illustrate, as noted earlier (see Footnote 7), for a subset ($n = 133$) of the reciprocal very best friendships in our sample, data on friendship quality were available from both partners. For these pairs, correlations between each partner's ratings ranged from .64 for companionship and recreation to .21 for conflict resolution, indicating considerable differences in the opinions of partners. Such differences may be due to real differences in the partners' experiences in the relationship. But, just as important, they may signal that the dyad has not progressed far toward a shared understanding of the meaning of each other's behavior. In future research, the concordance of the partners' perspectives on the relationship might be studied more systematically as a window on the quality of children's friendships.

Studies that rely on children's reports about their friendships also must allow that children's construals of their relationships do not represent objective accounts of their actual social interaction. It would be desirable in future research to supplement children's reports of their friendship's qualities with observational data on how qualities such as intimate disclosure, conflict resolution, help and guidance, and so on are expressed in the context of accepted and unaccepted children's interactions with their very best friends. Doubtless, further differences in the friendships of highly accepted and poorly accepted children will be observed.

The emphasis given to children's feelings of loneliness and social dissatisfaction in relation to friendship adjustment and peer acceptance in the present study is in keeping with the increasing interest within developmental psychology in the intersection of affect and social adjustment (Thompson, 1990). Moreover, because loneliness is already a well-established concomitant of problems of group acceptance, it represents a particularly good initial criterion against which to judge the magnitude of the predictive validity of measures of friendship and friendship quality in children. However, future research should consider the divergent as well as the convergent correlates of friendship adjustment and peer acceptance. For the most part, scholars who have stressed the importance of positive peer experiences in childhood have not sharply differentiated between the benefits associated with friendship as opposed to general peer acceptance. Thus, considerable conceptual groundwork remains to be established. However, as Furman and Robbins (1985) have compellingly argued, it seems reasonable that friendship and group acceptance would contribute in distinctive ways to children's socialization. The close, accepting context of friendship, for example, may permit children greater latitude in the behavior that they explore and the attitudes that they express. In addition, the voluntary nature of friendship may make it an extremely important context for understanding the skills and requirements of commitment, personal responsibility, and loyalty. And friendships may meet specific needs of children, including needs for intimacy, social support, instrumental aid, and a reliable ally. On the other hand, peer acceptance may be an important prerequisite for and outgrowth of children's leadership and assertive skills and may meet children's needs to feel that they are a part of a larger community, something that a particular friendship relationship is less likely to provide.

REFERENCES

Asher, S. R., & Coie, J. D. (Eds.). (1990). *Peer rejection in childhood.* Cambridge, England: Cambridge University Press.

Asher, S. R., & Hymel, S. (1981). Children's social competence in peer relations: Sociometric and behavioral assessment. In J. D. Wine & M. D. Smye (Eds.), *Social competence* (pp. 125–157). New York: Guilford Press.

Asher, S. R., Hymel, S., & Renshaw, P. D. (1984). Loneliness in children. *Child Development, 55,* 1456–1464.

Asher, S. R., & Parker, J. G. (1989). The significance of peer relationship problems in childhood. In B. H. Schneider, G. Attili, J. Nadel, & R. P. Weissberg (Eds.), *Social competence in developmental perspective* (pp. 5–23). Amsterdam: Kluwer Academic.

Asher, S. R., Parkhurst, J. T., Hymel, S., & Williams, G. A. (1990). Peer rejection and loneliness in childhood. In S. R. Asher & J. D. Coie (Eds.), *Peer rejection in childhood* (pp. 253–273). Cambridge, England: Cambridge University Press.

Asher, S. R., Singleton, L. C., & Taylor, A. R. (1982, April). *Acceptance versus friendship: A longitudinal study of racial integration.* Paper presented at the annual meetings of the American Educational Research Association, New York.

Asher, S. R., & Wheeler, V. A. (1985). Children's loneliness: A comparison of rejected and neglected peer status. *Journal of Counseling and Clinical Psychology, 53,* 500–505.

Berghout-Austin, A. M. (1985). Young children's atteniton to dyadic conversation as modified by sociometric status. *Genetic, Social, and General Psychology Monographs, 111,* 151–165.

Berndt, T. J. (1984). Sociometric, social–cognitive, and behavioral measures for the study of friendship and popularity. In T. Field, J. L. Roopnarine, & M. Segal (Eds.), *Friendships in normal and handicapped children* (pp. 31–52). Norwood, NJ: Ablex.

Berndt, T.J., & Perry, T. B. (1986). Children's perceptions of friendships as supportive relationships. *Developmental Psychology, 22,* 640–648.

Bichard, S. L. Alden, L., Walker, L. J., & McMahon, R. J. (1988). Friendship understanding in socially accepted, rejected, and neglected children. *Merrill-Palmer Quarterly, 34,* 33–46.

Blyth, D. A. (1983). Surviving and thriving in the social world: A commentary on six new studies of popular, rejected, and neglected children. *Merrill-Palmer Quarterly, 29,* 449–458.

Buhrmester, D., & Furman, W. (1987). The development of companionship and intimacy. *Child Development, 58,* 1101–1113.

Bukowski, W. M., & Hoza, B. (1989). Popularity and friendship: Issues in theory, measurement, and outcome. In T. J. Berndt & G. W. Ladd (Eds.), *Peer relationships in child development* (pp. 15–45). New York: Wiley.

Bukowski, W. M., Hoza, B., & Newcomb, A. F. (1987). *Friendship, popularity, and the "self" during adolescence.* Unpublished manuscript, University of Maine, Department of Psychology.

Buzzelli, C. A. (1988). The development of trust in children's relations with peers. *Child Study Journal, 18,* 33–41.

Carlson-Jones, D. (1985). Persuasive appeals and responses to appeals among friends and acquaintances. *Child Development, 56,* 757–763.

Carlson-Jones, D., & Bowling, B. (1988, March). *Preschool friends and affective knowledge: A comparison on mutual and unilateral friends.* Paper presented at the Southwest Conference on Human Development, Charleston, SC.

Cassidy, J., & Asher, S. R. (1992). Loneliness and peer relations in young children. *Child Development, 63,* 350–365.

Crick, N. R., & Ladd, G. W. (1993). Children's perceptions of their peer experiences: Attributions, loneliness, social anxiety, and social avoidance. *Developmental Psychology, 29,* 244–254.

Drewry, D. L., & Clark, M. L. (1984). Factors important in the formation of preschooler's friendships. *Journal of Genetic Psychology, 146,* 37–44.

Epstein, J. L. (1986). Friendship selection: Developmental and environmental influences. In E. C. Mueller & C. R. Cooper (Eds.), *Process and outcome in peer relationships* (pp. 129–160). San Diego, CA: Academic Press.

Feltman, R. F., Doyle, A. B., Schwartzman, A. E., Serbin, L. A., & Ledingham, J. E. (1985). Friendship in normal and deviant children. *Journal of Early Adolescence, 5,* 371–382.

Furman, W. (1984a). Issues in the assessment of social skills of normal and handicapped children. In T. Field, J. L. Roopnarine, & M. Segal (Eds.), *Friendships in normal and handicapped children* (pp. 3–30). Norwood, NJ: Ablex.

Furman, W. (1984b). Some observations on the study of personal relationships. In J. C. Masters & K. Yarkin-Levin (Eds.), *Boundary areas in social and developmental psychology* (pp. 16–42). San Diego, CA: Academic Press.

Furman, W., & Buhrmester, D. (1985). Children's perceptions of the personal relationships in their social networks. *Developmental Psychology, 21,* 1016–1024.

Furman, W., & Robbins, P. (1985). What's the point?: Selection of treatment objectives. In B. Schneider, K. H. Rubin, & J. E. Ledingham (Eds.), *Children's peer relations: Issues in assessment and intervention* (pp. 41–54). New York: Springer-Verlag.

Gottman, J. M. (1983). How children become friends. *Monographs of the Society for Research in Child Development, 48* (3, Serial No. 201).

Gottman, J. M., Conso, J., & Rasmussen, B. (1975). Social interaction, social competence, and friendship in children. *Child Development, 46,* 709–718.

Gottman, J. M., & Parkhurst, J. (1980). A developmental theory of friendship and acquaintanceship processes. In W. A. Collins (Eds.), *Minnesota symposia on child development: Development of cognition, affect, and social relations* (Vol. 13, pp. 197–253). Hillsdale, NJ: Erlbaum.

Hartup, W. W. (1986). On relationships and development. In W. W. Hartup & Z. Rubin (Eds.), *Relationships and development* (pp. 1–26). Hillsdale, NJ: Erlbaum.

Hartup, W. W., & Laursen, B. (1989, April). *Contextual constraints and children's friendship relations.* Paper presented at the biennial meetings of the Society for Research in Child Development, Kansas City, MO.

Hinde, R. A. (1979). *Towards understanding relations.* San Diego, CA: Academic Press.

Howes, C. (1988). Peer interaction of young children. *Monographs of the Society for Research in Child Development, 53*(1, Serial No. 217).

Kurdek, L. A., & Krile, D. (1982). A developmental analyses of the relation between peer acceptance and both interpersonal understanding and perceived social self-competence. *Child Development, 53,* 1485–1491.

Maccoby, E. E. (1990). Gender and relationships: A developmental perspective. *American Psychologist, 45,* 513–520.

Mannarino, A. P. (1976). Friendship patterns and altruistic behavior in preadolescent males. *Developmental Psychology, 12,* 555–556.

McGuire, K. D., & Weisz, J. R. (1982). Social cognition and behavioral correlates of pre-adolescent chumship. *Child Development, 53,* 1478–1484.

Nicholls, J. G., Licht, B. G., & Pearl, R. A. (1982). Some dangers of using personality questionnaires to study personality. *Psychological Bulletin, 92,* 572–580.

Oden, S., & Asher, S. R. (1977). Coaching children in social skills for friendship making. *Child Development, 48,* 495–506.

Parker, J. G., & Asher, S. R. (1989, April). Peer relations and social adjustment: Are friendship and group acceptance distinct domains? In W. M. Bukowski (Chair), *Properties, processes, and effects of friendship relations during childhood and adolescence.* Symposium conducted at the biennial meeting of the Society for Research in Child Development, Kansas City, MO.

Parkhurst, J. T., & Asher, S. R. (1992). Peer rejection in middle school: Subgroup differences in behavior, loneliness, and interpersonal concerns. *Developmental Psychology, 28,* 231–241.

Rizzo, T. A. (1988). The relationship between friendship and sociometric judgments of peer acceptance and rejection. *Child Study Journal, 18,* 161–191.

Roopnarine, J. L., & Field, T. M. (1984). Play interactions of friends and acquaintances in nursery school. In T. Field, J. L. Roopnarine, & M. Segal (Eds.), *Friendships in normal and handicapped children* (pp. 89–98). Norwood, NJ: Ablex.

Sharabany, R., Gershoni, R., & Hofman, J. (1981). Girlfriend, boyfriend: Age and sex differences in intimate friendship. *Developmental Psychology, 17,* 800–808.

Singleton, L. C., & Asher, S. R. (1977). Peer preferences and social interaction among third-grade children in an integrated school district. *Journal of Educational Psychology, 69,* 330–336.

Sroufe, L. A., & Fleeson, J. (1986). Attachment and the construction of relationships. In W. W. Hartup & Z. Rubin (Eds.), *Relationships and development* (pp. 51–72). Hillsdale, NJ: Erlbaum.

Sullivan, H. S. (1953). *The interpersonal theory of psychiatry.* New York: Norton.

Thompson, R. A. (Ed.). (1990). *Socioemotional development: Nebraska symposium on motivation, 1988* (vol. 36). Lincoln: University of Nebraska Press.

Vespo, J. E., & Caplan, M. Z. (1988, March). *Preschoolers' differential conflict behaviors with friends and acquaintances.* Poster presented at the Southeast Conference on Human Development, Charleston, SC.

Williams, G. A., & Asher, S. R. (1987, April). *Peer and self perceptions of peer rejected children: Issues in classification and subgrouping.* Paper presented at the biennial meetings of the Society for Research in Child Development, Baltimore.

Weiss. R. S. (1973). *Loneliness: The experience of emotional and social isolation.* Cambridge, MA: MIT Press.

4

A Longitudinal Study of Consistency and Change in Self-Esteem from Early Adolescence to Early Adulthood

Jack Block and Richard W. Robins
University of California, Berkeley

In a longitudinal study of 47 girls and 44 boys, developmental change in self-esteem (SE) was examined from early adolescence through late adolescence to early adulthood. Males tended to increase and females tended to decrease in SE over time. There was appreciable rank-order consistency in SE over time. Within each gender, the considerable individual differences in developmental trajectories were coherently related to personality characteristics independently assessed in early adolescence. Boys and girls with high SE possessed quite different personality characteristics in early adolescence; by early adulthood, although important differences remained, the personality characteristics associated with high SE were similar for the 2 sexes. Discussion focuses on the implications of our findings for the "consistency versus change" debate, the influence of gender-role socialization on SE development, and the importance of examining normative, gender-specific, and individual developmental change in SE.

Adolescence is a developmental period marked by rapid maturational changes, shifting societal expectations, conflicting role demands, and increasingly complex relations with the opposite sex (see, e.g., Douvan & Adelson, 1966). Self-esteem plays a critical role in this developmental process (see, e.g., Harter, 1983).

Reprinted with permission from *Child Development*, 1993, Vol. 64, 909–923. Copyright © 1993 by the Society for Research in Child Development, Inc.

This research was supported by National Institute of Mental Health grant MH 16080 to Jack and Jeanne H. Block. The second author was supported by a National Science Foundation Graduate Fellowship.

Relatively little is known, however, about the developmental path of self-esteem across adolescence and in the transition to adulthood.

To date, a number of useful longitudinal studies of self-esteem development during adolescence have been conducted (Abramowitz, Petersen, & Schulenberg, 1984; Alsaker & Olweus, 1992; Carlson, 1965; Engel, 1959; McCarthy & Hoge, 1982; O'Malley & Bachman, 1983; Savin-Williams & Demo, 1984; Simmons & Blyth, 1987). In the present paper, we seek to add to understanding by describing the developmental change in self-esteem in a sample of girls and boys studied longitudinally from early adolescence (age 14) through late adolescence (age 18) and into early adulthood (age 23). We also examine individual differences in developmental change patterns and explore the correlates of these individual differences, focusing on which personality characteristics at age 14 predict subsequent increases and decreases in self-esteem from age 14 to 23. All analyses are conducted separately for the two sexes in order to evaluate how girls and boys may differ in the ways they develop during adolescence.

Development proceeds through a complex process that involves the mutual influences of a person's innate characteristics, family experiences, peer interactions, social roles, cultural environment, and the fortuities that impinge upon a life. It is during adolescence that the biosocial transition from childhood to adulthood occurs, is experienced, and further influences development. For many decades, developmental psychologists have regarded adolescence as a period of "storm and stress" (Hall, 1904), a time of crisis and psychological upheaval precipitated by biologically driven maturational changes and marked in particular by a questioning of the self and subsequent reformulation of perceptions and evaluations of self. However, the empirical findings of the last 2 decades have not supported the contention that development during adolescence is problematic (Coleman, 1978; Hill, 1985; Montemayor, 1983; Rutter, Graham, Chadwick, & Yule, 1976). As a corollary, it has been suggested that "adolescence is not a time of upheaval in the self-concept. The person who enters adolescence is basically the same as [the one] who exits it" (Dusek & Flaherty, 1981, p. 39; see also Offer & Offer, 1975; Offer, Ostrov, & Howard, 1981; Savin-Williams & Demo, 1984; Simmons & Blyth, 1987). The present study brings additional evidence to bear on this insufficiently resolved issue.

In the study of developmental change, several facets of this issue must be considered (Block, 1971; Caspi & Bem, 1990; Dusek & Flaherty, 1981; Mortimer, Finch & Kumka, 1982; Simmons & Blyth, 1987). One concern is the direction and amount of age-related change in the level of an attribute. This question typically is posed for the sample as a whole, and is evaluated empirically by examining change in group means over time. The question can also be addressed with regard to subsamples (e.g., males or females) and individual cases. Longitudinal studies of self-esteem development that have examined age-related change in the mean level of self-esteem have tended to find, for the sexes combined, a small, gradual increase in measures of global self-esteem across adolescence (see O'Malley & Bachman, 1983, for a review). Gender differences in age-related changes in self-esteem have been reported by Blyth, Simmons, and Carlton-Ford (1983), who found that, from sixth grade to tenth grade, the global self-esteem of girls decreases while the global self-esteem of boys increases. We know of no longitudinal study that has explored individual differences in developmental change in self-esteem across any time period.

A second developmental question concerns the longitudinal consistency of interindividual differences: to what degree is the ordering of individuals according to their level on a variable maintained over time? Global indices (see below) of self-esteem during adolescence have shown moderate levels of longitudinal ordering consistency. For example, O'Malley and Bachman (1983) found a correlation of .41 across a 3-year period beginning when the subjects were high school seniors. Alsaker and Olweus (1992) and Simmons and Blyth (1987) report similar correlations across similar intervals. These correlations suggest substantial ordering consistency and yet permit considerable individual variations as well. Longitudinal consistency of self-esteem has yet to be examined across a wider range of time, from early adolescence through late adolescence and into young adulthood.

A third, largely unexamined question regarding the development of self-esteem focuses on the consistency of the pattern of relations between self-esteem and other conceptually relevant variables (e.g., personality characteristics). Little is known about the longitudinal consistency of the personality correlates of self-esteem. However, developmentally, it is of interest to examine whether the personality profile of individuals with high (vs. low) self-esteem in adolescence is similar to the personality profile of individuals with high (vs. low) self-esteem in early adulthood.

The three approaches to developmental change described thus far do not provide a complete account of *intra*individual development. Studies of self-esteem change that focus on mean-level changes and on the longitudinal ordering consistency of self-esteem reveal whether variables "behave" consistently across time rather than whether individuals are behaviorally consistent. However, "it is individuals who are stable [or unstable] across time, not variables" (Magnusson, 1990, p. 210), and there has been relatively little inquiry into the variation and the abidingness *within individuals* of their sense of self-worth. Given the myriad influences on self-esteem development during adolescence, it becomes important to examine the extent to which adolescents follow the same developmental path.

Assessing change within individuals therefore also requires a more "person-centered" approach to development (Block, 1961, 1971). Whereas a "variable-centered" perspective presumes that developmental change is much the same for all individuals, a "person-centered" perspective recognizes that individuals may not and often do not all develop in the same way; while some individuals may increase in self-esteem during adolescence, others may decrease in self-esteem, and others may show relatively little change. These observed differences in developmental paths require closer evaluation as to their reliability and significance. In the few instances where different developmental paths taken by individuals have been studied, social-contextual factors and prior personal characteristics have proven influential (e.g., Block, 1971).

In the person-centered study of different developmental paths, the role of gender requires special scrutiny. The characteristics underlying individual differences in self-esteem change in males may differ from the characteristics underlying self-esteem change in females. Although we know of no prior studies that specifically have examined the antecedent correlates of self-esteem change, Ozer and Block (1987) found that males increasing in IQ from age 11 to 18 tended to be shy, anxiety-prone, and non-competitive as children, while females showing IQ increases tended to be socially competent as children. Similarly, Block, Gjerde, and Block (1991) found gender differences in the early childhood antecedents of depression in late adolescence. Mortimer et al. (1982) have identified certain life experiences that *reciprocally* influence the self-concept. Mortimer and Lorence (1981), in an interesting study of males entering college, found that over the subsequent 14-year period a continuing sense of well-being that early was predicated on affectional family support later on was based on the quality of the relationship these men developed with their wives.

In the analyses to be presented, we examine: (*a*) mean-level changes in self-esteem through time; (*b*) the ordering consistency of self-esteem through time, and (*c*) the consistency of the personality correlates of self-esteem through time. To provide a more differentiated, more person-centered account of self-esteem development, all analyses in the present study were conducted separately for females and males and, within each sex, individual differences in age-related changes in self-esteem were examined to identify the personality characteristics predicting appreciable increase versus appreciable decrease in self-esteem from age 14 to age 23.

CONCEPTUALIZATION AND MEASUREMENT OF SELF-ESTEEM

The measurement of self-esteem is inextricably linked to its conceptualization. Not uniquely, we view self-esteem as *the extent to which one perceives oneself as relatively close to being the person one wants to be and/or as relatively distant from being the kind of person one does not want to be, with respect to person-qualities one positively and negatively values.* It follows that the study of self-esteem requires two kinds of assessment: (1) evaluation of the degree of congruence in an individual between the perceived self and the aspired self, and (2) consideration of the specific valued elements or valued criteria in terms of which self-evaluation is referenced. William James (1890), in his seminal formulation, said that self-evaluations depend on the degree to which actual successes coincide with one's goals and aspirations; self-esteem can be defined as "success divided by pretensions" (p. 310). Rosenberg (1965, pp. 243–245) strongly affirms the Jamesian view that it is crucial to know the specific self-values, and their weightings, on which an individual predicates self-esteem. In alternative psychoanalytic terms, an individual's "ego-ideal" provides a polestar—a personal value system—that permits and even compels self-evaluation. Thus, although it is crucial to know the extent to which an individual likes the self perceived, it is also the case that without knowing the particular personal qualities on which an individual "stakes" his or her characterological aspirations, we cannot truly know the meaning or psychological basis of an individual's "claim" to self-esteem.

In the present study, the Q-sort procedure (Block, 1961; Stephenson, 1953)—a different but long-employed approach to the operationalization of self-esteem (e.g., Block & Thomas, 1955; Rogers & Dymond, 1954; Turner & Vanderlippe, 1958)—was employed to assess self/ideal congruence.[1] In the Q-sort procedure, one considers the descriptiveness of a large set of statements, ordering the statements from those most to those least salient or characteristic of oneself or whoever is being described. The number of categories and the number of statements that can be sorted into each category are fixed, and so each respondent offers the same number of discriminations. The procedure is "ipsative," that is, the salience or descriptiveness of each item is evaluated relative to each other item *within* the particular individual being described rather than being evaluated separately, as is the case with most assessment procedures. Because the Q-items "compete" with each other, this approach brings subjects to offer reliable discriminations among attributes that often would not be offered via other procedures, such as Likert scales or via checklists (Block, 1956; 1961, chap. 6). To develop a self-ideal congruence index, a subject must do a Q-sort description of his or her self and, separately (usually at another time), a Q-sort description of his or her ideal self. The congruence between these two Q-sort descriptions subsequently is calculated by the investigator, and this congruence score becomes the subject's index of self-esteem.

We believe a Q-sort-based self-ideal congruence index, although more cumbersome to implement, has several advantages over the more widely used global self-esteem scales. First, such self-ideal indices are not confounded with individual

---

[1]A number of other investigators representing a variety of theoretical perspectives have worked with self-ideal indices but did not use the ipsative, forced-sort Q-sort approach (e.g., Blatt, Quinlan, Chevron, McDonald, & Zuroff, 1982; Higgins, 1987; Hoge & McCarthy, 1983; Lazzari, Fioravanti, & Gough, 1978; Pelham & Swann, 1989).

differences in scale usage because the procedure makes all subjects use the underlying metric commensurately. Incommensurate usage of the underlying dimension because of differences in response tendencies, present in most other self-esteem measures, can be a significant source of bias that renders such self-esteem scores and self-ideal congruence indices not based on Q-sort data sometimes difficult to interpret.

Second, compared with direct approaches to the indexing of self-esteem, Q-sort-based self-ideal indices are indirect and therefore more difficult for subjects to intentionally manipulate in the direction of favorable responses because the self data and the ideal data are collected in more complicated ways, usually on separate occasions, and the subject is unaware of the way these data subsequently will be employed. In contrast, the items used in the direct measurement of self-esteem are patent, even blatant in their content. Individuals can readily discern the underlying measurement intentions and may, ad libitum, manipulate their responses to achieve desired standings on the self-esteem continuum. Although low self-esteem, as reflected by such direct measures, can probably be accepted as such, high self-esteem so measured may not be a genuine expression of the individual's self-view or level of psychological health—contextual circumstances may be motivating and controlling, or the individual, for psychodynamic reasons, may be introspectively unaware (Block & Thomas, 1955).

Third, the self-ideal index provides an operationalization of self-esteem that is consistent with the phenomenological conception of self-esteem advanced by most self-theorists; normative judgments of self-worth are explicitly avoided because the index is based on the congruence between each subject's perceptions of self and his or her personal value system as expressed via the individual's aspirations for an ideal self.

Fourth, besides providing a conceptually satisfactory self-esteem index, the Q-sort approach also permits an analysis of the specific content of the perceived-self and ideal-self perceptions that underlie an individual's self-esteem or lack thereof. Access to the nature of the psychological building blocks on which the edifice of self-esteem is based provides crucial additional information. Besides wanting to know *whether* one likes oneself, it is important to know *why* one likes oneself.

METHOD

Subjects

The subjects are participants in the Block and Block longitudinal study of personality and cognitive development initiated in 1968 (see J. H. Block & J. Block, 1980, for a comprehensive description of the study). Initially, 128 3-year-olds were studied, coming from two successive cohorts at each of two nursery schools. Subsequently, sample attrition has been low (104 subjects were assessed at age 23). The subjects live primarily in urban settings and are heterogeneous with respect to the social class and educational level of their parents. Approximately two-thirds are Caucasian, one-fourth are African-American, and one-twentieth are Asian-American. There were no significant associations, or even trends toward associations, of our measure of self-esteem with either social class or ethnicity. Although we cannot claim full generalizability of the findings we will report, the sample we have employed, although not strictly representative of the national population, is not special in its characteristics.

The analyses reported in this paper are based on the 44 males and 47 females ($N = 91$) who, during intensive assessments at about the first year of high school (mean age $= 14.80$, SD $= .54$), the last year of high school (mean age $= 17.85$, SD $= .50$), and 5 years subsequent to high school (mean age $= 23.23$, SD $= .74$), provided complete self- and ideal-self descriptions. It should be noted that, because the same subjects were studied at each assessment period, the developmental changes during adolescence to be reported cannot be attributed to changes in sample composition.

Measuring Self-Esteem: The Self-Descriptive Q-Set

At ages 14, 18, and 23, subjects described themselves (i.e., their perceived-self) and, on another day a week or more later, the person they would ideally like to be (i.e., their ideal-self) using the 43-item Self-Descriptive Q-Set (SQ; J. H. Block & J. Block, 1980). Items on the SQ contain personality-descriptive adjectives and short phrases that are easily understood by adolescents (e.g., "competitive," "affectionate," "responsible," "gets upset easily," "creative"). For both the perceived-self and the ideal-self Q-sorts, subjects sorted the SQ-items into seven categories ranging from Most Undescriptive (1) to Most Descriptive (7), according to a fixed, discrimination-maximizing rectangular distribution (i.e., seven items in the middle category and six items in the remaining six categories).

To index self-esteem, and in accord with our conceptual definition of self-esteem, the congruence between each subject's perceived-self and ideal-self descriptions across the 43 SQ-items was calculated, using the correlation formula to create this score. Higher scores reflect greater congruence and therefore indicate higher levels of self-esteem.[2] The reliability of this self-ideal index was eval-

---

[2] The reader should note that self-esteem, an introspective condition that requires evaluation through self-report measures, stands in no necessary relation to psychological adjustment or mental health. Only when psychological health is evaluated by indices of adjustment not based on self-reports can the empirical connection between self-esteem and psychological health be established (Block & Thomas, 1955).

uated by applying the Spearman-Brown formula to split-half correlations computed between randomly generated equivalent halves of the 43 adjectives that comprise the SQ (this procedure was repeated three times, and the mean of the three estimates was used). Reliability estimates were computed separately for females and males at each age. The split-half reliability of the self-ideal index at ages 14, 18, and 23 was .88, .81, and .83 for the female sample and .63, .56, and .75 for the male sample, respectively.

Measuring Personality: Encoding Observer Descriptions with the California Adult Q-Set

At ages 14, 18, and 23, the personality characteristics of the subjects were independently described by four psychologists using the California Adult Q-set (CAQ) (Block, 1961). These psychologist judges (doctorates and graduate students in clinical and personality psychology) had each separately and independently observed and interacted with the subjects in the course of administering a wide variety of interviews, cognitive and personality tests, and other assessment procedures, formal and informal. However, they were entirely unaware of the self-esteem scores of the subjects. Each judge sorted the 100 widely ranging descriptive statements of the Q-set into a forced, quasi-normal distribution using nine categories, from *not at all characteristic or salient* to *highly characteristic or salient* of the subject being described. The multiple Q-sort formulations available for each subject were then averaged across corresponding items to form the composite Q-sort descriptions used for the present analyses. The estimated internal consistency reliabilities of the Q Items, based on correlations among observers, averaged .72, .59, and .70, at ages 14, 18, and 23, respectively. This approach to personality description previously has demonstrated its usefulness and validity in a variety of contexts (e.g., Block, Block, & Keyes, 1988; Block et al., 1991; Funder & Block, 1989; Kogan & Block, 1991).

RESULTS

Does Self-Esteem Increase or Decrease from Early Adolescence to Early Adulthood?

Mean-level change. For the combined sample, no age-related changes in the mean level of self-esteem were observed. However, males tended to have higher self-esteem scores than females at every age, and this disparity increased over time. For the males, the self-esteem means (and standard deviations) at ages 14, 18, and 23 were .56 (.20), .59 (.15), and .60 (.19); for the females, the corresponding figures were .53 (.26), .52 (.26), and .48 (.26). Analyses of the simple effects of sex at each age indicate a slight difference favoring the boys at age 14 which does not warrant interpretation ($F < 1$); by age 18, this difference has increased ($p < .07$, one-tailed test); and by age 23, the difference between the sexes in self-esteem has become statistically significant ($p < .005$, one-tailed test). In this developmental divergence, males on average increased in self-esteem from age 14 to 23 by about one-fifth of a standard deviation, whereas females on average decreased in self-esteem by about one-fifth of a standard deviation. We evaluated the reliability of this gender divergence in self-esteem using three different analytical strategies: (a) a Mann-Whitney analysis of sex differences in raw change scores (self-esteem at age 23 minus self-esteem at age 14) ($p < .03$), (b) correlating the sex dichotomy with residualized self-esteem change scores (see below) ($p < .01$), and (c) testing the interaction between sex and linear trends in age ($p < .04$) based on the method of orthogonal polynomial contrasts (Keppel & Zedeck, 1989). By all three approaches, the gender divergence in self-esteem levels across time proved to be statistically significant. Blyth et al. (1983) have reported a similar self-esteem divergence in their longitudinal study of sixth graders becoming tenth graders.

The longitudinal consistency of self-esteem. The longitudinal consistency of individual differences in self-esteem was assessed, for the sexes separately, by intercorrelating the self-esteem scores available at ages 14, 18, and 23 (see Table 1). Because these correlations are attenuated by inevitable measurement error, they provide an underestimate of the true longitudinal consistency of self-esteem. Therefore, the correlations were corrected for unreliability in the self-esteem measures, and these adjusted, theoretically more accurate figures are also shown in Table 1.

Across the 4-year period from age 14 to 18, the adjusted correlations were about .60 for both females and males (.57 and .63, respectively); across the 5-year period from age 18 to 23, the adjusted correlations were .65 for females and .50

TABLE 1
Longitudinal Consistency of Self-Esteem: Correlations
(and Corrected Correlations) Across Ages 14, 18, and 23

	INTERVAL ACROSS WHICH SELF-ESTEEM WAS CORRELATED		
	Age 14–18	Age 18–23	Age 14–23
Females	.48 (.57)	.55 (.65)	.55 (.65)
Males	.37 (.63)	.32 (.50)	.25 (.36)
Total sample	.45 (.59)	.50 (.65)	.44 (.55)

NOTE.—For females, $n = 47$; for males, $n = 44$. The correlations in parentheses were corrected for unreliability using Spearman-Brown reliability estimates, computed separately for females and males at each age.

for males. Across the entire 9-year period from age 14 to 23, the corrected correlations were .65 for females and .36 for males.

Across the 9-year period from age 14 to 23, the sex difference in the uncorrected correlations (.55 for females, .25 for males) is also quite large, corresponding to a ratio of almost 5 to 1 in variance terms ($p < .05$). The equivalent findings using both the adjusted and uncorrected figures obviates an interpretation that the observed gender difference is a statistical consequence of gender differences in the reliability of our self-esteem measure.

Another possible explanation for the gender difference in longitudinal consistency involves restriction of sample range; the self-esteem measure has less variance in the male sample than in the female sample (which had several outlying self-deprecators), and this difference conceivably may account for the difference between the across-time correlations of the two sexes. To evaluate this possibility, the across-time correlation in the male sample was corrected for range restriction (Hunter & Schmidt, 1990). This correction provides an estimate of what the correlation would have been for the males if the variance in the sample of males had been the same as in the female sample. The corrected correlation estimate was .55 for the females and .40 for the males—a difference of 2:1 in variance terms, which is still substantial considering that the restriction of range correction formula tends to overestimate the true correlation for sample sizes smaller than 50 (Mendoza, Hart, & Powell, 1991).

Thus, the greater longitudinal ordering consistency of self-esteem for females across adolescence and the transition to adulthood does not appear to be a statistical artifact. Rather, the greater ordering consistency within the sample of girls implies that, for many girls, personal levels of self-esteem are relatively well established by adolescence, while in our sample of adolescent boys, personal self views are relatively malleable throughout the teen years.

Patterns of individual-level change. The trends observed in the aggregate analyses reported thus far may not represent the patterns of change existing at the individual level; that is, they may mask individual differences in the direction and magnitude of developmental change. In the following analyses, we examine individual differences in self-esteem change from age 14 to 23.

The nomothetic expectation would be that the trends observed at the sample mean level typify the developmental change patterns exhibited by most of the subjects in the sample. However, substantial individual differences were observed in both the direction and the magnitude of self-esteem change from age 14 to 23. For the males, individual differences in self-esteem change ranged from an increase of .65 to a decrease of −.52 (note that the self-esteem measure has a possible range of −1.00 to +1.00). For the females, individual differences in self-esteem change ranged from an increase of .49 to a decrease of −.60.

In the male sample, from age 14 to 23, 34% decreased in self-esteem (20% by more than one-half a standard deviation, a relatively substantial change), and 64% increased in self-esteem (34% by more than one-half a standard deviation). In the female sample, 57% of the females decreased in self-esteem (49% by more than one-half a standard deviation), and 43% increased in self-esteem (21% by more than one-half a standard deviation). (In the combined sample, more than 60% of the subjects either increased or decreased by more than one-half a standard deviation during the period from age 14 to 23.) For the male and female samples, the proportions decreasing and increasing more than one-half a standard deviation differed significantly ($p < .02$).

These findings indicate substantial individual differences in self-esteem development, with different patterns of change characterizing females and males. They do not, however, provide insight into why some individuals increase in self-esteem from early adolescence to young adulthood while others decrease. Indeed, from a nomothetic viewpoint, these findings might be ascribed simply to random error superimposed upon the increasing gender differences observed over time. But another interpretive possibility is that these individual differences are systematic and are lawfully related to personality characteristics. To address this issue, the relations between personality characteristics existing at age 14 and individual differences in self-esteem change from age 14 to 23 were examined.

Personality Correlates of Self-Esteem Change

The personality correlates of self-esteem change were evaluated using a residualized change index, computed by regressing self-esteem at age 14 onto self-esteem at age 23 and retaining the residuals.[3] This residual index provides a directional measure of individual differences in self-esteem change from age 14 to 23 that is independent of each subject's initial level of self-esteem at age 14 (Cronbach & Furby, 1970; Lord, 1956). The index has a reliability of .70 in the male sample and .71 in the female sample (see Formula 49 in O'Connor, 1972). We correlated this self-esteem change index with each of the 100 CAQ items observers had evaluated as characterizing the subjects at age 14. A positive correlation with a CAQ item indicates that 14-year-olds who were high on the Q-characteristic were more likely to increase in self-esteem from age 14 to 23 than those who were low on the characteristic. Because the observers evaluated these personality characteristics when the subjects were 14 years old, they of course could not have been influenced by the changes in self-evaluation subsequently manifested by the subjects.

---

[3]We replicated these analyses using a raw change score (self-esteem at age 23 minus self-esteem at age 14) and obtained essentially the same pattern of results but with somewhat weaker relations.

Of the 100 CAQ items, 22 were significantly correlated with self-esteem change for females and six were significant for males at the .05 alpha level. The number of correlations well exceeds that expected by chance for females but not for males, suggesting that self-esteem change from adolescence to early adulthood may be more lawfully related to personality characteristics for girls than for boys. Although few in number, however, the Q-item correlates of self-esteem change in males display a coherent constellation. Because of the uniqueness and the difficulty of replicating the present longitudinal data and because in an exploratory study such as the present one it makes more sense to increase somewhat the risk of a Type 1 error in order to avoid the more consequential, irretrievable effects of a Type 2 error, we list the Q-items correlating at the .10 alpha level with subsequent self-esteem change for both females and males (see Table 2).

Females who were protective, humorous, sympathetic, and generous at age 14 tended to increase in self-esteem, whereas females who were critical, hostile, irritable, and negative at age 14 tended to decrease in self-esteem. Males who were calm, relaxed, not socially anxious, and who already felt satisfied with themselves at age 14 tended to increase in self-esteem, whereas males who were anxious and who fantasized and daydreamed tended to decrease in self-esteem. Overall, subsequent change in self-esteem among adolescent females seems to be related to an other-orientation, that is, to interpersonal characteristics reflecting warmth and a communal orientation. In contrast, subsequent change in self-esteem in adolescent males seems to derive from a self- rather than an other-orientation, and reflects differential tendencies to experience the personal discomforts of social anxiety.

How Similar Are the Personality Correlates of Self-Esteem Across Time?

In the previous set of analyses, we examined the personality antecedents of *self-esteem change,* rather than the correlates of *self-esteem per se.* We focus here on a different question: Do the character qualities surrounding self-esteem vary from early to late adolescence and into young adulthood or do they remain essentially the same? That is, do observers ascribe the same personality characteristics to individuals with high (vs. low) self-esteem at different developmental periods?

Self-esteem scores at each age were correlated with the 100 CAQ items measured *concurrently,* yielding three sets of 100 Q-item correlations; these three sets or vectors of correlations convey the concomitant relations between self-esteem and personality qualities at ages 14, 18, and 23. We then correlated the vector of 100 Q-item correlation values obtained at one age with the vector of 100 Q-item correlation values obtained at each other age. The resulting correlations between these sets of correlations provide an index of the congruence, or pattern similarity,

TABLE 2

Predicting Self-Esteem Change: Personality Characteristics Measured at Age 14 That Predict Increases in Self-Esteem from Age 14 to 23

Observer Judgments of Personality at Age 14	Correlation with *Increase* in Self-Esteem[a]
Females:	
Is moralistic	.47**
Responds to and appreciates humor	.46**
Is protective of those close to him/her	.42**
Is turned to or sought out for advice and reassurance	.38**
Is cheerful, happy	.37**
Has a clear-cut personality; is relatively easy to understand	.36**
Behaves in a sympathetic and considerate manner	.36**
Initiates humor; makes spontaneous funny remarks	.34**
Is giving, generous toward others	.34**
Is a talkative person	.30**
Has a high aspiration level for self; is ambitious	.30**
Has warmth; has the capacity for close relationships; compassionate	.28*
Compares self to others	.27*
Values intellectual and cognitive matters	.27*
Is productive; gets things done	.25*
Behaves in an ethically consistent manner	.25*
Is critical, skeptical, not easily impressed	− .36**
Has fluctuating moods; moods go up and down	− .34**
Expresses hostility, angry feelings directly	− .34**
Is irritable; overreacts to minor frustrations	− .34**
Is physically attractive; is good looking	− .34**
Is subtly negativistic; tends to sabotage other people	− .33**
Is unpredictable and changeable in attitudes and behavior	− .33**
Communicates through actions rather than words	− .32**
Is condescending to others; acts superior to others	− .31**
Gives up and withdraws in the face of frustration and adversity	− .30**
Has hostility toward others	− .29**
Tends to ruminate and have persistent, preoccupying thoughts	− .28*
Values own independence and autonomy	− .28*
Distrusts people; questions their motivations	− .28*
Feels a lack of meaning in life	− .28*
Keeps people at a distance; avoids close relationships	− .28*
Creates and exploits dependency in people	− .28*
Has a brittle ego-defense system; maladaptive under stress	− .27*
Is guileful and deceitful, manipulative, opportunistic	− .26*
Pushes and tries to stretch limits	− .26*
Is self-defeating	− .25*
Males:	
Socially at ease; has social poise and presence	.36**
Feels satisfied with self; is unaware of self-concern	.34**
Regards self as physically attractive	.33**
Is calm, relaxed in manner	.30**
Behaves in masculine style	.27*
Tends to fantasize, daydream, engage in fictional speculations	− .35**
Is basically anxious	− .30**
Anxiety and stress find outlet in bodily symptoms	− .29*
Tends to ruminate and have persistent, preoccupying thoughts	− .28*
Tends to be self-defensive	− .26*

NOTE.—For females, *n* = 47; for males, *n* = 44.

[a] Correlation between CAQ item at age 14 and residualized change in self-esteem. Positive correlations indicate that the item is more characteristic of individuals whose self-esteem increased from age 14 to 23, controlling for their initial level of self-esteem at age 14.

* $p < .10$ (two-tailed).

** $p < .05$ (two-tailed).

of the CAQ correlates of self-esteem for the ages being related. A high correlation between two vectors indicates that Q-items more strongly positively (or more strongly negatively) related to self-esteem at one age tend to be more strongly positively (or more strongly negatively) related to self-esteem at the other age. More generally, the correlations between vectors provide an estimate of the similarity at different ages of the personality attributes ascribed by observers to individuals with high (vs. low) self-esteem.

For the female sample, the patterns of Q-correlates of self-esteem were quite similar at ages 14 and 18 ($r = .67$), age 18 and 23 ($r = .68$), and across the entire period from 14 to 23 ($r = .81$).[4] For the male sample, in contrast, the pattern of Q-correlates of self-esteem at age 14 was quite different from the pattern of Q-correlates at age 18 ($r = .19$) or at age 23 ($r = .14$); however, the pattern of Q-correlates of self-esteem at age 18 closely resembles the pattern of Q-correlates at age 23 ($r = .69$). The independently assessed personality profile of a 14-year-old adolescent girl with high self-esteem appears to be already well established because it is quite similar to the personality profile of an 18- or 23-year-old young woman with high self-esteem. In contrast, the personality profile of a 14-year-old adolescent boy with high self-esteem seems not yet firmly formed and is radically different from the personality profile of an 18- or 23-year-old young man with high self-esteem. The transformation in the personality characteristics associated with self-esteem in males appears to occur between age 14 and age 18; by age 18, the pattern of Q-correlates established essentially continues to age 23.

We also evaluated gender similarities at corresponding ages in the Q-item personality patterns surrounding self-esteem. At age 14, the girls and boys showed quite different patterns of Q-correlates ($r = -.05$). However, as the girls and boys proceeded through adolescence to early adulthood, the personality patterns associated with self-esteem became progressively more similar for the two sexes ($r = .41$ at age 18; $r = .76$ at age 23). Thus, the personality profile of a 14-year-old girl with high self-esteem is quite different from the personality profile of a 14-year-old boy with high self-esteem, but there is a convergence over time in the personality profiles associated with self-esteem for the two sexes, although some important differences still remain at early adulthood.

To infuse psychological content into these somewhat abstract congruence coefficients, we report in Table 3 the CAQ items significantly correlated with self-esteem at age 23 for *both* young women and young men. As portrayed by psychologist-observers, and regardless of gender, 23-year-olds with high self-esteem tend to be satisfied with themselves, cheerful, assertive, poised, productive, quick to act, and turned to for advice. They do not delay or avoid action, they

---

[4]These correlations between vectors of correlations can only be interpreted descriptively; they cannot be referred to sampling distributions for evaluations of their statistical significance.

TABLE 3
Personality Correlates of Self-Esteem at Age 23

OBSERVER JUDGMENTS OF PERSONALITY AT AGE 23	CORRELATION WITH SELF-ESTEEM AT AGE 23	
	Females	Males
CAQ items correlated positively with self-esteem:[a]		
Assertive; not afraid to express opinions	.54**	.33**
Is cheerful, happy	.52**	.39**
Feels satisfied with self; is unaware of self-concern	.48**	.54**
Is turned to or sought out for advice and reassurance	.48**	.35**
Socially at ease; has social poise and presence	.46**	.39**
Is productive, gets things done	.38**	.45**
Has a rapid personal tempo; behaves and acts quickly	.36**	.33**
CAQ items correlated negatively with self-esteem:[a]		
Reluctant to commit self; delays or avoids making decisions	− .60**	− .53**
Feels a lack of meaning in life	− .56**	− .47**
Gives up and withdraws in the face of frustration	− .55**	− .46**
Has doubts about adequacy as a person	− .51**	− .44**
Is self-defeating	− .49**	− .50**
Vulnerable to real or fancied threat; generally fearful	− .49**	− .45**
Is basically anxious	− .46**	− .50**
Tends to ruminate; has persistent, preoccupying thoughts	− .45**	− .42**
Has a brittle ego defense system; maladaptive under stress	− .44**	− .49**
Feels cheated and victimized by life; self-pitying	− .43**	− .37**
Has fluctuating moods; moods go up and down	− .39**	− .45**
Is unpredictable and changeable in attitudes and behavior	− .35**	− .30**
Is subtly negativistic; tends to sabotage other people	− .34**	− .30**
CAQ items correlated differently with self-esteem for the two sexes:[b]		
Is a talkative person	.53**	.05
Is sociable, gregarious; emphasizes being with others	.47**	.16
Gives advice; concerns self with other people's business	.46**	.11
Has warmth; has the capacity for close relationships	.43**	.09
Is giving, generous toward others	.31**	− .08
Creates and exploits dependency in others	.27*	− .30**
Is self-dramatizing; histrionic	.21	− .18
Seeks reassurance from others	.01	− .35**
Is physically attractive; is good looking	− .07	.53**
Is an unemotional person; is emotionally bland	− .22	.21
Keeps people at a distance; avoids close relationships	− .49**	− .18

NOTE.—For females, $n = 47$; for males, $n = 44$.
[a] CAQ items that correlate above $|.30|$ ($p < .05$, two-tailed) with self-esteem for both females and males.
[b] CAQ items that have significantly different correlations ($p < .10$, two-tailed) with self-esteem in the female and male samples.
* $p < .10$ (two-tailed).
** $p < .05$ (two-tailed).

do not give up when frustrated, they do not ruminate or have fluctuating moods, they do not feel cheated and victimized by life, and they are not fearful. This is a coherent set of characteristics and there is no conceptual problem in seeing how these personality qualities are conducive to or expressive of a solid sense of self-worth and identity in either sex. This personality core, common to both sexes, underlies the impressive correspondence (.76) between their personality profiles at age 23.

However, it merits mention that, despite their appreciable characterological similarities, young women with high self-esteem also differ from young men with high self-esteem. Reported also in Table 3 are the CAQ items correlating significantly differently with self-esteem for the two sexes. These items suggest that young women with high self-esteem emphasize interpersonal connectedness far more than young men of high self-esteem. They tend to be warm, gregarious, talkative, giving, closely concerned individuals, whereas young men with high self-esteem are relatively unemotional, uninvolved, and independent in distancing ways.

DISCUSSION

In the present paper, developmental change in self-esteem was examined in a cohort of individuals followed longitudinally from age 14 through age 18 to age 23, a period spanning adolescence and the transition to young adulthood. During this cultural time (the decade of the 80s), our subjects confronted a number of important developmental tasks. From age 14 to 18, they were compelled to cope with the pressures and possibilities associated with becoming an adolescent. Puberty had opened the world to them in many alluring but also threatening ways; in junior and senior high school, more was being expected of them cognitively, and how they responded to this press, positively or evasively, had great immediate (and long-term) consequence; deeper and different peer relations were being formed, with many beginning dating; and the possibility of experimentation with sex and drugs was in the atmosphere. From age 18 to 23, our subjects necessarily moved on to begin to meet other demands and expectations associated with becoming an adult: most had finished high school; a fair number had gone to and through college, while others had begun jobs or careers; one was in prison. Some had married or otherwise established enduring relationships; others were in interpersonal limbo. We know of no other study that has longitudinally charted developmental change in self-esteem in the same group of individuals through a time period so long and so developmentally consequential.

What can we now conclude or interpret from our analyses regarding the development of self-esteem during adolescence? Is an individual's sense of self-worth consistent through adolescence or does it exhibit substantial changes?

For the combined sample, the mean level of self-esteem did not change appreciably. Further, there was appreciable longitudinal ordering consistency of self-esteem across the ages 14 to 18, ages 18 to 23, and across the entire 9-year period; individuals relatively high (or low) in self-esteem at age 14 tend to be relatively high (or low) in self-esteem at ages 18 and 23 as well. The notable absence of appreciable age changes in self-esteem, coupled with evidence of considerable levels of longitudinal consistency, might suggest that self-esteem follows the developmental pattern of "sameness," defined by Block (1971) as strong across-time ordering correspondence together with no indication of changes in mean level (p. 62). For the combined sample, then, the results might be said to support the position that the social, emotional, and biological changes occurring during adolescence do not produce normative psychological disturbance.

The magnitude of the across-time correlations was far from unity, however. When more closely analyzed, the "sameness" observed in the combined sample over time did not characterize the developmental trajectories followed by very many of the individuals within the sample or when the combined sample was partitioned according to gender. Although the "average" individual in the total sample showed virtually no change whatsoever, the majority of subjects changed in self-esteem by more than one-half a standard deviation. Moreover, there was a decided tendency for males to increase and females to decrease in self-esteem from early adolescence to young adulthood. These gender differences in self-esteem change were significantly and meaningfully related to coherent patterns of personality in both the sample of girls and the sample of boys. These findings highlight the importance of *not presuming*, without explicit evaluation, that reliable individual differences in development do not exist or are not important.

The findings revealed a number of theoretically provocative differences between females and males. First, longitudinal consistency was appreciably less for males than for females across ages 14 to 23. One conjectural explanation for this observed sex difference stems from the differential socialization experienced by girls and by boys. J. H. Block (1973) noted that socialization processes tend to restrict the range of experience for girls but broaden it for boys. For example, boys are given autonomy earlier than girls and have less constrained opportunities for play outside the home (Hoffman, 1977; Saegert & Hart, 1976). These differences in socialization emphases may produce or permit more diversity in the developmental change patterns of boys as compared to girls. These developmental diversities would produce more changes in the rank-ordering of boys within their peer group, thus decreasing the longitudinal ordering consistency of their self-esteem over time.

Our longitudinal finding that boys tend to increase and girls to decrease in self-esteem during adolescence is consistent with cross-sectional research showing that there are more girls than boys with low self-esteem in early adolescence, and that this difference grows larger by late adolescence (Simmons & Rosenberg, 1975). Further supporting this pattern, girls tend to increase in depressive affect during adolescence, so that by late adolescence they exhibit more depressive affect than boys (Petersen, 1988). Future research, necessarily longitudinal, should attempt to clarify when and why these gender-divergent trends occur. Our own continuing analyses, which will identify, for the sexes separately, the contentual changes from early adolescence to early adulthood in self-images and ideal-self aspirations, may well help our understanding.

Within each gender group, we also examined the relation of prior personality characteristics to the subsequent direction and magnitude of developmental change. Overall, self-esteem change among females seems to be related to prior interpersonal qualities such as warmth and nurturance, whereas self-esteem change among males seems to be more strongly linked to prior self-focused characteristics such as ability to control personal anxiety level.

More generally, our findings suggest that self-esteem development is integrally related to gender differences in the way the cultural press of adolescence is responded to. Sex-role development has been characterized as the process of socializing females to be more communal and males to be more agentic (J. H. Block, 1973); in crasser terms, females are socialized to get along in society and males are socialized to get ahead. Our findings suggest that the ability to relate to others in an interpersonally positive way promotes self-esteem for females. For males, achieving positive interpersonal connections seems less critical; their sense of positive identity seems, instead, to centrally depend on the ability to control social anxiety, thereby enabling them to function effectively.

Finally, we examined whether self-esteem has the same personological implications at early adolescence, late adolescence, and early adulthood. The personality profile associated with self-esteem was quite consistent over time for females but changed dramatically for males. Although the personality characteristics associated with self-esteem in females and males were quite distinct at age 14, these characteristics became progressively more similar over time. Together, these two findings suggest that the introspective criteria for positive self-evaluation are appreciably transformed in the males over the following decade. Thus, in early adolescence and based on analyses to be reported in detail in a later article, boys who regarded themselves highly were characterized by observers as stern, meticulous, humorless, unexpressive individuals lacking in warmth, while the girls with self-esteem were evaluated as cheerful, sociable, expressive, assertive, decisive individuals. By age 23, the young men are radically reordered with regard to their sense of self-worth. The young men now with high self-esteem are much like the young women with high self-esteem in being internally and externally cheerful, interpersonally poised and functionally effective, and consequently somewhat dominant individuals. And yet, despite these impressive personality equivalences in the two sexes during a later and presumably developmentally more mature stage of self-esteem, young women still manifest a greater concern for and effectiveness in achieving intimate interpersonal ties than do young men. Informally, and for ages, women (and men) have had (and have rued) this perception of gender differences. The present study only demonstrates this long-recognized interpersonal asymmetry (Josselson, 1992, chap. 11).

CONCLUSION

In this study of self-esteem in adolescence and early adulthood, we have examined multiple types of normative developmental change, assessed developmental trends separately for females and males, and conducted person-centered analyses that elucidate the nature of and influences on individual developmental trajectories. Of course, the usual caveats regarding our longitudinal findings apply: our samples of males and of females, although more closely studied than is the case in most psychological inquiries, are nevertheless still relatively small and, conceivably, may be unrepresentative. We do not think our findings are especially sample-dependent, but only subsequent research with other samples can respond to this ineluctable concern.

These reservations having been expressed, the levels of consistency in self-esteem manifested by our longitudinally followed sample impress us as quite remarkable. We are equally impressed by the considerable evidence of developmental change. What then can be concluded about "consistency" and "change"? Like almost any psychological attribute, self-esteem changes in some ways and is continuous in other ways throughout the life course. However, it is too easy to resort to the homily that there is continuity amidst change and change amidst continuity. To go beyond this trivially true, blandly wise response to a simplistically posed question regarding consistency *versus* change, it is necessary to approach the problem in deeper, more differentiated ways. What is needed is further study of the ways in which individuals maintain continuity or change at different periods of their life and the concomitants, consequences, and antecedents of these continuities and changes.

Adolescent self-esteem has important ramifications, both for the developing individual and for society, and therefore warrants further research into the myriad influences—universal, gender-specific, and unique—that lead some individuals to feel good about themselves and others to feel worthless.

REFERENCES

Abramowitz, R. H., Petersen, A. C., & Schulenberg, J. E. (1984). Changes in self-image during early adolescence. *New Directions for Mental Health Services, 22,* 19–28.

Alsaker, F. D., & Olweus, D. (1992). Stability of global self-evaluations in early adolescence: A cohort longitudinal study. *Journal of Research on Adolescence, 2,* 123–145.

Blatt, S. J., Quinlan, D. M., Chevron, E. S., McDonald, C., & Zuroff, D. (1982). Dependency and self-criticism: Psychological dimensions of depression. *Journal of Consulting and Clinical Psychology, 50,* 113–124.

Block, J. (1956). A comparison of the forced and unforced Q-sorting procedures. *Educational and Psychological Measurement, 16,* 481–493.

Block, J. (1961). *The Q-sort method in personality assessment and psychiatric research* (reprint ed. 1978). Palo Alto, CA: Consulting Psychologists Press.

Block, J. (1971). *Lives through time.* Berkeley, CA: Bancroft.

Block, J., Block, J. H., & Keyes, S. (1988). Longitudinally foretelling drug use in adolescence: Early childhood personality and environmental precursors. *Child Development,* **59,** 336–355.

Block, J., Gjerde, P. F., & Block, J. H. (1991). Personality antecedents of depressive tendencies in 18-year-olds: A prospective study. *Journal of Personality and Social Psychology,* **60,** 726–738.

Block, J., & Thomas, H. (1955). Is satisfaction with self a measure of adjustment? *Journal of Abnormal and Clinical Psychology,* **51,** 254–259.

Block, J. H. (1973). Conceptions of sex-roles: Some cross-cultural and longitudinal perspectives. *American Psychologist,* **28,** 512–526.

Block, J. H., & Block, J. (1980). The role of ego-control and ego-resiliency in the organization of behavior. In W. A. Collins (Ed.), *Minnesota symposium on child psychology* (Vol. **13,** pp. 39–101). Hillsdale, NJ: Erlbaum.

Blyth, D. A., Simmons, R. G., & Carlton-Ford, S. (1983). The adjustment of early adolescents to school transitions. *Journal of Early Adolescence,* **3,** 105–120.

Carlson, R. (1965). Stability and change in the adolescent's self-image. *Child Development,* **35,** 659–666.

Caspi, A., & Bern, D. (1990). Personality continuity and change across the life course. In L. A. Pervin (Ed.), *Handbook of personality theory and research* (pp. 549–575). New York: Guilford.

Coleman, J. C. (1978). Current contradictions in adolescent theory. *Journal of Youth and Adolescence,* **7,** 1–11.

Cronbach, L. J., & Furby, L. (1970). How should we measure "change"—or should we? *Psychological Bulletin,* **74,** 68–80.

Douvan, E., & Adelson, J. (1966). *The adolescent experience.* New York: Wiley.

Dusek, J. B., & Flaherty, J. F. (1981). The development of the self-concept during adolescent years. *Monographs of the Society for Research in Child Development,* **46**(4, Serial No. 191).

Engel, M. (1959). The stability of the self-concept in adolescence. *Journal of Abnormal and Social Psychology,* **58,** 211–215.

Funder, D. C., & Block, J. (1989). The role of ego-control, ego-resiliency, and IQ in delay of gratification in adolescence. *Journal of Personality and Social Psychology,* **57,** 1041–1050.

Hall, G. S. (1904). *Adolescence* (2 vols.). New York: Appleton.

Harter, S. (1983). Developmental perspectives on the self-system. In E. M. Hetherington (Ed.), P. H. Mussen (Series Ed.) *Handbook of child psychology: Vol. 4. Socialization, personality, and social development* (pp. 275–385). New York: Wiley.

Higgins, E. T. (1987). Self-discrepancy: A theory relating self and affect. *Psychological Review,* **94,** 319–340.

Hill, J. P. (1985). Family relations in adolescence: Myths, realities, and new directions. *Genetic, Social, and General Psychology Monographs,* **111,** 233–248.

Hoffman, L. W. (1977). Changes in family roles, socialization, and sex differences. *American Psychologist,* **32,** 644–657.

Hoge, D. R., & McCarthy, J. D. (1983). Issues of validity and reliability in the use of real-ideal discrepancy scores to measure self-regard. *Journal of Personality and Social Psychology,* **44,** 1048–1055.

Hunter, J. E., & Schmidt, F. L. (1990). *Methods of meta-analysis: Correcting error and bias in research findings.* Newbury Park, CA: Sage.

James, W. (1890). *Principles of psychology.* New York: Holt.

Josselson, R. (1992). *The space between us: Exploring the dimensions of human relationships.* San Francisco: Jossey-Bass.

Keppel, G., & Zedeck, S. (1989). *Data analysis for research designs: Analysis of variance and multiple regression/correlation approaches.* New York: Freeman.

Kogan, N., & Block, J. (1991). Field dependence-independence from early childhood through adolescence: Personality and socialization aspects. In S. Wapner & J. Demick (Eds.), *Biopsycho-social factors in the field dependence-independence cognitive style across the life span* (pp. 177–207). Hillsdale, NJ: Erlbaum.

Lazzari, R., Fioravanti, M., & Gough, H. G. (1978). A new scale for the adjective check list based on self versus ideal-self discrepancies. *Journal of Clinical Psychology,* **34,** 361–365.

Lord, F. M. (1956). The measurement of growth. *Educational and Psychological Measurement,* **16,** 421–437.

Magnusson, D. (1990). Personality development from an interactional perspective. In L. A. Pervin (Ed.), *Handbook of personality theory and research* (pp. 193–222). New York: Guilford.

McCarthy, J. D., & Hoge, D. R. (1982). Analysis of age effects in longitudinal studies of adolescent self-esteem. *Developmental Psychology,* **18,** 372–379.

Mendoza, J. L., Hart, D. E., & Powell, A. (1991). A bootstrap confidence interval based on a correlation corrected for range restriction. *Multivariate Behavioral Research,* **26,** 255–269.

Montemayor, R. (1983). Parents and adolescents in conflict: All families some of the time and some families most of the time. *Journal of Early Adolescence,* **3,** 83–103.

Mortimer, J. T., Finch, M. D., & Kumka, D. (1982). Persistence and change in development: The multidimensional self-concept. In P. B. Baltes & O. G. Brim, Jr. (Eds.), *Life span development and behavior* (Vol. **4,** pp. 263–313). New York: Academic Press.

Mortimer, J. T., & Lorence, J. (1981). Self-concept stability and change from late adolescence to adulthood. *Research in Community and Mental Health,* **2,** 5–42.

O'Connor, E. F., Jr. (1972). Extending classical test theory to the measurement of change. *Review of Educational Research,* **42,** 73–97.

Offer, D., & Offer, J. B. (1975). *From teenage to young manhood: A psychological study.* New York: Basic.

Offer, D., Ostrov, E., & Howard, K. (1981). *The adolescent: A psychological self-report.* New York: Basic.

O'Malley, P. M., & Bachman, J. G. (1983). Self-esteem: Change and stability between ages 13 and 23. *Developmental Psychology, 19, 257–268.*

Ozer, D., & Block, J. (1987, April). *Personality and IQ change from childhood through adolescence.* Paper presented at the meetings of the Society for Research in Child Development, Baltimore, MD.

Pelham, B. W., & Swann, W. B. (1989). From self-conceptions to self-worth: On the sources and structure of global self-esteem. *Journal of Personality and Social Psychology, 57, 672–680.*

Petersen, A. C. (1988). Adolescent development. *Annual Review of Psychology, 39, 583–607.*

Rogers, C. R., & Dymond, R. F. (1954). *Psychotherapy and personality change.* Chicago: University of Chicago Press.

Rosenberg, M. (1965). *Society and the adolescent self-image.* Princeton, NJ: Princeton University Press.

Rutter, M., Graham, P., Chadwick, O. F. D., & Yule, W. (1976). Adolescent turmoil: Fact or fiction? *Journal of Child Psychology and Psychiatry, 17, 35–36.*

Saegert, S., & Hart, R. (1976). The development of sex differences in the environmental competence of children. In P. Burnett (Ed.), *Women in society* (pp. 87–116). Chicago: Maaroufa.

Savin-Williams, R. C., & Demo, D. H. (1984). Developmental change and stability in adolescent self-concept. *Developmental Psychology, 20, 1100–1110.*

Simmons, R. G., & Blyth, D. A. (1987). *Moving into adolescence.* New York: Aldine De Gruyter.

Simmons, R. G., & Rosenberg, F. (1975). Sex, sex roles, and self-image. *Journal of Youth and Adolescence, 4, 229–258.*

Stephenson, W. (1953). *The study of behavior: Q-technique and its methodology.* Chicago: University of Chicago Press.

Turner, R. H., & Vanderlippe, R. H. (1958). Self-ideal congruence as an index of adjustment. *Journal of Abnormal and Social Psychology, 57, 494–498.*

Part II

GENDER ISSUES

The articles in this section focus on issues of gender. The first paper is a normative study of gender differences and the latter two papers examine atypical behaviors in nonclinical samples.

There has always been much interest in sex differences across the lifespan. Prior and colleagues present data from the Australian Temperament Project, a large longitudinal study that surveyed 2443 families beginning in the first year of the child's life. This paper uses a subsample of 300 families interviewed from infancy to eight years of age to examine sex differences in temperament, socioemotional development, and adjustment. A wide range of reliable measures were used including temperament scales, an intelligence test, adaptive behavior scales, behavior problem scales, and questionnaires for marital adjustment and childrearing practices and children's perceived competence.

The similarities among boys and girls were more striking than the differences. Contrary to other studies, boys were not biologically disadvantaged based on birth history or developmental defects. Before the age of three there were few gender differences in temperament. During the preschool years, there were some sex differences. Girls were rated by mothers as higher on adaptive behavior and daily living skills and boys were rated as having more acting-out behavior problems. Teachers rated boys as less ready for school on items such as concentration and self-reliance. Path analyses were used to assess gender-specific developmental pathways. For boys, behavior problems were more related to temperamental characteristics, specifically persistence and inflexibility, than environmental factors. In this study, girls appeared more sensitive to environmental and parental influences, although temperament was still a significant predictor. The data replicate and extend findings from Chess and Thomas' New York Longitudinal Study, in which temperamental inflexibility was the most powerful contributor to behavioral maladjustment for boys and girls at all prediction points.

The second paper in this section investigates the association of nonnormative gender behavior with boys' and girls' adaptation. A salient developmental task for preadolescents is expressing interest in and learning about the other gender while maintaining clear gender boundaries. Gender boundary is a psychological construct. It refers to preventing intimacy or identification with the other gender. Specific behaviors have to be viewed in context to determine whether they are boundary maintaining or violating. Sroufe and colleagues used subjects from the Minnesota Mother-Child Project who were enrolled in a specially designed sum-

119

mer camp. Observations based on both child sampling and event sampling were used to note the frequency of nongender boundary-violating behavior such as proximity, onlooking, or group interaction, and gender boundary-violating behaviors such as hovering, one child joining an opposite gender group, flirting, or physical contact. A counselor rating of social skill, an observational measure of friendship, and a peer measure of popularity were used as indices of competence. As predicted, maintenance of gender boundaries is an important developmental issue in the middle childhood years. Those who crossed gender boundaries at this age were less socially competent than precociously competent. The authors also found a link between attachment history and gender boundary maintenance. They propose that through the early child-caregiver relationship the child develops a sense of self, including gender identity and a capacity for boundaries.

The third paper in this section by Sandberg and colleagues is a community survey of the prevalence of gender-atypical behaviors. Gender-atypical behavior is defined as behavior that is thought to be uncommon in one gender but very common in the other gender. This includes doll-playing or dress-up by boys or taking the role of the other sex in games. A list of gender-related items for boys and girls was developed for this study. Parents rated the existence of gender-atypical behavior in a sample of 687 boys and girls aged six to 10 years. Gender-atypical behaviors were rare in both boys and girls, although rates were slightly higher for girls. Age, across the limited span studied, and ethnicity were not significant factors in the expression of most gender-atypical behaviors. Although the rate of individual items was low, most children expressed more than one gender-atypical behavior. Approximately one-fifth of the boys and one-third of the girls showed at least 10 different gender-atypical behaviors occasionally. These results are useful for parents who are often concerned when children, particularly boys, express gender-atypical behaviors. The authors suggest that only children who frequently and persistently express gender-atypical behaviors and limited gender-typical behavior should be evaluated for a gender identity disorder.

5

Sex Differences in Psychological Adjustment from Infancy to Eight Years

Margot Prior

La Trobe University, Bundoora, Australia
Royal Children's Hospital, Melbourne

Diana Smart

La Trobe University, Bundoora
University of Melbourne

Ann Sanson

University of Melbourne

Frank Oberklaid

Royal Children's Hospital, Melbourne

The objective of this study was to explore sex differences in development from infancy to 8 years of age in a community sample. Measures of biological, social, interactive, and parental functioning as well as teacher reports were obtained. There were minimal differences in infancy, but major psychosocial differences emerged with increasing age. In the biological sphere boys were disadvantaged only in ratings of language and motor skills at 3 to 4 years old. They showed greater temperamental "difficulty" and low persistence factor scores from 5 years onward. Boys were significantly more likely to have problems with adaptive behavior and social competence and to show behavior problems of the hyperactive and aggressive type, as rated by mothers. Parent and family functioning measures did not differentiate between the sexes. Teachers rated boys as having more problems in academic

Reprinted with permission from *Journal of the American Academy of Child and Adolescent Psychiatry*, 1993, Vol. 32(2), 291–304. Copyright © 1993 by the American Academy of Child and Adolescent Psychiatry.

This research was supported by grants from the National Health and Medical Research Council Australia.

and behavioral domains the first 3 years of school. Path analyses combining data sets gathered when the children were 3 to 8 years old demonstrated the differential courses of development for boys and girls although temperamental flexibility was the best predictor of behavioral adjustment for both sexes. A social learning explanation of the increased incidence of problems among males is supported, although biological influences are not ruled out.

The topic of sex differences across the life span is endlessly fascinating and controversial. Changes in social mores in the Western world, the emergence of the feminist movement, along with the increased attention paid to equality of educational opportunities for boys and for girls, have imbued the topic with considerable emotionality, which is reflected in the psychological literature on this topic. Debate over the relative weight of biological versus social learning explanations for reported sex differences (e.g., Benbow, 1990; Huston, 1983) generates considerable heat and little consensus in data interpretation (Block 1976; Maccoby and Jacklin, 1974, 1980; Tieger, 1980).

In the cognitive area, recent meta analyses suggest that sex differences are slight and perhaps diminishing (e.g., Shibley-Hyde and Linn, 1988). In the sphere of social and emotional development, males continue to be at a disadvantage at least until the adolescent years and perhaps also in adult life (Chess and Thomas, 1984). In the earliest developmental period, boys are at greater risk than girls for almost the entire range of developmental problems (Jacklin, 1989). Clinical studies attest to the higher referral rate of boys in the preadolescent years (Earls, 1987), and the few normal population studies available tend to support the clinical data (Achenbach et al., 1990; Esser et al., 1990; McGee et al., 1984; Offord et al., 1987; Weisz et al., 1989).

During the first few years, a gradually increasing proportion of boys are reported to have a difficult temperament, to be harder for their mothers to manage, and to show more behavior problems (Maziade et al., 1984; Prior et al., 1989). This is particularly the case for hostile-aggressive "acting-out" behavior and for hyperactive, distractible behavior. There is some debate about how early these differences appear, with some workers claiming distinct differential patterns of aggression in toddlerhood, and others finding no sex effects before the age of about 4 years (Richman et al., 1982). Bates (1980) reported that at 18 months boys were not more difficult or fussy in temperament than girls. However by the age of 2 years, difficult girls were more likely to have moderated their behavior and to have settled into comfortable relationships, whereas boys remained difficult. Toddler boys are more likely to get into mischief than are girls in the home setting (Maccoby, 1986), and it seems that boys may be generally more at risk for conflict with parents by contrast with girls who establish closer family ties in early childhood. It has been claimed that parents are more punitive toward boys and more likely to exhibit marital discord in front of boys (Earls, 1987).

Sex differences in temperament have been reported relatively rarely, and there is no consensus in the area although the rare differences found have generally indicated disadvantage for boys (see e.g., Oberklaid et al., 1990; Porter & Collins, 1982). There is a general belief that boys are more active than girls (Eaton & Enns, 1986; Maziade et al., 1984; Stevenson and Fielding, 1985) and harder to manage as they get older (Persson-Blennow & McNeil, 1981) (see Kohnstamm, 1989, for recent review of sex differences in child temperament). Sociocultural expectations for temperamental expressions differ for boys and for girls (Buss, 1989) emphasizing the importance of environmental effects on developing behavioral styles. For example, sex-differentiated relationships between child temperament and caregiver behavior have been reported in a number of studies (e.g., Radke-Yarrow et al., 1988; Stevenson and Fielding, 1985). Earls and Jung (1987) reported a differential pattern of correlations between temperament factors and behavior problems in 3-year-old boys and girls and showed that boys' behavior problems were much more strongly related to home environment characteristics than were those of girls (see also Scholom et al., 1979).

One of the problems of ascertaining the extent and significance of sex differences in this developmental period had been the overreliance on clinical data from children referred for learning and behavioral difficulties (Eme, 1979) with conclusions undermined by the unrepresentative nature of samples of boys and girls used. This is particularly the case for antisocial behavior problems where boys are much more likely to be reported as showing troubling or acting-out behaviors. For "troubled" behavior, or internalizing problems, sex differences are less likely to be reported and, therefore, less can be claimed with confidence concerning the nature and prevalence of this class of disorders. An additional problem has been that cross-sectional studies have provided only a single snapshot view of development in which differences in sampling (and even the era in which the testing was completed) severely limit conclusions about the emergence, development, and consistency of childhood sex differences. Only a longitudinal study, with the advantage of a constant subject base (e.g., Thomas and Chess, 1977), can provide the continuity to investigate these questions.

The purpose of this paper is to provide data on sex differences in temperament, socioemotional development, and behavioral and learning adjustment from a large-scale community sample studied prospectively from infancy to 8 years of age, The Australian Temperament Project (Prior et al., 1989). The prospective longitudinal design of the study lent itself to examination of sex differences and to hypothesizing about their origins and about differential pathways to adjustment and maladjustment. First, we had early biological data so that we could test for any initial disadvantage in boys or girls in our sample. Second, we had data on temperament and behavioral adjustment gathered at approximately 18-month intervals until the children were almost 8 years old. Hence we could watch the unfolding of sex differences using a set of measures with continuity across time. Third, we had data on the socioeconomic conditions and the psychological health of the parents, and their attitudes toward childrearing. Fourth, data obtained from teachers of the children provided an independent assessment of their academic and behavioral adjustment and interpersonal skills. In addition, we obtained standardized measures of the child's cognitive ability and reading achievement as well as his or her attitude toward cognitive and learning tasks in the second year of school.

The data for this paper are organized so that biological, social interactive, parenting, and school adjustment factors can be compared for the existence of systematic sex differences. The simplest prediction that could be made from longitudinal data such as ours is that if innate, early biological factors are important, sex differences should be apparent from very early in life. If socialization practices are more salient, sex differences should increase with age as the child becomes more influenced by external factors. Neither possibility precludes the most likely course of development, which is that nature and nurture interact inextricably to produce differences in boys and girls in the early period that in turn will influence future developmental pathways in gender-specific ways. We acknowledge too that genetic and hormonal effects are not steady or predictable in their influences across ages, so it cannot be shown conclusively that sex differences are the product of a specific biological or environmental factor.

In the final part of the paper we take advantage of our longitudinal data to report path analyses from age 3 to 4 to 7 to 8 years looking at the different factors that are predictive of adjustment for boys and for girls.

METHOD

Subjects

Children were drawn from the cohort of 2,443 Victorian children enrolled in the Australian Temperament Project in 1983 at the age of 4 to 9 months. These subjects came from 67 Local Government Areas (LGAs) that were randomly selected, with the advice of the Australian Bureau of Statistics, to provide an unbiased sample of the 203 Victorian LGAs. Forty-seven of the selected LGAs were rural (839 children), and 20 were urban (1,604 children) (Sanson et al., 1985). Immigrant families who constitute approximately 25% of the Australian population are proportionally represented. Most of these are of European origin. The children and their families have been mail surveyed every 18 months from 1983 to 1990 (i.e., five times) using age-appropriate questionnaires and rating scales for temperament, developmental and behavioral adjustment, sociodemographic indices, and health. In infancy, data were obtained through the estate Maternal and Child Health Centers attended by all families on the pregnancy, birth history, and early biological history of the child. During school age, teachers also have provided ratings of temperament, and social and academic development.

With such a large sample it was not possible to obtain detailed family and child data in personal interviews for the entire group. However, in 1986 when the children were between 3 and 4 years old, we selected a random subsample of 300 families who were *fully representative* of the total sample on all previously assessed characteristics and carried out more detailed, in-depth interviews and assessments to extend and complement the survey data. Data from this subsample provide the basis of this report. Subject numbers vary slightly across measures and across years of assessment from a low of 225 (total of father questionnaire responses in the last phase) to a high of 294 (144 boys, 150 girls) in the first phase. Teacher compliance was somewhat lower and varied from a low of 216 to a high of 258. Reported statistics allow for these variations.

All children lived in a metropolitan or outer-metropolitan area, but previous analyses of the large statewide sample had shown no significant differences in adjustment between urban and rural children (Sanson et al., 1985). The mean socioeconomic status rating for the sample was 3.63 (corresponding to middle socioeconomic status levels) with a range of 1.00 to 6.75. We combined information from the mail surveys as well as from family interviews involving mother, father, and child in this investigation of sex differences.

Measures

Biological development and "intrinsic" characteristics. Standard data were available from the Maternal and Child Health Nurses on pregnancy and birth history, prenatal and perinatal conditions, etc., in the infancy period. Temperament of the child is included here, although it is conceded that this is not a purely biological measure but involves some social interactive factors that affect the mother's responses to temperament questionnaires. However, the concept of temperament is that it is an organismic, relatively stable, individual characteristic that has a demonstrable inherited component (Buss and Plomin, 1984; Saudino and Eaton, 1991). The mother or primary caregiver at each survey point rated characteristic stylistic responses of the child in a variety of everyday situations (such as feeding, bathing, sleeping), reaction to new people and events, intensity of reactions, ease of soothability, activity level, mood, etc. (Thomas and Chess, 1977).

Temperament was measured in infancy (4 to 8 months) using the Australian version of the Carey and McDevitt Revised Infant Temperament Questionnaire (1978); at 1 to 2 and at 2 to 3 years using the Australian version of the Toddler

Temperament Scale of Fullard et al., (1984); at 3 to 4, 5 to 6, 6 to 7, and 7 to 8 years using the Childhood Temperament Questionnaire of Thomas and Chess (1977). Separate factor analyses of the temperament data obtained at each survey point yielded a number of reliable and continuous factors across the years (Sanson et al., 1991) i.e., sociability, flexibility, persistence, irritability, intensity, reactivity, and activity. In addition, we developed a continuous "Easy Difficult Scale" as a measure of the overall position of the child in the sample from the most easy to the most difficult (Prior et al., 1989). Although the temperament data came from mothers' ratings on the temperament questionnaires, observational studies using "blind" raters in the project have confirmed significant behavior differences between temperamentally easy and difficult children (Allen & Prior, unpublished).

Language development (slowness in talking, stuttering and articulation problems, referral to a speech pathologist) was rated by the mother when the child was 3 to 4 years of age. It was also assessed via administration of the Binet Intelligence Scale at 5 to 6 years (see below).

Motor Skills were assessed at 3 to 4 years of age via the Vineland Adaptive Behaviour Scales (Sparrow et al., 1984) administered by a trained psychologist to the mother. When the child was 6 to 7 years, and again at 7 to 8 years, a "coordination skills scale" (manipulative skills, coordination, handwriting, and orienting letters), formed one of six scales derived from factor analysis of teacher ratings of school performance and behavior.

Child Health indices were obtained at each time point using a structured questionnaire to report common illnesses, number of visits to doctors, hospitals, use of medication, etc. as reported by the mother.

As with temperament, it is conceded that IQ is not a purely biological factor, but it is included here as a stable, genetically influenced, intrinsic characteristic of the individual. A short form of the Binet Intelligence Scale (4th edition) (Thorndike et al., 1986) was administered to each child at the age of 5 to 6 years.

Interactive factors. At each survey point, mothers were asked to rate the temperament of their child compared with the average child, on a five-point scale ranging from "much more difficult than average" to "much easier than average." Although this measure is related to our easy-difficult temperament scale, which is empirically derived, it has validity as a measure of mother and child relationship and contributes independently to measures of adjustment (Sanson et al., 1991).

We incorporated four scores from the Vineland Adaptive Behavior Scales in this interactive measures group (Communication, Daily Living Skills and Socialization Subscales, and Overall Adaptive Behavior Composite Score), inasmuch as competence scores on this test depend not only on the child's abilities and maturity levels but also on the daily interactions within the family environment allowing the opportunity for such abilities to be manifested. By this argument, Motor Skills also could be part of this group, however, that score was argued to be more appropriate as a biological maturity measure.

Developmental and behavioral problems were rated by the mother on a four-point scale from "none" to "severe," at each year of survey in these ways: infancy, problems with colic, excessive crying, sleep; 1 to 4 years, temper tantrums, excessive shyness, mood swings, accident proneness, excessive crying, dependency; together these provide a composite behavior problems score. At 2 to 3, and 3 to 4 years, we obtained a measure of mother-rated aggression that has been shown to be reliable and highly predictive of later aggression (G. Arnold, unpublished master's thesis). Mothers also completed the Richman and Graham (1971) Behavior Checklist (2 to 3 years); the Behar Pre-school Behavior Questionnaire (PBQ) (3 to 4, and 5 to 6 years) (Behar and Stringfield, 1974), which gives an overall score as well as scores on Hostile Aggressive, Hyperactive Distractible, and Anxious Fearful factors; the Achenbach Child Behavior Checklist (CBCL) (Achenbach and Edelbrock, 1983), which gives scores for total behavior problems, externalizing and internalizing behavior problems, as well as specific sub-scale scores and a score for social competence (6 to 7 years). Raw scores for the CBCL rather than *T* scores were used. Behavior problems of both externalizing and internalizing types were measured at 7 to 8 years with the Child Behaviour Scale (Rutter et al., 1970), which provides similar subscale and total scores to the Behar and Stringfield PBQ. Mothers provided ratings of the relationships between the target child and any siblings in the family using a five-point rating scale from "very warm and friendly" to "very hostile and unfriendly" at 3 to 4 and 6 to 7 years.

Independent ratings of interactive factors came from three sources. The Maternal and Child Health Nurse rated the infant's overall temperament and the adjustment of the mother and baby pair in infancy; at 5 to 6 years the Binet administrator rated the child on task orientation, personal and social orientation, and language skills as shown during the testing session. Data provided by the third independent source, teachers, will be dealt with in more detail below.

Parental functioning and child rearing practices. When the child was 3 to 4 years and again at 6 to 7 years old, mother and fathers completed the General Health Questionnaire (Goldberg, 1978), which includes self-rated scales of Anxiety/Insomnia, Somatic Symptoms, Social Dysfunction, and Depression, and provides an overall adjustment score. At 3 to 4 years, mothers completed the Spanier Marital Adjustment Scale (Spanier, 1976); at 6 to 7 years both parents completed this scale. The mother's experiences of family stress and her coping abilities were self-rated using a scale developed for use in the Australian Temperament Project (J. C. Smith, unpublished data) and of family supports using the Social Support Scale of Henderson et al., (1978) at 3 to 4 and 6 to 7 years. Fathers' ratings of their experience of stress and coping were obtained when the child was 6 to 7 years.

A modified version of the Cohen et al. (1977) Child Rearing Practices Report (completed by mothers when the children were 3 to 4 years old and by both parents when the child was 6 to 7 years of age) assessed attitudes and professed practices in this area. Factor analyses computed for mother and father data revealed five factors in common: child centeredness, control through guilt and anxiety, use of punishment, encouragement of child autonomy, and degree of consistency.

Social and academic adjustment at school. Teachers of the children at 5 to 6 years, 6 to 7 years, and 7 to 8 years rated the child's temperament on the Keogh Teacher Temperament Scale (Keogh et al., 1982), which has three factors, task orientation, flexibility and reactivity. At 5 to 6 years, teachers completed the Behar and Stringfield PBQ to rate adjustment at school, providing parallel scores as noted above for mothers. They also rated the child on a school readiness scale. At 6 to 7 years, teachers completed the Teacher's Report Form (Achenbach and Edelbrock, 1980), a parallel form of the CBCL. Items common to both sexes formed the basis for comparison. Teachers also completed the Australian Temperament Project School Function Questionnaire (available from the authors), which gives ratings on general language skills, specific academic and language skills, creative and artistic abilities, coordination skills, attitudes toward work, temporal sequential processing ability, classroom adaptation, and variability of performance. During this year a trained psychologist administered the Revised Neale Analysis of Reading Ability (Neale, 1988) to all children, during a home visit.

Relationships with peers were assessed at the 7 to 8 year age period via the Interpersonal Competence Scale-T (IPC-T) (Cairns and Cairns, 1984), a 15-item rating scale completed by teachers, yielding four factors of aggression, popularity, affiliation, and academic competence.

At 7 to 8 years the children completed a grade-appropriate teacher administered reading test, the Australian Council for Educational Research Word Knowledge Survey, and they were rated again by their teachers on Keogh's Teacher Temperament Scale, the Rutter Child Behaviour Scale, and the School Function Questionnaire.

Child self-report. The most suitable measure available for such young children at the time of this study was the Harter and Pike (1984) Pictorial Scale of Perceived Competence and Social Acceptance, which provides a number of subscale scores including self-perceived cognitive, social, and physical skills, and maternal acceptance.

Procedure

Each family in the study reported here was visited at home three times, when the children were 3 to 4, 5 to 6, and 7 to 8 years old (at approximately 15-month intervals). The Vineland Adaptive Behaviour Scales was completed at 3 to 4 years of age, the Binet at 5 to 6 years of age, and the Neale Reading Test and the Harter Scales were given at 6 to 7 years of age. Parent questionnaires were completed independently during or just after each visit. Teachers were requested to complete questionnaires on the child in their class and to return them in the stamped addressed envelope provided. For the 7 to 8 year age level, data were obtained via Australian Temperament Project mail survey, both from home and from school.

RESULTS

The first set of results provides a series of *t* tests of chi-squared tests to assess differences between boys and girls at each age level assessed. In the second part, longitudinal data is presented via the inclusion of path analyses. With so many comparisons, the risk of obtaining significant differences by chance is high. Therefore, we adopted the strategy of assessing which of the obtained significant differences were meaningful by reference to Cohen's *d,* an estimate of effect size (Cohen, 1988). Cohen has developed a system of cutoff points to define differences between groups as "small," "medium," or "large"; these vary slightly depending on the statistical test used. With regard to the *t* test, a difference between the group means of 0.20 of a SD is defined as small, 0.50 as medium, and 0.80 as large. This is a stringent standard for significant differences, with a "medium" difference generally being beyond the 0.000 level of significance. In this study, medium or large effect sizes will be taken as substantial and those close to criterion for medium size (effect size 0.40 and above) also will be identified as meaningful.

Tables 1 through 5 provide a summary of *t*-test differences with effect sizes, along with results of chi-squared tests used with categorical data. For these latter tests, an adjusted α level of 0.001 was required as an indication of substantive differences. Results are arranged in categories reflecting the conceptual clusters noted in the introduction to the study, i.e., biological, interactive, etc. For reader interest we include in these tables those differences meeting conventional (nonrigorous) criteria for significance.

Comparisons on all other measures described above but not tabulated were nonsignificant. It should be noted that those differences not reaching criteria for meaningful effect size were consistent with the trend for greater problems being evident among boys.

TABLE 1
Biological Differences Between Boys and Girls

Variable	Boys		Girls		t Value	p <	Cohen's d
	X̄	SD	X̄	SD			
Physical development							
Birth weight (g)	3430.68	612.36	328.10	522.39	2.20	0.028	0.26
Weight (kg) 4–8 months	7.90	1.08	7.18	0.95	5.91	0.000	0.71[b]
3–4 years							
No. of medical problems	1.38	1.96	0.71	1.18	3.46	0.001	0.43
No. of medical treatments	5.85	1.86	5.39	1.70	2.23	0.026	0.26
Temperament factors[a]							
4–8 months							
Irritability	3.04	0.91	2.68	0.92	3.44	0.001	0.40
1–2 years							
Irritability	3.03	0.88	2.78	0.91	2.07	0.040	0.27
Intensity	4.43	0.90	4.12	0.87	2.63	0.009	0.35
Reactivity	3.73	0.74	3.45	0.75	2.79	0.006	0.37
Easy-Difficult Scale	3.61	0.64	3.43	0.66	2.15	0.032	0.28
2–3 years							
Cooperation/manageability	3.13	0.91	2.90	0.89	2.12	0.035	0.26
Persistence	3.04	0.79	2.83	0.84	2.17	0.031	0.27
Activity	4.72	0.89	4.43	1.01	2.42	0.016	0.29
3–4 years							
Cooperation/manageability	3.32	0.87	2.96	0.88	2.25	0.025	0.27
Persistence	3.42	0.91	3.03	0.81	3.76	0.000	0.44
Easy-Difficult Scale	3.23	0.56	2.99	0.60	2.78	0.006	0.33
5–6 years							
Cooperation/manageability	3.05	0.79	2.84	0.82	2.00	0.047	0.25
Persistence	3.09	0.81	2.75	0.79	4.95	0.000	0.61[b]
Easy-Difficult Scale	3.00	0.58	2.74	0.54	3.66	0.000	0.45

6–7 years							
Cooperation/manageability	2.91	0.82	2.64	0.70	2.78	0.006	0.35
Persistence	2.97	0.78	2.70	0.82	2.77	0.006	0.35
Easy-Difficult Scale	2.87	0.60	2.67	0.54	2.78	0.006	0.34
7–8 years							
Cooperation/manageability	2.97	0.84	2.66	0.75	3.11	0.002	0.39
Persistence	3.03	0.83	2.62	0.77	4.04	0.000	0.51[b]
Easy-Difficult Scale	2.90	0.59	2.64	0.55	3.55	0.000	0.46
Motor skills							
3–4 years							
Vineland Motor Skills Scale Score	93.21	13.41	99.64	10.78	−4.59	0.000	0.53[b]

Chi-square Test

	value	df	$p <$
3–4 years			
Slow to talk	11.58	1	0.001[c]
6+ words by 18 months	4.45	1	0.35
Language problems now	13.68	1	0.000[c]
Stutters/stammers	11.73	1	0.001[c]
Understandable speech	9.72	1	0.002
5–6 years			
Asthma/bronchitis	4.95	1	0.026
Kidney/bladder/urine infection	4.85	1	0.028
Handwriting skills	17.69	2	0.000[c]
7–8 years			
Kidney/bladder/urine infection	5.70	1	0.017
Hayfever	5.79	1	0.014

[a] Higher score = greater problems.
[b] Medium effect size; *t* test.
[c] Substantive chi-square difference ($p < 0.001$).

DISCUSSION

Biological Indices

Boys and girls did not differ in infancy on any biological or birth history indices, hence this cohort of boys did not begin life at any disadvantage. In fact, they had a weight advantage. They did have a higher rate of reported overall medical problems at 3 to 4 years of age, but at all other survey points did not suffer from a higher overall rate of illnesses or developmental defects (other than language problems, see below).

Girls were rated on the Vineland Adaptive Behaviour Scales as more advanced in motor skills at the age of 3 to 4. Boys were more likely to be slow to talk, to stutter or stammer at 3 to 4 years, and to be rated by their mothers as having real or suspected language problems at this age. Boys and girls scored equivalently on total Binet IQ and all subscales of this test, thus, apart from reported motor skills and language immaturity, boys did not seem to be "intrinsically" more at risk than girls.

Until the age of 3 years, sex differences in temperament were minor. Boys were less persistent than girls from 3 years onward and at 5 to 6 and 7 to 8 years, boys showed an overall more difficult temperament than girls. Other temperamental differences at school age, all of them consistent with the above, existed, but none reached our criteria for meaningful differences (Table 1).

Interactive Measures

In infancy, more mothers rated their daughters at the easy or very easy end of the scale, although they did not rate their sons as at the more difficult end. At 7 to 8 years there were more boys in the average to difficult levels and more girls at the easy end of the scale. However, only nine boys versus two girls were actually rated as difficult or very difficult by their mothers. At the two other measurement points, the trend was always similar but nonsignificant. Thus mothers showed relatively little differentiation between their boys and girls in their assessment of their overall relationships, despite the differences that emerged on other measures of temperament and behavior problems.

Medium effect sizes in favor of girls were shown on the Total Adaptive Behavior score of the Vineland and on the Daily Living Skills scale score, suggesting earlier maturing in these areas for girls. However, it is also likely that mothers foster these adaptive behaviors in their daughters and expect more from them. Such an interpretation is consistent with Goodnow and Delaney's (1989) findings with older children, that girls take a greater share of the daily living and family work responsibilities in the family home.

Behavior problem measures across all survey times showed mothers reporting more developmental behavior problems (colic, sleep, and crying) in their infant boys, greater aggression in toddlerhood and at 3 to 4 years, more hostile and aggressive behavior at 3 to 4 years, and a higher level of total behavior problems via the Preschool Behaviour Questionnaire. At 7 to 8 years, boys were more hostile-aggressive and hyperactive. The overall picture here was for more behavior disorder in boys of the aggressive or hyperactive, acting-out variety, from the early years of life. Greater aggression was apparent by the age of 2 to 3 years and remained a large and consistent difference across the time span of the study (Table 2). At no time were there any sex differences for ratings of anxious-fearful or internalizing problems.

Parental Functioning

None of the childrearing differences reached criteria for significance, although the findings concerning punishment for boys by both mothers and fathers are notable for their consistency. There is evidence in other literature that sons may be punished more than daughters (Dunn and Kendrick, 1982) and that this can contribute to escalation of conflict. None of the parental or family functioning measures or the sibling relationships scale showed differences by child sex. However, as most families had more than one child, little can be made of these data that can hardly be called gender specific. The findings suggest that the differences observed in mothers' ratings of their children's temperament and behavior problems are not the result of differences in their own personal psychological functioning (Table 3).

Teacher Data

There were substantial effect sizes for teacher-reported hyperactivity and total behavior problems in boys at 5 to 6 years. At 6 to 7 years old, boys were rated as having a higher level of total behavior problems, externalizing problems, and aggressive, nervous/overactive, and inattentive symptoms. At 7 to 8 years teachers again reported more hyperactive and total behavior problems in boys. There were no differences on internalizing behavior problems. Teacher ratings on the IPC-T showed boys as more aggressive (Table 4).

Teacher temperament measures showed that boys were less positively rated at all three school measurement times on task orientation where the effect size was consistent and medium to large; and on flexibility at 6 to 8 years. Task orientation is the temperament factor showing greatest associations with learning and behavioral adjustment (Prior et al., 1991). Its consistency with the parent-rated lower persistence in boys at 5 to 6 and 7 to 8 years is noteworthy. These latter problems

TABLE 2
Interactive Differences Between Boys and Girls

Variable	Boys		Girls		t value	p <	Cohen's d
	X̄	SD	X̄	SD			
Child's Social Maturity							
3–4 years							
Vineland Communication Scale Score	103.14	11.73	106.10	9.34	−2.54	0.016	0.28
Vineland Daily Living Scale Score	96.51	11.89	103.44	10.72	−5.33	0.000	0.61[b]
Vineland Socialization Scale Score	92.34	10.14	94.74	8.39	−2.24	0.026	0.26
Vineland Adaptive Behavior Composite	94.74	11.03	100.88	8.85	−5.35	0.000	0.62[b]
Binet Administrators' Ratings—5–6 years							
Language skills[a]	1.49	0.68	1.30	0.59	2.47	0.014	0.29
Task orientation[a]	1.60	0.72	1.43	0.62	2.11	0.036	0.25
6–7 years							
Achenbach Social Competence	20.59	3.60	21.56	2.04	−3.14	0.002	0.42
Behavior problems[a]							
4–8 months							
Behavior Problems Composite	1.90	0.68	1.61	0.66	3.80	0.000	0.44
2–3 years							
Behavior Problems Composite	1.98	0.48	1.86	0.49	2.05	0.042	0.25
Behavior Checklist (BCL)	19.99	3.23	19.01	3.05	2.50	0.013	0.31
Aggression Score	2.92	0.54	2.64	0.48	4.46	0.000	0.55[b]
3–4 years							
Behar Hostile-Aggressive	16.75	3.16	15.31	3.08	3.95	0.000	0.46
Behar Hyperactivity	6.71	1.75	6.13	1.64	2.92	0.004	0.34
Behar Total Behavior Problems	46.68	6.66	43.93	6.76	3.53	0.000	0.41
Aggression Score	2.83	0.70	2.44	0.51	5.28	0.000	0.64[b]

5–6 years							
Behar Hostile-Aggressive	15.92	3.02	14.80	2.93	3.05	0.003	0.38
Behar Hyperactivity	6.35	1.70	5.71	1.61	3.13	0.002	0.39
Behar Total Behavior Problems	44.13	6.75	42.64	6.69	2.52	0.012	0.31
6–7 years							
Achenbach Total Behavior Problems	28.28	18.29	22.56	15.21	2.75	0.006	0.35
Achenbach Externalizing	11.28	7.30	8.37	5.48	3.48	0.001	0.44
Achenbach Aggressive	5.90	4.23	3.87	3.27	4.35	0.000	0.54[b]
Achenbach Schizoid	1.33	0.93	0.97	0.80	3.35	0.001	0.42
7–8 years							
Rutter Hostile-Aggressive	0.41	0.34	0.25	0.29	3.77	0.000	0.51[b]
Rutter Hyperactive	0.47	0.47	0.25	0.35	4.21	0.000	0.54[b]
Rutter Total Behavior Problems	6.81	4.96	5.12	4.23	0.286	0.005	0.37

Variable	Chi-square test			Mantel-Haenszel Test		
	Value	df	$p <$	Value	df	$p <$
4–8 months						
Mother's overall rating of temperament	14.21	4	.007	11.34	1	.001[c]
1–2 years						
Mother's overall ratings of temperament	9.42	4	.051	8.56	1	.003
7–8 years						
Mother's overall rating of temperament	19.42	3	.000[c]	18.70	1	.000[c]

[a] Higher score = greater problems.
[b] Medium effect size; t test.
[c] Substantive chi-square difference ($p < 0.001$).

TABLE 3
Parental/Family Differences Between Boys and Girls

Variable	Boys		Girls		t Value	p <	Cohen's d
	X̄	SD	X̄	SD			
Parental functioning[a]							
Mother's psychological Health (6–7 years)							
Social Dysfunction	6.82	2.56	6.16	2.02	2.33	0.021	0.29
Fathers' psychological health (3–4 years)							
Depression	0.47	1.05	1.04	2.10	−2.79	0.006	0.36
Childrearing practices[a]							
6–7 years							
Mothers' use of punishment	14.83	3.95	13.60	3.86	2.68	0.008	0.33
Mothers' degree of autonomy	10.87	2.29	10.31	2.30	1.98	0.048	0.25
Father's use of punishment	14.34	4.58	12.89	3.74	2.58	0.011	0.35
Fathers' control through guilt/anxiety	13.21	5.03	11.76	4.47	2.28	0.024	0.30

[a] Higher score = greater problems.

are consonant with the lower school readiness scores for boys at 5 to 6 years, and with the lower Achenbach School Performance scores.

Boys and girls were rated by teachers as equivalent on the scale of "general language skills," "variability of performance," and in intellectual capacity at 7 to 8 years. The separate components of the school readiness measure, i.e., concentration, self-reliance, coping with personal needs, and fine motor control, all showed significant differences. The remaining components, cooperativeness, relationship with teacher, use of materials, following instructions, sociability, and overall coping did not reach this criterion but were consistent in indicating more positive ratings by teachers for girls. One year later, ratings made by a different set of teachers on classroom-related skills showed similar differences. At 6 to 7 years, coordination skills and overall school performance were poorer in boys, whereas at 7 to 8 years, boys were poorer on a variety of classroom adaptation and performance factors.

The only child self-report measure to show a significant difference was physical competence on the Harter scale. Here, although both groups were very positive in their self-evaluations (a mean score of > 3 within a range of 1 to 4), boys reported themselves as less physically competent than girls.

Despite this striking pattern of overall sex differences, there is considerable overlap in the distributions for boys and for girls. Hence, it is important to ascertain that the differences are not the product of a bias induced by the presence of a small number of very disturbed boys in the sample. We examined the data for evidence of problem cases, i.e. those children falling in the top 10 to 15% of the distribution on parent and teacher ratings. Based on commonly reported prevalence figures of approximately 12 to 18% of children with a significant disorder (depending on age, sex, type of informant, and type of disorder), we took those children falling above the first standard deviation (SD) of our total behavior problem distributions. This gave a prevalence of 16.7% for mother-reported overall behavior problems at 6 to 7 and 7 to 8 years. For these children, i.e., putative clinical cases (e.g., Offord et al., 1987), two thirds were boys and one third were girls at both age periods. For comparable teacher data, where 13% of the total group were above 1 SD at 6 to 7 years, 71% of behavior problem cases were boys and 29% were girls. At 7 to 8 years (12.4% of group above 1 SD) 62% were boys and 38% were girls. These findings were mirrored in the results for externalizing behavior problem scales for both mother and teacher report. Our data affirm claims (e.g., Cairns and Cairns, 1986; Maccoby, 1986) that the greater numbers of behavior problem boys contribute to findings of overall sex differences. Aggressive girls may be equally aggressive but are rarer.

The evidence provided by this normative longitudinal community survey of sociobehavioral development suggests little evidence for a male disadvantage on early biological measures, with the sexes also rated by teachers as and psycho-

TABLE 4
Teacher Rated Behavioral Differences Between Boys and Girls

Variable	Boys		Girls		t Value	p <	Cohen's d
	X̄	SD	X̄	SD			
Behavior problems[a]							
5–6 years							
Behar hostile-aggressive	12.64	3.12	11.67	2.54	2.51	0.013	0.32
Behar hyperactivity	5.90	2.04	4.78	1.42	5.15	0.000	0.67[b]
Behar anxious-fearful	12.80	2.87	12.10	2.53	2.15	0.033	0.27
Behar total behavior problems	39.83	7.63	36.56	5.37	3.90	0.000	0.51[b]
6–7 years							
Achenbach total behavior probs	20.01	15.90	12.98	15.76	3.40	0.001	0.46
Achenbach externalizing	12.45	12.05	5.64	9.98	4.51	0.000	0.62[b]
Achenbach aggression	6.10	7.37	3.13	6.86	3.06	0.003	0.42
Achenbach inattentive	5.92	6.44	2.54	4.26	4.53	0.000	0.63[b]
Achenbach nervous/overactive	1.38	1.41	0.60	1.10	4.48	0.000	0.62[b]
7–8 years							
Rutter hostile-aggressive	0.23	0.34	0.13	0.32	2.30	0.023	0.30
Rutter hyperactive	0.44	0.55	0.11	0.29	5.29	0.000	0.79[b]
Rutter total behavior problems	0.23	0.23	0.12	0.18	3.56	0.000	0.54[b]
Temperament[a]							
5–6 years							
Task orientation	2.79	1.05	2.25	0.90	4.41	0.000	0.69[b]
Flexibility	2.56	0.87	2.31	0.82	2.39	0.018	0.30
6–7 years							
Task orientation	2.87	1.10	2.23	0.88	4.99	0.000	0.69[b]
Flexibility	2.60	0.78	2.30	0.73	2.99	0.003	0.41

7–8 years						
Task orientation	3.02	1.11	2.13	0.87	6.27	0.000	0.90[c]
Flexibility	2.69	0.80	2.34	0.75	3.13	0.002	0.45
Social competence						
6–7 years						
Achenbach adaptive functioning	17.88	3.80	19.33	3.97	−2.68	0.008	0.33
7–8 years						
Cairns Affiliation Skills[a]	2.58	1.05	2.27	1.03	2.06	0.041	0.30
Cairns Academic Competence[a]	2.97	0.74	2.72	0.73	2.37	0.019	0.34
Cairns Aggression[a]	2.81	1.10	2.15	1.16	4.03	0.000	0.58[b]

[a] Higher score = greater problems.
[b] Medium effect size; *t* test.
[c] Large effect size; *t* test.

TABLE 5
Teacher Rated Differences Between Boys and Girls in Academic Performance

Variable	Boys		Girls		t Value	$p <$	Cohen's d
	$\bar{X}$	SD	$\bar{X}$	SD			
Reading skills							
6–7 years							
Neale accuracy percentile	50.85	28.83	59.03	26.82	−2.45	0.015	0.29
Neale comprehension percentile	57.76	27.50	66.89	25.39	−2.87	0.004	0.34
Neale combined accuracy comprehension percentile	54.31	27.45	62.96	25.47	−2.72	0.007	0.33
School performance and behavior							
5–6 years							
School readiness composite[a]	2.05	0.82	1.72	0.65	3.44	0.001	0.45
6–7 years							
Specific academic/language skills[a]	1.79	0.64	1.59	0.53	2.44	0.016	0.34
Temporal sequential organization[a]	1.73	0.65	1.50	0.52	2.82	0.005	0.39
Coordination skills[a]	1.91	0.59	1.64	0.44	3.90	0.000	0.54[b]
Attitude in class[a]	1.72	0.56	1.52	0.50	2.76	0.006	0.38
Creative skills[a]	1.94	0.39	1.77	0.66	2.33	0.021	0.33
Achenbach school performance	3.26	0.69	3.54	0.64	−3.06	0.003	0.42

7-8 years

Variable	Mean	SD	Mean	SD	t	p <	Effect size
Specific academic/language skills[a]	1.79	0.62	1.57	0.58	−2.37	0.019	0.37
Temporal sequential organization[a]	1.75	0.65	1.51	0.51	2.65	0.009	0.42
Coordination skills[a]	1.83	0.51	1.63	0.45	2.66	0.009	0.42
Attitude in class[a]	1.87	0.50	1.51	0.48	4.66	0.000	0.73[b]
Creative skills[a]	1.96	0.44	1.70	0.48	3.62	0.000	0.56[b]
Variability of Performance[a]	8.24	8.16	4.54	5.96	3.33	0.001	0.52[b]

	Chi-square Test			Mantel-Haenszel Test		
Variable	Value	df	p <	value	df	p <
5-6 years						
Self-reliance	19.50	4	0.001[c]	10.54	1	0.001[c]
Coping with personal needs	14.06	2	0.001[c]	10.16	1	0.000[c]
Concentration	16.74	4	0.002	13.90	1	0.000[c]
Fine motor control	19.58	4	0.001[c]	13.91	1	0.000[c]
Use of materials	6.20	2	0.045	5.53	1	0.019
Overall coping at school	8.03	3	0.045	5.52	1	0.019

[a] Higher score = greater problems.
[b] Medium effect size; t test.
[c] Substantive chi-square difference ($p < 0.001$).

metrically tested as equivalent on ability measures. Hence, there was consistency in findings of potential equivalence in these "intrinsic" factors, with the possible exception of language development capacities. Differences emerged when interpersonal issues became salient and when application to learning and classroom socialization was called for. Boys are, undoubtedly, more prone to the development of behavioral problems especially of the acting-out antisocial type, with aggression particularly prominent. Parents and teachers agreed on this despite their differing roles, values, and standards and the fact that they are rating behavior in different contexts. Signs of male aggression are evident as early as toddlerhood where the seeds of later conduct disorder may be observed. It could however be argued that such an early appearance of aggression may support the view that it is strongly biologically influenced (Rutter and Garmezy, 1983).

Boys seem to be less ready psychologically for the school learning situation and have greater problems in becoming task oriented and in adapting to classroom requirements during the early school years. They were only slightly more at risk for reading problems (effect sizes did not reach criterion). There are two possible interpretations for this somewhat weak effect which is not consistent with the almost universally reported preponderance of boys in the ranks of the reading disabled. It may be that reading difficulties are not firmly enough established by the age of 7 to 8 years to make this a reliable finding. However, our own follow-up data of the children who had especially poor reading skills (and here there was a majority of male "cases"), suggests that at least two thirds of them remain reading disabled by the end of their 3rd year of school (Prior et al., 1991). Alternatively, clinical referral of children for reading problems is much more likely when there is co-existing behavior disorder. As this is more prevalent in boys in the early school years, it may lead to a gender-biased ascertainment rate for reading disability. From this point of view, the availability of data from a community sample is particularly useful.

Generally, teachers report more differences to the disadvantage of boys than do other informants (McGee et al., 1983). Given that teachers are likely to underreport behavior problems in their pupils by comparison with mothers (Achenbach et al., 1987), our findings relating to poorer classroom and learning adjustment must be a cause for concern. Early language deficiencies and slower development of motor skills in boys are suggested in this study, reflecting perhaps slower maturation of these skills in males and again increasing their vulnerability to difficulties in adapting to school entry.

The increase in sex differences in behavior over time, with increasing exposure to social experiences, suggests that a social learning explanation may fit our data best. Even the temperamental differences that are open to interpretation as either biologically driven (organismic factors) or biosocially developed (interactive factors) support this argument. Substantial and consistent differences were found in those areas where social learning is important, i.e., ease or difficulty of temperament (comprising the factors of sociability, irritability, and cooperation or manageability). The approach or sociability factor on its own, the dimension of temperament for which there is greatest evidence for heritability (Goldsmith, 1983), showed no tendency to differentiate between boys and girls. Moreover, the temperament factor of activity, which may have strong biological components (Eaton and Enns, 1986), did not differentiate between the sexes here. *Problematic* or uncontrolled levels of activity did show strong effects, with boys rated by both mothers and teachers as more likely to be hyperactive.

The poorer early language skills found in boys may contribute to lower or delayed capacity for social problem-solving skill development in the early years. This is almost certainly relevant to the greater level of hyperactive and hostile aggressive behavior in boys. Although boys appear to recover from early language delay, as seen in the minimal differences in verbal ability later in life (Shibley-Hyde and Linn, 1988), it may be that some do not compensate for problems in social communication and interaction developed in earlier and more critical developmental stages. Instead, ineffective and inappropriate styles of interaction and social problem solving may become entrenched.

Two major concerns emerge from these data. Boys are seriously disadvantaged at school entry in those capacities that facilitate learning and social adjustment and may be at greater risk for long-term learning and behavioral difficulties with "a bad start" in an environment of great importance in their lives. Girls appear to develop closer cooperative relationships with their mothers in the early years than do boys (Maccoby, 1986), and to be more likely to comply with requests and rules (Rothbart, 1989). This may translate adaptively to classroom environments, aiding the greater success of girls in the early school years.

The second concern is that it is in the social interaction areas where boys begin to run into problems quite early in life. Uncooperative, difficult, aggressive, hyperactive behavior emerges in their encounters with other people as they develop beyond the early dependent stages bringing them into conflict with the environment. Maccoby (1986; 1990) has provided persuasive accounts of how gender-typed behaviors develop in male peer groups and how competitive and uncooperative behavior becomes normative. By comparison, girls' interactions seem to elicit and reinforce the empathic, nurturant roles assigned to them in society. Their greater maturity, attentional skills, and cooperative approach reduce risk for learning and behavior problems. In delinquency and crime statistics one sees clear evidence of the continuation of these "conflict with the environment" problems in offending males, almost all of whom have had antisocial behavior problems from early school age (Robins, 1978).

McGuire and Earls (1991) suggest that "gender-specific developmental pathways may be sufficiently well established in the first few years to interact with environmental contingencies in profoundly different ways" (p. 147). In the final part of this paper we report analyses that assess these pathways using the data collected when the child was between 3 and 8 years old and selecting variables that theory and our previous analyses indicated might be particularly influential.

Path Analyses

For these analyses, the sample consisted of 227 subjects for whom we had complete data sets during the period 3 to 4 years to 7 to 8 years (112 boys and 115 girls). The child variables selected were the temperament factors of inflexibility or cooperation/manageability (an uncooperative, inflexible, and overreactive style of response) and persistence (reflecting persistence at tasks, sitting quietly during activities) at 3 to 4 and 6 to 7 years; social maturity assessed at 3 to 4 years; intelligence at 5 to 6 years; and reading achievement at 6 to 7 years. The parental variables were mother's psychological adjustment (assessed at 3 to 4 and 6 to 7 years), mother's marital adjustment and level of social supports (3 to 4 and 6 to 7 years), and a stress factor comprising total number of stresses, degree of difficulty experienced, and expressed ability to cope with life (3 to 4 and 6 to 7 years). The interactional variables selected were the two child-rearing factors of child centeredness and disciplinary or punishment techniques (3 to 4 and 6 to 7 years) (high scores represent low child centeredness and high use of punishment). Total behavior problems at 3 to 4, 5 to 6, 6 to 7, and 7 to 8 years provided the outcome variables. Earlier behavior problems were not included as predictor variables in the longitudinal paths as their stability was very high, with correlations across the years ranging between 0.64 and 0.73. Hence, they exerted a powerful predictive effect that was similar for both sexes and that obscured the contribution of the other variables, which we see as of greater heuristic interest.

While a number of models were tested and compared, we report here the most explanatory and parsimonious models in which all paths contributed significantly by F test. It should be noted that the models are exploratory and need to be replicated. Standardized β coefficients, which indicate the direct effect of the variable, are shown next to the numbers in parentheses; pearson correlations, which indicate the total effect, are shown inside parentheses (decimal points have been omitted.) The variance accounted for is shown in a square box beneath the variable.

Figure 1 shows that two of the four variables with direct links to boys' behavior problems at 3 to 4 years were the child factors of persistence and temperamental inflexibility. Social maturity and use of punishment also contributed directly, and the other variables had indirect links only. Maternal characteristics appeared to exert their influence through the childrearing factor of punishment. The same variables had direct links to boys' behavior problems at 5 to 6 years, with mothers'

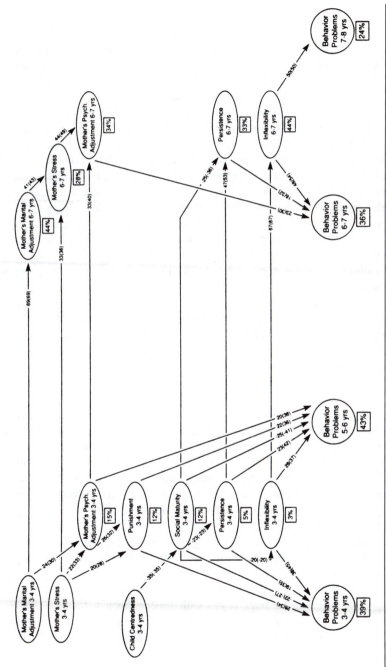

Figure 1. Path model predicting boys' behavior problems from three to eight years.

psychological adjustment now having a direct path. At 6 to 7 years, the temperament factors of inflexibility and persistence continued to have direct links to boys' behavior, and inflexibility was particularly powerful. Mother's psychological adjustment also contributed directly with maternal stress, and marital adjustment contributed through this variable. By 7 to 8 years, only inflexibility was directly and strongly linked to behavior problems.

The model shown in Figure 2 is more complex and reflects the fact that girls' behavior problems were consistently related to a range of child, maternal, and interactional factors. At 3 to 4 years, temperamental inflexibility, mother's psychological adjustment, and the two childrearing factors of child centeredness and punishment had direct links to behavior problems. Maternal stress and marital adjustment were expressed through maternal psychological adjustment, and there was also a path from marital adjustment to child centeredness. Temperamental inflexibility also contributed indirectly through punishment. At 5 to 6 years there were direct links between behavior problems and temperamental inflexibility, punishment, maternal stress, and marital adjustment.

Inflexibility punishment, and marital adjustment continued to have direct links to girls' behavior problems at 6 to 7 and 7 to 8 years, with maternal stress, and persistence also having direct paths at 6 to 7 years. In contrast to the boys' model, only at 6 to 7 was persistence directly linked to behavior problems for girls, and this was the only time that girls' social maturity at 3 to 4 years appeared in the model, where it contributed to later persistence. The greater degree of *consistent* influence of maternal interactional factors running from 3 to 4 through to 7 to 8 in paths for girls suggests greater sensitivity to family influences. Neither IQ nor reading achievement featured in either model.

Although there is a fair degree of consistency in the two path models, there are some intriguing points of contrast. There were gender differences whereby the boys' models were a little more powerful at the two earlier time points, and girls' models were more powerful at the two later time points. Temperamental inflexibility was clearly the most powerful contributor to behavioral maladjustment at all time points for boys and girls. However this trend seemed to grow stronger over time for boys, and by ages 7 to 8 years, inflexibility was the only variable with explanatory power in the boys' model.

An additional point of contrast is the greater relevance of temperamental persistence to the boys' model where there were significant paths to behavior problems at all times except 7 to 8 years. For girls, persistence was directly linked to behavior problems only at 6 to 7 years. Level of social maturity at 3 to 4 years was an important feature of the boys' model with direct paths to behavior problems at 3 to 4 and 5 to 6 years and an indirect effect moderated by persistence at 6 to 7 years; however, it contributed only indirectly via persistence at 6 to 7 years for girls.

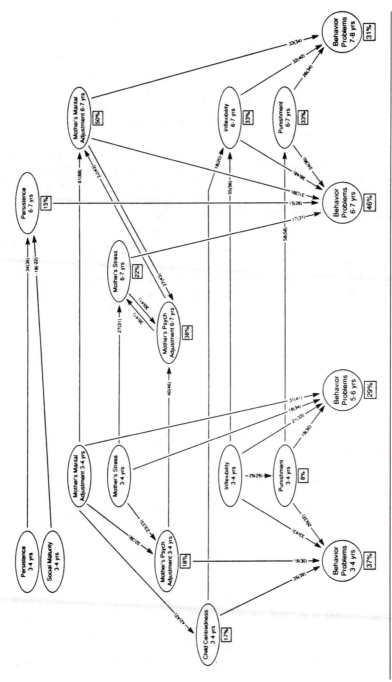

Figure 2. Path model predicting girls' behavior problems from three to eight years.

Interactional factors appeared to be more salient for girls than for boys. Punishment or disciplinary techniques were significantly linked to adjustment at every stage in the girls' model but featured only at the earlier ages for boys. Child centeredness was directly linked to behavior at 3 to 4 years and contributed indirectly through later inflexibility for girls whereas its influence was indirect for boys via social maturity at 3 to 4 years. Whereas maternal characteristics consistently were linked to girls' behavior, they had direct links for boys only at 5 to 6 and 6 to 7 years (psychological adjustment).

By the age of 7 to 8, boys' behavior problems seem more strongly related to intrinsic child characteristics; girls show more sensitivity to environmental and parental influences. These differences in the paths to behavioral adjustment for boys and girls provide some support for the recent suggestions of McGuire and Earls (1991), (see also Kellam and Brown, 1986).

Analyses combining both sexes produced paths that included all the variables shown in Figures 1 and 2 and obscured the fact that their influences operated differentially in theoretically significant ways. Quite inaccurate conclusions about the paths for boys or girls would have resulted from these analyses. We believe our findings emphasize the importance of separate analyses by sex in investigating paths to adjustment and maladjustment.

REFERENCES

Achenbach, T. & Edelbrock, C. (1983), *Manual for the Child Behaviour Checklist and Revised Child Behaviour Profile.* Burlington, VT, University of Vermont, Department of Psychiatry.

Achenbach, T. & Edelbrock, C. (1980), *Manual for the Teacher's Report Form and Teacher Version of the Child Behaviour Profile.* Burlington, VT, University of Vermont, Department of Psychiatry.

Achenbach, T. M., Hensley, V. R., Phares, V. & Grayson, D. (1990), Problems and competencies reported by parents of Australian and American children. *J. Child Psychol. Psychiatry,* 31:265–286.

Achenbach, T. M., McConaughy, S. H. & Howell, C. T. (1987), Child/adolescent behavioural and emotional problems: Implications of cross-informant correlations for situational specifity. *Psychol. Bull.* 101:213–232.

Bates, J. (1980), The concept of difficult temperament. *Merrill Palmer Quarterly,* 26:299–319.

Behar, L. & Stringfield, S. A. (1974), Behaviour Rating Scale for the Preschool Child. *Developmental Psychology,* 10:601–610.

Benbow, C. (1990), Gender differences: Searching for facts. *Am. Psychol.,* 45:988.

Block, J. H. (1976), Issues, problems, and pitfalls in assessing sex differences: A critical review of the psychology of sex differences. *Merrill-Palmer Quarterly,* 22:283–308.

Buss, A. (1989), Temperament as personality traits. In G. A. Kohnstamm, J. E. Bates &

M. K. Rothbart (Eds.). *Temperament in Childhood.* New York: John Wiley, pp. 49–58.

Buss, A. & Plomin, R. (1984), *Temperament: Early Developing Personality Traits.* Hillsdale, NJ: Erlbaum.

Cairns, R. & Cairns, B. (1984), Predicting aggressive patterns in girls and boys: a developmental study. *Aggressive Behavior,* 11:227–242.

Cairns, R. B. & Cairns, B. D. (1986), The developmental interactional view of social behaviour: four issues of adolescent aggression. In: *Development of Antisocial and Prosocial Behavior. Research Theories and Issues,* eds: D. Olweus, J. Block and M. Radke-Yarrow. London: London Academic Press, pp. 315–342.

Carey, W. & McDevitt, S. (1978), Revision of the infant temperament questionnaire. *Pediatrics,* 61:735–739.

Chess, S. & Thomas, A. (1984), *Origins and Evolution of Behavior Disorders.* New York: Brunner/Mazel.

Cohen, D. J., Dibble, E. & Grawe, J. M. (1977), Parental style: Mothers' and fathers' perceptions of their relations with twin children. *Arch. Gen. Psychiatry,* 34:445–451.

Cohen, J. (1988), *Statistical Power Analysis for the Behavioral Sciences,* 2nd ed. New York: Academic Press.

Dunn, J. & Kendrick, C. (1982), *Siblings: Love, Envy, and Understanding.* London: Grant McIntyre.

Earls, F. (1987), Sex differences in psychiatric disorders: origins and developmental influences. *Psychiatr. Dev.,* 1:1–23.

Earls, F. & Jung, K. G. (1987), Temperament and home environment characteristics as causal factors in the early development of childhood psychopathology. *J. Am. Acad. Child Adolesc. Psychiatry,* 26:491–498.

Eaton, W. & Enns, R. (1986), Sex differences in human motor activity level. *Psychological Bulletin,* 100:19–28.

Eme, R. F. (1979), Sex differences in childhood psychopathology: a review. *Psychological Bulletin,* 86:574–595.

Esser, G., Schmidt, M. H. & Woerner, W. (1990), Epidemiology and course of psychiatric disorders in school-age children—results of a longitudinal study. *J. Child Psychol. Psychiatry,* 31:243–264.

Fullard, W., McDevitt, S. C. & Carey, W. B. (1984), Assessing temperament in one-to-three year old children. *J. Pediatr. Psychol.,* 9:205–216.

Goldberg, G. (1978), *Manual of the General Health Questionnaire,* Windsor, United Kingdom: N.F.E.R. Publishing Company.

Goldsmith, H. (1983), Genetic influences on personality from infancy to adulthood. *Child Dev.,* 54:31–355.

Goodnow, J. & Delaney, O. (1989), Children's household work: differentiating types of work and styles of assignment. *Journal of Applied Developmental Psychology,* 10:209–226.

Harter, S. & Pike, R. (1984), The Pictorial Scale of Perceived Competence and Social Acceptance for young children. *Child Dev.,* 55:1969–1982.

Henderson, S., Duncan-Jones, P., McAuley, H. & Ritchie, K. (1978), The patient's primary group. *Br. J. Psychiatry,* 132:74–86.

Huston, A. C. (1983), Sex typing. In: *Handbook of Child Psychology,* ed: P. H. Mussen. 4th edition, Vol. 4. New York: Wiley, pp. 387–468.

Jacklin, C. N. (1989), Female and male: issues of gender. *Am. Psychol.,* 44:127–133.

Kellam, S. G. & Brown, C. H. (1986), Social adaptational and psychological antecedents in the first grade of adolescent psychopathology ten years later. In: *Suicide and Depression among Adolescents and Young Adults,* eds: G. L. Klerman. Washington, DC: American Psychiatric Press, pp. 147–184.

Keogh, B. K., Pullis, M. E. & Cadwell, J. (1982), A short form of the Teacher Temperament Questionnaire. *Journal of Educational Measurement,* 19:323–329.

Kohnstamm, G. A. (1989), Temperament in childhood: cross-cultural and sex differences. In: *Temperament in Childhood,* eds: G. A. Kohnstamm, J. E. Bates & M. K. Rothbart. New York: John Wiley, pp. 483–508.

Maccoby, E. E. (1986), Social groupings in childhood: their relationship to prosocial and antisocial behavior in boys and girls. In: *Development of Antisocial and Prosocial Behavior. Research, Theories and Issues,* D. Olweus, J. Block and M. Radke-Yarrow (Eds.) London: London Academic Press, pp. 263–284.

Maccoby, E. E. (1990), Gender and relationships: a developmental account. *Am. Psychol.,* 45:513–520.

Maccoby, E. E. & Jacklin, C. N. (1974), *The Psychology of Sex Differences.* Stanford, CA: Stanford University Press.

McGee, R., Silva, P. A. & Williams, S. (1983), Parents' and teachers' perceptions of behavior problems in seven year old children. *Except. Child,* 30:151–161.

McGee, R., Silva, P. A. & Williams, S. (1984), Behavior problems in a population of seven year old children: prevalence, stability and types of disorder. *J. Child Psychol. Psychiatry,* 25:251–259.

McGuire, J. & Earls, F. (1991), Prevention of psychiatric disorders in early childhood. *J. Child Psychol. Psychiatry,* 32:129–154.

Maziade, M., Cote, R., Boudreault, M., Thivierge, J. & Caperaa, P. (1984), The New York longitudinal studies model of temperament: gender differences and demographic correlate in a French-speaking population. *J. Am. Acad. Child Adolesc. Psychiatry,* 23:582–587.

Neale, M. D. (1988), *Neale Analysis of Reading Ability-Revised: Manual.* Melbourne, Australia: Australian Council for Educational Research.

Oberklaid, F., Prior, M., Sanson, A., Sewell, J. & Kyrios, M. (1990), The assessment of temperament in the toddler age group. *Pediatrics,* 85:559–566.

Offord, D. R., Boyle, M. H., Szatmari, P. et al. (1987). Ontario Child Health Study II Six-month prevalence of disorder and rates of service utilization. *Arch. Gen. Psychiatry,* 44:832–836.

Pellegrini, D. (1990), Psychosocial risk and protective factors in childhood. *J. Dev. Behav. Pediatr.* 11:201–209.

Persson-Blennow, I. & McNeil, T. (1981), Temperament characteristics of children in relation to gender, birth order and social class. *Am. J. Orthopsychiatry,* 51:710–714.

Porter, R. & Collins, G. M. (1982), *Temperament differences in infants and young children.* Ciba Foundation Symposium 89. London: Pitman.

Prior, M., Sanson, A. V. & Oberklaid, F. (1989). The Australian Temperament Project. In: *Temperament in Childhood,* eds: G. A. Kohnstamm, J. E. Bates, M. K. Rothbart. New York: John Wiley, pp. 537–556.

Prior, M., Smart, D., Nursey, J., Sanson, A., & Oberklaid, F. (1991), Behaviour problems and reading disability—which comes first? Paper presented at the International Society for Research in Child & Adolescent Psychopathology, Zaandvoort, Netherlands, June.

Radke-Yarrow, M., Richters, J. & Wilson, W. (1988), Child development in a network of relationships. In: *Relationships within Families: Mutual Influences,* eds: M. Hinde & J. Stevenson-Hinde. Oxford: Clarendon Press, pp. 48–67.

Richman, N. & Graham, P. J. (1971), A Behavioural screening questionnaire for use with three-year-old children. Preliminary findings. *J. Child Psychol. Psychiatry,* 12:5–33.

Richman, N., Stevenson, J. & Graham, P. J. (1982), *From Pre-school to School: A Behavioural Study.* London, UK: Academic Press.

Robins, L. N. (1978). Sturdy childhood predictors of adult antisocial behavior: replications from longitudinal studies. *Psychol. Med.* 8:611–622.

Rothbart, M. (1989), Temperament and development. In G. A. Kohnstamm, J. E. Bates, & M. K. Rothbart (Eds.), *Temperament in Childhood.* New York: John Wiley, pp. 187–247.

Rutter, M. & Garmezy, N. (1983), Developmental psychopathology. In: P. H. Mussen (Ed.), *Handbook of Child Psychology,* Vol. 4, 4th edition. New York: John Wiley, pp. 775–912.

Rutter, M., Tizard, J. & Whitmore, K. (1970), *Education, Health and Behaviour.* London: Longman.

Sameroff, A. J., Seifer, R. & Elias, P. K. (1982), Sociocultural variability in infant temperament ratings. *Child Dev.* 53:164–173.

Sanson, A. V., Prior, M. & Oberklaid, F. (1985), Normative data on temperament in Australian infants. *Australian Journal of Psychology,* 37:185–195.

Sanson, A., Prior, M. & Oberklaid, F. (1991), *Structure and stability of temperament in the Australian Temperament Project.* Paper presented at the Society for Research in Child Development Conference, Seattle, April.

Sanson, A. V., Oberklaid, F., Pedlow, R. & Prior, M. (1991), Risk indicators: assessment of infancy predictors of preschool behavioural maladjustment. *J. Child Psychol. Psychiatry,* 32:609–626.

Saudino, K. J. & Eaton, W. O. (1991), Infant temperament and genetics: an objective twin study of motor activity level. *Child Dev.,* 155:1167–1174.

Scholom, A., Zucker, R. A. & Stollak, G. E. (1979), Relating early child adjustment to infant and parent temperament. *J. Abnorm. Child Psychol.* 3:41–56.

Shibley-Hyde, J. S. & Linn, M. C. (1988), Gender differences in verbal ability: a meta-analysis. *Psychol. Bull.,* 104:53–69.

Spanier, G. B. (1976), Measuring dyadic adjustment: new scales for assessing the quality of marriage and similar dyads. *Journal of Marriage and the Family,* 38:15–28.

Sparrow, S. S., Balla, D. A. & Cichetti, D. V. (1984), *Vineland Adaptive Behaviour Scales Interview Edition Survey Form Manual.* Circle Pines: MN: American Guidance Service.

Stevenson, J. & Fielding, J. (1985), Ratings of temperament in families of young twins. *Br. J. Dev. Psychol.,* 3:143–152.

Thomas, A. & Chess, S. (1977), *Temperament and Development.* New York: Brunner/Mazel.

Thorndike, R. L., Hagan, E. P. & Sattler, J. M. (1986), *Stanford Binet Intelligence Scale,* 4th edition. Chicago: Riverside Publishing Company.

Tieger, T. (1980), On the biological basis of sex differences in aggression. *Child Dev.,* 51:943–963.

Weisz, J. R., Suwanlert, S., Chaiyasit, W., Weiss, B., Achenbach, T. M. & Trevathan, D. (1989). Epidemiology of behavioural and emotional problems among Thai and American children: Teacher reports for ages 6–11. *J. Child Psychol. Psychiatry,* 30:471–484.

6

The Significance of Gender Boundaries in Preadolescence: Contemporary Correlates and Antecedents of Boundary Violation and Maintenance

L. Alan Sroufe, Christopher Bennett,
Michelle Englund, and Joan Urban
University of Minnesota, Minneapolis

Shmuel Shulman
Tel Aviv University

Previous research has established the importance of gender boundaries as a normative aspect of development in middle childhood. Here, the nature and importance of gender boundaries as an individual differences construct was explored. Ratings of gender boundary violation and gender boundary maintenance were made of 47 10–11-year-old children participating in a series of summer day camps. These ratings were supported by videotape-based behavior codings of gender boundary violating behaviors and by live observations of sheer number of associations with members of the opposite gender. In addition, considerable external validation of these individual differences was obtained. Children low on gender boundary violation and (especially) children high on boundary maintenance were independently judged by camp counselors to be socially competent. They also were found to be higher on a friendship variable, based on observation. Those who violated boundaries were especially unpopular with peers, based on a child interview. Finally, boundary violation and maintenance were

Reprinted with permission from *Child Development*, 1993, Vol. 64, 455–466. Copyright © 1993 by the Society for Research in Child Development, Inc.

This research has been supported by a grant from the National Institute of Mental Health (MH 40864-05).

related to attachment history and to early measures of parent-child
generational boundary distortions.

The literature on peers in middle childhood and preadolescence has been focused largely on interactions and friendships within gender groups (Hartup, in press). This, no doubt, is due to the characteristic and culturally universal segregation of the genders that occurs prior to adolescence (e.g., Maccoby & Jacklin, 1987; Schofield, 1981; Whiting & Edwards, 1988). However, this relative neglect of cross-gender phenomena has been unfortunate for a number of reasons. What boys and girls do together, as well as how they do it and what they do not do, seem likely to be of developmental significance (Maccoby, 1990).

As Thorne (1986) points out in her article, "Girls and Boys Together . . . but Mostly Apart," gender cleavage is not total even in the preadolescent period. Moreover, although direct interactions are rare, members of the opposite gender are often of great interest to children during this period. Ten and eleven-year-old boys and girls talk about each other a great deal (including assertions about who likes whom), and, at times, observe the actions of one another closely. Also, when social commerce does cross gender boundaries, the interactions are often marked by high arousal and displays of affect.

The salience of cross-gender interactions also may be inferred from the elaborate system of rules and rituals that surround them (Thorne & Luria, 1986). At no other age do boys and girls behave as though one may be contaminated by mere interaction or proximity with members of the other gender. Claimed fear of "cooties" and "boy germs" conveys in a playful way the seriousness of the issues involved. So too do the swift and certain consequences that occur when gender boundaries are crossed. For example, a boy is seen leaving a girls' tent (where he went to get his radio). All boys who witness this begin to tease and taunt him ("Uuh, he's with the girls!", "Did you kiss anyone Charlie?", etc.). He has to chase and hit each boy, in turn, to reestablish his place in the group. Like Thorne and Luria (1986) we observed this and countless such examples in our summer camp research (e.g., Elicker, Englund, & Sroufe, 1992).

In general, contact by children with members of the other gender in public settings is disallowed, yet there are numerous exceptions to this "law," all of which are widely understood by children (Maccoby, 1990). These include protection when accompanied by a same-gender peer, immunity when there is active disavowal of interest or when there is some form of "cover" or excuse. Such hypothesized rules, abstracted from our own experience and the work of Thorne and Luria (1986), have been summarized in Table 1. Were cross-gender interactions of minimal importance or of little interest to children, such an elaborate system of rules and rituals would hardly be necessary.

It is our contention that preadolescents face a complex developmental task.

TABLE 1

Knowing the Rules: Under What Circumstances Is It Permissible to Have Contact with the Other Gender in Middle Childhood?

Rule:	The contact is accidental.
Example:	You're not looking where you are going and you bump into someone.
Rule:	The contact is incidental.
Example:	You go to get some lemonade and wait while two children of the other gender get some. (There should be no conversation.)
Rule:	The contact is in the guise of some clear and necessary purpose.
Example:	You may say, "Pass the lemonade," to persons of the other gender at the next table. No interest in them is expressed.
Rule:	An adult compels you to have contact.
Example:	"Go get that map from X and Y and bring it to me."
Rule:	You are accompanied by someone of your own gender.
Example:	Two girls may talk to two boys though physical closeness with your own partner must be maintained and intimacy with the others is disallowed.
Rule:	The interaction or contact is accompanied by disavowal.
Example:	You say someone is ugly or hurl some other insult or (more commonly for boys) push or throw something at them as you pass by.

They must harmonize two seemingly contradictory goals. On the one hand, they must maintain a clear gender boundary, and, on the other hand, they must find opportunities to express their interest in, and learn about, members of the other gender. We believe both goals are important. Maintaining gender boundaries likely functions to enhance loyalty in same-gender friendships and to promote acquisition of skills for group functioning, as well as preventing premature efforts at heterosexual intimacy. Thus, intimacy and capacity for functioning in groups are first mastered in the less complex, same-gender peer group, as suggested by Sullivan (1953). Yet, exposure to, and learning about, members of the other gender during this period should reduce the challenges of heterosexual friendship or intimacy in adolescence (Thorne & Luria, 1986).

Herein lies the importance of the rule system that governs cross-gender social contacts. By adhering to this system preadolescents can acquire experience with the other gender, while still maintaining a distinct boundary between genders; that is, they can be together while still being apart. The rule system serves a regulatory function. By prescribing when contact may occur, in what circumstances, and in what manner, it assures that contact which serves development may take place. It is for these reasons that we emphasize assessments of gender boundary violation and maintenance in the report to follow.

The concept of a "gender boundary," while having physical manifestations, is a psychological construct. Maintaining the gender boundary does not prohibit mere physical proximity or even interaction but, rather, psychological intimacy or identification with the other gender. Whether particular behavior violates or maintains the gender boundary depends on context. Two children may be right next to each other, but if sitting back to back at separate lunch tables and taking no notice of one another, there is little risk of boundary violation even though they are only inches apart. Even physical contact may occur in certain circumstances; yet the boundary may be maintained, if certain actions are taken. Risk of boundary violation and boundary maintenance activities must both be considered in seeking to understand the boundary construct.

Prototypic of "engagement with protection" is what Thorne and Luria (1986) call "borderwork." This term applies to the ubiquitous taunting, teasing, name calling, and chase games between boys' and girls' groups seen on playgrounds. Such high energy contacts not only are generally brief, hit-and-run missions but are also accompanied by outspoken disavowal of interest. They occur at the boundary between groups and serve to proclaim the boundary through verbal assertions and physical definition of "sides." Yet, anyone who observes such transactions cannot miss the high level of interest and excitement that characterizes them. Measures of mere frequency of contact underestimate the importance of such behavior.

Almost all past work on gender boundaries in childhood has been normative, examining behavior of boys and girls in general. Maccoby and Jacklin (1987) did explore the stability and correlates of individual preference for same-sex playmates, finding little support for this individual differences construct. But these were 4½–6½-year-olds. Perhaps gender boundary maintenance is not yet a salient developmental issue at that age.

If maintenance of gender boundaries is, indeed, a salient issue for the preadolescent period, then it should be an important arena for assessing individual differences. Reciprocally, should individual differences with regard to gender boundary maintenance (or violation) have meaningful contemporary, antecedent, and outcome correlates, this would affirm the importance of the construct (Sroufe, 1991; Sroufe, Carlson, & Shulman, in press). In our view, maintaining gender boundaries is an important aspect of social competence during preadolescence. Therefore, we would predict that it would correlate positively with other contemporary assessments of social competence, such as counselor rankings, sociometric popularity, and capacity to form friendships, and with key antecedents of social competence (Waters & Sroufe, 1983). These predictions are in sharp distinction to the alternative hypothesis that preadolescents who frequently cross gender boundaries are the precocious leaders of the peer group.

The purpose of this paper is to present procedures for assessing gender boundary maintenance (and violation) in individual children and to validate this construct against antecedent and contemporary correlates, drawing on the data base of a longitudinal study. The antecedents included assessment of attachment in infancy and assessments of parent-child boundary problems at 24 and 42 months. Attachment classification is a robust predictor of later social competence (e.g., Elicker et al., 1992) and has been implicated in self-development (e.g., Sroufe, 1990). The *generational* boundary assessments were specifically selected as potential antecedents of gender boundary violation. This prediction was based on a presumed role of parent-child relationships in promoting firm ego boundaries in the child and the tendency for boundaries to be violated across genders in families where it occurs (Sroufe & Fleeson, 1988; Sroufe, Jacobvitz, Mangelsdorf, DeAngelo, & Ward, 1985). Correlates of these individual differences in adolescent behavior await later data collection, although this issue has been studied indirectly by Kagan and Moss (1962) and, more recently, by Feldman, Rosenthal, Brown, and Canning (in press).

METHOD

Subjects

Subjects were selected from the Mother-Child Project at the University of Minnesota, a 15-year longitudinal study of children at risk for developmental problems, due to poverty at the time of the child's birth (Egeland & Brunnquell, 1979). Mothers of the children were primiparous and were recruited during the third trimester of their pregnancy from public health clinics in Minneapolis. At the time of delivery, the mothers were young (range $= 12-37$ years, $M = 20.52$, SD $= 3.65$) and mostly single (62%). Forty percent had not completed high school. Eighty percent of the mothers were Caucasian, 14% were Black, and the remaining 6% were Native American or Hispanic. At the time of the 10–11-year-old assessment 20% of the heads of household in the subsample described below had professional, technical, or managerial jobs; 62% were in clerical, crafts person, service or labor jobs; 16% were unemployed, and 2% were students.

Forty-eight children were selected from the larger sample for participation in three 4-week summer camps held in consecutive years on the university campus. Sixteen children participated each year; one child in the third camp returned to his out-of-state home after 5 days, leaving 47 subjects for the study. Children for each camp were selected on the basis of several criteria: attachment classification (approximately equal numbers of children with secure and anxious histories and, as much as possible, children with resistant and avoidant histories in each camp); gender (equal numbers of boys and girls in each camp and within secure and anxious groups); race (approximately equal numbers of Caucasian children in secure and anxious groups); and age (to reduce age variation across camps, the younger subjects in the sample were selected for participation in the last year). Mean age of the subjects at the time of camp participation was 10 years, 11 months (range $= 9$ years, 7 months to 11 years, 8 months; SD $= 7$ months).

Procedure

Setting and camp routine. Children attended the Minnesota Summer Camps 5 days a week, 4½ hours each day for 4 weeks. They were transported daily by van or car between home and camp. The attendance of the children was very consistent ($M = 18.3$ days, SD $= 1.8$), and there were few absences. The daily program of activities was varied and interesting, including group circle times, singing, snacks and lunch, swimming, arts and crafts, and outdoor games and sports. Weekly day trips were taken to local recreation parks, and one overnight camp-out was held at the camp headquarters on the university campus. Many of the camp activities involved all of the children as a group, but there were also opportunities for children to choose among two or more activities and to select their own companions. Observations took place during all of these activities.

Each year's camp counselor staff was composed of four or five master's level graduate students and one or two advanced undergraduate assistants, all experienced in working with school-aged children.

Live observational data. The relative frequency of cross-gender interaction was determined from live observations made during the camp. A child sampling procedure was used, with observations being made in all activities except for counselor-structured activities. Frequency of observation of each child was approximately equal in each activity within each camp. Because of some slight variations and occasional larger variations (due to absences), proportion scores were used. Each child was observed, in turn, just long enough to determine whether the child was engaged with anyone and the identity of the partner(s). An average of 317 observations were made per child over the course of the 4-week camps. For each child several scores were derived. The "cross-gender" score is the proportion of times that each child, when observed, was engaged with only members of the opposite gender.

Videotape data. A total of 138 hours of videotape were available for this study, primarily high-quality, close-in color video recordings. These were edited to extract examples of interaction or proximity between boys and girls, excluding activities structured by counselors, resulting in 438 events on approximately 7 hours of tape. An event sampling method was used; therefore children were not equally represented on the tapes. Isolated children would be seen less frequently, for example, though every child appeared numerous times. These tapes were the basis of behavioral codings and ratings of gender boundary violation and boundary maintenance (described below). Two independent coders did all codings and ratings. Coders viewed the tapes as often as they wished before making their judgments. The two ratings were made for children in all camps; the behavioral codings, which are time consuming and difficult, were made only in the first camp. Although the ratings represent the principal data, we believe that effort in doing the behavioral coding helped insure reliability on the ratings. Also, the ratings are based on the behaviors in the coding scheme.

Measures

Behavioral codes (camp 1).

Nonviolating behavior. Non-gender-boundary violating codes included proximity or interaction which contained no element of personal interest, was casual, entailed active disavowal of interest, and/or was in the context of some form of protection. Brief sketches of the specific codes are as follows:

1. Proximity: The child is merely near members of the opposite gender; no interest, interaction or desire for interaction is apparent.

2. Onlooking: Here the child in fact watches (but only watches) members of the other gender. Interest in the activity may be apparent, but there is no expressed interest in the group per se. Such episodes must be brief, and the child does not follow the group from place to place (in contrast, see "hovering" below).

3. Relaxed interaction: This often entails multiple members of each gender ("safety in numbers"). If there is one-on-one interaction, it must be brief, casual, demanded by a counselor or have some clear purpose, other than interaction per se (e.g., "Pass the lemonade"). It can only rarely be one on more-than-one; then some form of protection is needed. It is called "relaxed" because tension is rare in such interaction.

4. Border work: This is interaction where the apparent motive is to disclaim interest (see Thorne & Luria, 1986). It is often brief and filled with tension (teasing, insults, taunts, shoving, etc.). It may involve an individual child but is often done in groups.

Gender boundary violating codes. These disparate codes have in common a threat to the boundary, either because interest in intimacy is expressed or one remains too long in a vulnerable position. Codes are as follows:

1. Hovering: The child stays oriented to and near a group of the opposite gender more than briefly, perhaps communicating with them, and perhaps changing locations with them. In some way interest in them per se is conveyed and no protection (e.g., from a same-gender counselor or peer) is present. The child is not necessarily attempting to join the group and rarely appears to be doing so.

2. Joining: A single child actually becomes part of an opposite gender group. This would include moving into a certain area (e.g., sitting at a lunch table with only members of the other gender) or engaging in interaction or an activity without protection.

3. Heterosexual meaning: This includes intimate physical contact, flirting, sexual gestures, or verbal sexual innuendoes expressed to members of the other gender. It does not include statements made when in the presence of only

same-gender peers. Boys and girls this age generally do not touch, except as part of border work, and sexual comments usually are made when no members of the other gender are present. This category does not include statements about another party's interests (e.g., "Jennifer likes you Greg") or even expressions of liking deliberately sent through an emissary (although we never observed this behavior).

One other category, "participating with members of the other gender" was considered ambiguous. Here the child is involved with only members of the other gender in some activity (e.g., waiting for a turn to dive) but is not interacting with them. They may be in "dangerous" territory, but the interest seems to be in the activity. This was coded but not included in the analyses. A complete manual for these codings is available from the authors.

Ratings of violation and maintenance (camps 1–3). The seven-point Gender Boundary Violation and Boundary Maintenance Scales are found in the Appendix. These scales are not simply opposites, although one would expect a modest negative correlation. To get the highest scores on maintenance, the child must engage in behaviors that *actively* define the gender boundary, such as taking immediate action to leave a threatening area, calling in reinforcements when needed, asserting disinterest or dislike of opposite-gender members, or assuming a protective physical stance (as witnessed by one girl who kept her elbows up when in close proximity to boys). A child gets the highest score on violation if he or she frequently violates boundaries and expressed intimacy with the other gender, regardless of whether also showing maintenance behaviors at times. On the other hand, a child may get a low boundary violation score simply by having no cross-gender contact. Some may have a lot of contact but always maintain; an occasional child may show a lot of each category of behavior. Still, children showing high violation and low maintenance should be the least competent children. The two scales together define the boundary construct.

Social competence indices. The rationale for selecting social competence indices had two parts: (1) given the limited sample size we limited the number of variables used and (2) we wanted to sample the domain broadly. Therefore, rather than using multiple counselor ratings, observational indices, or child nomination measures, we drew one measure from each of these sources and sought to tap a different aspect of competence with each. We used a counselor rating of social skill, an observational measure of friendship, and a peer-interview-based measure of "popularity." It was the case that each of these measures was supported by data from the other domains; for example, the observational friendship measure (to be described) was strongly related to counselor judgments of friendship and to reciprocated peer nominations of friends (Elicker et al., 1992). We believed a convergence of measures from different sources would be the most adequate test of our hypotheses.

Counselor judgments. Each of four counselors made ratings of each child on a seven-point Social Skills with Peers Scale. High scores on this scale involve more than merely being socially active. Children receiving high scores skillfully modulate their behavior to enhance interaction and to sustain interest in activities. They enjoy social relationships, establish close friendships, and are comfortable in a wide variety of social settings. Data were composited across counselors, yielding a highly reliable index.

Peer popularity. A camp "exit" interview was used to index the overall popularity of each child. While the interview had as primary foci the child's models of relationships and social awareness, it also was possible to derive a within-gender popularity index (Elicker et al., 1992). In our procedure each child was asked whom they especially liked and disliked. Then, they also were asked specifically about unnamed children of the same gender. For each interview a given child received a score of $+2$, if spontaneously named as liked, $+1$ if described as liked under questioning, 0 if regarded in neutral terms, -1 if described as not liked under questioning, and -2, if spontaneously named as disliked. These are then summed for each child across all interviews with children of the same gender.

Observation "friendship" score. We had records of the proportion of times each child was with every other child. The highest of these was taken as the friendship score, under the assumption that associations would pile up between friends, whereas children without close friends would have more scattering of associations. This measure is strongly related to both counselor and peer judgments of friendship (Elicker et al., 1992). We used this as our behavioral measure of competence, rather than total peer contact or total same gender contact, because it is more independent of the frequency of cross-gender association score and controls for amount of sheer social activity.

Early childhood measures.

Attachment pattern. At 12 and 18 months, all subjects were assessed in Ainsworth's Strange Situation procedure with their primary caregivers. Cases were classified as anxious/avoidant (A), secure (B), or anxious/resistant (C) by trained pairs of coders following Ainsworth's procedures (Ainsworth, Blehar, Waters, & Wall, 1978). In those cases where the 12- and 18-month assessments were not consistent (25%), a profile of behavior in a tool problem assessment at 24 months, previously validated against attachment classification, was used to resolve the case (Gove, 1983). In the end all of these subjects were given a single classification, A, B, or C.

Seductive care (24 months). During a clean-up task at 24 months, approximately 10% of the mothers in the total sample were seen to exhibit some form of seductive behavior with the child. Behaviors included sensual whispering or touching, touching of genitals, and attempted bribes with affection. These are described more fully in Sroufe and Ward (1980). A total of seven children across the three camps had mothers who behaved seductively at 24 months.

Generational boundary dissolution (42 months). In a series of teaching tasks, caregivers were rated on two scales: (1) Nonresponsive Physical Intimacy, which overlapped somewhat with the seductive category at 24 months (including any efforts at physical intimacy that was for the mother's gratification rather than for support of the child); (2) Generational Boundary Dissolution, which focused on blurring of boundaries between parent and child (e.g., the child is pressed toward the parental role; parent engages in provocative teasing and taunting or otherwise behaves as though a peer with the child). Both scales, and the rationale for combining them into a more molar scale ("Boundary Dissolution Composite"), are described in a prior publication (Sroufe et al., 1985). Both the 24-month and the 42-month scales were broadly considered as assessments of parent-child generational boundaries.

RESULTS

Reliability and Convergent Validity

Cross-gender behavior codes. Percent agreement of the two coders for the cross-gender behavior codes ranged from .41 to .71. Despite extensive training, certain categories proved difficult to differentially code; for example, hovering (.41) versus joining (.54). Reliabilities for frequently occurring categories were more adequate; for example, border work (.71) and relaxed interaction (.68). When boundary violating and nonviolating categories were collapsed, reliability improved to .83. Agreement on violating behaviors was .80, on nonviolating behaviors .84. This collapsed score, the proportion of violating behaviors observed, was used in the analyses below. (All disagreements were conferenced to consensus.)

Ratings. Across the three camps, reliability for the Gender Boundary Violation Scale was .79 and for the Boundary Maintenance Scale .67 (Pearson *r*'s). The composite of the two coders served as data, and the estimated reliability of these composites (Spearman-Brown formula) is .88 and .80, respectively, for the two scales.

Correlations of ratings and behaviorally based indices. The Boundary Maintenance Scale scores and Boundary Violation Scale scores, which were as predicted modestly negatively correlated ($r = -.20, p < .10$), were combined by subtracting the latter from the former. The correlation of this index with the violation behavioral code index in the first camp was .68 ($p < .01$). The correlations of the behavioral index with each of the two scale scores taken individually were .69 ($p < .01$) for boundary violation and .36 ($p < .10$) for maintenance; that is, the boundary violation behavioral code index correlated better with the Boundary

Violation Scale. Overall, this convergence attests to the meaningfulness and behavioral base of the ratings used as primary data below.

Frequency of cross-gender association. In accord with the previous literature, preadolescents in our camp rarely associated exclusively with members of the other gender. Based on extensive child sampling, with an average of 317 observations per child, there was a mean of 17.2 instances of cross-gender association or 6% of the observations. However, there was ample variation to allow this index to be used in other analyses.

Contemporary correlates of boundary violation and maintenance. The major index of social competence available was the composited social skill rating of the four counselors. Both the Gender Boundary Violation Scale and the Boundary Maintenance Scale correlated significantly and in the expected direction with this measure (see Table 2). The composite of the scales (Maintenance Scale score minus Violation Scale score) correlated .53 with the counselor judgments of competence ($p < .001$). Those who frequently violated gender boundaries were independently judged by counselors to be lower on social competence ($r = -.33$); those who actively maintained boundaries were judged to be higher ($r = .53$). Likewise, for Camp 1, those higher on the behavioral index of boundary violation were judged as less competent ($r = -.36$), although this does not reach the .05 level of confidence with 16 subjects. Even the crude index of sheer frequency of association with the other gender was negatively correlated with counselor judgments of social competence ($-.32$ and .30, respectively, for the two competence indices; $p < .02$).

The counselor data are supported by corroborating observational data, namely, the friendship score. Correlations with the violation and maintenance scales were $-.18$ and .55, respectively, and for the composite of these ratings .44 ($p < .001$). The violation behavior index from Camp 1 ($N = 16$) also correlated significantly with the camp friendship measure ($r = -.43$, $p < .05$), and the more specific "joining" score approached significance ($r = -.41$, $p < .06$).[1]

Finally, children themselves indicated that those who violate gender boundaries and show little evidence of maintaining them (our composited index) are less popular, based on our camp interview ($r = .37$, $p < .005$). Again, this index of competence also correlated negatively with sheer frequency of contact ($r = -.30$, $p < .05$). For Camp 1, the correlation with the violation behavioral index was $-.60$ ($p < .01$) and with "joining" was $-.38$ ($p < .10$).

Sex differences. While it was found that boys received both higher boundary violation and boundary maintenance scale scores than girls (presented below in the "antecedents" section), there was no difference in the patterns of correlations for

---

[1]While the reliability of the "joining" index was only .54, the conferenced scores used can be assumed to be more reliable. Still, the low reliability constrains the relationship with other variables.

TABLE 2

Correlations (Pearson r) Between Gender Boundary Indicators and Social Competence and Early Parent-Child Generational Boundary Assessments

	GENDER BOUNDARY INDICATORS					
	Boundary Violation Rating[a]	Boundary Maintenance Rating	BM-BV Composite	Opposite Gender Association Score	Violation Behaviors	"Joining" Behaviors
Social skills rating	-.33*	.53***	.53***	-.33*	-.36	-.30
Sociometric status	-.34**	.22	.37**	-.30**	-.60**	-.38
Friendship score	-.18	.55***	.44***	-.42**	-.43*	-.41*
Generational boundary dissolution rating—42 months	.38**	-.29*	-.44***	.19	.48*	.29
Nonresponsive intimacy	.38**	.08	-.23	.01	.38	.11
Composite (GBD and NPI)	.44***	-.16	-.41**	.14	.51*	.26

[a] For the ratings and opposite gender association data, $N = 46$–47; for the two behavioral codes, $N = 16$.

* $p < .05$.
** $p < .01$.
*** $p < .001$.

boys and girls. For example, the correlation between the counselor social skills rating and the composite Boundary Violation–Boundary Maintenance Scale was exactly .53 for boys and for girls. Moreover, regression analyses in which gender was entered first still consistently showed significant effects for the competence variables when predicting boundary violation and boundary maintenance. Moreover, the interaction effect between gender and the social competence indices never approached significance in these regressions.

Controlling for social activity. We doubted that our competence measures were merely reflections of social activity, even though proportion of time spent with other children did correlate significantly and positively with the social skill rating (.63, $p < .001$) and modestly with peer-based popularity (.21, $p < .10$). Nonetheless, it was possible to control for amount of child contact using partial correlations. Proportion of time spent with other children was used in these analyses for the social skill rating and the peer popularity variable. A partial correlation was not necessary for the friendship score, since this is already a proportion score and thus accounts for individual differences in activity. This approach is very conservative, because meaningful variance is being partialled out. Social competence does involve being with other children. Nonetheless, for the social skills variable, the resulting partial correlation was significant for the Boundary Violation Scale ($-.35$, $p < .01$), the Boundary Maintenance Scale (.26, $p < .05$) and the combined scales (.40, $p < .01$). For popularity, the violation and combined scales were significant ($-.33$ and .32, respectively, $p < .02$). The result was not significant with the maintenance scale. It also should be mentioned that proportion of time spent with the opposite gender correlated negatively ($-.26$, $p < .05$) with boundary maintenance, while proportion of time in isolation correlated positively with boundary violation (.22, $p < .10$). Neither of these results would follow from a social activity interpretation.

Antecedents of Boundary Violation and Maintenance

Attachment history. Since attachment history has proven to be a robust predictor of later social competence (e.g., Elicker et al., 1992) and because it has been viewed as integral in development of the self (e.g., Sroufe, 1990), it was used as another external correlate for assessing the validity of the gender boundary construct. All camp children had previously been grouped into secure and anxious attachment categories. For this analysis A and C anxious patterns were combined in carrying out posttests.

Analyses of variance were carried out on the violation and maintenance scale scores and the composite index (maintenance – violation), in each case yielding significant main effects for attachment history, $F = 5.287$, $p < .002$;

$F = 12.507, p < .001; F = 14.389, p < .001$; respectively. Posttesting revealed no significant differences between the two anxious attachment groups, which were, taken together, significantly different from the secure group for each scale ($p < .005$ for the Boundary Violation Scale, $p < .001$ for the Boundary Maintenance and Composite Scales). Those with secure histories more likely maintained, and less likely violated, gender boundaries. In addition, for each of the two scales there was a main effect for sex: boys showed significantly more boundary violation *and* boundary maintenance.

Generational boundary violation. Each measure of generational boundary violation available from our longitudinal assessments in early childhood was related to later gender boundary violation and maintenance, always in the expected direction.

For the categorical "seductive behavior" index at 24 months, a chi-square analysis was carried out. In the camps seven children were present whose mothers had behaved seductively in the clean-up task at 24 months; five of these children were among the 10 children (of 47) who had scores of 5 or higher on the boundary violation scale. The resulting chi square was $12.35, p < .001$.

The two scales from the 42-month teaching task (Generational Boundary Dissolution and Nonresponsive Physical Intimacy), and the combination of these, all are continuous variables, so correlational analyses were carried out. The Generational Boundary Dissolution Scale at 42 months correlated significantly, and in the expected direction, with both gender boundary scales at age 10–11 years and their composite (range .29–.44). The Nonresponsive Physical Intimacy Scale correlated significantly with the later Gender Boundary Violation Scale ($r = .38$). This patterning may be seen in Table 2.

DISCUSSION

Substantial validation for the gender boundary construct was obtained in this study, in accord with the previous literature. Support for the idea of gender boundaries as a normative developmental issue derives from the finding of predominantly within-gender associations during free choice time. It seems likely that all of the children observed have some understanding of this norm and the rules governing it, including contexts in which cross-gender association would be appropriate (Maccoby, 1990). No child associated predominantly with the other gender. From a normative point of view it was also noteworthy that boys showed both more boundary maintenance and boundary violation than girls. Past literature has suggested greater sanctions against boys for boundary violation, as well as greater stigma for doing so (Thorne & Luria, 1986). We do not view our data as inconsistent with this. Rather, we take the set of findings as implying that gender boundary issues are of great salience for boys and that boys may do more work at the boundaries. It is important to note that past studies have not documented less violation of boundaries by boys, only more sanctions.

Beyond these normative issues, we view these data as strongly validating gender boundary violation/maintenance as an individual differences construct as well. Both gender boundary violation and gender boundary maintenance were reliably rated. It was difficult to achieve reliability for some of the specific behavioral codes, but these too were reliable when collapsed across categories. Moreover, the ratings and collapsed behavioral codes were in good agreement, attesting to the behavioral basis of the ratings. More important, external validity was demonstrated for all assessments of gender boundary violation or maintenance. Both a broad range of contemporary competence correlates and meaningful antecedents were demonstrated. With the most robust external correlates—the composited counselor rating of social skill and the composited generational boundary dissolution index—impressive correlations were obtained with the combined Gender Boundary Maintenance Scale (.53 and −.41, respectively).

Our strong support for boundary violation/maintenance as an individual differences construct may at first seem inconsistent with an earlier claim by Maccoby and Jacklin (1987) that differences in cross-gender interaction are not stable. Without such stability one would never have expected external correlates of such a measure. However, their subjects were 4½–6½ years old, an age when boundary maintenance may not yet be a salient issue. Moreover, they did not directly assess boundary maintenance and violation but gender segregation per se.

The correlations with social competence, popularity, and friendship suggest that those who cross gender boundaries are lacking in social competence, rather than being precociously competent, and support the hypothesis that maintenance of gender boundaries is an important sign of positive adaptation in late middle childhood. Our interpretation of these findings follows from the notion that acquiring peer group norms is an important task in middle childhood and preadolescence. One such norm may concern the maintenance of gender boundaries. Children who violate such boundaries are generally unpopular with peers. In addition, such violation is one marker of social incompetence. Even more strongly, maintenance of gender boundaries is a marker of social competence; as such, it correlates with other indices of social competence.

The link between attachment history and the gender boundary assessments can be explained in several ways. It may again be interpreted in terms of all measures being from the competence domain. Since attachment security predicts broad indices of competence, so too it predicts these particular indicators in preadolescence. Along these lines, one reason children may cross gender boundaries is failure within the same-gender peer group. Being unsuccessful with same-gender peers, they may spend more time with members of the other gender. This would not seem to be the total picture, however, since behaviors in the boundary violation category imply more than de facto interaction with members of the opposite gender.

Another interpretation of the attachment-gender boundary linkage is more deeply theoretical and centers on the notion of self-development. Identity and, as part of that, gender identity may have important roots in the dyadic child-caregiver relationship. Boundaries are an important aspect of self-development, as the young child learns to be both autonomous and connected. A secure attachment relationship, in which the child achieves a smooth balance between exploring away from the caregiver and seeking contact when threatened or distressed, may mark the early origins of a clear sense of self or identity.

Such theoretical concerns led us to examine aspects of our data set targeted at the boundaries between parent (mothers in our risk sample) and child. These measures showed clear associations with the gender boundary outcome measures. The fact that the parent-child boundary dissolution measures also correlated with other aspects of later social competence, as well as the correlational nature of this study, suggests that conclusions must be tempered at this point. However, the patterning of the findings, with seductiveness at 24 months and non-responsive physical intimacy at 42 months correlating with later gender boundary violating and the broader generational boundary dissolution scale correlating (negatively) with boundary maintenance, are suggestive. We believe that two things may be involved: first, through clear parent-child boundaries clear self or ego boundaries may be evolved, and, second, such parent-child boundary dissolution may in many cases be gender based. Unfortunately, with our predominantly single mother sample we are not able adequately to investigate differential boundary dissolution across parents. At the least, these findings again attest to the meaningfulness of gender boundary maintenance as a developmental construct.

An important task for future research will be to relate individual differences on gender boundary violation and maintenance in preadolescence to peer relationship variables in adolescence. If we are correct that adhering to the gender boundary norm promotes acquisition of the experiences and skills that will promote later successful functioning in the adolescent peer group, numerous predictions follow. In an earlier study Kagan and Moss (1962) reported that boys who were centrally involved in the male peer group in preadolescence were less avoidant of sexual activity in early adolescence. More recently, Feldman et al. (in press) reported different pathways to adolescent heterosexual functioning for boys who had been popular or rejected in middle childhood. Both of these studies defined preadolescent competence in broad terms. We would propose more specifically that individuals following the culturally normative pathway of cross-gender engagement with boundaries maintained in later middle childhood should as adolescents be able to deal well with the social complexities of that period; namely, coordinate same-gender friendships and group functioning with cross-gender relationships and functioning in the mixed-gender crowd. In particular, maintenance of cross-gender boundaries in preadolescence may predict successful cross-gender relationships in adolescence.

APPENDIX

Rating Scale for Boundary-violating Behaviors

1. This child never violates gender boundaries (0%). When interactions occur, the child is always with gender mates, and cross-gender behaviors are always in the service of boundary maintenance (show some disavowal of interest). It may be that this child is never seen interacting with the other gender.

2. Child seldom violates boundaries and typically does so by either hovering or by showing ambiguous behavior.

3. Occasionally violates boundaries—there may be a mixture of hovering and joining.

4. Child has a moderate amount of low-intensity violations (hovering, joining, participating).

5. Boundary violations may be rare but are strong when they occur, involving sexualized comments or inappropriate physical contact, or these may occur in addition to what happens in 4. Or, the child spends a great deal of time hovering, joining, or participating.

6. The child occasionally makes intimate physical contact of a sensual or aggressive nature, or the child makes frequent sexualized comments/gestures toward the opposite gender, but they are not so intense or found in the diversity of settings as 7. Or, the child spends an inordinate amount of time hovering, joining, or participating and seems to associate more readily with the other gender than their own.

7. Child regularly violates boundaries under a variety of circumstances. The majority of these occur in the absence of gender mates. The child often makes intimate physical contact of a sensual or aggressive nature.

Rating Scale for Boundary Maintenance Behaviors

1. Child never maintains boundaries during cross-gender encounters. They seem to associate more readily with the opposite gender than their own. This is true whether the child is alone with the other gender or part of a mixed group. Or, this child is never seen interacting with the other gender.

2. Child uses only passive maintenance, on an occasional basis.

3. Passive maintenance only, in a moderate amount.

4. Child engages in passive maintenance nearly all the time. Or, does a small amount of active maintenance.

5. Moderately active at maintaining boundaries. May do some passive maintenance.

6. Boundary is maintained nearly all of the time, through a mixture of active (mainly) and passive maintenance.

7. Boundary is always maintained. Child uses most or all opportunities for active maintenance. Child is quick to leave situations where alone with the other gender.

DEFINITIONS

Active maintenance: border work and escape strategies, such as calling for support from gender mates or leaving the scene when none are available.

Passive maintenance: relaxed interaction, onlooking, contexts where boundary is provided by "cover," for example, being in a group or with an adult.

REFERENCES

Ainsworth, M., Blehar, M., Waters, E., & Wall, S. (1978). *Patterns of attachment.* Hillsdale, NJ: Erlbaum.

Egeland, B., & Brunnquell, D. (1979). An at-risk approach to the study of child abuse: Some preliminary findings. *Journal of the American Academy of Child Psychiatry,* **18,** 219–225.

Elicker, J., Englund, M., & Sroufe, L. A. (1992). Predicting peer competence and peer relationships in childhood from early parent-child relationships. In R. Parke & G. Ladd (Eds.), *Family-peer relationships: Modes of linkage.* Hillsdale, NJ: Erlbaum.

Feldman, S., Rosenthal, D., Brown, N., & Canning, R. (in press). Predicting sexual experience in adolescent boys from peer rejection and acceptance during childhood. *Child Development.*

Gove, F. (1983). *Patterns and organizations of behavior and affective expression during the second year of life.* Unpublished doctoral dissertation, University of Minnesota.

Hartup, W. (in press). Peer relations in early and middle childhood. In V. VanHasselt & M. Hersen (Eds.), *Handbook of social development: A lifespan perspective.* New York: Plenum.

Kagan, J., & Moss, H. (1962). *Birth to maturity.* New York: Wiley.

Maccoby, E. (1990). Gender and relationships. *American Psychologist,* **45,** 513–520.

Maccoby, E., & Jacklin, C. (1987). Gender segregation in childhood. In H. W. Reese (Ed.), *Advances in child development and behavior* (Vol. **20,** pp. 239–288). New York: Academic Press.

Schofield, J. (1981). Complementary and conflicting identities: Images and interaction in an interracial school. In S. Asher & J. Gottman (Eds.), *The development of children's friendships* (pp. 53–90). Cambridge: Cambridge University Press.

Sroufe, L. A. (1990). An organizational perspective on the self. In D. Cicchetti & M. Beeghly (Eds.), *The self in transition: Infancy to childhood* (pp. 281–307). Chicago: University of Chicago Press.

Sroufe, L. A. (1991). Considering normal and abnormal together: The essence of developmental psychopathology. *Development and Psychopathology, 2,* 335–347.

Sroufe, L. A., Carlson, E., & Shulman, S. (in press). The development of individuals in relationships: From infancy through adolescence. In D. C. Funder, R. D. Parke, C. Tomlinson-Keasey, & K. Widaman (Eds.), *Studying lives through time: Approaches to personality and development.* Washington, DC: American Psychological Association.

Sroufe, L. A., & Fleeson, J. (1988). The coherence of family relationships. In R. A. Hinde & J. Stevenson-Hinde (Eds.), *Relationships within families: Mutual influences* (pp. 27–47). Oxford: Oxford University Press.

Sroufe, L. A., Jacobvitz, J., Mangelsdorf, S., DeAngelo, E., & Ward, M. J. (1985). Generational boundary dissolution between mothers and their preschool children: A relationships systems approach. *Child Development, 56,* 317–325.

Sroufe, L. A., & Ward, M. J. (1980). Seductive behavior of mothers of toddlers: Occurrence, correlates, and family origins. *Child Development, 51,* 1222–1229.

Sullivan, H. S. (1953). *The interpersonal theory of psychiatry.* New York: Norton.

Thorne, B. (1986), Girls and boys together . . . but mostly apart: Gender arrangements in elementary schools. In W. Hartup & Z. Rubin (Eds.), *Relationships and development* (pp. 167–184). Hillsdale, NJ: Erlbaum.

Thorne, B., & Luria, Z. (1986). Sexuality and gender in children's daily worlds. *Social Problems, 33,* 176–190.

Waters, E., & Sroufe, L. A. (1983). Social competence as a developmental construct. *Developmental Review, 3,* 79–97.

Whiting, B. B., & Edwards, C. P. (1988). *Children of different worlds.* Cambridge, MA: Harvard University Press.

7

The Prevalence of Gender-Atypical Behavior in Elementary School Children

David E. Sandberg
Children's Hospital of Buffalo, New York
State University of New York at Buffalo

Heino F. L. Meyer-Bahlburg,
Anke A. Ehrhardt, and Thomas J. Yager
College of Physicians and Surgeons of
Columbia University, New York City

Objective: *To supplement the few small-scale studies on convenience samples of boys with an epidemiological study on the prevalence of gender-atypical behaviors (GABs) in boys and girls and to assess the influence of variation of age, ethnicity, and socioeconomic status.* **Method:** *The present study, a postal questionnaire survey, used an existing pool of GAB items for boys, developed comparable GAB items for girls, and analyzed parent-reported frequencies of GABs in a demographically heterogeneous community sample of 687 boys and girls age 6 to 10 years.* **Results:** *The majority of GABs were quite rare, but there was considerable variability in their prevalence. Nevertheless, many children show multiple GABs although each individual GAB at low frequency; for instance, 10 or more different GABs were exhibited by 22.8% of boys and 38.6% of girls. Only few GABs*

Reprinted with permission from the *Journal of the American Academy of Child and Adolescent Psychiatry,* 1993, Vol. 32(2), 306–314. Copyright © 1993 by the American Academy of Child and Adolescent Psychiatry.

We thank the children and parents who participated in the study. This research was conducted while David Sandberg was a postdoctoral fellow of the National Institute of Child Health and Human Development (National Research Service Award HD06726). In addition, this work was supported in part by grants to Drs. Ehrhardt and Meyer-Bahlburg from the Spencer Foundation, the William T. Grant Foundation, and the Ford Foundation, National Institute of Mental Health Clinical Research Center Grant MH-30906, and National Institute of Mental Health Research Grant MH-34635.

varied significantly with age, ethnicity, or socioeconomic status.
Conclusions: *These data are of relevance to clinicians counseling parents who are worried about the occurrence of GABs in their children.*

The sex typing of behavior begins at birth and, from preschool age on, children have well-formed notions of what constitutes "typical" behavior for each gender, as do adults (Huston, 1983). When discordance between the gender stereotype and a child's actual behavior is observed, it can elicit negative appraisals by both peers and adults (Zucker, 1985) and may lead to referral for clinical evaluation. In this context, "gender-atypical behavior" (GAB) denotes a behavior that is thought to be relatively uncommon in one gender but very common in (or "typical of") the other gender. In some cases, developmental concerns are elicited by a single, isolated, GAB (e.g., doll playing in a boy). This is likely because our society sets narrow limits of tolerance for GABs, in particular for boys; many parents show a high sensitivity to any indication of deviations from stereotypical gender-role behavior in their children.

Implicit in parents' concerns about the presence of even a single GAB is the suspicion that the presence of one GAB implies the presence of additional ones (for example, in addition to doll playing in boys, playing dress-up or house). In addition, there is the widespread belief that GABs in childhood foreshadow the development of homosexuality in adolescence and adulthood. Although there exists reasonably compelling data indicating, at least for boys, that a history of gender identity disorder of childhood (American Psychiatric Association, 1987) which implies the pervasive and persistent expression of multiple GABs is strongly predictive of a homosexual or bisexual orientation in late adolescence or young adulthood (Green, 1987; Zucker, 1985), little is known about the predictive significance of lesser forms of cross-gender behavior.

How common are GABs in childhood? A crude estimate can be obtained from the proportion of parents responding positively to two items on the Child Behavior Checklist (CBCL) (Achenbach, 1991) that tap cross-gender identification. The CBCL recently has been restandardized using a nonclinical sample chosen to be representative of the 48 contiguous states with respect to socioeconomic status, ethnicity, region, and urban-suburban-rural residence. Between the ages of 4 to 11 years, 4% of boys and 10% of girls are reported to "behave like opposite sex," and 1% of both boys and girls "wishes to be of opposite sex" (Achenbach, 1991, Appendix D, pp. 260–284). Because the CBCL was designed as a screening checklist for a wide range of child and adolescent behavioral and emotional problems, details regarding the specific manifestations of cross-gender behavior or identification are necessarily lacking.

Three surveys provide much greater detail concerning GABs, but this has been accomplished by using relatively small, demographically limited, and possibly highly self-selected samples of boys only. Zuger and Taylor (1969) interviewed the mothers of 95 second-grade school boys regarding the presence of six GABs (feminine dressing, wearing lipstick or other makeup, preference for girl playmates, desire to be female, doll playing, and aversion to boys' games). These items were chosen on the basis of their frequent presence in boys with gender identity disturbance. Any behavior falling into these categories that was currently being exhibited, regardless of its frequency or duration, was rated as positive. Of the 95 boys, 69 (73%) were reported by their mothers to have never engaged in these behaviors. Positive occurrences of currently exhibited GABs ranged from 2% (preference for girl playmates) to 15% (doll playing). In addition to the fact that GABs were generally uncommon in these psychiatric-nonreferred middle-childhood boys, the number of different GABs shown by an individual child was small; of 26 boys currently showing any one GAB, 20 (77%) were positive on no more than two of the behaviors. In marked contrast, 25 of 26 (96%) boys in the gender-disturbed sample in this study were positive on four or more items.

Bates, et al. (1973) reported on the development of their parent-report-based Child Behavior and Attitude Questionnaire (CBAQ) for the purpose of screening for gender-disturbed boys of middle childhood age. (The CBAQ is the name used on the questionnaire form we received from the authors, whereas the name used in the corresponding publication is the Gender Behavior Inventory for Boys.) Questionnaires were distributed to mothers of 5- to 10-year-old boys attending Parent Teacher Association meetings. The representativeness of the sample was affected by a poor participation rate: completed questionnaires were obtained for only 175 of 485 distributed (36%). Although the Parent Teacher Associations were chosen to be representative of the full range of socioeconomic levels, the final sample was biased toward lower-middle- and upper-middle-class mothers. Within these limits to representativeness, the study essentially replicated the findings of Zuger and Taylor (1969); GABs occurred infrequently throughout middle childhood, even among children as young as age 5 years. There was an indication of a decline of feminine behaviors with age.

Assessing the question of the prevalence of GABs in early childhood, Zucker et al. (1980) administered a questionnaire to the parents of 162 boys between 20 months and 5 years of age. The majority of the parents (90%) were apparently recruited based on previous participation in research studies at a local university. The return rate of completed questionnaires was 73% for this subsample. The questionnaire contained many of the same GAB items included in the Bates et al. (1973) inventory with the addition of items pertaining to same-gender and cross-gender identity statements and fantasies. The findings indicated that GABs are uncommon throughout early childhood and that gender-typical behaviors steadily increase in frequency with age.

Inasmuch as gender-role behavior is thought to be strongly influenced by socialization factors (Huston, 1983), it would be useful to know to what extent GABs vary as a function of socioeconomic status and race or ethnicity. Significant subcultural differences in the prevalence of GABs obviously would influence the interpretations regarding their presence. To the best of our knowledge, this question has not been researched.

Even more significantly, studies of individual GABs in girls have not been conducted. Although studies have suggested that girls are afforded greater latitude in the expression of GABs (for review, see Zucker, 1985), no studies have looked specifically at the prevalence of GABs in girls and compared these rates with those observed in boys.

The purpose of the present study is to develop corresponding sets of GAB items for boys and girls and to answer the following questions using a demographically heterogeneous, community sample:

1. How common are individual GABs during middle childhood (ages 6 to 10 years) in either gender?

2. How common is it for boys and girls to engage in more than one GAB?

3. How much do GABs in boys and girls vary with subjects' age, race/ethnicity, and socioeconomic status?

METHOD

Subjects

All children ranging in age from 6 to 10 years at the time of the study and who attended any of the four elementary schools comprising a complete school district of a northern New Jersey city were eligible for inclusion in the study. The study was conducted over 2 academic years (1986 to 1988). School rosters were used to target eligible children, and their parents or guardians were asked to serve as informants. The only exclusion criterion was the absence of an English-speaking parent/guardian living in the home who would be able to complete the questionnaires.

There was a total of 927 children of the ages 6 to 10 years at the start of the survey whose families met the English-language criterion. The parents of 193 children (21%) refused to participate, and the parents of 46 (5%) either could not be contacted by repeated phone calls or home visits, or the child left the school district after the survey had begun but before the parent had an opportunity to participate, or the child's guardian had insufficient information on the child to participate in the survey. The parents of 688 children (74% of the eligible sample) agreed to participate. Completed questionnaires were obtained from the parents of 687 children (332 boys and 355 girls). The respective sample sizes at ages 6 to

10 years for boys were 59, 64, 85, 74, and 50, and the sample sizes for girls were 65, 74, 68, 75, and 73.

The mean ($\pm$ SD) grade placement in school was 2.2 ($\pm$ 1.5) and 2.4 ($\pm$ 1.6) for boys and girls, respectively, with a range from kindergarten to grade 5. The racial or ethnic background for the total sample was 41.3% white, 36.8% African-American, 13.8% Hispanic, and 8.1% Other (Asian, native American, or biracial). Educational attainment of the parents was used as an index of socioeconomic status and rated on a 7-point scale (Hollingshead, 1975). Where educational level was given for both parents, the higher level was used. The mean ($\pm$ SD) parental education for the total sample was 4.7 ($\pm$ 1.2), which falls at approximately the midpoint for the ratings of high school graduate (4) and partial college or specialized training (5). Of one or both of the parents 36.9% had completed high school, and 14.6% had completed a standard college or university degree.

Procedure

Details of the procedure have been previously described (Sandberg et al., 1991). Briefly, the survey was conducted in two stages: first, a cover letter from the school principal and a more detailed letter from the authors' research unit were sent together to the parents of all children fulfilling the age criterion. The letters explained the purpose of the study, namely, to obtain an overview of general behavioral development and problem behaviors among children with varied medical backgrounds. A brief answer sheet (with a stamped return envelope addressed to the school) was included in which the parents were asked about family characteristics including race or ethnic background, occupation and education of the parents, the language spoken at home, and whether or not they agreed to participate in the postal questionnaire survey. In the second stage, parents agreeing to participate in the survey were mailed the questionnaires (with a return envelope addressed to the investigators). They were ensured in a cover letter that survey information was confidential and would be made available to the schools only in the aggregate without personal identifying information. After the return of the questionnaires, missing items were completed and ambiguous responses were clarified by phone or home visit, if necessary. The findings presented here are part of a larger study focusing on the relation between gender-role behavior and psychosocial adjustment in children with various medical backgrounds. The survey included several questionnaires, all of which were parent or guardian completed. Only the data pertaining to one of the gender-behavior questionnaires, the male and female versions of the *Child Behavior and Attitude Questionnaire (CBAQ-M, CBAQ-F)*, are the focus of this paper.

Gender-role behavior. Gender-related items for boys were derived from three sources: (1) all items of the original CBAQ (Bates et al., 1973), including both boy-typical and boy-atypical items that discriminated between effeminate boys and controls and nongender items assessing positive social adjustment and behavior disturbance; (2) a review of the gender identity disorder literature, in particular the works of John Money, Richard Green, and Kenneth Zucker, and the authors' own clinical experience working with gender-disordered children and individuals born with anomalies of the sex organs in whom shifts in the typical pattern of gender-role behavior are occasionally observed; and, (3) items adapted from the *Gender Role Assessment Schedule* (Meyer-Bahlburg et al., 1984), a half-structured gender interview covering a variety of behaviors. As in the original CBAQ, GAB items were intermixed with gender-typical items and nongender items to reduce their salience. The parent rated the frequency of the occurrence of the specific behavior on verbally anchored five-point ("never" to "always") or eight-point ("once every 6 months or less" to "daily") response scales. The response scales were the same as those used for the original form of the CBAQ (Bates et al., 1973). This (modified) male version of the CBAQ (CBAQ-M) contained 71 items.

Gender-related items for girls were obtained in part through conversion of the boys' items (above). The development of a girls' questionnaire to parallel the one for boys turned out to be a more complex endeavor than first expected because simple pronoun changes (from "he did" to "she did"), sufficient for the gender conversion of items covering most types of behaviors, are suitable only for a subset of items covering gender-related behaviors. Another set of gender items requires changes of both the pronoun and a gendered object (e.g., from "he imitated a female" to "she imitated a male"). A third set includes gender items that require additional reformulations or do not have direct parallels in both genders. Examples are "He wears things like wigs, towels, and shirts on his head"; "he 'swishes' and swings his hips when he walks"; "she dislikes wearing attractive girls' clothes"; "she is called a 'tomboy' by other people." For the girls, such items were drafted as described for boys above. Nongender items in the male version of the questionnaire were converted for use in the female version by pronoun change only and were intermixed with the gender-related items. The response scales for the girls were the same as those used for the boys. The female version of the CBAQ (CBAQ-F) contained 68 items.

Classification of gender-behavior items. The gender-related items of the CBAQ-M and CBAQ-F were classified into three groups based on wording, specific content, and the inspection of item frequency distributions for this sample.

1. Opposite-gender object (OGO): this group included items in which the gender opposite to that of the study subject was specifically mentioned. An example of an item for boys in this category is "he is good at imitating females," and the parallel version for girls is "she is good at imitating males." Items indicative of cross-gender role-taking or identification also were included in the OGO category although the opposite gender was not specifically mentioned. An example of this

subtype of item for boys is "he wears things like wigs, towels, and shirts on his head."

2. Boy-typical (B > G): this group included items other than OGO in which the behavior described is performed more frequently by boys than by girls, e.g., "he plays with boy-type dolls such as 'G.I. Joe' or 'He-Man.'"

3. Girl-typical (G > B): items other than OGO that are performed more frequently by girls than by boys, e.g., "she plays with girl-type dolls such as baby or 'Barbie' dolls." A listing of all of the gender-behavior items according to this classification scheme is provided in Table 1. Within each class there were two subcategories of items: (1) items for which parallel versions existed for both genders (shared), and (2) items that were specific to one gender (specific). In three cases, the parallel female and male versions of the same item were categorized as gender-specific because they fell into different classes according to the classification scheme above: "He plays sports with boys" (B > G) versus "She plays sports with boys" (OGO); "He imitates male characters seen on T.V. or in the movies" (B > G) versus "She imitates female characters seen on T.V. or in the movies" (G > B); and "He plays with boy-type dolls such as 'G.I. Joe' or 'He-Man'" (B > G) versus "She plays with girl-type dolls such as baby or 'Barbie' dolls" (G > B).

Data analysis. The frequency distributions for each item by gender (either overall or further broken down by demographic variables) provided the prevalence data. The analysis of co-occurrence of items for each child also was done descriptively. Developmental trends in the expression of individual gender behaviors were assessed within each gender by one-way analyses of variance with age as the independent factor. The nonoverlapping and combined contributions of several demographic variables to variability in the expression of gender-role behavior was assessed by three parallel, multiple regressions conducted on each item separately. In the first model, designed to assess the unique contribution of subject's age, the variables of parents' education and race/ethnicity were entered into the model at the first step. A set of dummy variables (white, black, and Hispanic) were created to characterize the four levels of race or ethnicity in the sample; the fourth racial or ethnic group, "other," which was the "constant" in the model, included Asian, native American, and biracial subjects). Subject's age was then entered into the model at the second step. In the second model (race/ethnicity), subject's age and parents' education were entered first and race or ethnicity last. Finally, in the third model (parents' education), subject's age and race or ethnicity were entered first and parents' education last.

TABLE 1

Child Behavior and Attitude Questionnaire—Male/Female (CBAQ-M, CBAQ-F) Gender Behavior Items

Response Scale	Boys (B)	Girls (G)
	Opposite-Gender Items Shared	
5	He is good at imitating females.	She is good at imitating males.
5	In dress-up games he likes to dress-up in women's clothing.	In dress-up games she likes to dress-up in men's clothing.
5	He has stated the wish to be a girl or a woman.	She has stated the wish to be a boy or a man.
5	He does things with female relatives.	She does things with male relatives.
5	He is called a "sissy" or similar names by other people.	She is called a "tomboy" or similar names by other people.
5	In playing "mother/father," "house," or "school" games he takes the role of a girl or woman.	In playing "mother/father," "house," or "school" games she takes the role of a boy or man.
8	He imitates females.	She imitates males.
8	He dresses in female clothing.	She dresses in male clothing.
8	He imitates *female* characters seen on T.V. or in the movies.	She imitates *male* characters seen on T.V. or in the movies.
8	At school he plays with girls.	At school she plays with boys.
8	At home he plays with girls.	At home she plays with boys.
8	He plays with girl-type dolls, such as baby or "Barbie" dolls.	She plays with boy-type dolls such as "G.I. Joe" or "He-man."
	Opposite-Gender Items Specific	
5	He uses feminine gestures with his hands when talking.	She plays sports with boys.
5	He prefers the company of adult women.	She prefers the company of boys.
5	He "swishes" and swings his hips when he walks.	She dislikes wearing attractive girls clothes.
8	He wears a shirt or towel around his waist as a skirt.	
8	He wears things like wigs, towels, and shirts on his head.	
	B > G Items Shared	
5	He is interested in real automobiles.	She is interested in real automobiles.
8	He dresses sloppily.	She dresses sloppily.
8	He likes to rough-house (play-wrestle, play-fight) with other children.	She likes to rough-house (play-wrestle, play-fight) with other children.
8	He plays games such as baseball, football, soccer or hockey.	She plays games such as baseball, football, soccer or hockey.
8	He reads books about dinosaurs and space.	She reads books about dinosaurs and space.

Continued

TABLE 1 (*cont.*)

Child Behavior and Attitude Questionnaire—Male/Female (CBAQ-M, CBAQ-F) Gender Behavior Items

Response Scale	Boys (B)	Girls (G)
	B > G Items Specific	
5	He plays sports with boys.	
8	He imitates *male* characters seen in the movies.	
8	He plays with boy-type dolls such as "G.I. Joe" or "He-Man."	
	G > B Items Shared	
5	He likes to dance.	She likes to dance.
5	He likes fairy tales like Snow White.	She likes fairy tales like Snow White.
8	He plays house.	She plays house.
8	He plays games such as jacks and jump-rope.	She plays games such as jacks and jump-rope.
8	He play-acts, puts on little dramas.	She play-acts, puts on little dramas.
8	He plays with dolls.	She plays with dolls.
8	He experiments with cosmetics.	She experiments with cosmetics.
	G > B Items Specific	
8		She imitates *female* characters seen on T.V. or in the movies.
8		She plays with girl-type dolls such as baby or "Barbie" dolls.

RESULTS

Prevalence of GABs and Gender-typical Behaviors

Table 2 provides the frequency distributions (reported in percentage of the male/female subsample) for all gender-related items of the CBAQ-M and CBAQ-F. The items are categorized according to the classification scheme in Table 1. The majority of OGO behaviors were exhibited at very low rates. Notable exceptions for both sexes included items concerning affiliation with the opposite sex: "He/She does things with female/male relatives," "At school he/she plays with girls/boys," "At home he/she plays with girls/boys," "He prefers the company of adult women," "She plays sports with boys," and, "She prefers the company of boys." In contrast to the majority of OGO items, greater variability in frequency ratings was observed for both genders in the expression of most behaviors classified as either B > G or G > B (Table 2). There were three G > B behaviors, however, that boys only very rarely exhibited: "He plays house," "He plays with dolls," and, "He experiments with cosmetics." In the case of both B > G and G > B items, the expected gender differences in the frequency ratings for these items were observed. With respect to gender differences in the expression of GABs, an inspection of the frequency distributions reveals that girls generally show slightly higher rates of GABs than do boys.

Coexistence of Multiple GABs

Although an inspection of the frequency distributions for individual GAB items (Table 2) indicates that these behaviors occur only rarely in middle childhood boys and girls, it is of interest to know how common it is for children to concurrently exhibit multiple types of GAB. The frequency distributions for boy and girl subjects who scored positive to any degree (i.e., scored "2" or higher; "2" denotes "seldom" or "once every 3 months" on the 5- and 8-point response scales, respectively) on the GAB items (OGO or G > B / B > G) are summarized in Table 3. Differences between boys and girls are readily discernible. The frequency distribution for GABs was more positively skewed for boys (skewness = 0.752), i.e., asymmetric with a larger tail to the right, than the parallel distribution for girls (skewness = 0.174). For boys, the median number of GABs reported was seven (or 29.2% of a total of 24 GAB items defined for boys). Of the boys, 22.8% showed 10 or more different GABs, at least at low frequencies ("seldom" or "once every 3 months"). For girls, the median number of GABs reported was eight (or 40.0% of a total of 20 GAB items defined for girls). Of the girls, 38.6% scored positive on 10 or more items.

Because of the relatively high rate of positive responses of both boys and girls

TABLE 2
Frequency of CBAQ-M/F Behaviors

CBAQ-M/F Item	Response Scale[b]		1	2	3	4	5	6	7	8
OGO (Shared)										
He/She is good at imitating females/males.	5	Boys	58.7	31.3	5.7	3.0	1.2			
		Girls	51.8	32.7	8.2	4.5	2.8			
In dress-up games he/she likes to dress-up in women's/men's clothing.	5	Boys	90.1	8.1	1.2	0.3	0.3			
		Girls	96.5	12.1	0.6	0	0.8			
He/She has stated the wish to be a girl/boy or a woman/man.	5	Boys	94.9	4.5	0.6	0	0			
		Girls	92.7	6.2	0	0.6	0.6			
He/She does things with female/male relatives.	5	Boys	22.6	36.7	28.3	10.8	1.5			
		Girls	28.8	40.7	21.8	7.3	1.4			
He/She is called a "sissy/tomboy" or similar names by other people.	5	Boys	78.3	17.8	3.6	0	0.3			
		Girls	74.9	15.5	4.5	3.1	2.0			
In playing "mother/father," "house," or "school" games he/she takes the role of a girl/boy or woman/man.	5	Boys	92.8	6.9	0	0	0.3			
		Girls	78.3	19.2	0.8	1.4	0.3			
He/She imitates females/males.	8	Boys	94.6	1.8	1.5	0.9	0.6	0.6	0	0
		Girls	87.9	4.5	4.5	1.1	1.4	0	0.3	0.3
He/She dresses in female/male clothing.	8	Boys	99.1	0.3	0.3	0.3	0	0	0.6	0
		Girls	95.8	0.8	2.3	0.3	1.2	0.3	0	0
He/She imitates *female/male* characters seen on TV or in the movies.	8	Boys	84.2	3.4	4.8	2.0	3.1	1.1	0.8	0.6
At school he/she plays with girls/boys.	8	Boys	30.1	6.0	7.5	5.1	13.0	12.0	10.2	16.0
		Girls	16.4	5.4	4.8	3.1	16.7	18.6	14.1	20.9
At home he/she plays with girls/boys.	8	Boys	33.4	5.7	6.0	7.5	13.6	7.8	9.9	16.0
		Girls	26.8	6.5	6.5	3.4	17.2	12.4	9.3	18.0
He/She plays with girl/boy type dolls.	8	Boys	89.8	3.0	3.9	0.6	1.8	0.6	0.3	0
		Girls	78.2	4.5	4.5	3.1	5.1	2.0	2.0	0.6
OGO (Specific; Boys)										
He uses feminine gestures with his hands while talking.	5	Boys	92.2	6.3	0.9	0.6	0			
He prefers the company of adult women.	5	Boys	38.1	45.6	10.9	3.3	2.1			
He "swishes" and swings his hips when he walks.	5	Boys	87.0	9.9	1.8	0.9	0.3			
He wears a shirt or towel around his waist as a skirt.	8	Boys	92.5	0.9	1.2	0	1.5	0	1.2	2.7
He wears things like wigs, towels, and shirts on his head.	8	Boys	96.1	1.5	1.8	0	0.3	0	0	0.3
OGO (Specific; Girls)										
She plays sports with boys.	5	Girls	16.1	38.9	25.4	13.0	6.8			
She prefers the company of boys.	5	Girls	27.6	52.4	17.2	2.0	0.8			
She dislikes wearing attractive girl's clothing.	5	Girls	74.1	15.2	3.1	2.8	4.8			

TABLE 2 (*cont.*)

Frequency of CBAQ-M/F Behaviors

Item	Scale	Sex	1	2	3	4	5	6	7	8
B > G (Shared)										
He/She is interested in real automobiles.	5	Boys	8.1	16.9	20.5	23.5	31.0			
		Girls	34.2	36.4	15.0	6.8	7.6			
He/She dresses sloppily.	8	Boys	5.1	8.4	8.7	15.7	4.8	6.0	7.5	43.7
		Girls	59.4	7.0	8.2	7.0	7.3	6.5	3.1	1.4
He/She likes to rough-house (play-wrestle, play-fight) with other children.	8	Boys	9.9	2.7	5.1	6.3	11.7	13.6	18.4	32.2
		Girls	49.2	7.9	7.3	9.0	6.2	5.6	7.3	7.3
He/She plays games such as baseball, football, soccer or hockey.	8	Boys	3.9	1.5	3.0	5.1	12.7	11.7	25.6	36.4
		Girls	54.9	7.9	8.7	4.8	10.4	5.1	5.6	2.5
He/She reads books about dinosaurs and space.	8	Boys	4.8	3.9	12.0	15.4	15.4	11.4	19.3	17.8
		Girls	49.9	14.1	10.1	7.3	5.4	5.4	3.1	4.8
B > G (Specific; Boys)										
He plays sports with boys.	5	Boys	1.2	3.3	12.7	31.6	51.2			
He imitates *male* characters seen in the movies.	8	Boys	19.3	6.3	6.6	10.8	16.0	11.7	16.6	12.7
He plays with boy-type dolls such as "G.I. Joe" or "He-Man."	8	Boys	9.3	3.9	3.0	6.9	8.7	13.6	16.9	37.7
G > B (Shared)										
He/She likes to dance.	5	Boys	14.5	33.4	23.5	14.8	13.9			
		Girls	0	7.9	13.0	22.5	56.6			
He/She likes fairy tales like "Snow White."	5	Boys	16.3	33.7	24.7	13.3	12.0			
		Girls	1.4	15.2	20.6	24.8	38.0			
He/She plays house.	8	Boys	72.9	9.0	10.2	2.1	3.9	1.2	0.3	0.3
		Girls	8.2	7.3	7.0	6.8	18.9	14.6	24.2	13.0
OGO (Shared)										
He/She plays games such as jacks and jump-rope.	8	Boys	63.6	14.5	7.2	4.2	4.8	3.0	2.4	0.3
		Girls	6.5	3.7	6.2	6.8	14.1	18.3	22.3	22.3
He/She play-acts, puts on little dramas.	8	Boys	51.7	18.4	9.7	7.3	5.1	1.8	3.6	2.4
		Girls	14.9	11.3	10.1	9.3	15.2	12.4	14.6	12.1
He/She plays with dolls.	8	Boys	82.5	4.8	2.7	1.5	2.7	1.5	3.0	1.2
		Girls	3.4	1.7	3.4	3.7	9.3	9.9	24.6	44.1
He/She experiments with cosmetics.	8	Boys	97.3	1.5	0.9	0.3	0	0	0	0
		Girls	16.1	9.3	14.6	11.8	16.1	10.4	13.0	8.7
G > B (Specific; Girls)										
She imitates *female* characters seen on TV or in the movies.	8	Girls	23.4	8.5	9.3	11.6	15.8	10.5	11.3	9.6
She plays with girl-type dolls such as baby or "Barbie" dolls.	8	Girls	2.5	2.0	2.3	5.4	11.0	9.3	23.2	44.4

Note: CBAQ = Child Behavior and Attitude Questionnaire, OGO = opposite-gender object.

[a] Percentage of male/female subsample showing behavior at specified frequency.[b]

[b] 5-point response scale: 1 = never, 2 = seldom, 3 = frequently, 4 = very often, 5 = always. 8-point response scale: 1 = once every 6 months or less, 2 = once every 3 months, 3 = once a month, 4 = twice a month, 5 = once a week, 6 = twice a week, 7 = 3 or 4 times a week, 8 = daily.

TABLE 3
Frequency of Positive Rating for All GAB (OGO and G › B/B › G) Items in Boys and Girls

	Boys (N = 333)				Girls (N = 355)		
Number of Items Scored Positive[a]	Frequency	%	Cumulative %	Number of Items Scored Positive[a]	Frequency	%	Cumulative %
0	1	0.3	0.3	0	1	0.3	0.3
1	2	0.6	0.9	1	8	2.3	2.5
2	11	3.3	4.2	2	6	1.7	4.2
3	22	6.6	10.8	3	12	3.4	7.6
4	38	11.4	22.2	4	25	7.0	14.6
5	35	10.5	32.7	5	37	10.4	25.1
6	46	13.8	46.5	6	28	7.9	33.0
7	51	15.3	61.9	7	31	8.7	41.7
8	27	8.1	70.0	8	37	10.4	52.1
9	24	7.2	77.2	9	33	9.3	61.4
10	27	8.1	85.3	10	46	13.0	74.4
11	18	5.4	90.7	11	25	7.0	81.4
12	12	3.6	94.3	12	20	5.6	87.0
13	8	2.4	96.7	13	20	5.6	92.7
14	3	0.9	97.6	14	7	2.0	94.6
15	3	0.9	98.5	15	8	2.3	96.9
16	1	0.3	98.8	16	10	2.8	99.7
17	2	0.6	99.4	17	0	0	99.7
18	0	0	99.4	18	0	0	99.7
19	1	0.3	99.7	19	0	0	99.7
20	1	0.3	100.0	20	1	0.3	100.0
21	0	0	—	Skewness = 0.174			
22	0	0	—				
23	0	0	—				
24	0	0	—				

Skewness = 0.752

Note: GAB = gender-atypical behaviors, OGO = opposite-gender object.
[a] Item counted as positive when rating was scored "2" or higher, meaning "Seldom" or "Once every 3 months" on the 5- and 8-point scales respectively.

to those GAB items that refer to affiliation with the other gender (Table 2), a second frequency distribution for GABs that excluded these items ("He/She does things with female/male relatives," "At school he/she plays with girls/boys," "At home he/she plays with girls/boys," "He prefers the company of adult women," "She plays sports with boys," and, "She prefers the company of boys") was constructed. The result for both genders was to make the distributions substantially more positively skewed than when these items remained in the list, while preserving the gender difference in skewness.

Developmental Trends in GABs

To assess the presence of age trends for individual GAB items, simple one-way analyses of variance were performed on OGO, G > B (in the case of boys), and B > G items (in the case of girls). A statistically significant ($p < 0.05$) decline with increasing age was shown by only three behaviors for boys ("At school he plays with girls," "He likes fairy tales like Snow White," and "He plays house") and one for girls ("She plays with boy-type dolls such as 'G.I. Joe' or 'He-Man'"). (A complete set of tables showing the mean [± SD] frequency of GABs by subject's sex and age is available from the corresponding author.)

Variation of GABs with Demographic Characteristics

Multiple regression analyses were used to determine the unique contributions of several demographic factors to variability in the expression of GABs (see Data Analysis for details of regression model building). Relatively few items were significantly related to the combined influences of subject's age, race/ethnicity, and parents' educational level. Table 4 summarizes the findings for those regression models for which the percent of variance accounted for by the complete model was statistically significant ($p < 0.05$).

For boys, there were only four items (one OGO item, three G > B items) that showed variability with the various demographic variables. The complete regression model including all demographic variables accounted for between 4.3% and 11.4% (R^2) of the variance in these four GABs. The largest share of variance was accounted for by age for two items, by socioeconomic status for one item, and by ethnicity for one item. For girls, there were seven items for which the complete model was statistically significant (five OGO and two B > G items). In the case of all seven items, the variable race or ethnicity accounted for the largest share of variability in the GABs (between 2.4% and 8.4%) after controlling for the influences of subject's age and parents' educational level. The complete regression model including all demographic variables for girls accounted for between 3.3% and 10.5% (R^2) of the variance in GAB scores.

TABLE 4
The Influence of Demographic Variables on the Expression of GABs in Boys and Girls

| | Unique Percentage Variance Accounted for by Subject's ... | | | | | | | | | | |
| | ... Age [a] | | | ... Parents' Education [d] | | | ... Race or Ethnicity [e] | | Complete Model [f] | |
	β [b]	% [c]	p	β	%	p	%	p	%	p
Boys											
OGO Items											
He plays with girl-type dolls such as baby or "Barbie" dolls.	−0.097	0.9	0.077	0.178	2.7	0.003	0.9	0.392	4.3	0.0143
G > B Items											
He likes to dance.	−0.141	2.0	0.008	−0.047	0.2	0.408	8.2	0.000	11.4	0.0000
He likes fairy tales like Snow White.	−0.229	5.2	0.000	−0.101	0.9	0.086	0.1	0.949	6.5	0.0006
He plays house.	−0.243	5.9	0.000	0.027	0.1	0.646	0.6	0.561	6.4	0.0006
Girls											
OGO Items											
She does things with male relatives.	−0.055	0.3	0.281	0.047	0.2	0.401	8.4	0.000	10.5	0.0000
At school she plays with boys.	−0.111	1.2	0.037	−0.063	0.3	0.275	3.8	0.004	5.4	0.0018
At home she plays with boys.	−0.095	0.9	0.074	0.018	0.0	0.750	3.4	0.007	4.8	0.0051
She plays with boy-type dolls such as "G.I. Joe" or "He-Man."	−0.163	2.6	0.002	−0.132	1.5	0.021	3.1	0.010	6.5	0.0003

She plays sports with boys.	−0.027	0.1	0.614	−0.066	0.4	0.257	3.8	0.004	3.9	0.0189
B > G Items									
She dresses sloppily.	0.090	0.8	0.088	0.108	1.0	0.060	2.6	0.027	6.2	0.0005
She likes to rough-house (play-wrestle, play-fight) with other children.	−0.088	0.8	0.101	−0.052	0.2	0.368	2.4	0.040	3.3	0.0442

Note: GAB = gender-atypical behaviors, OGO = opposite-gender object.

[a] Results from second step of stepwise multiple regression in which the variables of race/ethnicity and parents' education were entered first and subject's age last.

[b] β = standardized regression coefficient.

[c] % = change in R^2 associated with variable (entered at last step) after controlling for the other two variables (entered at first step).

[d] Stepwise multiple regression: parents' education entered after other two demographic variables.

[e] Stepwise multiple regression: race or ethnicity entered after other two demographic variables.

[f] Percent of variance and probability associated with complete multiple regression model.

DISCUSSION

Item validation was not the focus of the current project. However, the items investigated here derive content validity from the fact that they have been selected from item pools reflecting differences either between the genders or between gender-atypical and gender-typical children. The sex differences contained in Table 2 attest to the discriminant validity of the items. Finally, there is ample evidence that interview or questionnaire-based reports on observable gender-related behaviors such as the ones covered by our items correspond well to the findings of behavior observations (e.g., Huston, 1983). Thus, we can be confident that our findings do not just reflect parental gender stereotypes.

The present study shows that not only boys but also girls exhibit GABs at low rates during middle childhood. For boys, this finding replicates the observations of both Zuger and Taylor (1969) and of Bates et al. (1973) and extends them by demonstrating this phenomenon with a more diverse pool of GAB items and in a large and demographically heterogeneous community sample.

Although GABs, in particular OGO-type items, are typically rarely observed, both this study and that of Bates et al. (1973) indicate that, for boys, play with girls (i.e., "At school he plays with girls," "At home he plays with girls," and "He does things with female relatives") is not that uncommon. Similarly common in girls were the parallel OGO items concerning affiliation with boys. In contrast, Zuger and Taylor's (1969) study of second-grade boys suggests very low rates of affiliation of boys with girls. This apparent discrepancy is most likely accounted for by differences in the precise wording of items. Whereas the relevant items used in the present study, which were adopted without modification from the original Bates et al. (1973) inventory, assess actual affiliation with the opposite gender and do not imply a "preference" for opposite gender over same gender, the item from the Zuger and Taylor (1969) interview concerning gender of playmates specifically refers to a "preference for girl playmates."

The observation that subject's age in the middle childhood age range (6 to 10 years) is only rarely related to the expression of GABs is consistent with the findings of Bates et al. (1973). These data in conjunction with that of Zucker et al. (1980) suggest that GABs are rare at any point during childhood, including early childhood, even though there are some GABs that decline even further in frequency with age.

Girls, almost without exception, showed more types of GABs and exhibited these more frequently than did boys. This observation supports the consensus view that our society is more tolerant of the expression of GABs in girls than it is in boys thus allowing for greater variability in its expression in girls.

Finally, demographic variables such as race or ethnicity and parents' educational background accounted for a statistically significant proportion of the variance in only a small number of GAB items. With the Bonferroni correction for the number of statistical analyses performed, the number would be even smaller. Although cultural factors are thought to be important in the conditioning of gender-role behavior, the particular family background factors investigated here do not appear to have a marked influence on the expression of GABs. Thus, the clinician does not have to be overly concerned about identifying differences in gender-atypical behaviors that are specific for white, African-American, or Hispanic subcultures, or for different levels of socioeconomic status.

It is remarkable that despite the low prevalence of individual GABs, most children express more than one. A review of Table 3 shows that only 0.3% of boys and 0.3% of girls are reported to show practically no GABs (including the cross-gender affiliation items). That 22.8% of boys and 38.6% of girls show 10 or more different GABs ("seldom" or "once every 3 months") is important to keep in mind when counseling parents who are worried about the occurrence of GABs in their children. In our experience, it is helpful to many parents if one quotes such figures. Only the child who frequently and persistently expresses many such GABs relative to little gender-typical behavior needs to be evaluated for a gender identity disorder.

REFERENCES

Achenbach, T. M. (1991), *Manual for the Child Behavior Checklist/4–18 and 1991 Profile.* Burlington, VT: University of Vermont Department of Psychiatry.

American Psychiatric Association (1987), *Diagnostic and Statistical Manual of Mental Disorders, 3rd edition–revised (DSM-III-R).* Washington, DC: American Psychiatric Association.

Bates, J. E., Bentler, P. M. & Thompson, S. K. (1973). Measurement of deviant gender development. *Child Dev.,* 44:591–598.

Green, R. (1987), *The "Sissy Boy Syndrome" and the Development of Homosexuality.* New Haven, CT: Yale University Press.

Hollingshead, A. B. (1975), *Four Factor Index of Social Status.* New Haven, CT: Yale University Sociology Department.

Huston, A. C. (1983), Sex-typing. In: *Handbook of Child Psychology,* ed: P. H. Mussen. New York: John Wiley & Sons, pp. 387–467.

Meyer-Bahlburg, H. F. L., Feldman, J. F, Ehrhardt, A. A. & Cohen, P. (1984), Effects of prenatal hormone exposure versus pregnancy complications on sex-dimorphic behavior. *Arch. of Sex. Behav.,* 13:479–495.

Sandberg, D. E., Meyer-Bahlburg, H. F. L. & Yager, T. J. (1991), The child behavior checklist nonclinical standardization samples: should they be utilized as norms? *J. Am. Acad. Child Adolesc. Psychiatry,* 30:124–134.

Zucker, K. J. (1985), Cross-gender-identified children. In *Gender Dysphoria:*

Development, Research, Management, ed: B. W. Steiner. New York: Plenum Press, pp. 75–174.

Zucker, K. J., Bradley. S. J., Corter, C. M., Doering, R. W. & Finegan, J-A. K. (1980), Cross-gender behavior in very young boys: a normative study. In *Childhood and Sexuality,* ed: J. Samson. Montreal: Editions Etudes Vivantes, pp. 599–622.

Zuger, B. & Taylor, P. (1969), Effeminate behavior present in boys from early childhood. II. Comparison with similar symptoms in non-effeminate boys. *Pediatrics,* 44:375–380.

Part III

CHILD SEXUAL ABUSE: PSYCHOLOGICAL AND LEGAL ISSUES

The articles in this section revolve around the common theme of childhood trauma, specifically sexual abuse. In the last decade, estimates of the frequency of childhood sexual abuse have increased dramatically. The rise is in part due to several highly publicized cases of alleged abuse in day care centers and of repressed memories of abuse returning in adulthood. Reports of these incidents have led people to suspect that childhood sexual abuse is more widespread than previously suspected and have led many adults to claim histories of abuse. This has also led to an increase in research on the effects of abuse and on the capacity of children to testify. The first article focuses on children's capacities to serve as legal witnesses to traumatic events, particularly sexual abuse. The second article deals with the concept of repression for childhood memories of abuse. The third article reviews the impact of sexual abuse on children.

In the first paper in this section, Ceci and Bruck present a thorough review of the literature on suggestibility as it relates to children's capacity to serve as witnesses. They integrate a significant body of research, most of which has been conducted in the last decade. In an effort to reconcile the contradictory findings on children's suggestibility, they repose the questions. For example, "Are children suggestible?" is redefined as, "Under what conditions are children more suggestible than adults?" The early studies of children's suggestibility are reviewed. Then, various social and cognitive factors that could influence suggestibility are described. Cognitive factors include language ability, attainments in memory such as encoding and retrieval, and the capacity to distinguish reality from fantasy. Social factors such as the desire to be cooperative and to comply with authority figures are described. Normative and clinical studies of the use of anatomical dolls are also summarized. The authors conclude that even very young children are capable of serving as witnesses, although there are obviously developmental trends in suggestibility. Children are especially capable of providing reliable testimony when an event is of personal significance. They also note that there are situations under which children, as well as adults, can be suggestible and that the interview techniques

191

allowed in many legal cases lead to inaccurate testimony. This is an important paper for legal and mental health professionals.

In the second paper in this section, Loftus discusses the notion of repression and the likelihood that many adults have repressed memories of abuse. She begins by describing a highly publicized case of repressed memory that led to a murder conviction. She then presents evidence to indicate that some instances of repressed memories may be accurate but that repressed memories can be the result of suggestion. She notes the difficulties inherent in studying repressed memories. Studies indicate that many people fail to remember significant life events as recent as one year after they have occurred. Furthermore, forgetting is not always thought to involve repression. There are numerous reasons to doubt claims of repressed memories. For example, claims of memories from infancy are unlikely since few people have recollections before the age of three or four. Construction of false memories could be due to popular literature and therapist suggestion. Loftus also describes studies that indicate that memories of genuinely experienced traumatic events become altered with time and that memories of an event that never happened can be "injected." Thus, we do not know how to distinguish real memories of abuse from false memories. Nonetheless, results of simulated juror reaction studies indicate that people believe claims of repressed memory. The literature reviewed leads to several conclusions. There is a need to reexamine the notion that people with severe mental illness necessarily have experienced early childhood trauma. Researchers need to challenge the reality of memories of abuse. Finally, Loftus suggests that therapists and law enforcement personnel should be careful in how they probe for traumatic event memories.

In the third paper in this section, Kendall-Tackett, Williams, and Finkelhor review the recent literature on the psychological effects of sexual abuse. Studies of child victims of sexual abuse primarily use comparison groups of either nonabused clinical or nonclinical children. Results indicate that sexually abused children were more symptomatic on a variety of measures than nonclinical children. Symptoms included sexualized behavior as well as a range of global symptoms such as depression, aggression, and withdrawal. However, compared to clinical nonabused children, sexually abused children were less symptomatic, except for sexualized behavior and post traumatic stress disorder. Sexualized behaviors were most prominent for preschool-age children.

The authors highlight the fact that 20 to 50 percent of children studied were asymptomatic or within the normal range on the measures studied. To determine why effects of abuse vary, models and intervening variables including child's age at the time of assessment, age of onset of abuse, gender, penetration, identity of the perpetrator, and time elapsed since the abuse are considered. Longitudinal studies indicate improvement in many children over time. Internalizing symptoms tend to lessen while externalizing symptoms tend to increase. Instrumental in recovery was family support, though court case involvement yielded mixed results. Kendall-Tackett et al. conclude that no specific pattern of symptoms is associated with childhood abuse. Therefore, symptoms alone cannot be used to confirm the presence of sexual abuse, and the absence of symptoms cannot rule out sexual abuse. Suggestions for future research to understand the course of symptomatology and recovery over time include expanding the instruments used to measure the trauma of abuse, dividing children into age ranges, and using a longitudinal developmental framework.

8

Suggestibility of the Child Witness: A Historical Review and Synthesis

Stephen J. Ceci

Cornell University, Ithaca, New York

Maggie Bruck

McGill University, Montréal, Quebec, Canada

The field of children's testimony is in turmoil, but a resolution to seemingly intractable debates now appears attainable. In this review, we place the current disagreement in historical context and describe psychological and legal views of child witnesses held by scholars since the turn of the 20th century. Although there has been consistent interest in children's suggestibility over the past century, the past 15 years have been the most active in terms of the number of published studies and novel theorizing about the causal mechanisms that underpin the observed findings. A synthesis of this research posits three "families" of factors—cognitive, social, and biological—that must be considered if one is to understand seemingly contradictory interpretations of the findings. We conclude that there are reliable age differences in suggestibility but that even very young children are capable of recalling much that is forensically relevant. Findings are discussed in terms of the role of expert witnesses.

Reprinted with permission from *Psychological Bulletin*, 1993, Vol. 113(3), 403–439. Copyright © 1993 by the American Psychological Association, Inc.

This research article was supported by a National Health and Welfare Scholar Award to Maggie Bruck, by Natural Sciences and Engineering Research Council Grant 0GP000 A1181 to Maggie Bruck, and by National Institutes of Child Health and Human Development Grant RO1 HD 25775 to Stephen J. Ceci.

We are particularly indebted to the thorough, thoughtful, and helpful comments provided by the four reviewers of this article, Stephen Lindsay, Peter Ornstein. Amye Warren, and Maria Zaragoza—as well as by the comments and advice of other colleagues: Chuck Brainerd, Beth Loftus, John Doris, Steve Golding, and Urie Bronfenbrenner.

Since the turn of the century, psycholegal scholars have examined the suggestibility of children's testimony in an effort to determine whether they would be credible witnesses. A major issue in this research concerns the degree to which heightened levels of suggestibility may affect children's ability to accurately report what they have witnessed.

In this article, we review and integrate the entire corpus of 20th-century social science research concerning young children's presumed suggestibility. In the past 10 years, more research has been conducted on the suggestibility of child witnesses than in all of the prior decades combined. This increased research has been motivated by practical concerns: Young children are increasingly being called to testify in court, particularly in sexual abuse cases. Because the earlier literature was criticized for its lack of methodological sophistication and poor ecological validity, it was deemed unsatisfactory for addressing the issue of children's testimonial competence. However, as we show, although contemporary cognitive, social, and developmental psychologists have attempted to provide insights into the intricacies of children's testimonial competence in ecologically relevant settings, the literature is riddled with contradictory interpretations of results. On the one hand, children are described as highly resistant to suggestion, as unlikely to lie, and as reliable as adult witnesses about acts perpetrated on their own bodies (e.g., Berliner, 1985; Goodman, Rudy, Bottoms, & Aman, 1990; Jones & McGraw, 1987). On the other hand, children are described as having difficulty distinguishing reality from fantasy, as being susceptible to coaching by powerful authority figures, and therefore as potentially being less reliable than adults (e.g., Feher, 1988; Gardner, 1989; Schuman, 1986; Underwager & Wakefield, 1990).[1]

The purpose of this review is to provide a historical integration of the research in this area. We attempt to show how the research has reflected cultural, legal, and psychological concerns of the day. Although our review shows that there is still controversy regarding some aspects of children's suggestibility, we try to reconcile this controversy by taking issue with extreme views regarding children's competence. We argue that although there is controversy, it is less the result of inconsistent data than of how these data are interpreted. To resolve this apparent controversy, we reorient this debate to one concerning the causal mechanisms underlying suggestibility in order to understand under what conditions children are or are not more suggestible than adults.

We begin this review by describing two recent court cases in which child witnesses provided critical eyewitness testimony. These cases serve as "windows" through which the points we make later can be viewed; namely, how accurate are

---

[1]We did not mean to imply that proponents of these opposing positions have wholeheartedly endorsed extreme views of the child witness because both camps express the belief that children are capable of high levels of accuracy, provided that adults who have access to them do not attempt to bias their reports.

children's recollections of everyday events? How suggestible is the child witness? How much difficulty does the child have distinguishing reality from fantasy? How honest are children?

THE WEE CARE NURSERY CASE

Margaret Kelly Michaels, a 26-year-old nursery school teacher, was accused of sexually abusing children at the Wee Care Nursery School. She was said to have licked peanut butter off children's genitals; played the piano while nude; made children drink her urine and eat her feces; and raped and assaulted them with knives, forks, spoons, and Lego blocks. She was accused of performing these acts during school hours over a period of 7 months. No alleged act was noticed by staff or reported by children to their parents. No parent noticed signs of strange behavior or genital soreness in their children or smelled urine or feces on them.

The first suspicion that Kelly Michaels abused her charges occurred 4 days after she had left the Wee Care Nursery School. A 4-year-old former student of Kelly's was having his temperature taken rectally at his pediatrician's office and said to the nurse, "That's what my teacher does to me at school." When asked to explain, he replied, "Her takes my temperature" (Manshel, 1990, p. 8). On the advice of the pediatrician, the child's mother notified the state's child protective agency. Two days later, when the child was interviewed by the assistant prosecutor, he inserted his finger into the rectum of an anatomical doll and reported that two other boys also had their temperatures taken. When questioned later, these two boys denied the claim, but one indicated that Kelly Michaels had touched his penis. The first child's mother then told a parent, who was a board member, of her son's disclosures. This board member interrogated his son about Kelly Michaels touching him inappropriately, remarking that "he was his best friend and that he could tell him anything" (Manshel, 1990, p. 126). His son said that Kelly had touched his penis with a spoon. The Wee Care Nursery School sent out a letter to parents, informing them of an investigation of a former employee "regarding serious allegations." In a subsequent meeting, a social worker explained to the parents that sexual abuse of children is very common, with one out of three children being victims of an "inappropriate sexual experience" by the age of 18 years. She encouraged parents to examine their children for genital soreness, nightmares, bed-wetting, masturbation, or any noticeable changes in behavior and to have them examined by pediatricians for injury. Soon, there were many more allegations against Kelly Michaels. Two and one half years later, she was convicted of 115 counts of sexual abuse against twenty 3- to 5-year-old children. She is serving a 47-year sentence.

THE COUNTRY WALK BABYSITTING SERVICE

Frank Furster, a 36-year-old small-business owner and his 17-year-old wife, Iliana, operated the Country Walk Babysitting Service out of their Miami home. Parents became concerned because of numerous problems with their children. One parent believed her child had been drugged and abused by the Fursters; other children claimed that Frank and Iliana kissed their penises, inserted fingers into their rectums, and paraded nude in front of them. Interweaved among the credible allegations that the children made were ones that seemed fabulous, such as riding on sharks and eating the head of another person. The children claimed that Frank Furster videotaped their sexual abuse, although the alleged tapes were never found. In 1986, 3 years after parents first voiced their concerns, Frank and Iliana Furster were tried on multiple counts of child abuse, rape (sexual battery), sodomy, terrorism, and lewdness with a child. The children told interviewers about events that allegedly had taken place several years earlier, when they were aged 1–5 years. After nearly 15 months of denials, Iliana Furster turned state's evidence against her husband. She revealed that she too had been a victim of Frank's abuse and corroborated many of the claims the children made. Frank Furster was convicted of 14 counts of sodomy, rape, and abuse and was sentenced to the equivalent of several life sentences. Iliana was sentenced to 10 years, with 10 additional years of probation.

FROM CASE STUDIES TO SYSTEMATIC RESEARCH

These two cases highlight different aspects of children's credibility that have been the focus of research. The first aspect involves the accuracy of recalling events over long periods of time. In the Country Walk case, the children sometimes described events that allegedly occurred several years before they gave their testimony. Hundreds of studies have examined the degree to which children are able to accurately encode, store, and retrieve different types of information. Most of these studies, however, have examined short-term recollections of objects (as opposed to actions) and of peripheral (as opposed to central) events. Despite these limitations, on the basis of this literature it is safe to conclude that memory skills do improve with age (e.g., see reviews by Kail, 1989; Ornstein, 1978; Schneider & Pressley, 1989).

Notwithstanding this age-related improvement in recall, even very young children's memory is accurate over long delays if the materials and procedures make sense to them (Flavell, 1985) or if the object to be remembered is a salient action or a personally meaningful event (Cutts & Ceci, 1988; Fivush & Hamond, 1990; Jones, Swift, & Johnson, 1988; Perris, Myers, & Clifton, 1990). Recall of action-related events is highly reliable, even in preschoolers (e.g., Davies, Tarrant, &

Flin, 1989; Jones et al., 1988), particularly when they are participants in an event (Rudy & Goodman, 1991).

Furthermore, age differences in *recognition* memory are far less pronounced than age differences in *free recall,* and at times these are nonexistent (Ceci, Ross, & Toglia, 1987; Cole & Loftus, 1987; Jones et al., 1988; List, 1986; Saywitz, 1987). For example, preschoolers remember as much as adults when the task does not emphasize verbal recall (Nurcombe, 1986) and in response to specific questions. Even 3-year-olds recognize as many familiar drawings as 12-year-olds (Ceci et al., 1987). Studies such as these indicate that preschoolers' recognition memory can be remarkably accurate (Kail, 1989).

The second aspect of children's testimonial credibility concerns their "suggestibility," and it is this aspect that is the focus of our review. According to its broadest definition, *suggestibility* concerns the degree to which children's encoding, storage, retrieval, and reporting of events can be influenced by a range of social and psychological factors. This broad definition contrasts with the narrower and more traditional definition of suggestibility, which asserts that it is "the extent to which individuals come to accept and subsequently incorporate post-event information into their memory recollections" (Gudjonsson, 1986, p. 195; see also Powers, Andriks, & Loftus, 1979). This narrower definition implies that suggestibility can only be unconscious (i.e., interfering information is unwittingly incorporated into memory); suggestibility results from the provision of information following an event as opposed to preceding it; and suggestibility is a memory-based, as opposed to a social, phenomenon. We adopt the broader definition of suggestibility because it implies that (a) it is possible to accept information and yet be fully aware of its divergence from some originally perceived event, as in the case of "confabulation" (such as is shown by brain-injured patients; see Johnson, 1991), acquiescence to social demands, or lying (see footnote 5); thus, these forms of suggestibility do not involve the alteration of memory. (b) Suggestibility can result from the provision of information preceding *or* following an event. (c) Suggestibility can result from social as well as cognitive factors. Thus, this broader view of suggestibility is consistent with the legal use of this term to connote how easily one is influenced by both subtle suggestions and leading questions, as well as by explicit bribes, threats, and other forms of inducement.

Within this framework, one can examine how much children's testimonies reflect their desire to protect themselves, the cultural and personal beliefs that also influence adults' willingness to accept children's testimony, and the nature of the interrogations that induce children to make certain statements or accusations. For example, in our two sample cases, expert witnesses and prosecutors insisted that the children must be believed because children do not lie and they cannot be mistaken about sexualized claims. In the Country Walk case, there was repeated provision of an atmosphere of accusation, with interviewers informing children, "It's okay to tell . . . You'll feel better once you tell." Finally, in the Wee Care Nursery School case, most of the children were told by interviewers prior to their own disclosures that their peers had already disclosed that Kelly Michaels was a bad person who had hurt them. These are issues that we return to in evaluating the research on children's incorporation of adult beliefs and the creation of an "atmosphere of accusation" in interviews.

By broadening the definition of suggestibility to entail nonmnemonic influences, we summarize the literature on the following two questions: First, are younger children more suggestible than older children? Second, to what degree does suggestibility reflect cognitive, social, and biological factors? The examination of these questions allows for a more precise understanding not only of the conditions under which children are suggestible but more generally of the causal mechanisms that underlie their suggestibility.

Before turning to these issues, it is important to emphasize that we do not mean to imply that adults are not suggestible, that their memories are always reliable, or that their testimonies are highly accurate. These statements are clearly false. There is a sizable literature on the suggestibility of adults' memory (e.g., Belli, 1989; Gudjonsson, 1986; Lindsay, 1990; Loftus, 1979). In this article we examine factors that may influence witnesses of all ages but that may exert a disproportionate influence on children.

HISTORICAL REVIEW

Early Research: 1900–1914

Historically, interest in children's testimonial competence, both by the legal profession and by social scientists, has reflected specific judicial events, the structure of the judicial system, and general social conditions of the era. In the United States, there was little interest in this field until the last half of the 20th century. To some degree this reflected the Salem Witch Trials of 1692. At that time a group of children gave false testimony in the witchcraft trials of more than 20 residents of Salem Village and Salem Farms. The girls made fantastic claims (Ceci, Toglia, & Ross, 1990). Several years after the execution of defendants, some of the child witnesses publicly recanted their testimonies. For the most part, the prevailing legal attitude for the following 300 years has been one of skepticism about the testimony of child witnesses (e.g., Wigmore, 1935). Repeatedly, legal scholars have cited the excesses of Salem as a basis for their views of child witnesses.

Although there was little if any interest among psychologists in children's testimonial competence in the United States at the start of the 20th century, this was not the case in Europe, where systematic research on adults' and children's testimony flourished, especially in the Federal Republic of Germany and France. To a large degree, differences in the adjudication procedures in the two continents can account for these differences in research in this area. An inquisitorial system of justice prevails in many European countries in which the judge is responsible for calling and questioning witnesses. Because there is often no jury, the European judge is more likely to call on expert witnesses to testify about the competence of witnesses (Loh, 1981). In the early part of this century, these expert witnesses were often psychologists who carried out experiments to examine the veracity of the children's testimony. By contrast, in an adversarial system, such as the one used in the United States, the use of opposing attorneys and a jury was considered sufficient to evaluate witness credibility (see Loftus, 1986, for additional details).

Because few of the early studies on testimonial competence were published in English, unilingual Anglophones have had to rely on reviews of this research for its details. The most influential of these were published in the *Psychological Bulletin* by Whipple (1909, 1911, 1912, 1913). These reviews were notable for their coverage of the child suggestibility research by European psychologists and medical experts. In the course of these reviews, Whipple became increasingly convinced that young children are highly suggestible and capable of making serious errors in their testimony, even when they testify about matters of great personal importance. Although these reviews are still cited as definitive summaries of early research (e.g., Baxter, 1990; Goodman, 1984a), they provide few details of the actual procedures or results of the studies. This is unfortunate for today's reader because some of the methodologies used in modern research were developed by these early scientists who also had sophisticated views on issues that are currently debated. In order to introduce the reader to some of these methodologies and issues, we provide some details on the work of four pioneering European scientists: Binet, Stern, Varendonck, and Lipmann. The following summaries are based on our translations or published translations of primary source materials.

A. Binet. On the basis of a series of studies of children between the ages of 7 and 14 years, Binet (1900) claimed that suggestibility reflected the operation of two classes of factors. The first class concerns the influence of a prominent thought (autosuggestion) that develops within the individual, and is not the result of another's influence, but that paralyzes the critical senses. The second class of factors is external to the individual and reflects mental obedience to other individuals.

Although Binet's (1900) autosuggestion techniques were adapted by the next generation of researchers, they are rarely used in modern studies. The best known of these involved showing children a series of lines and then asking them to draw the final one. The first five lines progressively increased in length. The sixth line, however, was the same length as the fifth. Children tended to be swayed by the perceptual or internal suggestion of ever-increasing lines; thus, their drawings of the sixth line were too long. However, the influence of the suggestion was not long-lasting; children could easily regain control of themselves and accurately redraw the target line when asked to do so at the end of the experiment.

In contrast to Binet's (1900) paradigms for examining internal forces, his paradigms to examine external forces are still used today. In one study, children saw five objects for 10 s (e.g., a button glued to poster board). Some were told to write down everything they saw. Others were asked direct questions (e.g., "How was the button attached to the board?"). Others were asked mildly leading questions (e.g., "Wasn't the button attached by a thread?"). Some were asked highly misleading questions (e.g., "What was the color of the thread that attached the button to the board?"). The major finding was that free recall resulted in the most accurate statements and that highly misleading questions resulted in the most inaccurate statements. As we discuss later, this pattern of results has since been replicated in dozens of studies. Children's answers to Binet's questions were characterized by an exactness and certainty, regardless of their accuracy. Because children did not correct their inaccurate responses, Binet concluded that their erroneous responses reflected gaps in their memories; they attempted to fill in these gaps to please the experimenter. However, once an erroneous response was given, Binet proposed that it became incorporated into memory. In other experimental contexts, Binet directly ascribed children's suggestibility to social factors, namely, children's eagerness to comply with adult suggestions rather than to memorial factors. In those cases, Binet discovered that children's suggestibility was not long-lasting; they quickly realized their errors.

In sum, Binet was prescient in three ways: First, he distinguished between errors of reporting caused by actual memory changes versus those caused by social conformity, arguing that the latter include attempts to please adult authority figures and do not always reflect incorporation of the suggestion into the memory record. Later, we review modern evidence on the debate over the supremacy of cognitive versus social mechanisms. Second, Binet foreshadowed the current debate over whether the original memory trace is itself impaired or simply allowed to "coexist" with traces of the erroneous suggestion (Loftus, 1979). Third, Binet alerted researchers to the weak relation between confidence and accuracy (see Bothwell, Deffenbacher, & Brigham, 1987, for current data). *W. Stern.* Stern (1910) developed two types of experiments that are still in use today. In the first paradigm, subjects were shown a picture and asked to study it for a short period of time. Immediately after its presentation, they were asked to recall what they had seen. They were then asked a series of direct questions, requesting information that was in the picture, and a series of misleading questions, requesting information about nonexistent objects. In one study that included

7- to 18-year-olds, free recall produced the fewest errors, whereas misleading questions produced the most errors (Stern, 1910). Although younger children were the most suggestible, even the 18-year-olds occasionally were misled by the suggestive questions.

The second paradigm, the "reality" experiment, was developed to mimic situations that were closer to real life. Here, naive subjects observed staged incidents. In a typical experiment, an argument occurred during a seminar between two students, one of whom drew a revolver. The other students in the class were then questioned about the scenario.

Stern made several observations that continue to be important. He warned about repeated questioning of the same event, claiming that a subject's original verbal answers are better remembered than the actual events themselves (Stern, 1910). He also talked about the "force" that questions have in determining answers, claiming that many children answer questions because they view them as imperatives. Stern argued that the questioner, by virtue of the nature of the questions asked, is often responsible for the unreliable testimony of witnesses. Finally, Stern (1910) believed that children are especially suggestible at certain times of their lives when they merge fiction and reality. Children, particularly girls, were said to be suggestible around puberty as the result of hormonal changes. Stern is to be credited for illuminating the notion of "reality monitoring judgments," an area of continued activity (Johnson, 1991; Johnson & Raye, 1981), although his predictions concerning both age and sex effects were subsequently shown to be wrong.

J. Varendonck. Varendonck, a Belgian psychologist, was an expert witness in a trial involving allegations by several children that a young girl named Cecile was murdered by a local man (Varendonck, 1911). Two of Cecile's friends who had played with her on the day of her murder were awakened that night by Cecile's mother to ask of her whereabouts. One of the children replied that she did not know. Later that night, she led the police to the spot where the children had played, not far from where Cecile's body was found. In the next month, the two children were repeatedly interviewed by authorities who asked many suggestive questions. The children quickly changed their original testimony of not knowing about Cecile's actions on the day of her murder. They provided details of the appearance of the murderer as well as his name. Because of an anonymous letter, the police arrested the father of one of the playmates for the murder of Cecile. On the basis of the details of the case, Varendonck was convinced of the defendant's innocence. He quickly conducted a series of studies with the specific intent of demonstrating the unreliability of children's testimony.

In one study, Varendonck (1911) asked the children in his class to describe a person who had approached him in the school yard that morning. Although there was no such person, most of the children fell sway to his suggestion, with 17 out of 22 giving a name for the person, the color of his clothes, and so on. Varendonck claimed that the types of questions he used were parallel to those that the examining magistrate used with one of the child witnesses.

Varendonck concluded from his demonstrations that the two children's statements to the police were false, the result of suggestions provided by influential adults. He carefully documented how the children changed their testimonies between the first and second interrogations and how other social factors conspired to produce their testimony. He concluded that children cannot observe accurately and that their suggestibility is inexhaustible ("We cannot set the least value in their declarations"; Varendonck, 1911, p. 168). His work is noteworthy because of the direct forensic applications of his empirical data.

O. Lipmann. The work of Lipmann, a German psychologist, is of interest because many of his hypotheses are the focus of modern research. Consistent with Binet, he concluded that cognitive as well as social factors accounted for children's greater suggestibility. Children were thought to have different, not fewer, memories than adults because they were sensitive to different attributes of stimuli than adults. When children are questioned by adults, who have authority over them, about events that are neither essential nor salient to the child, the child will attempt to revise his or her memory, making the report consistent with the question. "If the respected person who is questioning me expects such an answer then it must be the right one" (Lipmann, 1911, p. 253). Thus, rather than answering "I do not know," the child accepts any material that comes to mind to fill in these gaps, whether it is imaginary or real. Eventually everything that is imagined becomes real (i.e., the child fails to differentiate fantasy from reality). Modern researchers would return to the issue of the young child's ability to separate the sources of their information, including whether it was imagined or perceived (Foley & Johnson, 1985; Foley, Johnson, & Raye, 1983; Lindsay, Johnson, & Kwon, 1991). Modern researchers would also return to the idea that children have different perceptions (or scripts) of the world than adults and that these can also affect the nature of their memories.

Summary of research during the early European period. Two important elements of the early European work on children's suggestibility deserve mention. First, all of the researchers during this early period were interested in applications of children's memory research to the legal system. Second, multifactorial mechanisms underlying suggestibility were posited. These involved cognitive factors related to children's encoding, storage, and retrieval of events as well as social factors related to children's compliance with authority figures. It should also be noted that this early work foreshadowed a large number of findings that were to appear in the modern literature, such as the idea that repeated questioning is detrimental, that questions are interpreted as "imperatives" by young children, that free recall produces fewer errors than yes-no questioning, that fantasy-reality distinctions are problematic for very young children, and that even adults are suggestible.

The Dry Middle Years: 1924–1963

Overview. Although European courts were eager consumers of the psychological research on children's suggestibility, the same could not be said of American courts. According to Loh (1981), similar studies of the reliability of witnesses in the United States were rejected by the legal profession. Münsternberg (1907a, 1907b), a Harvard psychologist, summarized the European literature on the unreliability of adult witnesses and made a strong case for using psychological methods in U.S. courts of law. His position, however, was ruthlessly criticized by jurists such as Moore (1907, 1908) and Wigmore (1909) on the grounds that psychology had nothing useful to offer law. Wigmore claimed that psychological experimentation produced results based on group averages, whereas in a court of law the relevant issue concerns the reliability of a specific witness in a specific situation. (Wigmore did soften his stance against psychology later in his career.) This rejection of psychological research by leading members of the U.S. legal community resulted in a long hiatus, during which little work was carried out by psychologists on the accuracy of witnesses' testimony. Until the reemergence of this genre of research in the late 1970s, there was only a handful of studies on children's suggestibility, most carried out in the 1920s and 1930s and, for the most part, marked by their unoriginality. The major focus of these studies was to examine the relations of age, intelligence, and sex to suggestibility or to examine the correlations among different suggestibility measures, most of which were adaptations of tasks devised by Binet and Stern. The interesting questions raised by Binet, Stern, Varendonck, and Lipmann went unaddressed. For this reason, we do not devote as much space to these studies.

Otis (1924) examined the development of children's ability to rely on their own judgments. Her test included many items similar to those devised by Binet to assess autosuggestion. Other questions, which were phrased in a leading manner, assessed the influence of external forces. Students in Grade 3 through college were tested. Suggestibility decreased as a function of age and intelligence. Using a similar measure, Hurlock (1930) replicated these results with a sample of 10- to 17-year-olds. Burtt and Gaskill (1932) showed students in Grade 4 and college a movie and asked them leading and nonleading questions about what they had witnessed. College students' errors on the suggestive questions were much lower than those of the fourth graders.

Sherman (1925) examined the association of suggestibility with chronological and mental age in normal and mentally challenged children. The children were given eight different tasks that involved "direct" questions and "autosuggestions." In general, suggestibility decreased with age in both samples. In addition, suggestibility also decreased as mental age increased in the mentally challenged sample. By contrast, Messerschmidt (1933) tested 6- to 16-year-olds on a battery of similar tests and found a strong association between age and performance that was consistent across tasks. The youngest children were the most suggestible across tasks, and the oldest children were the least suggestible.

The next suggestibility study involving children did not appear in the literature until 30 years later (McConnell, 1963). Several measures of visual perceptual suggestibility were given to children in Grades 1–12. For example, they were shown two equal objects and asked to circle the one that looked the biggest. Next, the experimenter told them that one of the circles really was larger than the other and to circle the largest. They were given the option of marking "neither." On all tasks suggestibility correlated with age.

Summary of research during the dry middle years (1924–1963). Two consistent findings emerge from this set of studies. First, younger children were more suggestible than older children and adults. Second, there was a negative correlation between suggestibility and IQ, with those possessing lower IQs being less able to resist suggestion. However, it must be kept in mind that in most cases, many of these memory measures were paper-and-pencil tests; thus, the correlations with IQ may reflect the fact that the poorer students had more difficulty dealing with written materials, or keeping their attention focused during long written tasks, rather than with suggestibility of the experimental manipulations.

In contrast to the earlier European studies, the studies conducted by American researchers during the 1924–1964 period were not couched in legally relevant terms. For reasons stated earlier, there was never any mention of the applicability of these findings to the issue of children's testimony. One is also struck by their atheoretical nature. No new principles or paradigms were discovered, and there was little theorizing about the underlying causes of developmental differences in suggestibility. One issue that does recur is the degree to which suggestibility is a trait. However, not only are the data inconsistent across studies, but even on those occasions when the same patterns of data were reported, they led to different interpretations. One view was that susceptibility to suggestive questioning resulted from a traitlike tendency (e.g., Aveling & Hargreaves, 1921). Children were more suggestible because of immature but developing mechanisms that made them more susceptible to external factors. According to this view, suggestibility was an individual-differences variable along which people could be differentiated and along which children as a group were relatively deficient. Others (e.g., Remmers, Cutler, & Jones, 1940; Sherman, 1925) viewed suggestibility not as a trait but as a function of task-specific factors, including characteristics of the experimenter and laboratory.

Our review suggests that a consensus was building about children's testimonial incompetence, reflected in Burtt's (1948) description of children as "dangerously vulnerable to coaching and erroneous leading questions: Suggestion is especially apt to play a role in the testimony of children because they are more suggestible than adults" (p. 307).

The Modern Period: 1979–1992

Following a 16-year hiatus in research on children's suggestibility, the late 1970s marked a resurgence of interest among developmental researchers in the reliability of children's reports. Since 1979, more than 100 studies on children's suggestibility have been reported. Four interrelated factors account for this dramatic increase in empirical work.

First, there has been a broadening of admissibility of expert psychological testimony in recent years, particularly with regard to issues concerning mental disorders, pretrial publicity, and civil rights (see Loh, 1981). Thus, social science research, after a long period of being ignored or rejected by judicial policymakers, has come to be viewed, at least on occasion, as being relevant to the legal system. Second, in part fueled by the sociopolitical *zeitgeist* of the late 1960s, social scientists attempted to apply their scientific training to socially relevant issues, particularly those concerning children's rights and the protection of minors. Third, many studies were motivated by or influenced by methods and theories emanating from studies on eyewitness testimony of adults, which, for the reasons just mentioned, were also increasing in number.

The fourth and undoubtedly the biggest stimulus for the explosion of research on children's suggestibility is the legal community's heightened interest in behavioral science data related to specific innovations for dealing with child witnesses. For example, until recently, there has been a reluctance to accept the uncorroborated statements of child witnesses in courts of law in all English-speaking countries (Chadbourn, 1978). This reluctance is reflected in competency hearings, corroboration requirements, and cautionary instructions that some North American judges give to juries concerning the inherent reliability risks of convictions based solely on the testimony of child witnesses (Andrews, 1964; Cohen, 1975). However, since the 1980s, more children are being admitted as witnesses as a result of dramatic increases in reports of crimes involving sexual abuse and physical abuse in which the child has been a victim or a witness. In 1989, there were 2.4 million reports of suspected child maltreatment in the United States; 900,000 were substantiated (Daro & Mitchel, 1990).

As a result of the ineffective prosecution of child abuse cases, in the past decade the legal system has been forced to change some of its rules concerning the admissibility of child witnesses' testimony. During the 1980s all states dropped their corroboration requirement for children involved in sex abuse cases, a crime that by its nature is often without corroboration. Seventeen states now allow children to testify regardless of the nature of the crime, permitting the jury to determine how much weight to give to the child witness. As more and more children are allowed to provide uncorroborated testimony, courts begin turning to psychological research to inform their proceedings.

Because children are increasing being admitted as courtroom witnesses, courtroom procedures have also been modified. Of particular pertinence to this article, most states have evidentiary codes that permit asking the child leading questions in sex abuse cases. Other procedures, such as shield laws and hearsay exclusions, have been instituted to assist child witnesses (see McGough, in press). In light of claims that such modifications challenge the constitutional rights of defendants (*Maryland v. Craig,* 1990), it is important to obtain empirical data that such procedures do in fact enhance the court's truth-seeking function.

This increased demand for scientific data on children's credibility has resulted in a large number of recent studies that are methodologically superior to the older work and that aim for greater external validity through the use of experimental procedures that seem more realistic. Thus, in contrast to many of the older studies that required children to make perceptual judgments (e.g., Which line is longer?) or to recall neutral stories or pictures, many of the newer studies have examined the manner in which children process and recall important, personally experienced, highly salient, affectively loaded events in the context of strong preevent or postevent suggestions. However, although much of this research on children's recollections is being carried out in more naturalistic contexts, this does not in itself make it generalizable to a particular court case unless the research context closely mirrors the factors "at bar" (see Ceci, 1991; Loftus & Ceci, 1991).

The current research is also beginning to reexamine (and in some cases reinvent) hypotheses that were first raised by the early European scientists. The focus has thus shifted from simply examining whether children are suggestible to determining under what conditions they are suggestible. To some degree this shift has been influenced by current work on the testimonial competence of adults (e.g., Melton & Thomson, 1987), as well as by recent basic research on the cognitive and social development of children.

A final feature of the newer studies concerns the ages of the children studied. In contrast to previous studies, which focused on school-aged children, modern researchers often include preschoolers. Because preschoolers are increasingly being called to testify, the need for a greater understanding of their testimonial accuracy is urgently needed. Approximately 25 of the studies described in this article involved preschoolers; by contrast, during the first 80 years of this century, there was not a single study, to our knowledge, that included children this young.

We turn next to a review of the modern child suggestibility literature. During the modern period, some investigators, like their predecessors, have emphasized evidence of children's special vulnerability to suggestions. Other investigators, however, have emphasized evidence of children's ability to resist suggestions and to give accurate testimony. We describe five representative studies from each of these positions. We selected these studies because each has been cited in support of the claim that there are or are not developmental changes in children's suggestibility. As we show, studies published by both camps often contain mixed results (i.e., there is evidence of age-related changes under some conditions but not under others). Furthermore, there are inconsistencies in the pattern of results between some studies. Such inconsistencies illustrate our earlier claim that despite the superior methodology and greater ecological realism, these modern studies have initiated and fueled, rather than resolved, disagreements among researchers over the suggestibility of children's statements.

Children are more suggestible than adults. Our review of the studies conducted during the first 70 years of this century indicated that almost without exception, researchers believed children were more suggestible than adults. The following five examples of recent research, which used more sophisticated methodologies and ecologically realistic settings, showed results similar to the earlier work.

1. Cohen and Harnick (1980) presented a 12-min film about a petty theft to 9-year-olds, 12-year-olds, and college students and tested their memory for the details of the film immediately afterward and 1 week later. For the first interview, half of the 22 probe questions were misleading (e.g., "The young woman was carrying a newspaper when she entered the bus, wasn't she?"), and the other 11 questions were not phrased in a misleading manner. The youngest subjects produced the least accurate responses to both nonmisleading and misleading questions, indicating that they were more suggestible than the older subjects. These age differences were not reliable, however, when the subjects were tested 1 week later, using a multiple-choice question format. The authors concluded that younger children were more likely to consciously submit to suggestions than older subjects but that the suggestions did not differentially affect their memory for the event.

2. King and Yuille (1987) staged a live event for 6-, 9-, 11-, and 16-year-olds. The subjects were seated in a room when a stranger entered to care for some plants. Prior to leaving the room, the stranger noted the time and indicated it was late. When the children were subsequently interviewed, they were asked for a description of what they could recall as well as some leading questions such as "On which arm did the man wear his watch?" (He had not worn a watch.) The 6-years-olds were significantly more suggestible than 9- to 16-year-olds, and they also recalled less.

3. Ceci et al. (1987, Experiment 1) presented short stories accompanied by illustrations to 3- to 12-year-olds. One day after the presentation, they provided misleading information about aspects of the stories to half of the subjects. Two

days later, they tested the children's memories of the stories by having them select from a series of four pictures the two that had actually appeared in the story. Age differences were obtained only for children who were given misleading information. Preschoolers were more likely than the older children to select pictures that were described in the misleading session than pictures that appeared in the actual story.

4. Ornstein, Gordon, and Larus (1992) tested 3- and 6-year-olds' memories of a pediatric examination. Approximately half of the children at each age were tested immediately following the examination and 1 week later, and the others were tested immediately and 3 weeks later. Most of the children were asked some misleading questions. At each test session, the older children's memories were better than the younger children's as assessed by free-recall and objective questions. Furthermore, the 3-year-olds gave fewer correct answers to the misleading questions than did the 6-year-olds during the first two testing periods. These age differences were not reliable after 3 weeks; this reflected the fact that 6-year-olds' accuracy on misleading questions was greatly reduced between the first and last session relative to that of the 3-year-olds.

5. Oates and Shrimpton (1991) studied the effect of questioning on the memories of two groups of 4- to 12-year-olds. One group received a blood test and the second group encountered a friendly stranger in their school library who put a loose cotton shirt over the child's clothes and then removed it. The children's memory of the event was assessed 4–10 days following the event or 3–6 weeks later. On all measures, children in the blood group performed comparably to children in the library group. Also, children were more accurate when tested after the short delay than after the long delay. Of particular importance, older children (aged 7–12 years) performed better than younger children (aged 4–6 years) on free-recall, direct questions, and some types of misleading questions. Compared with younger children, older children were less misled about actions, but there were no age differences on resistance to being misled about the person with whom they interacted. Finally, the effect of the delay of interview was especially consequential for the misleading *action* questions; children interviewed after a long delay were more susceptible to suggestion than those interviewed after a short delay. Recently, Poole (in press) has found that long delays (nearly 2 years) are disproportionately more detrimental to the memories of 4-year-olds than older children and adults.

Younger children are not less suggestible than older children. In view of the findings presented to date, it is surprising to discover that there are those who argue that there is no evidence of age differences in suggestibility. For example, three years ago Gary Melton, the past president of the American Psychological Association's Division on Psychology and the Law, expressed concern over the fact that the dissenting Supreme Court justices in the case of the *State of Maryland v. Sandra Ann Craig* maintained that children were substantially more suggestible than adults. Melton asserted that "the dissent's discriminate plucking of such material from the psychological literature doesn't reflect the broad findings within the field" (cited in DeAngelis, 1990, p. 1). More recently, Melton (1992) reaffirmed (and seemingly strengthened) this assertion:

> There is now no real question that the law and many developmentalists were wrong in their assumption that children are highly vulnerable to suggestion, at least in regard to salient details. Although some developmentalists may be challenged to find developmental differences in suggestibility in increasingly arcane circumstances, as a practical matter who really cares whether 3-year-old children are less suggestible about peripheral details in events that they witnessed than are 4-year-old children? Perhaps the question has some significance for developmental theory, but surely it has little or no meaning for policy and practice in child protection and law. (Melton, 1992, p. 154)

Melton's dismay reflects the fact that there are studies to support the view that children are no more suggestible than adults. The following five studies are examples of this literature.

1. Marin, Holmes, Guth, and Kovac (1979) exposed 5-, 8-, and 12-year-olds and college students to a live staged argument between two adults. After a brief delay, subjects were asked 20 objective questions and an additional misleading question. The impact of the misleading question was assessed 2 weeks later, when all 21 questions were asked in a nonleading form. Children did not differ from college students on objective questions asked immediately after the event. Furthermore, although the introduction of the misleading question produced a significant increase in inaccurate answers on the corresponding objective question asked 2 weeks later, the size of this suggestibility effect was similar across all ages. Thus, children were no more suggestible than adults.

2. Duncan, Whitney, and Kunen (1982, Experiment 2) showed 7-, 9-, and 11-year-olds and college students slides depicting scenes from the movie *Star Wars*. Following the presentation of the slides, subjects received related, unrelated, and neutral information that was either consistent with the slides they had just seen or was consistent with distractor slides that were shown at the time of testing. In a complex analysis that entailed having subjects' d' recognition scores contingent on their memory criterion (i.e., using only the stories on which children demonstrated good memory for follow-up questions), they showed that the older subjects were *more* likely than younger subjects to incorporate misleading verbal information into their visual memories for slides.

3. Flin, Boon, Knox, and Bull (1992) exposed 6-year-olds, 10-year-olds, and

adults to a realistically staged argument during a presentation on foot hygiene by a nurse in the school auditorium. Half of the subjects were questioned about the event 1 day later, and all subjects were questioned 5 months later. Three of the questions contained erroneous suggestions. In both interviews, responses to these questions were highly accurate across all age groups; few subjects of any age accepted the erroneous information.

4. Perhaps no researcher has done more to redress the historical imbalance in favor of child witnesses than Gail Goodman. After almost a century of research criticizing and belittling the accuracy and suggestibility of child witnesses, Goodman has presented a far more optimistic picture of children's abilities. Her work is animated in part by a desire to know whether nonabused children will make false claims of abuse in response to erroneous suggestions by adults. In order to examine this question, her strategy has been to interview nonabused children about sexual as well as nonsexual experiences.

As one example, Rudy and Goodman (1991) studied pairs of 4- and 7-year-olds who were left in a trailer with a strange adult. One child played a game with the adult that involved being dressed in a clown's costume and being lifted and photographed while the other child was encouraged to carefully observe this interchange. Approximately 10 days later, the children were asked suggestive and nonsuggestive questions about the event. Some of these questions concerned actions that might lead to an accusation of child abuse, such as "He took your clothes off, didn't he?" Across all question types, there were few differences between participants' and bystanders' responses.[2] Older children were more accurate than younger children on nonsuggestive (abuse and non-abuse-related) questions. On misleading questions, these same age effects were obtained only for the nonabuse questions. Accuracy rates on the abuse misleading questions were similar for the younger and older children. A more detailed analysis of the incorrect answers to the suggestive abuse questions revealed only one false report of abuse; a 4-year-old bystander falsely claimed that he and the participant had been spanked.

---

[2]Note that this statement differs from the conclusions offered by Rudy and Goodman: "As predicted, participation in a real-life event heightened the children's resistance to suggestion. On misleading questions, participants were less suggestible than bystanders. On misleading questions concerning the confederate's appearance, 4-year-old participants were less suggestible than 4-year-old bystanders, and an age difference appeared only for bystander witnesses. This pattern indicates that participation can strengthen resistance to suggestion and that at least at times, the effects are especially evident for young children" (Rudy & Goodman, 1991, p. 534). Rudy and Goodman failed to consider in this discussion that when "don't know" answers were included in the data, only one of the four analyses of misleading questions yielded significant results for participation. When only the misleading abuse questions were considered (a fifth analysis), there was no significant effect for participation. Furthermore, the analysis of the nonmisleading direct questions and of the free-recall data failed to reveal any advantage for participation. Thus, their conclusions concerning the effects of participation seem overgenerous, given the actual pattern of results.

5. A second study conducted by Goodman and her colleagues (Goodman & Clarke-Stewart, 1991; Saywitz, Goodman, Nicholas, & Moan, 1991) examined 5- and 7-year-old girls' memories of medical examinations. Half of each age group had a scoliosis exam, and half had a genital exam. Children were tested 1–4 weeks following their exam. Children were asked suggestive and nonsuggestive questions that were abuse related or non-abuse-related. The older children's answers to the suggestive non-abuse questions and to the nonsuggestive abuse questions were more accurate than those of the younger children. However, there was essentially no difference in resistance to suggestibility for suggestive abuse questions (e.g., "How many times did the doctor kiss you?"), with few children giving incorrect responses. The 7-year-old children never made a false report of abuse, and this occurred only 3 out of 215 times for the 5-year-olds.

Weighing the pros and cons. Because there was so much variability in the methodologies used in the 10 studies, it was not possible to resolve the modern controversy concerning age differences in suggestibility by direct comparisons of them. That is, no two studies were alike on many of the relevant dimensions, such as the nature of the event to be remembered (e.g., verbal stories, slide shows, or physical examinations); the timing of the misleading information (prior to the memory test vs. during it); timing of the interview (shortly after the stimulus event vs. several weeks after it); and the type of data-analytic techniques (analysis of raw data vs. signal-detection techniques).

It also does not seem fruitful to resolve the existing controversy through a point-by-point criticism of the methodological weaknesses of each study. Methodological concerns can be raised with equal force at studies on both sides of the debate. We now provide a sampling of some the concerns that, although not exhaustive, demonstrates that interpretative problems plague studies on both sides of the debate. For example, the failure to find statistically reliable age differences on a number of the suggestibility measures may reflect the use of relatively small sample sizes, which masks real developmental differences. As an example, Cohen and Harnick's (1980) failure to find reliable age effects after a 2-week delay could have been caused by their having only 3 subjects in each cell of their analysis. This could have prevented observed age differences that were large in magnitude from reaching traditional levels of reliability. (Incorrect response rates to misleading questions were 51%, 33%, and 22%, respectively, for the three age groups.) Examination of the sample sizes and large variances reported in Duncan et al. (1982) and Flin et al. (1992) raise similar concerns.

A second concern is the number of suggestive questions included in the interviews. For example, the Marin et al. (1979) study included only one leading question. Because chance accuracy with a single yes–no question is .50, it is noteworthy that the rate of answering the suggestive question correctly after a 2-week delay was essentially this value for the four age groups (.50, .50, .46, and

.46, respectively). These data leave open the possibility that all subjects might have been influenced by the misleading question but that floor effects prevented a powerful test of any age difference. Concerns about the number of suggestive questions can also be raised for studies that showed age effects. In the Ornstein et al. (1992) study, the size of the question set changed for each child. It is possible that older children were less suggestible because they were asked more suggestive questions (producing a larger denominator and a smaller overall suggestibility ratio).

Perhaps age differences are obtained only when situations are highly artificial or irrelevant to forensically important issues. For example, in the Ceci et al. (1987) study, the experimental context was a nursery school story in which unfamiliar characters were described to children for brief periods and later described erroneously. That young children succumbed to such suggestions under those circumstances does not necessarily indicate that they will do so in response to more emotionally salient and powerful materials. Nevertheless, age trends in suggestibility effects have been reported for more stressful and naturalistic situations (e.g., Oates & Shrimpton, 1991; Ornstein et al., 1992). And, in their ecologically based studies of thefts, both Cassel and Bjorklund (1992) and Warren and Hagood (in press) found age differences in succumbing to suggestive questions even for central events, with younger children more suggestible.

The linguistic complexity of the misleading questions may be related to the appearance or nonappearance of age-related differences in suggestibility. Some of the questions used in various studies might have been too complex and beyond the comprehension of young children. An example of such a question is as follows: "What did the costume that he asked the other boy to wear look like?" (Rudy & Goodman, 1991, p. 538). In response to such questions, the children might have answered "I don't know" (which was counted as an accurate answer), not because they were resisting the suggestion but because they did not comprehend the question. This could obviate potential age-related differences, particularly if the "don't know" answers of the younger children reflect poor comprehension, whereas the "don't know" answers of the older subjects reflect resistance to suggestion. However, similarly difficult questions were also found in studies that did report age-related differences in suggestibility (e.g., from Oates & Shrimpton, 1991, p. 8): "The person who gave you the blood test put your arms behind your back, didn't she?"), forcing the alternative argument that perhaps high rates of acquiescence reflect poor comprehension of the questions.

One might also note that although each of the 10 studies cited are commonly used to provide evidence for or against age differences in children's suggestibility, within each study there are conflicting results. Thus, Rudy and Goodman (1991) consistently reported that there were age-related differences in children's answers to misleading questions, except for one special type of question. Similarly, Cohen

and Harnick's (1980) study is commonly used to support the age-difference position, but age-related differences were obtained only on the first, and not on the
second, testing.

This discussion demonstrates that any attempt to resolve these inconsistent
results by a point-by-point examination of whether researchers on the two sides
of the debate use different age groups, settings, and events still leaves many contradictory findings and does little to illuminate the nature of the age differences
when they do occur. Thus, rather than attempting to contrast each of these studies
on a microlevel, it seems more fruitful to explore the causal mechanisms that may
underlie obtained suggestibility effects and, in turn, to consider how these various
mechanisms might explain the appearance or nonoccurrence of age trends in suggestibility effects. With this goal in mind, we now explore three types of factors:
cognitive, social-motivational, and biological.

CAUSAL MECHANISMS: COGNITIVE FACTORS

Children become increasingly cognitively sophisticated with development as a
result of a confluence of attainments in memory, concept formation, reasoning,
language ability, and introspective awareness of the cognitive system's executive
functions (Ceci, 1990). In this section, we discuss the aspects of this research that
have the greatest relevance to understanding the potential causal mechanisms of
suggestibility.

Memory

One issue related to the underlying mechanisms of suggestibility involves the
extent to which erroneous postevent information interferes with the original memory. We describe the procedures developed by Loftus and her colleagues (e.g.,
Loftus, Miller, & Burns, 1978) to examine these effects first, because the developmental data on suggestibility are primarily based on these procedures or on
modifications of them. Subjects first view an event that consists of a number of
details (e.g., a man holding a hammer while drinking cola). They then receive
information about the event, some of which is misleading (e.g., the man was holding a wrench while drinking cola). Finally, their memories for the original events
are tested (e.g., Was the man holding a hammer or a wrench?). Commonly, subjects make more errors for items about which they were given incorrect information than for control items (e.g., Ceci et al., 1987; Loftus et al., 1978; Marin et
al., 1979). Thus, although they incorrectly reported that the man was holding a
wrench, they correctly remembered that he was drinking cola.

Although this demonstration of the phenomenon of suggestibility is highly reliable among children and adults, there is considerable debate concerning the mech-

anisms underlying the suggestibility effect. One view is that the original memory trace for the event was changed (overwritten) as a result of the suggestion. A second hypothesis is that the postevent suggestion interferes with recollection because it renders the original memory unretrievable but unchanged, as in the case of creating access competition. Whereas these first two hypotheses posit memory impairments (which reflect storage failures) as the basis of suggestibility effects, a third hypothesis is that suggestibility effects reflect gap-filling strategies rather than a memorial distortion of the original event (e.g., McCloskey & Zaragoza, 1985a); subjects accept the misleading information because they have no memory for the original event. A fourth hypothesis is that suggestibility effects result from retrieval difficulties that reflect source monitoring difficulties. According to this view, the subject has simultaneous access to representations of the original event as well as to the erroneous suggestion but has difficulty distinguishing which one *was* the original event. Source confusions might occur when only the erroneous suggestion comes to mind, that is, even when the original event cannot be retrieved (Lindsay, 1990). Source monitoring difficulties can reflect source monitoring decisions that are fast and made without conscious deliberation, or they can reflect conscious processes, such as when the subject realizes that two competing memories exist and therefore carries out a deliberate reflective analysis to determine which is the original source. Finally, some researchers (e.g., McCloskey & Zaragoza, 1985a) have posited that suggestibility effects arise out of social pressures: The subject accepts the misleading information to please the experimenter or because the experimenter is trusted. In this section, we focus on the first three hypotheses. The claims about source monitoring problems and social influences are discussed later.

In the course of encoding an event, the memorizer carries out a string of pattern recognition and interpretative analyses. The former entails the abstraction of the features of the event, such as its contrast, shape, contour, and size, whereas the latter entails attaching meaning to the event, such as naming it, assigning it an emotional valence, or forming semantic associations to it. According to trace theorists (e.g., Brainerd & Reyna, 1988; Tulving & Watkins, 1975; Zaragoza, Dahlgren, & Muench, 1992), a memory trace is the record of such pattern recognition and interpretative analyses that are carried out at the time of encoding.[3] Over time, and in response to erroneous suggestions, a trace's features may begin to loosen until they are nearly "disintegrated." At the time of retrieval, it is possible for its features to be reassembled. Thus, there are both encoding and retrieval opportunities for distortion. In addition, trace theorists (Brainerd, Reyna, Howe, & Kingma, 1990) assume that the more interpretative semantic features are less

---

[3]There are many subtle differences among trace theorists, and the description of these is beyond the scope of this article (the interested reader should consult Howe, 1991, for a description of the differences among various trace-strength approaches).

vulnerable to encoding and to retrieval manipulations of all types (e.g., delay, interference, modifiability).

Trace theorists assume that the incorporation of postevent information occurs as a function of the strength of the trace, with weak traces being especially vulnerable to featural dilution or blending (i.e., "destructive updating") or erasure (Ceci, Toglia, & Ross, 1988). Incorporation of postevent information also occurs as a function of the degree of the trace's "fuzziness," with interpretative or gistlike traces being more resistant to postevent suggestions than verbatim traces.

Two mechanisms have been invoked to account for the greater susceptibility of weak traces to being altered. One has to do with the nature of weak traces themselves, which tend to be loosely integrated, thus permitting greater intrusion from external sources (Brainerd, Kingma, & Howe, 1985; Brainerd et al., 1990). Because a trace is a concatenation of features that represents the original event, once these features begin to unravel it permits the incorporation of suggested features. This type of incorporation or blending of features is less likely when a trace's features are tightly bundled. On the other hand, a weak trace may provide a more hospitable encoding context for an erroneous suggestion to be admitted into memory as a *coexisting trace*. Thus, in addition to the incorporation of isolated features of the erroneous suggestion into the original trace, it is also possible that the entire erroneous trace is encoded and is allowed to attain a status on par with the original trace in terms of its strength. This happens because the contents of a weak original trace may be inaccessible at the time the erroneous suggestion is made, thereby making the intruding suggestion more likely to be subsequently recalled because there is no strong coexisting trace for the original event to compete with (Ceci et al., 1988; Howe, 1991; McCloskey & Zaragoza, 1985a; Zaragoza et al., 1992).

One important prediction of trace theory is that age differences in memory impairments will occur because younger children encode weaker traces, which are more vulnerable to featural disintegration or overwriting and also because young children encode more verbatim perceptual features and fewer interpretative or gistlike representations than older individuals. As mentioned earlier, verbatim representations should not survive as long as gist representations because they are more susceptible to disintegration. There is some support for these predictions (Toglia, 1991). Several researchers have reported that children with weaker memories of the original event are less likely to resist to suggestions about that event (King & Yuille, 1987; Warren, Hulse-Trotter, & Tubbs, 1991). Although these researchers did not directly show that the postevent suggestions overwrote an original trace, Warren et al. (1991) concluded that misinformation exerts its strongest effect on traces that were previously unreported (i.e., those traces that are presumably weakest). The converse of this position is that if a child has a strong memory trace for an event, he or she will be highly resistant to suggestion (e.g., Goodman, 1984b). Hence, it may be futile to try to overwrite a child's memory for traces that have become strengthened as a result of repetition, such as a child's name or sex.

Thus, trace theory models make a priori predictions about the conditions under which age differences in suggestibility may be pronounced or attenuated. For example, Lindberg (1991) showed that there are times when older children will actually be more suggestible than younger children, such as when the younger child's greater knowledge about some material permits stronger, gistlike encodings or when older subjects' greater knowledge leads them to make erroneous inferences that are impossible for the younger children to make because of their lack of the requisite knowledge. A good example of this latter situation can be found in the study by Duncan et al. (1982), mentioned earlier. When those researchers analyzed only the trials in which subjects correctly answered all of the control questions (i.e., the questions that were not related to the correct or incorrect postevent suggestions), they found that the youngest subjects were *less* likely to be influenced by erroneous postevent information than were the college students.[4]

However, barring the exceptional cases in which young children encode more enduring traces, the normal developmental path is from weak, verbatim traces to more durable gistlike traces. This more common pattern will ordinarily result in age-related differences favoring reduced suggestibility in older subjects.

One feature of the trace strength work that deserves special mention is the claim that some, perhaps even most, of the variance in the observed age differences in suggestibility resides at the time of *encoding* as opposed to during retrieval. On the basis of extensive analyses, some theorists conclude that age dif-

---

[4]Duncan, Whitney, and Kunen's (1982) procedure might have underestimated younger children's suggestibility in two ways: First, because it was based exclusively on trials in which the trace was strong, this might have favored immutability (Brainerd, Reyna, Howe, & Kingma, 1990). However, when Duncan et al. did not exclude weaker trace data from their analyses, age differences favoring younger children disappeared. Second, to the extent that there exist age-related differences in the contents of an encoding, the use of postevent semantic information to alter a visual memory might have worked in favor of first graders being less suggestible because they might have encoded primarily perceptual or *verbatim* features from the visually presented slides of the Duncan et al. *Star Wars* story, whereas the older subjects might have encoded the *gistlike* semantic features of the story. Hence, the use of verbal postevent information might have been encoded semantically (as gist) by the college students and integrated with their earlier semantic codes, whereas younger subjects might have encoded a verbatim trace that was never integrated with the postevent gistlike questioning. Duncan et al. acknowledged this possibility in their conclusion. This is the only study of which we are aware that has used a traditional suggestibility design and found greater suggestibility effects for adults than children. We did not describe in the text a study by Leippe, Romanczyk, and Manion (1991), which reported that adults "acquiesced" more than children, because the questions used in this study would not be considered nonsuggestive in most traditional suggestibility paradigms (see Goodman, Rudy, Bottoms, & Aman, 1990, p. 260). Moreover, the results of the Leippe et al. (1991) study can be interpreted differently depending on which questions are regarded as reflecting acquiescence. This makes it unclear if acquiescence is conceptually the same as suggestibility.

ferences in suggestibility arise primarily because younger children store traces that are more apt to be overwritten by subsequent suggestions (i.e., trace destruction), not because younger children have more difficulty retrieving traces, the so-called trace competition (Lindberg, 1991). In a developmental study, Howe (1991) found that when misinformation effects occurred, they were related to alterations in the original trace and not to trace competition. If replicated and extended, this would suggest that some of the susceptibility of younger children to postevent suggestion might involve actual trace destruction as opposed to trace coexistence or competition. To the extent that this is true, subsequent probing or context reinstatement cannot undo the damage caused by erroneous suggestions.

Some trace theorists have challenged the notion that memory impairment is related to trace strength and more generally that suggestibility reflects memory impairments. The Modified Test was introduced by McCloskey and Zaragoza (1985a) as a means of determining the degree to which suggestibility effects reflect memory impairments. This test is similar to the standard paradigm developed by Loftus et al. (1978), but instead of asking subjects to choose between the original event and the erroneous event (e.g., a hammer and a wrench in the example provided earlier), they are required to choose between the original event and a new event that has not been seen or suggested (e.g., a hammer and a screwdriver in the example provided earlier). If subjects' memory for the hammer has been impaired by the provision of the wrench suggestion, then when shown the hammer and the screwdriver, subjects should select the screwdriver more often compared with a nonmisled control group. However, if subjects select the screwdriver as frequently as a nonmisled control group, then suggestibility effects reported in standard procedures (i.e., selecting the wrench over the hammer) do not reflect memory impairment but social factors (which are discussed in a separate section) or gap-filling strategies. That is, the subject does not remember the original event but does remember the postevent information and uses this to "fill in the gap" of the missing memory. The gap-filling-strategy hypothesis seems particularly relevant for the elucidation of developmental differences in children's suggestibility in that there are reliable age differences in rates of forgetting (Brainerd et al., 1985, 1990). Thus, when asked to reconstruct the original event, younger children may readily accept misinformation to fill in missing memories.

The Modified Test has produced mixed results in the study of children's suggestibility. Zaragoza et al. (1992) found no evidence of memory-based impairment in four separate experiments. Ceci et al. (1987) reported evidence of memory impairment in their third and fourth experiments, and Delamothe and Taplin (1992) reported evidence of an impairment using the Modified Test, with both 5- and 10-year-olds. There are several procedural differences between these three sets of studies (e.g., the number of times the suggestion was given, whether it was a within- or a between-subjects design, the length of the retention interval), but it is not obvious a priori why these differences should have resulted in such different outcomes.

In a slightly different paradigm in which kindergarten and Grade 2 children were told a story, provided with misleading information and then several days later asked to recall the story, Howe (1991) found that the children showed little evidence of memory impairments. That is, although children added more intrusions to their recollections when their encoding of an event was weak, the content of these intrusions was not related to the erroneous suggestions. He concluded that

> the degree of trace strength . . . is not directly related to memory impairment effects. That is, although trace strength is directly related to the rate of forgetting and the number of schema- and misinformation-relevant intrusions, it does not impair recall of the original story details. . . . Overall, . . . weak traces are no more susceptible to misleading information than strong traces. (Howe, 1991, p. 760)

This is a view echoed by Zaragoza et al. (1992).

The resolution to this dispute may have to do with the "boundary conditions" on the memory impairment effect. It may be that memory impairment occurs only when certain conditions exist, such as the strength of the erroneous suggestion (a function of, among other things, the number of times that the erroneous suggestion is made) in interaction with the strength of the original trace. Certain events, such as dynamic ones that involve actions, may have more durable trace strengths that render them more resistant to alteration than other types of events, such as those containing static attributes. For instance, Schwartz-Kenney and Goodman (1991) found that although memory-based impairment does occur for 6- and 9-year-olds, it does so only for memories having to do with person and location information, not for memories of actions. On the other hand, Rovee-Collier and Borza (in press) conducted five experiments with 3-month-olds in which evidence for memory impairment seemed strong. Infants were trained to kick in order to make an overhead mobile move across their crib. Once they acquired this association between kicking and mobile movement, they were exposed to a novel mobile overhead that was unconnected to their kicking. During later tests of memory, features of the novel mobile impaired infants' memory for the original mobile. Rovee-Collier and Borza reasoned that their paradigm contained all of the ingredients of the Modified Test: First, infants witnessed an event (a mobile moving). Second, they were exposed to postevent information that conflicted with their original memory (a new mobile that did not move in conjunction with their foot kicking). Third, they were tested for their memory of the original event.

Of course, this area of study is still in its early stages. Although the Modified

Test procedure sometimes fails to produce evidence of memory impairment, these results by themselves do not indicate the source of children's (or adults') difficulties on standard misinformation paradigms; they merely indicate that acceptance of the postevent misinformation on some occasions does not reflect memory impairment. However, the results do not indicate whether social mechanisms or other cognitive mechanisms (e.g., filling-in-the-gap procedures) underpin suggestibility effects. It is also the case that the correlational data presented on the relation between children's memories and suggestibility may just as easily support a gap-filling position (no memories or unreported memories are associated with acceptance of the misleading information) as a memory impairment position. Finally, as must also be clear from this review of the literature, few of the studies were developmental. Thus, more research is required to examine the memorial bases of suggestibility effects in children as well as to determine the degree to which age-related increases in memorial skills are directly related to age-related increases in resistance to suggestive questioning.

Linguistic

Linguistic competence is also implicated in suggestibility. Because many of the studies of suggestibility include a wide age range of children of varying levels of language skill, it is reasonable to assume that there may be age differences in understanding the original events if they are verbally presented (see Garbarino & Stott, 1989; Nurcombe, 1986, for similar points). It is also possible that children's understanding of the lexical items and syntactic structures used to test their memories may differ as a function of age. (Children's understanding of the social intents of verbal interactions are discussed in a later section on social factors.) Finally, adults may incorrectly interpret children's verbal reports as a result of children's limited production skills.

Some researchers have documented children's limited understanding of legal concepts (Saywitz, 1989; Warren-Leubecker, Tate, Hinton, & Ozbek, 1989) or have examined the complexity of the language used within the courtroom setting (Walker, 1988) and children's actual comprehension of courtroom language (Brennan & Brennan, 1988). Although these data provide important glimpses into children's comprehension of legal language, these studies do not bear directly on the issue of suggestibility.

One of the few studies to examine the effects of linguistic structure on children's suggestibility was inspired by work with adults (Loftus & Zanni, 1975). After viewing a short film, adults were asked several questions about the events. They gave more false recognitions to questions with definite articles (e.g., Did you see *the* car?) versus indefinite articles (e.g., Did you see *a* car?). The same pattern was found for 4- and 5-year-olds (Dale, Loftus, & Rathbun, 1978). The use of definite articles in questions produced more answers to questions about nondepicted events. Thus, young children appear to have the same understanding of this particular linguistic marker as do adults.

A second study examined children's responses to questions containing marked and unmarked modifiers. An example of a pair of unmarked and marked modifiers is *fast* versus *slow*. The unmarked term *fast* carries no assumption concerning an upper or lower bound, whereas the marked term *slow* implies the absence of the property in question. Children generally acquired the unmarked form of a pair before the marked form (Clark & Clark, 1977). Lipscomb, Bregman, and McCallister (1984) showed first- through eighth-grade children and college students a film of an automobile collision. Subjects were then questioned about the speed of the car using marked or unmarked terms (e.g., "How slow/fast was the car going when it smashed/hit the other car?"). Subjects of all ages provided faster estimates to questions with the word *fast* than to questions with the word *slow*. However, only seventh and eighth graders provided faster speed estimates when the word *smashed* was used. These results are suggestive only of developmental differences because the adult subjects did not provide different estimates for *smashed* and *hit*, a result discrepant with that obtained by Loftus and Palmer (1974).

Hence, it is possible that the way questions are worded may affect age patterns in suggestibility. If young children do not have full syntactic or semantic understanding of linguistic features, they may not be biased in the same way as older children, thus canceling out any potential suggestibility effect. Therefore, the inconsistent results of some developmental studies may reflect subtle linguistic differences among stimuli.

Knowledge

Semantic. Semantic knowledge refers to an individual's repository of world knowledge about the declarative, procedural, and associative meanings of concepts. Memories of events reflect, among other things, how much was known about the event prior to its observation and how this knowledge is represented in memory. Thus, chess masters recall board positions of past games better than nonmasters, and baseball experts remember more details about baseball games than nonexperts (see Chi & Ceci, 1987). Occasionally, younger children possess superior knowledge to older children (e.g., about cartoons), and in these cases they often excel at remembering (Chi & Ceci, 1987; Lindberg, 1980).

In addition to the sheer amount of factual knowledge, the representation of this knowledge in long-term memory (i.e., its relational and implicational structure) plays an important role in recall. If a 7-year-old's knowledge about a character is that she is strong and smart, then an implication might be that she is also attractive. When children with such beliefs try to recall incongruous events about characters (e.g., a character is smart and strong yet unattractive), they often can do so if tested immediately, while the trace is still strong. However, when the trace has been weakened because of a 3-week delay, children make erroneous recalls that are consistent with their prior knowledge but inconsistent with what they actually saw (Ceci, Caves, & Howe, 1981). Similarly, 5- and 6-year-olds who have differentiated sex-based knowledge often incorrectly select the pictures seen 1 week previously of male and female actors performing sex-incongruent tasks (Martin & Halverson, 1983). They report having seen a picture of a male actor playing a traditional male role even though it was a female actor who was depicted in the picture.

Thus, developmental differences in the structure of semantic knowledge can lead to different inferences about witnessed events. Usually, increased knowledge facilitates recall, but not invariably. One qualification to this broad conclusion is warranted: When the event being recalled is so unlike a child's representation that it appears bizarre, then it is recalled more accurately (Davidson, 1991). Nonplausible details and events can actually facilitate memory if they are so different from the child's knowledge as to appear bizarre.

Scripted knowledge. Temporally organized, habitual, agent-actor-action routines are referred to as *scripts*. For example, a restaurant script includes the expectation that the customer is first seated by the waitress, given a menu, places his or her order, and so forth. Scripts serve to generate expectations, and when the expectations run counter to what occurred, the result can be that scripts produce an erroneous reconstruction of the events.

Although scripts develop with age, even very young children possess these for familiar events. These scripts influence the child's reconstruction of previously experienced events. In certain conditions scripted knowledge may exert positive effects on memory reconstruction. For example, if children have a script for the sequence of events that unfolds in a normal school day, they may unconsciously use scripts to fill in gaps when their actual memory has faded (Myles-Worsley, Cromer, & Dodd, 1986).

However, scripted knowledge may also exert negative effects on memory. If a girl has attended multiple gym classes, she is more likely than a child who has attended only one workshop to erroneously claim that a particular habitual act (e.g., stretching) occurred even when it did not (Hudson, 1990). This is because attending multiple gym classes or school events that share the same structure leads to the creation of generalized scripts, something that one-time attendees do not possess.

The relation between scripted knowledge and accurate recall may change as a function of age, depending on the level of children's scripted knowledge and the characteristics of the to-be-remembered event (Ceci et al., 1981). Once children have acquired scripts, preschoolers' recall may be more vulnerable to the negative effects of script-based knowledge than elementary school-aged children. Hudson and Nelson (1986) summarized their research in this area by concluding that pre-schoolers were less flexible than older children; they were more likely to read off scripts than to recall single episodes. When the information was discrepant or unexpected in relation to scripts, preschoolers had more trouble recalling this information than older children. Farrar and Goodman (1990) elaborated this posi-tion by examining recall in relation to children's development of scripted knowl-edge. Young (4-year-old) and older (7-year-old) children experienced an unfamiliar event in a laboratory on several different occasions. These repeated experiences were intended to allow the children to develop script-based knowl-edge for these "standard" events. The children then experienced a novel set of events called *deviation events.* One week later, the children were asked to recall the standard and deviation events. The older children were able to distinguish between their memories for the standard and deviation events. That is, they devel-oped a script for the standard events, and the deviation events were separately tagged in memory. By contrast, the younger children confused the events from the two different sets of experiences; they incorporated the deviation events into their developing schemata of the standard events. The results of these studies provide a theoretical basis for age differences in suggestibility. Younger children are more suggestible because they are overly dependent on scripted knowledge and incor-porate discrepant or novel events (which could be a suggestion) into their script of the event rather than keeping them tagged as separate events.

When younger children's scripted knowledge is insufficient or poorer than that of older children, older children might make more false inferences about events that are not witnessed but that are part of their scripts. Lindberg (1991) showed this to be the case. Because of their more elaborate scripts about how cheating could occur, sixth graders and college students made more false attributions than third graders about an ambiguous event. When subjects were erroneously told that the film they were viewing depicted cheaters, sixth graders and college students tended to report cheating that was based on innocent acts such as a student asking another for the time of day. Younger children's scripts for cheating did not contain this scenario as a pretext for cheating, so their limited script knowledge made them less prone to the erroneous suggestion. Along the same lines, adults are more likely than young children to assume that on meeting someone, they are to shake the person's hand because doing so is part of their script for new encounters (Goodman & Reed, 1986).

The finding of Duncan et al. (1982) of greater suggestibility on the part of older subjects may also reflect the interfering effects of scripted knowledge. Their task required the integration of high levels of scripted knowledge, which the youngest children probably did not possess, thereby precluding its effectiveness as a source of biasing. For example, the supposition embedded in the question, "Was the hunter's fishing pole broken by a bear?" (in reality, the hunter did not have a fishing pole but a spear), may be more easily integrated into a college student's "hunting" script than a first grader's, thus leading adults to integrate the misinformation with the original information more readily than younger children.

In summary, it seems reasonable to assume that a positive relation exists between the amount and structure of knowledge and children's resistance to suggestion, at least in cases in which an event is congruent with existing knowledge. In other situations, older children and adults may be more suggestible than young children because their greater knowledge might lead them to infer script-relevant details that were omitted from the actual event or to integrate postevent information with the original event.

Stereotypical knowledge. Stereotypes are naive theories about personal characteristics that organize and structure experience by directing individuals to look for certain types of information and advising them on how to interpret it. Stereotypes are a form of schematic knowledge that helps organize memory, sometimes distorting what is perceived by adding thematically congruent information that was not perceived (Martin & Halverson, 1983).

Little is known about whether there are reliable age differences in the tendency to extrapolate from stereotypical knowledge to provide erroneous but plausible accounts of nonwitnessed events. However, even 3- and 4-year-olds will sometimes be misled and claim to have witnessed events that did not occur but that are consistent with a stereotype. For instance, a character named Sam Stone was described over a 1-month period to 3- to 6-year-olds as someone who was very clumsy and who always broke things that did not belong to him (Ceci, Leichtman, & White, in press). After this stereotype-induction procedure, Sam Stone visited the children's nursery school, where he spent 2 min amiably interacting with the children during a group story-telling session. At that time he did not behave clumsily or break anything. The following day, the children were shown a ripped book and a soiled teddy bear. They were asked if they knew how the book had been ripped and the teddy bear soiled. Few children claimed to have seen Sam Stone do these things, but 25% said that *perhaps* he had done it—a reasonable statement given the stereotype-induction they had received. Next, the children were interviewed once per 2 weeks for 2 min each over the course of the next 10 weeks. During each interview, the children were asked two leading questions such as "I wonder whether Sam Stone was wearing long pants or short pants when he ripped the book?" or "I wonder if Sam Stone got the teddy bear dirty on purpose or by accident?" These suggestive questions were consistent with the stereotype that had been previously provided, and nearly all of the children answered them. At the end of this 10-week interrogation period, the children were interviewed by a new interviewer who told them she was not at their school the day Sam Stone visited and wanted to know everything that happened. When asked, 72% of the 3- and 4-year-olds said Sam Stone had ruined at least one of the items in question (the book or bear). When they were explicitly asked, 45% of the 3- and 4-year-olds replied that they actually had seen him do these things, as opposed to merely being told that he did. These false accounts often were embellished with perceptual details (e.g., Sam Stone took a paint brush and painted melted chocolate on the teddy bear, Sam took the book into the bathroom and soaked it in warm water until it fell apart) or emotional details (e.g., Sam was acting very silly when he spilled coffee on the bear, Sam was mad and ripped the book with his hands). In contrast to the 3- and 4-year-olds, only 11% of the 5- to 6-year-olds claimed to have actually observed Sam Stone damage the items. A control group, who received only the multiple suggestive interviews, with no prior stereotypical knowledge about Sam, made significantly fewer false claims than children who were given stereotypical knowledge. Thus, these results indicate that not only do young children form stereotypes but that stereotype formation interacts with suggestive questioning to a greater extent for younger than older children.

Much work remains to be carried out on the relation of semantic, scripted, and stereotypical knowledge to suggestibility. Nevertheless, the existing work indicates that the quality and quantity of memory representations influence subsequent recall and susceptibility to suggestibility. Although most of the time this works in favor of older children and adults, special circumstances can be found wherein younger children's lack of knowledge actually prevents them from succumbing to an erroneous suggestion.

Source Monitoring: Distinguishing Reality From Fantasy

An important but relatively unexplored cognitive variable is the extent to which suggestibility in children arises from an incapacity to distinguish between the various sources of their memory. Freud (1933/1966) postulated that claims of childhood sexual abuse by his female adult patients were false, reflecting their inability as children to distinguish between reality and fantasy (however, see Masson, 1984, for an alternate account). Freud thought it possible to retrieve original memories through the removal of symbolic transformations that "blockaded" them from consciousness. Piaget (1926), however, was less optimistic that early memories could be separated from fantasies, commenting that "the child's mind is full of these 'ludistic' (fantasy play) tendencies up to the age of seven or eight, which means before that age it is very difficult for him to distinguish the truth" (p. 34).

Outside of the classical work on animism by Piagetians, the topic of reality monitoring did not receive empirical scrutiny until the 1970s, when a number of researchers converged on the view that young children were able to distinguish between reality and fantasy (Flavell, Flavell, & Green, 1987; Morison & Gardner, 1978; Taylor & Howell, 1973). For example, Morison and Gardner (1978) presented 5- to 12-year-olds with three toys and asked them to group fantasy figures (e.g., a dragon and elf) and to exclude real figures (e.g., a frog). Even 5-year-olds were highly accurate, although errors decreased with age.

Harris, Brown, Marriott, Whittall, and Harmer's (1991) results modify these conclusions in important ways. As in previous studies, 4- and 6-year-olds reliably distinguished between fantasy and reality; most children rightfully stated that imagined ghosts, monsters, and witches were not real. However, when told to imagine a pretend character that was sitting in a box, after a short period of time many of the children began to act as though the pretend character was real. For example, half of the children were told that the pretend character was a rabbit and half were told that it was a monster. The experimenter then said she had to leave the room for a few minutes; four of the twelve 4-year-olds who were told that there was a pretend monster in the box would not let her leave the room even though they had just seen and stated that the box was empty. None of the other children acted this way. When the experimenter returned, almost half of the children in both age groups wondered whether perhaps three was an imaginary creature in the box. Questioning uncovered some magical and unrealistic thinking. Although almost all of the children admitted to pretense before the experimenter's departure, 25% of the children now thought that pretend creatures could become real. These data reflect the fragile boundaries of children's fantasy–reality distinctions. When situations become intense, children appear to easily give up these distinctions. Although the children were repeatedly assured that the creatures were imagined, it seems that the experimental procedure was mildly suggestive, breaking down their shaky differentiations, and the 4-year-olds had more fragile boundaries than did the 6-year-olds. In both case studies (summarized at the beginning of this article), children's disclosures became increasingly bizarre and incredible. This evolution could have been caused by the interviewers not drawing the children back to reality when they made "fantastic" claims and perhaps as a result, their allegations moved from fantasy to reality for the children who came to believe themselves.

Another area of research focuses in greater detail on young children's difficulty distinguishing between what they experienced through perception and what they only imagined they experienced. Johnson and her colleagues have been at the forefront of this area for a decade (see M. K. Johnson, 1991, for a review; Foley & Johnson, 1985; Lindsay et al., 1991). In the most comprehensive model, the "multiple-entry modular memory system," recollection is based on the interplay of two subsystems. The perceptual system records and stores the contents of perceptual processes such as seeing and hearing, whereas the reflective system records psychologically generated information such as imagining, thinking, and speculating. Developmental differences in reality–fantasy monitoring could reflect the earlier functional capability of the perceptual subsystems and the later development of the reflective systems. At issue is whether these subsystems are developmentally invariant or unfold over a long period of time (Lindsay et al., 1991).

When asked to judge whether they had said a word versus imagined saying it, 6-year-olds have more difficulty discriminating between these two sources of memories than 9-year-olds and adults (e.g., Foley et al., 1983). Apparently, the cues involved in differentiating between certain types of actual and imagined events may not be well developed before late childhood. Because young children do not have difficulty distinguishing between something they said (or did) and something that someone else said (or did), it seems that they can differentiate between these sources of their memories except in situations in which at least one of the sources is self-generated (Foley, Santini, & Sopasakis, in press). Specifically, younger children are more error prone at distinguishing between real versus imagined acts or words when both concern themselves, but they are no worse than adults when it comes to judging whether an act (or words) was performed (or spoken) or imagined by themselves versus someone else.

Recently, however, a more general source monitoring framework has been invoked to account for young children's source confusions. According to this account, young children find it especially difficult to separate sources of information that are perceptually and semantically similar. For example, 7- and 10-year-olds and adults were shown a videotape of a set of actions and were instructed to either perform, to watch others perform, to imagine themselves perform, or to imagine another perform these actions (e.g., "Please watch the girl touch her nose" vs. "Please imagine touching your nose"). Subjects were later asked to indicate for each of a list of actions which acts had actually been performed and which they had imagined and which were new. Compared with adults, children found it more difficult to distinguish between imagined and actual actions if the same actor was involved in both kinds of actions (e.g., watching vs. imagining the girl touch her nose). By contrast, young children performed as well as adults when the sources of information were relatively discriminable (self vs. girl). Thus, although all age groups reliably distinguished between the actions of two perceptually or semantically distinct actors, "children are more likely to confuse memories from different sources whenever those sources are highly similar to one another" (Lindsay et al., 1991, p. 18).

Source monitoring studies suggest that children could be vulnerable to a range of confusions between actual events and suggested events when they are perceptually and semantically similar. However, because the locus of children's greater misattributions is unclear, and there are no data that link children's suggestibility and source monitoring difficulties (see Lindsay, 1990, for adult data), these claims are speculative at this stage.

Summary: Cognitive Abilities

Although our review of cognitive factors does not include all of the cognitive variables that could conceivably be involved in age differences in suggestibility (e.g., inferential skills; abstract reasoning abilities; perspective-taking, metacognitive skills), it does describe the factors that have received the attention of researchers. In view of the previous discussion of the fundamental role that the development of these abilities plays in decreasing children's susceptibility to suggestion, it is not surprising that IQ tests that measure many of these cognitive skills correlate with children's levels of suggestibility (e.g., Hurlock, 1930; Otis, 1924). Recently, Haugaard and Repucci (1992) reported that although IQ was unrelated to children's accuracy in realizing that another child was inaccurate in claiming that her neighbor hit her, preschoolers with low IQ scores were more likely to erroneously attribute this inaccuracy to truthfulness on the part of the child. We now discuss social and motivational factors that need to be considered to explain age differences in suggestibility.

CAUSAL MECHANISMS: SOCIAL AND MOTIVATIONAL FACTORS

As originally suggested by early researchers such as Binet, Stern, Varendonck, and Lipmann, children's suggestibility is not purely a cognitive phenomenon but also reflects social and motivational factors. After a 70-year hiatus, modern researchers have begun to examine the potential effects of selected social and motivational factors on children's suggestibility. In this section, we focus on specific conditions within an interview that induce compliance to the interviewer's misleading questions.

An interview is successful when the interviewer obtains a complete and accurate account from the interviewee. In order to achieve this goal, more is required than the accurate comprehension and production of linguistic utterances. In addition, participants must understand a broader set of conversational rules that bind the questions and answers. Of particular importance to the present topic is the degree to which children's performance in an interview reflects their understanding of the social rules underlying conversations.

In an interview, the listener tries to figure out the speaker's intent; often, this involves going beyond the direct meaning and computing an indirect meaning. The number of interpretations of messages, however, is constrained by the social conventions and context of the interview. These social conventions include the "principle of cooperativity" (Grice, 1975), which states that listeners interpret speakers' utterances on the assumption that they are informative, true, relevant, and clear. These assumptions about cooperativity, which are used to infer the meaning and intent of utterances, may change as a function of the social relationships, perceived motivations, beliefs of the participants, and the actual setting of the conversation. Good listeners ask, "Given the context of this conversation, what is the intended meaning of the utterance?" If there is a disjunction between a questioner's goals and a listener's perceptions of these goals, the interaction will not be successful.

From an early age, children perceive their adult conversational partners as being cooperative, truthful, and not deceptive (Garvey, 1984; Nelson & Gruendel, 1979; Romaine, 1984). Children are also cooperative partners; they supply their adult questioner with the type of information they think is being requested (e.g., Ervin-Tripp, 1978; Read & Cherry, 1978). This pattern reflects children's desire to comply with a respected authority figure. As a result, when questioned by adults, children sometimes attempt to make their answers consistent with what they see as the intent of the questioner rather than consistent with their knowledge of the event. Several pieces of data support these contentions.

First, young children perceive adults as being highly credible and competent sources of information; they place more faith in the credibility of adults' statements than in those of their peers. Sonnenschein and Whitehurst (1980) reported that 6-year-olds became better referential speakers after listening to competent peers, but not after listening to incompetent adults, because they assumed that all adults are competent. Ackerman (1983) presented first and third graders and adults with paragraphs containing contradictory information between a contextual source that was either authoritative (e.g., a doctor) or nonauthoritative (e.g., a janitor) and a speaker that was either a child or an adult. Subjects were asked which source of information was the most believable. Adults based their judgments on the authority of the source, whereas first graders based their judgments on the age of the speaker, with adult speakers being rated as more believable than children regardless of authoritativeness. Third graders weighed both sources of information. These data suggest that young children are biased to believe adults and to accept their statements as credible.

Second, children attempt to answer adults' questions even if the questions are bizarre. When asked nonsensical questions such as "Is milk bigger than water?", most 5- and 7-year-olds replied "yes" or "no"; they rarely responded "I don't know" (Hughes & Grieve, 1980). These data suggest that children perceive adults as being cooperative conversationalists who ask honest and logical questions that must have an answer. Pratt (1991) reported that adults are not immune to such pressures; they (i.e., adults) also provide answers to some types of bizarre questions even if preschoolers are more pervasively willing to do so.

Finally, when children are asked the same question more than once, they often change their answers presumably because they interpret the repeated question as "I must not have given the correct response the first time; therefore, to comply and be a good conversational partner, I must try to provide new information." In Cassel and Bjorklund's (1992) study of children's memory for a bicycle theft, 42% of kindergarten children changed their mind on repeated questioning. Young children's responses to Piagetian conservation questions are more accurate when they are asked only once versus several times, as a result of their proclivity to change their answers in response to their impression of what the interviewer wants them to say (Gelman, Meck, & Merkin, 1986; Rose & Blank, 1974; Siegal, Waters, & Dinwiddy, 1988). Siegal et al. (1988) showed young children a videotape of a puppet being given a conservation test. After the puppet made a response, the children were asked if it had responded to please the adult or because that was what the puppet really thought was true. The children were more likely to say that the puppet pleased the experimenter when he gave an incorrect response in a two-question interview. By contrast, they were more likely to say that the puppet really thought the answer was true in the one-question procedure.

Although these results suggest that repeated questioning within the same session may decrease the consistency of children's performance, they do not address the potential effects of repeated questioning across (as opposed to within) sessions. Repeated questioning across sessions has at times facilitated memory, possibly because recalling an event is a form of rehearsal that serves to reactivate traces. This has been found in several studies in which children have recalled approximately 10% more information on repeated recall versus a single test (Baker-Ward, Hess, & Flannagan, 1990; Brainerd et al., 1990; Tucker, Merton, & Luszcz, 1990). In other studies, however, facilitation has not been found (Dent & Stephenson, 1979; Flin et al., 1992; Ornstein et al., 1992; Steward, 1989; Warren & Swartwood, in press). For example, Dent and Stephenson (1979) found that 10- and 11-year-olds gave virtually identical answers to the same questions that were posed on 2 consecutive days. Similarly, Steward (1989) found that repeated questioning of children between the ages of 3 and 7 years led to equivalent performance regardless of whether the children were questioned one, two, or three times over a 6-month period.

The data just reviewed about social factors are relevant to the issues of children's testimony and suggestibility because they point to the possibility that children provide incorrect answers to suggestive questions because they view the interviewer as asking credible questions and thus incorporate the content of the question into their answers. Unlike adults, children may rarely challenge the credibility of adult questioners. If true, then the following manipulations to an interview should result in reduced suggestibility. When children rather than adults provide misleading information to other children, suggestibility effects should be diminished because peers should be viewed as being less trustworthy and authoritative than adults. Also, if children are told that it is permissible to say "I don't know" or if they are warned that the experimenter may be trying to trick them, they should be less suggestible. Finally, if children are asked repeatedly to recall a specific event, their responses to the first question should be more accurate than their responses to repeated questions because the first question does not imply that a prior answer was incorrect or otherwise undesirable. Data supporting some of these hypotheses exist.

Ceci et al. (1987) presented short stories accompanied by illustrations to preschool children. One day following the presentation, an adult (Experiment 1) or a 7-year-old child (Experiment 2) provided misleading information about certain aspects of the stories. Two days later, the children were questioned. Children were less suggestible when they were given the same misleading information by a child than by an adult, indicating that they yielded the contents of their own memory to that of a more powerful adult authority figure—something they did less often when the misinformation was supplied by another child.

Moston (1987) questioned 6- to 10-year-olds about an event that was observed during a school assembly. Half the children were told that it was acceptable to give "I don't know" responses. Provision of the "don't know" instruction did not result in increased accuracy or in "don't know" responses. Contrary to other results, even children in the control group gave a number of "don't know" responses, and all children gave more "don't know" responses to misleading than to direct questions. Thus, the results of this study do not provide support for the hypothesis that children are unwilling to provide "don't know" answers, especially in response to misleading questions.

When children are given some warning about the potential for deceit or false suggestions by their questioner, they are more resistant to misleading questions. Warren et al. (1991) read a story to subjects (aged 7, 12, and adult) and then asked questions about the story, some of which were misleading. At the onset of the experiment, half of the subjects were warned that the questions were difficult or tricky and that they should try to answer only what they really remembered. At all ages, warned subjects correctly answered more misleading questions than unwarned subjects. It should be noted, however, that the effect was equally small across all age groups; the warning increased subjects' accuracy by approximately 5%.

The effect of repeated questions on children's recall has been the focus of several studies. In the Warren et al. (1991) study, subjects were told after answering the first round of questions that they did not do so well and that they should try again. When told this, children changed their answers more often than did adults. As part of Moston's (1987) study, subjects were asked the same questions twice within the same interview session. The number of correct responses significantly declined from the first question to the second question, in line with the Piagetian studies mentioned earlier. Although Moston found that accurate responses dropped overall, from 69% to 54%, the effect of repeating a question was especially dramatic for the youngest children (6-year-olds), whose accuracy fell from 60% to 39%. In contrast to their 21% drop, the two older groups' accuracy rate dropped 9%–16%. Moston interpreted the decline to have been caused by the children's belief that the experimenter was "telling" them that their first answer was wrong or unacceptable.

Poole and White (1991) examined the effects of repeated questioning within and across sessions. In this study, 4-, 6-, and 8-year-olds as well as adults witnessed an ambiguous event. Half of the subjects were interviewed immediately after the event and 1 week later. The remaining subjects were interviewed only once, 1 week after the event. Within each session, all questions were asked three times. Although Poole and White did not use leading questions, their repeated use of yes–no questions can be viewed as a subtle form of suggestion. As noted earlier, simply repeating a yes–no question could have the effect of suggesting to a child that the interviewer is unsatisfied with the initial answer.

Poole and White (1991) found that repeated questioning with open-ended questions, both within and across sessions, had little effect (positive or negative) on children's or adults' responses. However, on repeated yes–no questions, 4-year-olds were most likely to change their responses, both within and across sessions. Thus, the major finding of this study was that repeated questioning may affect very young children's responses to specific questions. Although repeating open-ended questions may merely signal a request for additional information, repeating specific questions that have a limited pool of responses (yes or no) may signal to young children that their first response was unacceptable. This finding is important because young children tend to give limited responses to open-ended questions, and therefore interviewers often resort to specific questions to elicit additional information. In order to confirm a child's answer, interviewers frequently repeat the question. In a 2-year follow-up study, Poole (in press) found that the youngest children were significantly less accurate between and within interviews.

The results of these modern studies are reminiscent of those of Binet, Lipmann, and Stern, all of whom spoke of the authority of the interviewer in the eyes of the child. According to their accounts, children view interviewers' questions as imperatives to answer, or else they attempt to revise or fill in memory gaps in order to please the experimenter. This is illustrated dramatically in some court cases. For example, in a highly publicized sexual abuse case in Jordan, Minnesota, in 1984, one child later confessed that he fabricated detailed stories of abuse because "I could tell what they wanted me to say by the way they asked the questions" (Benedek & Schetky, 1987, p. 915).

Although the studies just described highlight how particular aspects of an interview may influence children's reports, these experimental settings are pale versions of interviews carried out in legal settings (McGough, in press). In the latter context, children are questioned, on average, 11 times prior to testifying in court, often by a number of different interviewers (e.g., parents, police, therapists, child protection workers, lawyers) who usually do not have a specific set of written questions. Rather, interviewers generally use a variety of on-line strategies before and during the interview to obtain the most detailed and accurate information about events that a child might have witnessed.

Interview strategies are characterized not only by the types of questions asked (open ended vs. yes–no) but also by the emotional tone or disposition of the interviewer. It is also the case that interviewers often do not have complete or accurate information about the target events that are the basis of the interview. This is important because an absence of knowledge or incorrect knowledge about the target events may affect the style of the interview, which may affect children's suggestibility. Furthermore, some interviewers may have strong vested interests in a particular type of report.

Clinical psychologists place particular importance on building rapport with young clients so that they will feel relaxed and nonthreatened. To achieve this goal, they act positively toward the children by encouraging and reinforcing their answers and, on rare occasion, chastising their failure to disclose. Interviewers are sometimes criticized for reinforcing and encouraging children's responses (Raskin & Yuille, 1989). It is claimed that these strategies are not conducive to accurate reporting, as can be illustrated by a social worker's interview of Child 5C in the Kelly Michaels' Wee Care case study:

> do you want to sit on my lap? Come here. I am so proud of you. I love big girls like you that tell me what happened—that aren't afraid because I am here to protect you. . . . You got such pretty eyes. . . . I'm jealous, I'm too old for you. (7/3/85 at 12 in Point VII of the Appelate Court Brief)

A few studies have examined how the emotional tone of an interview influences children's recall, and these results are not entirely consistent. Goodman et al. (1990) interviewed 3- to 7-year-olds 2–4 weeks after they had received an inoculation. They were interviewed either by a "nice" person who gave them considerable support for their performance throughout the interview or by a neutral experimenter who provided little support for their performance by maintaining a detached manner of interacting. All children were asked a series of specific and misleading questions; in addition, they were asked a set of misleading abuse questions (e.g., "Did he take you into the bathroom?"). Data were reported only for the last set of questions. Although interview style had no effect on older children's false reports, younger children gave fewer false reports to "nice" interviewers, and in one subclass of leading questions, the age effect was eliminated entirely. Goodman et al. concluded that young children were most resistant to misleading abuse questions, and less likely to falsely claim their clothes had been removed, or their bottoms touched, when they felt comfortable with the interviewer.

In another study (Saywitz, Geiselman, & Bornstein, 1992), detectives from a sheriff's office used a variety of interviewing techniques and personal styles when questioning third and sixth graders about a staged event. Children who were engaged in the most rapport-building events before the interview produced the fewest errors. Collapsing across various interview conditions, children questioned by unenthusiastic, neutral detectives produced the fewest accurate details but also the fewest inaccurate statements. Children interviewed by condescending detectives, who purported to have little faith in children's answers, produced more accurate statements, but also more inaccurate statements, than children interviewed by unenthusiastic detectives. Finally, those interviewed by positive detectives, who were supportive throughout the interview, produced the most accurate details; however, they also produced as many incorrect details as children interviewed by condescending detectives.

Thus, whereas positive interviewers may elicit the most accurate details from children, results of one study suggest that they also tend to elicit more inaccurate statements than neutral interviewers. These data appear inconsistent with those reported by Goodman et al. (1990). However, it is important to note that Goodman et al. reported data only for "abuse" questions. It is not known how their children responded to nice and neutral interviewers' nonabuse questions.

In another study, 3- and 6-year-old children played with an unfamiliar male for 5 min while seated across the table from him. Four years later, Goodman, Wilson, Hazan, and Reed (1989; also described in Goodman & Clarke-Stewart, 1991) reinterviewed the children. At this time, the researchers created "an atmosphere of accusation" by telling the children that they were to be questioned about an important event and by saying things such as "Are you afraid to tell?" You'll feel better once you've told." Although few of the children remembered the original event from 4 years earlier, their performance on suggestive abuse questions was, according to the researchers, "mixed." Five of the 15 children incorrectly agreed with the interviewer's suggestive question that they had been hugged or kissed by the confederate, 2 of the 15 agreed that they had had their picture taken in the bathroom, and 1 child agreed that she had been given a bath. These data suggest that children can be influenced by an interviewer's tone and urgency to make erroneous claims about events for which they have *no* memory. Although Goodman found reason for optimism in these results (noting that none of the children claimed that their clothes had been removed or that they had been touched in a bad way or spanked), the results are damaging to the claim that children cannot be led by suggestive questions to make abuse-related claims. Furthermore, if those children were subjected to the kinds of prolonged and pressurized interviews that we describe later, it is conceivable that even more might eventually have alleged that they had been bathed or kissed in the bathtub. If a boy had told his parent that a babysitter took his picture or kissed him while in the bathroom, this could prompt the parent to pursue an aggressive and persistent line of questioning.

In a follow-up to the aforementioned study, Goodman (1990) found that 8% of college students and child protection workers who were shown videotaped interviews of the children's answers to the suggestive questions said that sexual abuse was "very likely," and an additional 10% said that abuse was "likely." Goodman (1990) was encouraged by the fact that only 18% of the adults felt that abuse had occurred, remarking that "lay persons, at least the ones in our study, were unlikely to think that the non-abused children had been abused. Had the same information been presented at a trial, it is likely that the (innocent) defendant would have gone free" (Freiberg, 1990, p. 32). This optimistic interpretation ignores three potential outcomes that could result in unjust prosecution. First, a single juror, highly convinced that abuse occurred, may be able to persuade the other 11 jurors who are less certain about its occurrence, just as it only takes a single juror who is convinced that no abuse occurred to persuade an entire jury that it has not. If a single juror can do this, then two jurors (16.67%) will have an even easier time. Second, if a boy alleges that a babysitter or stranger took his picture or kissed him in the bathroom, this could launch an investigation that, even if it did not result in a conviction, might still be personally devastating to the accused. Third, when these data are extrapolated to forensic settings, there is even less basis for optimism because the typical forensic case would have involved *multiple* prior attempts to create an "atmosphere of accusation," not just a single one several years after the event. If children will claim to have been kissed and photographed by strangers after a single enjoinder that "they will feel better once they tell," then repeated and stronger enjoinders (e.g., "Don't you want to help us keep him in jail?") may result in greater numbers of children making similar claims. The use of repeated atmospheres of accusation is exemplified in the Country Walk Baby Sitting Service case by the following interaction between a psychologist and one of the children.

> *Dr. Braga:* Did they [Frank and Iliana Furster] ever tell you at any time that anything would happen to you if you told the secret? . . . You see, if you tell us, then it will go away and you won't have to be scared any more.
> *Child:* I know, um.
> *Dr. Braga:* We can make it go away if you just tell us anything that they told you would scare us. By telling us, it will never be anything to worry about any more.
> (Hollingsworth, 1986, p. 69)

Usually, interviewers have varying amounts of information about the events under question. Pettit, Fegan, and Howie (1990) examined how an interviewer's information about events would affect the style of questioning and the accuracy of the child's reports. Three- to five-year-olds participated in a staged event and were questioned 2 weeks later. Some interviewers were given full, accurate knowledge of the event; some were given a report containing inaccurate information; and others were given no information about the event. All interviewers were told to question each child until they found out what happened and to avoid the use of leading questions.

Collapsing across interview groups, the children were asked an average of 50 questions during the 20- to 30-min interview; thus, they were put under a great deal of pressure to provide information. Despite the warning to avoid leading questions, 30% of all questions were leading, and half of these were misleading. Interviewers with inaccurate knowledge asked four to five times as many misleading questions as the other interviewers. Overall, children agreed with 41% of the misleading questions, and children who were interviewed by misled interviewers gave the most inaccurate information. Interviewers with no knowledge showed marked rises in their use of leading questions as additional children were interviewed; these interviewers extracted more inaccurate information from the children on later compared with earlier interviews. These results suggest that interviewers' knowledge influences their style of questioning, which in turn affects the accuracy of children's testimony.

It may be that inaccurate information is detrimental only when the interviewer is a stranger. When parents were given inaccurate information about an event, they were still able to elicit accurate information from their preschoolers (Goodman, Sharma, Golden, & Thomas, 1991). Replication of this result would provide an assurance of the reliability of children's disclosures to parents, as opposed to unfamiliar law-enforcement officials.

As we have seen, child witnesses are often questioned about events that may have several interpretations, at least for the child. In the legal setting, children are interviewed many times by a variety of interviewers before they ever testify in court. What happens when children are repeatedly questioned about an event that has different interpretations for different interviewers? On the basis of the data reviewed so far, one might expect young children to be most inconsistent and suggestible in this situation. The results of a study conducted by Clarke-Stewart, Thompson, and Lepore (1989; also reported in Goodman and Clarke-Stewart, 1991) support this hypothesis. In that study, 5- and 6-year-olds interacted with a confederate posing as a janitor who followed one of two scripts. In both scripts, the confederate, named Chester, cleaned the room and then began either cleaning the toys, including a doll, or handling the doll roughly and suggestively. Chester's dialogue reinforced the idea that he was either cleaning the doll or playing with it in a rough manner. The child was then questioned about this event several times by different interviewers who differed in their interpretations of the event. Their style of questioning mirrored their interpretations. The interviewer was either (a) accusatory in tone (suggesting that Chester had been inappropriately playing with the toys instead of working); (b) exculpatory in tone (suggesting that Chester was just cleaning the toys and not playing); or (c) neutral and nonsuggestive in tone. In the first two types of interviews, the questions changed from mildly to strongly suggestive as the interview progressed. Following this interview, each child was interrogated by a second interviewer who either reinforced or contradicted the first interviewer.

When questioned by the neutral interviewer or by an interviewer whose interrogations were consistent with what the child had witnessed, children's accounts were factually correct. However, when the first interviewer contradicted the script, children's stories quickly conformed to the suggestions of the interviewer; by the end of the interview, 75% of the children's remarks were consistent with the examiners' script, and 90% answered the interpretative questions in agreement with the interviewer, as opposed to what had actually happened. When questioned by parents immediately following the interview and 1-week later, children's answers reflected the interviewers' interpretation of the events.

When the second interviewer contradicted the first interviewer, the majority of children fit their stories to the suggestions of the second interviewer. Moreover, children's subsequent reports to their parents reflected a mixture of both interviewers' interpretations.

These results concerning children's reports to their parents are inconsistent with the Goodman, Sharma, et al. (1991) finding that children make accurate disclosures to their parents. Perhaps accurate disclosure to parents is obtained when the child is questioned only by the parent on one occasion.

The aforementioned studies show how emotional tone and interviewer beliefs mold the linguistic interactions of an interview and how these molded interactions may at times promote children's false reports. Because many of the authors of these studies did not make developmental comparisons, one cannot firmly conclude that these factors uniquely affect children's reports. However, it does seem plausible that adults would not be as affected by interviewer style. This hypothesis is based on other developmental evidence, presented earlier, that suggests that compared with adults, children do view adult questioners as being more authoritative and trustworthy and thus are more likely to comply with their intended requests (Moston, 1987; Poole & White, 1991; Pratt, 1991; Warren et al., 1991).

As studies on the effects of interviewing techniques become more realistic (e.g., by providing additional interviews, with interviewers differing in style), it seems likely that they will lead to the conclusion that earlier studies of the suggestibility of children's memories for neutral events in a single interview might have underestimated young children's suggestibility in real-life interviews. However, they also might have overestimated the amount of suggestibility that arises from interviews by parents and others who are highly familiar with the child. Clearly, more research is needed on this important topic before these conclusions can be accepted, even though many examples consistent with the claim that interview bias has large effects on children's reports can be found in legal case files. This can be seen explicitly in the Kelly Michaels case, which, as of this writing, is being appealed on the basis of the defendant's contention that most of the children were subjected to relentless and single-minded interviews that were suggestive and even threatening. The following interview of one of the alleged victims, Child 8C, was conducted jointly by Mr. Fonolleras, a social worker, and by Detective Mastrangelo of the local police department:

Fonolleras: Don't be so unfriendly. I thought we were buddies last time.

8C: Nope, not any more.

Fonolleras: We have gotten a lot of other kids to help us since I last saw you. . . . Did we tell you that Kelly is in jail?

8C: Yes. My mother already told me.

Fonolleras: Did I tell you that this is the guy (pointing to Mastrangelo) that arrested her? . . . Well, we can get out of here real quick if you just tell me what you told me the last time, when we met.

8C: I forgot.

Fonolleras: No you didn't. I know you didn't.

8C: I did! I did!

Fonolleras: I thought we were friends last time.

8C: I'm not your friend any more!

Fonolleras: How come?

8C: Because I hate you!

Fonolleras: You have no reason to hate me. We were buddies when you left.

8C: I hate you now!

Fonolleras: Oh, you do not, you secretly like me, I can tell.

8C: I hate you.

Fonolleras: Oh, come on. We talked to a few more of your buddies. And everyone told me about the nap room, and the bathroom stuff, and the music room stuff, and the choir stuff, and the peanut butter stuff, and everything. . . . All your buddies [talked]. . . . Come on, do you want to help us out? Do you want to keep her in jail? I'll let you hear your voice and play with the tape recorder; I need your help

again. Come on. . . . Real quick, will you just tell me what happened
with the wooden spoon? Let's go.

8C: I forgot.

Mastrangelo: Now listen, you have to behave.

Fonolleras: Do you want me to tell him to behave? Are you going
to be a good boy, huh? While you are here, did he [Det. Mastrangelo]
show you his badge and his handcuffs? . . . Back to what happened
to you with the wooden spoon. If you don't remember words, maybe
you can show me [with anatomical dolls present].

8C: I forgot what happened, too.

Fonolleras: You remember. You told your mommy about everything
about the music room and the nap room, and all that stuff. You want
to help her stay in jail, don't you? So she doesn't bother you anymore
and so she doesn't tell you any more scary stories.

(6/27/85 Appelate Court Brief)

This interview was characteristic of many of the state's interviews in the Kelly
Michaels's case, with highly suggestive use of props and a relentless pursuit of
only one hypothesis, often accompanied by bribes for disclosures and implied
threats in the face of nondisclosure. Similar patterns of threats, bribes, and insin-
uations that their friends had already told investigators of the defendant's abusive
behavior can also been seen in other cases (see Benedek & Schetky, 1987).
Finally, these sorts of threats and bribes are not unique to prosecution interviews;
similar examples can be found in defense interviews. For instance, in the Country
Walk case, the following interview occurred between Samek, Frank Furster's
attorney, and a 6-year-old child who had made multiple allegations:

Samek: You have been saying a lot of things about Frank and Iliana,
haven't you?

Child: Yes.

Samek: I'm Frank's friend, and I want to help Frank, and I think
you're lying. I think you're lying.

Child: No.

Samek: I don't think any of the things you are saying about Frank
are true. Do you know what a lie is?

Child: When you—

Samek: No, look at me! You know what a lie is. What's a lie?

Child: When you say something that's not true.

Samek: OK, that's right. That's exactly what a lie is. I think you've
been lying to me about Frank and Iliana. I don't think Frank and Iliana
ever did anything to you. Frank didn't do anything to you, did he?

Child: Yes he did.

Samek: Frank never put his mouth on your penis, *did he?*

(Hollingsworth, 1986, p. 76)

Clearly, the impact of that style of questioning, of being forced to look into the eyes of an angry and accusatory attorney in a strange and threatening courtroom, would seem threatening to a child. Yet, the child maintained his story that Frank Furster did have oral sex with him, a story that was later supported by Frank Furster's wife, Iliana. Thus, young children are apparently capable of accurately reporting what they witnessed at least some of the time, assuming that Iliana Furster's supporting testimony was itself truthful in this case.[5]

Anatomical dolls. Anatomical dolls are frequently used by professionals, including child therapists, police, child protection workers, and attorneys, when interviewing children about suspected sexual abuse. According to recent surveys, 90% of field professionals use anatomical dolls in their investigative interviews with children suspected of being sexually abused (Boat & Everson, 1988; Conte, Sorenson, Fogarty, & Rosa, 1991). Although we could find no national figures, it appears that expert testimony is often based on observations of children's interactions with these dolls (Mason, 1991). We discuss anatomical dolls in this section on interviews because issues regarding the degree to which dolls are suggestive have been raised by a number of commentators (e.g., McGough, in press; Moss, 1988; Raskin & Yuille, 1989).

One rationale for the use of anatomical dolls is that they allow children to manipulate objects reminiscent of a critical event, thereby cuing recall and overcoming language and memory problems. A second rationale for the use of these dolls is that they are thought to overcome motivational problems of embarrassment and shyness. Children may feel more comfortable enacting an abusive event using the dolls than verbally recounting it. The dolls have also been used as projective tests. Some professionals claim that if a child actively avoids these dolls, shows distress if the dolls are undressed, or shows unusual preoccupation with the dolls' genitalia, this is consistent with the hypothesis that the child has been abused.

The use of these dolls, however, has raised skepticism among researchers and professionals alike. There are two related arguments frequently made against their use. The first is that the dolls are suggestive; they encourage the child to engage in sexual play even if the child has not been sexually abused (e.g., Gardner, 1989;

---

[5]Since we wrote this section, we have learned of arguments that Iliana Furster's "confession" might not have reflected her true opinion. She was held in solitary confinement for 1 year following her arrest. During this time, she consistently denied any allegations of abuse. Then, for a period of 2 months, she was visited on a daily basis by a friend of her lawyer, a priest, and a therapist. The latter is claimed to have made every effort to persuade her to turn state's evidence to save herself from a much more severe sentence (Nathan, 1993).

Terr, 1988). For instance, a child may insert a finger into a doll's genitalia simply because of its novelty or "affordance." Another criticism is that it is impossible to make any firm judgments about children's abuse on the basis of their doll play because there are no normative data on nonabused children's doll play and no standardized procedures for their use (e.g., at which point in the interview they are introduced, whether they are introduced with their clothes on or off).

Because of these concerns, the use of dolls for the purpose of providing legal evidence has been banned in a few jurisdictions until scientific data can be produced to attest to their validity. That research is beginning to be conducted. Since 1985, five studies have examined the degree to which sexually abused children's interactions with the dolls differ from those of nonabused children. The findings of these studies are inconsistent.

August and Forman (1989) observed the spontaneous doll play of 5- to 8-year-old girls who were suspected of being abused or who were not abused; they used the dolls to retell a story. Two raters who were aware of the children's status conducted ratings of the children's behavior. Abused children showed more avoidance of the dolls when asked to tell a story, and they engaged in more sexual activities than did the nonabused children.

White, Strom, Santili, and Halpin (1986) conducted interviews using anatomical dolls with 2- to 6-year-old abused and nonabused children. Raters, unaware of the status of the children, were more likely to rate the abused children as showing abuse. The two groups of children also differed in the quality of doll play; sexually abused children showed excessive interest in the anatomical parts and in their demonstration of sexual acts. Nonabused children showed no unusual behavior in relation to sexual play with the dolls.

However, using a similar methodology, Realmuto, Jensen, and Wescoe (1990) reported that raters could not reliably distinguish between abused and nonabused children's play with anatomical dolls. Similarly, Cohn (1991) compared the doll play behaviors of children referred for assessment of sexual abuse with a nonabused group of children. All subjects were aged 2–6 years. The two groups did not differ on measures of frequency of sexually explicit behaviors. For example, 11% of the referred children and 17% of the nonabused children inserted their fingers into the dolls' private parts. Finally, although Jampole and Weber (1987) found that 90% of their abused sample engaged the dolls in sexual activity more than did a nonabused sample, these sexually explicit behaviors were also observed in 20% of the nonabused children.

The divergent findings of these studies may reflect two factors. First, in most studies, interviewers were aware of the status of the children, a condition that could have influenced their subsequent interactions with the children, especially when playing with the dolls (Wolfner, Faust, & Dawes, 1993). Second, in most studies, children "suspected" of being abused are compared with children "not referred" to sexual abuse clinics. Because there is rarely any validation of these diagnostic categories, it is likely that some of the children are misclassified in terms of group membership.

A second set of studies have examined in greater detail how children who are not suspected of being abused play with anatomical dolls. Sivan, Schor, Koeppl, and Noble (1988) observed a middle-class sample of 3- to 8-year-olds interact with anatomical dolls. Role playing with explicit sexual activity was not observed. Glaser and Collins (1989) conducted a similar study on middle-class children (aged 2–6 years). Five percent of the children refused to play with the dolls, and 35% showed some reticence or avoidance of the dolls. Five percent showed explicit sexual play. On further investigation, 3 of these 5 children had been exposed to either pornographic literature or had observed sexual activity. There were no apparent explanations for the interactions of the other 2 children. Thus, premature exposure to sexuality rather than sexual abuse could account for some children's explicitly sexual interaction with anatomical dolls.

A third study, conducted by Everson and Boat (1990), examined the interactions of a socially diverse sample of children. Their focus was on the degree to which 2- to 6-year-olds used the dolls to show suggestive or explicit sexual behavior when they played with anatomical dolls in the presence of an interviewer versus when they were alone. Although none of the 2-year-olds showed suggestive or clear intercourse positioning, this did occur for 9% of the 4-year-olds and 16% of the 5-year-olds. When the data were analyzed in terms of race and socioeconomic status (SES) of the child, only low-SES Black boys showed clear intercourse positioning in the interviewer-present condition.

In order to determine whether their subjects' initial exposure to the anatomical dolls had any long-lasting influences, Boat, Everson, and Holland (1990) interviewed a subsample of mothers of the 3- to 5-year-olds who had played with the dolls 2 weeks previously in the Everson and Boat (1990) study just described. None of the mothers of 5-year-olds reported any noticeable behaviors that might have been related to the doll play. However, 37% of mothers of 3- and 4-year-olds reported that there were behavioral sequelae to the doll play. This was mainly demonstrated in an increase in sexual interest that involved talking or asking about sexual parts. Furthermore, 50% of the mothers of 3- and 4-year-old children believed that their children's behaviors were more sexually focused. However, these were considered to be benign behaviors that would not lead to a later interpretation or question of sexual abuse. Nevertheless, these data do indicate that after one exposure to the dolls, preschool children's behaviors were noticeably different in the eyes of their mothers.

To our knowledge, there has been only one study in which dolls were used to probe children's memories for a neutral event that involved interacting with a male confederate (Goodman & Aman, 1990). Three- and five-year-olds were questioned 1 week after this interaction. Children were questioned under one of four conditions: anatomical dolls, regular dolls, regular dolls that the child could not touch, or no dolls. The children were encouraged to use the dolls to show what had happened. Recall of events and answers to objective and misleading questions were similar across all conditions. Although this study showed that children in the anatomical doll condition did not report more sexually related events, it is important to note that the dolls did not facilitate accurate memory recall of this neutral event, indicating that their mnemonic value may be limited.

To summarize, the data on anatomical dolls are equivocal. Some studies have shown clear differences between abused and nonabused children's interactions with the dolls. Some researchers claim that nonabused children rarely if ever show sexually explicit play with the dolls, whereas others argue that a small proportion do show such behaviors. Although these rates are low for middle-class samples, they increase in more socially diverse samples. Our reading of the literature suggests that the techniques for using anatomical dolls have not been developed to the level that they allow for a clear differentiation between abused and nonabused children. It seems that for a small number of nonabused children, the dolls are suggestive in that these children engage them in sexual play.

It is not clear why these studies have yielded such divergent findings, although they do differ in the age groups studied, the procedures used, and the demographic characteristics of the samples. This divergence points to the need for additional research as well as to the need for explicit procedures to govern the use of the dolls by interviewers. Until such time that research is available, the dolls ought to be used with great caution.

Caveat lector. In the debate over the suggestibility of dolls, one problem has been overlooked: One cannot generalize from studies of anatomical dolls to actual sexual abuse interviews because the contexts for the presentation of the dolls is much different in research settings than in forensic and clinical settings. Transcripts of therapy sessions with children suspected of being sexually abused reveal the following practices: naming the dolls after defendants, berating the dolls for alleged abuses against the children, assuming the role of fantasy characters in doll play, and creating a persistent atmosphere of accusation. In the experimental studies of anatomical dolls, nonabused children were not subjected to such highly suggestive experiences prior to being interviewed with the dolls; they were not given prior motivation to play with the dolls suggestively or aggressively. On the other hand, the children who were alleged to have been abused were exposed to the dolls repeatedly prior to coming to the research setting, often amid a stream of suggestions from parents and interviewers about various sexual themes. That they played with the dolls differently from nonabused children who lacked this prior experience could have been the result of the prior experience rather than anything inherent in the way an abused child would play with the dolls for the first time. Thus, the literature on anatomical dolls does not reveal whether nonabused children would interact with the dolls differently from abused children if the former were subjected to the same preexperimental experience of the abused children (i.e., multiple interviews with the dolls in the context of discussing sexual matters). This raises the possibility that a child behaved sexually with the dolls, not because he or she was abused but because of prior sexual discussions in conjunction with previous doll use—a possibility independently raised by Wolfner et al. (1993).

Summary of interviewing studies. The studies on interviewing provide evidence that suggestibility effects are influenced by the dynamics of the interview itself, the knowledge or beliefs possessed by the interviewer (especially one who is unfamiliar with the child), the emotional tone of the questioning, and the props used. Children attempt to be good conversational partners by complying with what they perceive to be the belief of their questioner. Their perceptions, and thus their suggestibility, may be influenced by subtle aspects of the interview such as the repetition of yes–no questions, but their compliance is evidenced most fully in naturalistic interview situations in which the interviewer is allowed to question the child freely; this gives the child the evidence to make the necessary attributions about the purposes of the interview and about the intents and beliefs of the interviewer.

Observations of interactions in the legal arena highlight the fact that children who testify in court are not interviewed in sterile conditions such as those found in many of the experiments we have reviewed. They are usually questioned repeatedly within and across sessions, sometimes about an ambiguous event by a variety of interviewers, each with their own agenda and beliefs. Children are sometimes interviewed formally and informally for many months preceding an official law-enforcement interview with anatomical dolls, providing an opportunity for the child to acquire scripted and stereotypical knowledge about what might have occurred.

SOCIAL AND COGNITIVE MECHANISMS IN LYING

An equally important consideration in evaluating the suggestibility of child witnesses concerns the conditions under which children *consciously* and deliberately distort the truth because of a variety of social and motivational factors that extend beyond the interview. Historically, it was felt that lying[6] was beyond a young

---

[6]Here, we use the term *lying* to refer to the deliberate, conscious production of a response that the child believes to be incorrect for the purpose of achieving a goal, namely, misleading the listener to believe it is correct. We do not assume any malintent on the part of the "liar" that the term sometimes connotes. Also, we do not assume when we use the term *lie* that the child has solved the philosophical problem of inferring the contents of the listener's mind (Chandler, 1989). Philosophers like Flanagan (1992) have assumed that to engage in a minimal lie, the perpetrator who believes *x* must do something or omit something with the intent of making the listener think *not x:* "A minimal lie requires understanding the complex relation between actions (pointing in the wrong direction, speaking falsely), and

child's cognitive capability because it required a greater degree of decentration than preschoolers exhibited (e.g., Piaget, 1926).

Since the time of Piaget, much progress has been made in understanding the development and definitional features of deception. It is beyond the scope of this review to chronicle this progress because much of it is not germane to the main theme here: young children's proneness to suggestion in response to powerful motives.[7]

With advances in the understanding of young children's cognitive sophistication, there is now evidence that even very young children sometimes do lie, with full appreciation of the differing perspectives of their listeners. For example, 88% of 3-year-olds who were instructed not to peek at a toy proceeded to peek. When asked if they had peeked, only 38% admitted to it, prompting the investigators to conclude that "thus, we have some evidence . . . that deception strategies are adopted at early ages" (Lewis, Stranger, & Sullivan, 1989, p. 442). Although some researchers have claimed that higher order deception (the child infers the state of mind of the people they are trying to deceive and tries to inculcate a false belief in them) does not appear prior to the elementary school years (see Perner, 1991), others have shown that most 4-year-olds have some degree of cognitive sophistication in attempting to deceive, whereas 3-year-olds do not (Leekam, 1992).

We now focus on studies that have examined preschoolers' deception, ignoring whether behaviors are more appropriately construed as "sabotage," "deceit," "tricking," "politeness," or "tact." Furthermore, we avoid delving into distinctions that have occupied "theory of mind" scholars, such as lying versus telling a lie and minimal lies versus deception.

Recent research has sought to examine the specific conditions that may foster lying. Five motivations to lie or tell the truth have been studied: avoiding punishment; sustaining a game; keeping a promise (e.g., to protect a loved one); achieving personal gains (e.g., rewards, being accepted in a group); and avoiding embarrassment. Existing data show that not all motivations produce comparable levels of lying and truth telling.

Lying and truth telling to avoid punishment. Children will lie about events when the operative motives are sufficiently salient, and they will do so at an earlier age than previously assumed to be the case. Mothers report that the most frequent

---

the production of false beliefs in one's audience" (Flanagan, 1992, p. 15). We merely use the term *lying* for ease of reference in discussing research that does not meet this high standard of cognitive awareness.

[7]For recent discussions of the definitional complexity of deception, see reviews and analyses by Leekam (1992), Perner (1991), and Sodian (1991). For an analysis of the link between emergent theories of mind and children's understanding of the beliefs of those they try to deceive, see Mitchell and Thompson (1986), Chandler, Fritz, and Hala (1989), Perner (1991), and the recently published book by Whiten (1991).

motivation for their 4-year-olds to lie is to avoid punishment (Stouthamer-Loeber, 1987), a finding echoed in the recent findings of Bussey (1992).

Lying and truth telling to sustain a game. Some children can be induced to tell a lie in the context of a game. For example, an adult experimenter pretended to find a watch left behind by the teacher (Ceci, DeSimone, Putnick, Lee, & Toglia, 1990). After showing the child the watch, the child was told they were going to play a game of hiding it from the teacher. The child was told the game was a secret and was instructed not talk to anybody about it. Later, the returning teacher asked the child who had taken her watch. Only 10% of the preschoolers lied to sustain this game. Tate and Warren-Leubecker (1990) and Pipe and Goodman (in press) have reported similar figures. However, when the motivational salience of the experimental procedure was increased by having a well-known adult coach the child to tell a lie about playing with a toy, 35% of 2- to 8-year-olds lied to sustain a secret game (Tate, Warren, & Hess, 1992). It appears that the degree to which children will lie to sustain a game is context dependent and that the use of stronger coaching will result in higher rates of deception.

Keeping promises. There is consistent evidence that children as young as 3 years of age will omit important information about transgressions and accidents if adults ask them to do so (see Pipe & Goodman, in press, for a recent review). For example, in one study an adult spilled ink on a pair of gloves the child was wearing and told the child that she (the adult) would "get into trouble" if anyone found out. Subsequently, 42% of the 5-year-olds claimed not to know who spilled the ink, and 25% maintained ignorance on repeated questioning 10 days and 2 months later (Wilson & Pipe, 1989). Peters (1991c) reported similar results. Four- to ten-year-olds witnessed a staged event of a stranger who stole a book and were asked to keep the theft a secret. When the children were asked by the owner of the book whether they had seen who took it, 82% either delayed reporting the theft or never reported it. The most common reason given by the children for not disclosing was to honor the stranger's secret and to avoid getting him into trouble. Finally, some of the children in the Clarke-Stewart et al. (1989) study were told by Chester that he would lose his job if his boss learned that he had played with the dolls. Sixty-nine percent kept the secret when they were interviewed by a neutral interviewer. However, they all eventually revealed the secret when asked suggestive questions.

If children will lie to protect a stranger, they should do so even more readily to protect a loved one. Results of one study support this hypothesis (Bottoms, Goodman, Schwartz-Kenney, Sachsenmaier, & Thomas, 1990). When mothers of 3- and 5-year-olds broke a Barbie doll, only 1 of the 49 children mentioned this to an interviewer who asked what happened. Furthermore, when asked specific questions about the event, 5-year-olds did not tell the secret, even when asked leading questions.

Lying and truth telling for personal gain. Sometimes children will lie to gain a material reward or to gain acceptance in a group. For example, in the Pettit et al. (1990) study, 7 children were absent from school on the day of the staged event but were in the same classrooms as the children who saw the event. Only 1 of the 7 children said that he was not present on the day the staged event occurred. Three of the 7 children gave accounts to the interviewers that were indistinguishable from those of children who had seen the event. These 7 children probably overheard discussion of the event and wanted to be part of the group.

Material and psychological rewards do not need to be of a large magnitude to be effective. Children as young as 3 years of age will engage in sabotage behaviors to gain some reward (e.g., covering up a treasure that is in jeopardy of being discovered by a puppet), but they will not engage in verbal deceit for another year (Leekam, 1992). In a study by Ceci and colleagues, more than 50% of nursery school subjects lied to obtain a gumball as a prize by falsely claiming that they had won a game while the interviewer was out of the room (Ceci, Leichtman, Putnick, & Nightingale, 1993). Control children who had played the game but were not offered any prizes accurately reported that they had not won the game, so simple memory failure can be ruled as an explanation of children's erroneous claims.

Lying and truth telling to avoid embarrassment. Not all behavior is regulated by external outcomes, rewards, and fears of reprisals. Self-regulatory mechanisms also effectively direct behaviors (Bandura, 1986). In the context of lies, the most relevant self-regulators are guilt, shame, and pride. Although children prior to the age of 7 (Bussey, 1992; Leekam, 1992) appear to be inferior to older children at inferring some of these self-regulatory states (e.g., appreciating that a sense of pride results from telling the truth), even 4-year-olds distinguish between statements meant to minimize the embarrassment of another (e.g., "I like your new hairdo") and those meant to cause distress (Bussey, 1992).

In an effort to study lying to avoid personal embarrassment, Ceci, Leichtman, Putnick, and Nightingale (1993) instructed two parents to kiss their 3-year-olds while bathing them the evening before being interviewed. During an interview in which their parents were absent, the children were told that it was naughty to let someone kiss them when they did not have any clothes on. They were then asked, "No one ever kissed you when you didn't have any clothes on, did they? . . . No one kissed you last night when you were in the bathtub, did they?" (Ceci et al., 1993). These instructions provided a motivation to make "errors of omission," or withhold information about an event portrayed as taboo, in order to avoid the embarrassment of having done something naughty. Immediately following the child's reply, he or she was told it was okay to be kissed by a parent or someone they knew. Later, the children were asked by their parents whether they had been kissed while being bathed. In a different condition, two children who had *not* been kissed during their baths were told at the start of the interview that parents who love their children often kiss and hug them while they are in the tub and asked them the following: "Your mommy kissed you when she bathed you last night, didn't she?" (Ceci et al., 1993). Later, their parents also asked this question. The purpose of this condition was to provide a motivation to make "errors of commission" in order to avoid embarrassment.

Initially, both children who were told that it was naughty to allow an adult to kiss them while being bathed replied that they had *not* been kissed. Later, when a parent interviewed them alone and asked if they had been kissed while being bathed, they affirmed that they had, offering specific and accurate details (e.g., "Yes, I think mommy kissed me three times in the tub last night"). Interestingly, the children quickly added a codicil that was nearly a verbatim restatement of the interviewer's assurance: "But it's OK because I know her" (Ceci et al., 1993). Of the 2 children who had not been kissed during the evening bath, 1 child reported that she had been but reversed her report when interviewed by a parent alone. The results of this case study indicate that occasionally, children will consciously distort the truth about events that were allegedly perpetrated to their bodies. Both errors of omission and errors of commission were produced by the strong motives used by these researchers.

It is imprudent to make too much of this research because of its limited sample size and scope. Yet, the fact that 1 out of 2 children made an error of commission about an abuse-relevant action raises doubts about claims that fewer than 1% of children can be led to report false touching (Goodman et al., 1990). Until now, researchers who have claimed that children cannot be coached to distort their testimony appear to have tilted the odds toward finding truthfulness among preschoolers by implicitly using motives that favor a truthful outcome (e.g., Goodman et al., 1990; Saywitz et al., 1991). There were no motives for the child to make false disclosures in these earlier studies. It might even be claimed that in such studies, there are implicit motives to correctly report because to do otherwise would bring embarrassment. If children were to distort what they had witnessed and claim to have been sexually touched when they were not, this could be expected to result in embarrassment, thus tilting the motivational structure toward truthful reporting. Contrast this approach with a child asked to make errors of commission to avoid embarrassment (e.g., "He kissed you because he loves you, didn't he?") or to an approach in which a child is asked to make errors of omission to avoid embarrassment (e.g., "No one ever touched you there, did they?"). Therefore, it is important in making sense of the disparate findings to be mindful of the operative motives, both implicit and explicit.

In sum, the most recent research on lying has attempted to approximate real-life crime contexts by weaving affect and motive into studies of recollection and by using highly familiar contexts such as observing loved ones break toys or being kissed while in the bathtub. Young children will consciously distort their reports of what they witnessed, and they will do so more in response to some motives (e.g., fear of reprisal and avoidance of embarrassment) than others (e.g., to sustain a game, gain rewards).

Earlier research has shown that children do not have the cognitive skills to engage in deception at early ages (see chapters in Ceci, Leichtman, & Putnick, 1992). However, these earlier studies used paradigms that required a high level of cognitive skill to carry out the ruse. For example, children were asked to pretend that they liked something that they did not in fact like (Ceci, Leichtman, & Putnick, 1992). Because of the sophisticated cognitive skills needed to engage in pretense play, such paradigms seem to have underestimated preschoolers' ability to use deception. Alternatively, it may be that even when young children have the requisite cognitive skills to engage in pretense play of the sort required by these paradigms, they will refuse to do so because it would conflict with their negative affect (i.e., claiming to like something that they do not like), something they are unwilling to admit at a young age for reasons having more to do with social than cognitive skills.

PRIMACY OF COGNITIVE VERSUS SOCIAL MECHANISMS

Our review of the literature indicates that there are a variety of cognitive as well as social and motivational mechanisms that influence children's suggestibility. The issue that we address in this section concerns which set of factors may best account for children's suggestibility and for age-related differences in children's suggestibility and how these factors may interact.[8]

There have been few studies that have directly contrasted the relative influence of social and cognitive factors on children's suggestibility. Ceci et al. (1987) showed that when an erroneous postevent suggestion was supplied by an adult, it resulted in significantly more incorrect recognitions of the original event than when it was supplied by another child, confirming the importance of social factors, such as interviewer prestige in the suggestibility effect. However, even when a child supplied the erroneous suggestion, it still resulted in more incorrect recognitions than was found for children in the nonmisled group. These data suggest that although social factors are clearly important, they do not fully account for suggestibility effects. Young children's memory is affected by erroneous suggestions over and above the problems created by social factors. Of course, it is possible that even a child interviewer who provides erroneous suggestions presents some degree of social influence.

---

[8]As we show, it is somewhat misleading to speak of social and cognitive factors as though they operate independently in producing suggestibility effects.

The degree to which social and cognitive factors influence suggestibility may be gleaned from a consideration of the methodology for assessing suggestibility. A review of the studies described in this article makes clear that there is much variability in the manner in which misinformation is provided and in the methods used to assess suggestibility. In some studies, misinformation was incorporated into the interview questions that occur after the subjects have viewed the critical event (e.g., Warren et al., 1991). In other investigations, misinformation was presented prior to testing (e.g., Ceci et al., 1987; Zaragoza, 1991; Zaragoza et al., 1992). In addition, the timing of the misinformation varied across studies: Misinformation could occur minutes to several hours or even days relative to the target event. Although all ways of assessing suggestibility may be related, they need not be. For example, a child who acquiesces to a leading question that is presented for the first time during the testing session may at a later time not exhibit suggestibility (e.g., Cohen & Harnick, 1980). This would be an example of a social factor affecting the report (e.g., going along with an interviewer's suggestion because of a perceived pressure to conform) rather than a cognitive factor (memory alteration). Thus, acquiescence to a leading question provided at the time of testing does not in itself imply that the misinformation contained in the leading question has been incorporated into the memory. Similarly, it is possible that a child who initially resisted misinformation during testing might on subsequent occasions show evidence of suggestibility. Memory impairment may require a delay interval in order for sufficient forgetting to occur before the erroneous suggestion can alter the original memory (Belli, Windschitl, McCarthy, & Winfrey, 1992). Thus, presenting information shortly after the original information may result in a different mechanism than when misinformation is presented much later.

Focusing on cognitive versus social factors in the suggestibility effect obscures the possibility that both factors interact in producing it. For instance, it is possible that the degree to which social factors play a role has a cognitive basis. When memory traces are weak (or when there is no memory for the original event), children may be more compliant and willing to accept suggestions because there is no competing trace to challenge the suggestion. On the other hand, when the traces are strong, the child (or adult) is less likely to incorporate misleading suggestions into memory. Thus, Warren et al. (1991) reported that lower recall was significantly related to greater suggestibility. Their subjects were most easily misled about the details that were omitted in their original recalls. Furthermore, there was a significant correlation between subjects' free recall of the event and the degree to which they changed their answers to their questions on the second round of questioning, a reflection of how cognitive factors affect social manipulations (i.e., children are most susceptible to suggestible influences when their memories for events are weakest).

In addition to cognitive factors underpinning the effectiveness of social factors, it is also possible that social factors underpin the effectiveness of cognitive mechanisms in producing suggestibility (e.g., a child may attend more to suggestions from authority figures), thus ensuring greater encoding. However, this is a hypothesis in need of data.

Finally, it is possible that a child's report may initially be the result of some social factor, but over time the report may become a part of the actual memory. Earlier, we described the "Sam Stone" study in which preschool children were given stereotypical knowledge about a clumsy character (Ceci, Leichtman, & White, in press). Children later used this knowledge to reconstruct what Sam Stone *might* have done. On repeated postevent questioning, however, the children often became more convinced that the clumsy events had actually occurred, as opposed to *might* have occurred. Over 70% of 3- and 4-year-olds incorporated some of these postevent suggestions into their reports, and nearly 20% of them refused to relinquish their claims when the interviewer tried to talk them out of it. In the legal arena, in response to strongly suggestive—even pressurized— interviews, children may initially realize that they are providing the interviewer with an erroneous account, but after repeated retellings to different interviewers, the erroneous account may become so deeply embedded as to be indistinguishable from an actual memory. This is precisely the point of contention between those who maintain that genuine memory impairment can result from persistent erroneous postevent suggestions (e.g., Ceci et al., 1987) and those who argue that the original memory of the event is unimpaired (e.g., McCloskey & Zaragoza, 1985a, 1985b; Zaragoza, 1991).

Although cognitive and social factors may both play a role in suggestibility effects, the important question is, When do social variables become important developmentally and to what degree do social or cognitive variables account for suggestibility effects? Of particular interest to our discussion is whether age-related changes in the relative importance of these social and cognitive factors can account for the situations when children show heightened levels of suggestibility. Clearly, much more research is needed to gain a fuller understanding of the boundary conditions.

Finally, it needs to be stressed that regardless of the outcome of the debate over cognitive versus social mechanisms, both camps agree that there are pronounced age differences in the accuracy of children's reporting in the face of misleading questions. The disagreement is confined to the causal mechanisms that underlie the observed suggestibility effects, not to whether suggestibility effects exist, a position that almost all endorse.

CAUSAL MECHANISMS: BIOLOGICAL FACTORS

No review of suggestibility would be complete without inquiring into the biological variables that have been posited to account for age differences in suggestibility. Here, we focus on the factor of arousal or stress. This issue is of importance in our discussion because children who provide testimony often recall events that occurred under highly stressful conditions, and often these children become stressed as a result of the interviewing contexts. Thus, it is useful to examine the degree to which children provide accurate reports under these conditions.

Stress, Memory, and Suggestibility

There is a growing but controversial literature on the relation between arousal and children's memory, and some of these studies have included tests of the relation between arousal and suggestibility. Some researchers claim that high levels of arousal are beneficial for children's testimonial accuracy as well as for their resistance to suggestions (e.g., Goodman, 1991); others maintain that high levels of stress are debilitating, resulting not only in less memory but also greater suggestibility (e.g., Peters, 1991a, 1991b, 1991c); and some researchers argue that stress and arousal are unrelated to memory or suggestibility effects (e.g., Oates & Shrimpton, 1991; Steward, 1989).

The position that stress facilitates recall is consistent with the phenomenon known as "flashbulb memories" (e.g., R. Brown & Kulik, 1977; Linton, 1982). The classic example of this is the claim that most people can remember where they were when they heard of President Kennedy's assassination. Events that are emotionally arousing are thought to receive privileged encoding; high emotional salience is associated with a "print now" mechanism that reputedly permits the core details of affectively valenced events to be automatically encoded (R. Brown & Kulik, 1977). A physiological explanation for flashbulb memories posits that shock releases hormones such as adrenaline that drive up the plasma glucose level, which may be the basis for the enduring memory (e.g., Gold, 1987).

There is some support for the hypothesis that high levels of emotional arousal are associated with accurate and consistent recall. High arousal among college subjects in the aftermath of the space shuttle *Challenger*'s explosion was associated with greater consistency of reporting over a 3-year interval (Bohannon, 1988). There are some child studies that are consistent with the concept of flashbulb memories. Terr (1983, 1990) has described numerous clinical cases in which individuals exposed to traumatic experiences in early childhood, such as a sibling's murder or their own rape, were able to recollect their experiences in detail. Children's reports of the *Challenger* disaster over a 2-year period were more consistent among those who reported higher emotional responses to the disaster than those who reported lower emotional responses (Warren & Swartwood, in press).

In line with these results, Goodman and her colleagues conducted four experiments to examine children's memory for stressful events involving inoculation and venopuncture (Goodman, Hirschman, Hepps, & Rudy, 1991). In two studies, stress was beneficial to recollections of children, and in one of the two, high stress was associated with resistance to suggestion. In the first of these studies, 3- to 6-year-olds received an inoculation; their emotional state during this procedure was categorized on a 6-point scale ranging from *very relaxed* to *very frightened*. The children's recollections of the inoculation were tested 3–9 days following the shot. The highest levels of arousal were associated with the most accurate recall and the lowest levels of suggestibility. In the second study, children who did not receive an inoculation but who went to the clinic to have a decal rubbed onto their arm and leg were also interviewed 3–9 days after this procedure. Their responses were compared with those of the inoculated children just described. Of the eight major analyses performed, one resulted in a significant difference between inoculated and noninoculated children: Noninoculated children (i.e., those with lower levels of stress) recalled more incorrect information than did the inoculated children.

There is another set of studies in which stress was associated either with no differences in subsequent memory or with detrimental effects on memories and their resistance to suggestion (Kramer, Buckhout, Fox, Widman, & Tusche, 1991). This literature has fueled the growing discontent over the flashbulb metaphor because of the presumed uniqueness of its mechanisms and the consequences related to completeness of report, accuracy, and immutability (see Bohannon, 1988; McCloskey, Wible, & Cohen, 1988; Pillemer, 1990; Winograd & Killinger, 1983).

Several studies in the child literature have also failed to show any association between stress and memory. Even though there was a relation between children's emotional response to the *Challenger* disaster and the consistency of their recalls over a 2-year period, there was no relation between emotional response and number of core details reported after 2 years (Warren & Swartwood, in press). Steward (1989) reported that in initial interviews, children who received a painful medical procedure disclosed significantly more information about being touched than did children who did not receive this procedure. However, 6 months later, there were no differences in the reports of the high-pain group and the group that did not receive this procedure (see Goodman, Hirschman, et al., 1991, Studies 1 and 4, for similar findings).

In some cases, stress is related to impoverished recall on some but not all measures. Vandermaas (1991) found that high levels of stress associated with dental procedures had no effect on the accuracy of 4- to 7-year-olds' responses to specific questions, although it did have a detrimental effect in terms of their free recall; it led to diminished recall among the youngest children. Ornstein et al. (1992) correlated children's distress (as rated by nurses, doctors, and parents) to children's immediate and delayed recall of their visit to their pediatrician. Of the nine possible correlations, only one was significant. Parental stress ratings of the older children were negatively correlated with delayed recall; the more stressed children recalled fewer details of their visit than did less stressed children.

Several studies have shown a more consistent association between high levels of stress and low levels of recall. Bugental, Blue, Cortez, Fleck, and Rodriguez (1992) have provided a direct test of the hypothesis that stress influences encoding by recording 5- to 10-year-olds' electrodermal responses and heart rate changes as they watched a mildly stressful video showing frightened faces. Details of the video that followed heightened arousal were remembered less well than details presented prior to the elevated arousal. Thus, if it is argued that higher levels of stress result in better encoding, the evidence does not seem to support this (Oates & Shrimpton, 1991; Warren & Swartwood, in press).

The most extensive evidence in favor of the hypothesis that stress impairs children's memory and increases their suggestibility has been provided by Peters (1991a, 1991b), who conducted five experiments of children's recollections of different stressful events. After testing close to 400 children in which several measures of arousal were used, he concluded that high arousal levels can at times impair the eyewitness performance of children and that high arousal levels are never associated with increased recall. Experiment 5 of Peters (1991a) is most pertinent to this review because it included a suggestibility manipulation.

Five- to 10-year-olds were performing a card-sorting task when they unexpectedly heard either a fire alarm (high-stress group) or a loud radio (low-stress group). Measure of blood pressure and pulse rate taken before and after the onset of the noise showed a significant elevation only for the fire-alarm group. When children's memory was tested, no differences were found between the two groups on free recall, but the radio listeners gave more accurate responses to the objective questions than did the fire-alarm group. Recall was distorted by misleading questions in both groups, but the difference was significantly greater in the alarm condition. Thus, the stress of the alarm condition coupled with exposure to misleading questions reliably reduced accuracy of children's recall.

Unfortunately, few other studies have examined the effect of stress on suggestibility. Four studies showed no relation between these variables. Oates and Shrimpton (1991) found no differences in suggestibility between children who had received a blood test (high-stress group) or children who had interacted with a friendly stranger (low-stress group). Furthermore, there were no correlations between children's self-rated stress and their performance on suggestive questions or any other memory measures. Finally, although Goodman, Hirschman, et al. (1991) found that stress led to resistance of suggestions, this was obtained only in one of the four studies reported. For the three other studies, all of which involved recall of events related to inoculations or to venopuncture, stress was unrelated to suggestibility.

Summary of Stress and Memory Studies

To summarize, 15 studies that examined the relation between stress and memory in children are reviewed in Table 1. In only two cases were there reports that high stress was beneficial to memory. In the remaining 13 studies, there was either no effect of stress on memory accuracy ($n = 5$) or high levels of stress were detrimental to memory ($n = 8$). Finally, only 6 of the 15 studies examined the effects of stress on suggestibility. Most ($n = 4$) studies reported no associations between stress and suggestibility. Two studies did show an association, but the direction of the correlation was different for each. It is difficult to resolve these inconsistent data, but we offer a few possible explanations.

First, there are clear differences among studies in the ways in which stress was measured and operationalized. Some studies relied on self-reports, whereas others

TABLE 1
Summary of Stress Studies

Study	Memory effect	Suggestibility effect
Goodman, Hirschman, et al. (1991. Exp 2)	+	0
Goodman, Hirschman, et al. (1991, Exp 3)	+	+
Peters (1991a. Exp 1)	−	
Peters (1991a. Exp 2)	−	
Bugental et al. (1992)	−	
Peters (1991a, Exp 3)	−	
Peters (1991a, Exp 4)	−	
Peters (1991a. Exp 5)	−	−
Vandermaas (1991)	−	
Ornstein et al. (1992)	−	
Goodman. Hirschman. et al. (1991, Exp 1)	0	0
Goodman, Hirschman, et al. (1991. Exp 4)	0	0
Warren and Swartwood (in press)	0	
Oates and Shrimpton (1991)	0	0
Steward (1989)	0	

Note. To save space. only the first author's or the first and second authors' last names appear in the table citations. Exp = experiment. + = significant positive associations between stress and either memory or suggestibility. − = significant negative associations between stress and either memory or suggestibility. 0 = no significant associations between stress and either memory or suggestibility.

relied on measures of physiological changes in arousal, such as salivary norepine-phrine and immunoglobin A levels. It is important to note that there were only moderate correlations between objective rating scales and various types of self-reports and that the correlations between different *subjective* reports of stress (parents', children's, and other observers') were often weak (Ornstein et al., 1992; Vandermaas, 1991). Thus, there were significant problems in terms of the validity of the classification of subjects according to stress. Even when these methods may be valid, however, there still is the problem of whether what is counted as a stressful event in one study is comparable to what is counted as a stressful event in another.

Interpretations of these results are also complicated because the accuracy and consistency of memory may be curvilinear across factors that are assumed to be correlated with levels of stress (Pillemer, Koff, Rhinehart, & Rierdan, 1987) as well as asymmetric across processing loci. Concerning the first claim, it may be that both the child who has received many prior inoculations and the child who has received no prior inoculations will differ from the child who has received a moderate number of prior inoculations. The former groups may have weaker emotional reactions to the inoculation experience, either because of an absence of prior experience that would result in little stress at the time of the first shot or so much experience receiving shots that the procedure has lost some of its fright. By contrast, the child who has experienced some, but not many, shots may be most stressed by the prospect of another shot. Pillemer et al. (1987) found that very strong as well as very weak emotional reactions may be associated with less subsequent recall among adults than moderate levels of stress (see also Deffenbacher, 1991, for a recent review of the adult memory–affect relationship and its consistency with the Yerkes-Dodson law).

Concerning the claim that stress may exert asymmetric effects on memory at different processing loci, it is possible that stress at the time of encoding *could* aid the storage of information, whereas stress at the time of retrieval could impair access to the contents of storage. For instance, Goodman, Levine, Melton, and Ogden (1991), in the amicus brief to the Supreme Court in *Craig v. Maryland,* noted that children's stress during testimony (i.e., during retrieval) could reduce willingness to articulate their memories. However, it is important to underscore the word *could* because the evidence that stress aids encoding is uncompelling.

One suggested resolution to the ongoing debate concerns a consideration of the type of information that is being erroneously suggested as well as the type of memory test used. Christianson and Loftus (1987) found that high arousal was associated with improved memory for central information in adults but that it was associated with a diminished ability to remember the specific details of the traumatic scenario. Similarly, Goodman et al. (1990) found that memory for central information is harder to bias through suggestive questioning. However, in the one study that examined suggestibility for central actions, high levels of arousal were also associated with heightened suggestibility. Oates and Shrimpton (1991) reported that children's suggestibility for actions or central information was greater than their suggestibility for the people with whom they interacted.

A compromise position may emerge on the basis of Pillemer's (1990) view that there is no mechanism inherently unique to the formation of flashbulb memories. Rather, the shock and salience of flashbulb experiences may result in their greater rehearsal and elaboration, which results in greater retention. A key determinant of whether arousal will be associated with subsequent age differences in memory and suggestibility may be moderated by how much the children know about the event. In two studies, children who had a fuller understanding of an emotionally arousing event remembered more than did children with less understanding of the event (Pillemer, in press; Warren & Swartwood, in press). According to this view, stressful experiences may be differentially rehearsed and elaborated by different age groups, and this could lead to different levels of memory and perhaps to differential suggestibility effects.

This interpretation may start to disambiguate some of the results previously reviewed. It is possible that stress levels are sometimes not associated with suggestibility effects or memory deficits because the stress manipulations are confounded with knowledge differences. In most studies, children who were classified as stressed usually received a procedure that was highly scripted and perhaps rehearsed with parents before and after the event (e.g., a visit to the doctor's office). This could have resulted in very high levels of recall, especially if the procedures were well known to the parents. By contrast, in many of these same studies, children in the control group received less stressful procedures, but they also were asked to recall highly unfamiliar events for which there was no script and no chance for preevent rehearsal (e.g., meeting a stranger in the school library). Therefore, the recall of the stressed children might have been artificially high and that of the control children artificially low. Even when children received the same procedure, it is possible that few relationships were found because the children were so familiar with these events that there were ceiling effects. In this light, the results of Peters's (1991a, 1991b, 1991c) studies become particularly interesting because some of his procedures were novel for both stressed and unstressed children, and these events were not known to their parents before participation (e.g., a surprise fire alarm). Thus, the existing literature may conflate the effects of stress with the effects of highly scripted versus unfamiliar events. In terms of age differences in suggestibility, these results indicate that perhaps younger children may be more suggestible than older children in the stressful situations for which they have little understanding of or experience in that situation. At this point in time, these are merely hypotheses in search of data.

CONCLUSIONS

In her analyses of appellate court decisions involving expert witnesses' statements about the accuracy of children's testimony, Mason (1991) argued that "courts are unconcerned about scientific knowledge, but are willing to accept the testimony of expert witnesses as long as they have had significant clinical experience" (p. 20). The result is that so-called experts often make claims that are not in accord with—or are even diametrically opposed to—the research we have just reviewed. Experts in psychology, social work, pediatrics, and psychiatry frequently claim in court that children are incapable of lying or are not suggestible (Mason, 1991; McGough, in press). Experts rarely present a careful summary of the research because doing so would probably force them to attenuate their often-strident claims. This can result in distrust of social scientists on grounds that their testimony is speculative at best (Myers, 1987; Zacharias, 1990).

As a way of avoiding this problem, legal jurisdictions traditionally adopted a "Frye test," stipulating that expert testimony is permitted when the research underpinning the expert's testimony is "sufficiently established to have gained general acceptance in the particular field in which it belongs" (*Frye v. the United States*, 1923). Federal Rule 703 has diluted the Frye test standard somewhat, allowing that the database expert witnesses used must be reasonably relied on by experts in the field in forming opinions or inferences on the subject. Hence, it is permissible for experts to disagree about the meaning of research as long as they are aware of it. Because we assume that this review will serve as a basis for the opinions of some who venture into court as expert witnesses, the following three conclusions would seem to meet a traditional Frye test standard.

First and foremost, contrary to the claims made by some (e.g., Melton, 1992), there do appear to be significant age differences in suggestibility, with preschool-aged children being disproportionately more vulnerable to suggestion than either school-aged children or adults. This conclusion follows from a synopsis of the reviewed literature. In approximately 83% (15 out of 18) of the developmental studies that have compared preschoolers with older children or adults, preschoolers were the most suggestible group (see Table 2). To many, this figure of 83% may sound like an overestimate, given the belief that many studies of preschoolers have *not* shown age decrements in suggestibility (e.g., Goodman et al., 1990; Saywitz et al., 1991).[9] However, reliable age differences in suggestibility *were*

---

[9]The figure, 83%, is most likely an underestimate of the extent of actual age differences in suggestibility for three reasons. First, it does not reflect the inclusion of studies that report age differences but are not viewed as traditional suggestibility studies. Poole and White's (1991) finding that preschoolers were disproportionately likely to change their answers in response to repeated yes/no questions falls into this class of excluded studies. Second, the 83% estimate reflects a measurement bias, namely, that some studies may have failed to find age differences because of ceiling effects or low statistical power. Third, the denominator for calculating the 83% estimate includes studies that did not

TABLE 2
Summary of Studies That Compared Suggestibility of Preschoolers
to Older Children or to Adults

Study	Reliable age effects for suggestibility
Ceci et al. (in press)	+
Ceci et al. (1987, Exp 1)	+
Ceci et al. (1987, Exp 2)	+
Gordon et al. (1991)	+
Goodman and Aman (1990)	+
Goodman et al. (1990, Exp 4)	+
Goodman, Hirschman, et al. (1991, Exp 3)	+
Goodman, Hirschman, et al. (1991, Exp 2)	+
Goodman, Hirschman, et al. (1991, Exp 4)	⁴ +
Goodman and Reed (1986)	+
Oates and Shrimpton (1991)	+
Ornstein et al. (1992)	+
Rudy and Goodman (1991)	+
Saywitz et al. (1991)	+
Marin et al. (1979)	0
Howe (1991)	0
Delamothe and Taplin (1992)	0
Cassel and Bjorklund (1992)	+

Note. To save space, only the first author's or the first and second author's last names appear in the table citations. Exp = experiment. A plus sign denotes that preschoolers were significantly more impaired by misleading questions than older subjects. A zero denotes no significant age differences in the suggestibility effect.

found in nearly all of these studies despite impressions to the contrary. The reason for this misunderstanding is that those authors sometimes did not focus on age differences in overall suggestibility but instead emphasized a subset of items for which there were no developmental differences in suggestibility, or they focused on a theoretical issue that was independent of the suggestibility debate. For example, although Goodman and her colleagues chose to focus on segments of their data that did not contain age differences (e.g., abuse-related suggestions, stress

use a traditional contrast between a group of children who received misleading information and a control group but instead reported only the far more conservative contrast between the control group performance and a group that received the modified testing procedure (e.g., Delamothe & Taplin, 1992). From all that we know (e.g., Ceci, Ross, & Toglia, 1987), had the traditional contrast been included, such studies probably would have found reliable age differences. Having noted these three factors that may have led to an underestimate of age differences, it is only fair to point out again that we excluded one study (Leippe, Romanczyk, & Manion, 1991) that reported reverse age differences in acquiescence to specific questions (e.g., "Were there flowers on the wall?"), on the ground that such questions traditionally have not been viewed as suggestive, even though they include information not spontaneously provided by the child (Goodman, Rudy, Bottoms, & Aman, 1990, p. 260).

induction), it should be kept in mind that they almost always found age differences in overall suggestibility, with the youngest preschoolers being disproportionately more suggestible than older children.

Although the literature clearly reveals age differences in overall suggestibility, the exact mechanisms involved in producing distortion in young children's reports are still being debated by researchers. Until there is a consensus, nothing like a Frye test standard can be met to account for the mechanism by which age differences in suggestibility arise. Some believe that young children's faulty reports are partly the result of an "erasure" mechanism by which erroneous postevent suggestions overwrite or replace the original memory trace (Ceci et al., 1987, 1988; Delamothe & Taplin, 1992; Goodman, Sharma, et al., 1991). By contrast, others believe that social processes lead to distortion in children's reports (Zaragoza et al., 1992). However, all of these researchers agree that regardless of the underlying mechanism, preschoolers' reports *are* distorted by erroneous suggestions.

Controversy exists as to the boundary conditions for younger children's greater suggestibility. Some argue that suggestibility is diminished or even nonexistent when the act in question concerns a central action, when the child is a participant, or when the report is a free narrative (e.g., Fivush, in press; Goodman et al., 1990). The strongest claim of this position is that children are not suggestible concerning central actions, personally experienced, and especially those that involve their own bodies:

> Experiments in which children are given misleading information about personally experienced events, as opposed to misinformation about stories, tend to find less of an effect of misleading information. . . . Events which are extremely personally important are probably less prone to suggestion than are less important events. . . . Finally, misleading information is more likely to influence future recall when it is about peripheral details of an event rather than more central aspects. (Fivush, in press, p. 25)

Others, however, have failed to provide support for these claims. Our review of the literature indicates that children can indeed be led to make false or inaccurate reports about very crucial, personally experienced, central events. In Oates and Shrimpton's (1991) study, 4- to 6-year-olds were disproportionately impaired by misleading questions having to do with actions (e.g., having their arms held behind them) compared with older children. By contrast, these investigators failed to find age differences on suggestive questions having to do with nonactions (e.g., a stranger's identity). Similarly, other studies have shown that personally experienced actions are not immune to suggestion. For example, Ceci, Leichtman, Putnick, and Nightingale (1993) have shown that children can be led to falsely report whether they had been kissed while being bathed, and Lindberg (1991) reported that children were suggestible about actions involved in cheating. Recently, Ornstein and his colleagues (Gordon, Ornstein, Clubb, & Nida, 1991) replicated their previous study (Ornstein et al., 1992) on children's memories of their visits to their pediatrician and found that 3-year-old children were prone to making false claims about "silly events" that involved bodily contact (e.g., Did the nurse lick your knee? Did she blow in your ear?) and that these false claims persisted in repeated interviewing over a 3-month period. Finally, both Cassel and Bjorklund (1992) and Warren and Hagood (in press) found younger children reliably more suggestible about salient, central actions, with fully 42% altering their answer in response to repeated questioning in the former study.

Ironically, studies by Goodman and her colleagues provide some of the most compelling evidence that young children do in fact make false claims about actions, central events, and even events that could be construed as being sexually abusive (see Goodman et al., 1990). For example, in their anatomical doll study, Goodman and Aman (1990) found that 3- and 5-year-old children frequently gave false answers to abuse-related questions such as "Did he touch your private parts?" (i.e., 32% of 3-year-olds and 24% of 5-year-olds gave inaccurate answers to these types of questions) and to misleading abuse-related questions such as "How many times did he spank you?" (i.e., 24% of 3-year-olds and 3% of 5-year-olds gave inaccurate answers to these types of questions). In addition, these effects are not limited to this one study. In the Rudy and Goodman (1991) study of children's memories of playing with a stranger in a trailer, children made false reports to both misleading abuse questions (i.e., 12% for 4-year-olds and 6% for 7-year-olds) as well as to direct abuse questions (i.e., 18% for 4-year-olds and 10% for 7-year-olds). The age effects were significant only for the direct questions. In the Saywitz et al. (1991) study of children's memories of physical examinations, when all abuse-related questions (nonmisleading and misleading) were pooled, there were significant age differences between 5- and 7-year-old children's reports, and these figures again showed that children do misreport central events, particularly those that involve their own bodies (i.e., error rates were 13% for 5-year-olds and 7% for 7-year-olds). Finally, when 3- to 4-year-olds were interviewed by a neutral interviewer about events surrounding an inoculation, there was an error rate of 23% on questions such as "How many times did she kiss you?" and "She touched your bottom didn't she?" (Goodman et al., 1990, p. 278). That is, many of these children answered yes even though the events did not occur.

The second major conclusion is that contrary to the claims of some, children sometimes lie when the motivational structure is tilted toward lying (e.g., Peters, 1990). In this sense they are probably no different from adults. Because most of the existing data are not developmental, no age comparisons in willingness to lie in response to various motives can be made with confidence at this time, although there is some indication that 5-year-olds are more likely than 3-year-olds to keep secrets (e.g., Bussey, 1992; Pipe & Goodman, in press).

Extreme statements that some have proferred in the media (e.g., children never lie vs. children are incapable of getting it right because they cannot distinguish between reality and fantasy) are not supported by the findings reviewed here. That children are found to lie at times should not surprise anyone except the extreme advocates who have made such baseless claims. More research is needed on age-related shifts in motivational salience to better understand whether different motives, such as fear of reprisals, honoring a promise, or resisting a bribe, are more or less influential for a given age group. Until such research becomes available, it is safe to conclude that sometimes children will lie, but certainly not all of the time or uniformly in response to all motivational forces.

Third, notwithstanding the aforementioned two points, it is clear that children—even preschoolers—are capable of recalling much that is forensically relevant. That their reports are more vulnerable to distortion than those of older individuals, and that they can be induced to lie in response to certain motives, is not meant to imply that they are incapable of providing accurate testimony. In fact, in most of the studies that have been reported during the past decade, young children were able to accurately recollect the majority of the information they observed, even though they did not recall as much as older children. They may be more likely to succumb to erroneous suggestions than older children, but their vulnerability is a matter of degree only. As was pointed out in the overview, even adults are suggestible (e.g., Belli, 1989; Gudjonsson, 1986; Lindsay, 1990; Loftus, 1979).

Therefore, the question ought not to be whether children are suggestible but whether their level of suggestibility is so much greater than that of an adult as to (a) render them an obstacle to the court's truth-seeking process when they serve as witnesses, (b) require competency hearings to determine whether they ought to be allowed to provide testimony to juries, or (c) require judges to give juries cautionary instructions about their special reliability risks. On the basis of the evidence reviewed in this article, the answer to the first two of these questions appears to be a qualified "no" because, as our review shows, although there are many conditions under which children can report much that is accurate, there are a variety of conditions under which young children appear to be reliably as well as substantively more suggestible than older subjects. Therefore, it is of the utmost importance to examine the conditions prevalent at the time of a child's original report about a criminal event in order to judge the suitability of using that child as a witness in the court. It seems particularly important to know the circumstances under which the initial report of concern was made, how many times the child was questioned, the hypotheses of the interviewers who questioned the child, the kinds of questions the child was asked, and the consistency of the child's report over a period of time. If the child's disclosure was made in a nonthreatening, nonsuggestible atmosphere, if the disclosure was not made after repeated interviews, if the adults who had access to the child prior to his or her testimony are not motivated to distort the child's recollections through relentless and potent suggestions and outright coaching, and if the child's original report remains highly consistent over a period of time, then the young child would be judged to be capable of providing much that is forensically relevant. The absence of any of these conditions would not in and of itself invalidate a child's testimony, but it ought to raise cautions in the mind of the court.

The answer to the third question will depend on whether the courts believe that cautionary instructions about children's reliability risks will serve the useful purpose of taming jurors' unbridled enthusiasm for the young child's credibility (Ross, Dunning, Toglia, & Ceci, 1990; Spencer & Flin, 1990) or whether the courts believe that such cautionary instructions may exaggerate jurors' preexisting skepticism of children's competencies to a point that is undesirable (Vasek, 1986; also see McCloskey & Egeth, 1983, for a similar point regarding adult witnesses).

In view of our conclusions, extreme negative opinions about the young child's ability to resist leading questions that have been proferred throughout this century are unwarranted. Assertions from the earlier historical periods, such as "Create, if you will, an idea of what the child is to hear or see, and the child is very likely to see or hear what you desire" (M. R. Brown, 1926, p. 133), are needlessly ungenerous views of children's abilities. Similarly, modern surveys indicating that 91% of psychologists believe that an 8-year-old witness will respond in a way the questioner wished or else say they did not know (Yarmey & Jones, 1983), or the typical college student who believes that children under 6 years of age are "highly prone to be liars, second only to politicians" (Vasek, 1986, p. 157), are also inaccurate.

In light of the full corpus of data that we have reviewed, these extreme opinions are not supported by the available research. This research shows that children are able to encode and retrieve large amounts of information, especially when it is personally experienced and highly meaningful. Equally true, however, is that no good will be served by ignoring that part of the research that demonstrates potentially serious social and cognitive hazards to young child witnesses if adults who have access to them attempt to usurp their memories. Inattention to the full corpus of empirical data will only forestall efforts to improve the way child witnesses are treated and delay needed research to ways of optimizing young children's testimonial accuracy through better interviewing techniques and judicial reform.

REFERENCES

Ackerman, B. (1983). Speaker bias in children's evaluation of the external consistency of statements. *Journal of Experimental Child Psychology, 35,* 111–127.

Andrews, J. A. (1964). The evidence of children. *Criminal Law Review, 64,* 769–777.

August, R. L., & Forman, B. D. (1989). A comparison of sexually abused and nonsexually abused children's behavioral responses to anatomically correct dolls. *Child Psychiatry and Human Development, 20,* 39–47.

Aveling, F., & Hargreaves, H. (1921). Suggestibility with and without prestige in children. *British Journal of Psychology, 11,* 53–75.

Baker-Ward, L., Hess, T., & Flannagan, D. (1990). The effects of involvement on children's memory for events. *Cognitive Development, 5,* 55–69.

Bandura, A. (1986). *Social foundations of thought and action: A social cognitive theory.* Englewood Cliffs, NJ: Prentice-Hall.

Baxter, J. (1990). The suggestibility of child witnesses: A review. *Journal of Applied Cognitive Psychology, 3,* 1–15.

Belli, R. F. (1989). Influences of misleading postevent information: Misinformation interference and acceptance. *Journal of Experimental Psychology: General, 118,* 72–85.

Belli, R. F., Windschitl, P., McCarthy, T., & Winfrey, S. (1992). Detecting memory impairment with a modified test procedure: Manipulating retention interval with centrally presented event items. *Journal of Experimental Psychology: Learning, Memory, and Cognition, 18,* 356–367.

Benedek, E. P., & Schetky, D. H. (1987). Problems in validating allegations of sexual abuse: Parts 1 and 2. Factors affecting perception and recall of events. *Journal of the American Academy of Child and Adolescent Psychiatry, 26,* 915–922.

Berliner, L. (1985). The child and the criminal justice system. In A. W. Burgess (Ed.), *Rape and sexual assault* (pp. 199–208). New York: Garland Publishing.

Binet, A. (1900). *La suggestibilité.* Paris: Schleicher Freres.

Boat, B., & Everson, M. (1988). The use of anatomical dolls among professionals in sexual abuse evaluations. *Child Abuse and Neglect, 12,* 171–186.

Boat, B., Everson, M., & Holland, J. (1990). Maternal perceptions of nonabused young children's behaviors after the children's exposure to anatomical dolls. *Child Welfare, 64,* 389–399.

Bohannon, J. N. (1988). Flashbulb memories for the space shuttle disaster: A tale of two theories. *Cognition, 29,* 179–196.

Bothwell, R., Deffenbacher, K., & Brigham, J. (1987). Correlation of eyewitness accuracy and confidence: Optimality hypothesis revised. *Journal of Applied Psychology, 72,* 691–695.

Bottoms, B., Goodman, G., Schwartz-Kenney, B., Sachsenmaier, T., & Thomas, S. (1990, March). *Keeping secrets: Implications for children's testimony.* Paper presented at the biennial meeting of the American Psychology/Law Society, Williamsburg, VA.

Brainerd, C. J., Kingma, J., & Howe, M. L. (1985). On the development of forgetting. *Child Development, 56,* 1103–1119.

Brainerd, C. J., & Reyna, V. (1988). Memory loci of suggestibility development: Comment on Ceci, Ross, and Toglia. *Journal of Experimental Psychology: General, 118,* 197–200.

Brainerd, C. J., Reyna, V. F., Howe, M. L., & Kingma, J. (1990). The development of forgetting and reminiscence. *Monographs of the Society for Research in Child Development, 55*, (3–4, Serial No. 222).

Brennan, M., & Brennan, R. (1988). *Strange language.* Wagga Wagga, New South Wales, Australia: Riverina Murry Institute of Higher Education.

Brown, M. R. (1926). *Legal psychology.* New York: Bobbs-Merrill.

Brown, R., & Kulik, J. (1977). Flashbulb memories. *Cognition, 5*, 73–99.

Bugental, D., Blue, J., Cortez, V., Fleck, K., & Rodriguez, A. (1992). Influences of witnessed affect on information processing in children. *Child Development, 63*, 774–786.

Burtt, H. E. (1948). *Applied psychology.* Englewood Cliffs, NJ: Prentice Hall.

Burtt, H., & Gaskill, H. (1932). Suggestibility and the form of the question. *Journal of Applied Psychology, 16*, 358–373.

Bussey, K. (1992). Children's lying and truthfulness: Implications for children's testimony. In S. J. Ceci, M. Leichtman, & M. Putnick (Eds.), *Cognitive and social factors in preschoolers' deception* (pp. 89–110). Hillsdale, NJ: Erlbaum.

Cassel, W. S., & Bjorklund, D. F. (1992, April). *Age differences and suggestibility of eyewitnesses.* In D. F. Bjorklund & P. A. Ornstein (Cochairs), *Children's memory for real world events: Implications for testimony.* Symposium conducted at the annual meeting of the Conference on Human Development, Atlanta.

Ceci, S. J. (1990). *On intelligence . . . more or less: A bio-ecological treatise on intellectual development.* Englewood Cliffs, NJ: Prentice-Hall.

Ceci, S. J. (1991). Some overarching issues in the child suggestibility debate. In J. L. Doris (Ed.), *The suggestibility of children's recollections* (pp. 1–9). Washington, DC: American Psychological Association.

Ceci, S. J., Caves, R., & Howe, M. J. A. (1981). Children's long term memory for information incongruent with their knowledge. *British Journal of Psychology, 72*, 443–450.

Ceci, S. J., DeSimone, M., Putnick, M., Lee, J. M., & Toglia, M. (1990, March). *Motives to lie.* Paper presented at the biennial meeting of the American Psychology/Law Society, Williamsburg, VA.

Ceci, S. J., Leichtman, M., & Putnick, M. (Eds.). (1992). *Cognitive and social factors in early deception.* Hillsdale, NJ: Erlbaum.

Ceci, S. J., Leichtman, M., Putnick, M., & Nightingale, N. (1993). Age differences in suggestibility. In D. Cicchetti & S. Toth (Eds.), *Child abuse, child development, and social policy.* (pp. 117–137). Norwood, NJ: Ablex.

Ceci, S. J., Leichtman, M., & White, T. (in press). Interviewing preschoolers: Remembrance of things planted. In D. P. Peters (Ed.) *The child witness: Cognitive, social, and legal issues.* Netherlands: Kluwer.

Ceci, S. J., Ross, D., & Toglia, M. (1987). Age differences in suggestibility: Psycholegal implications. *Journal of Experimental Psychology: General, 117*, 38–49.

Ceci, S. J., Toglia, M., & Ross, D. (1988). On remembering . . . more or less. *Journal of Experimental Psychology: General, 118*, 250–262.

Ceci, S. J., Toglia, M., & Ross, D. (1990). The suggestibility of preschoolers' recollections:

Historical perspectives on current problems. In R. Fivush & J. Hudson (Eds.), *Knowing and remembering in young children.* (pp. 285–300). New York: Cambridge University Press.

Chadbourn, J. (1978). *Wigmore on evidence.* Boston: Little, Brown.

Chandler, M. (1989). Doubt and developing theories of mind. In J. W. Astington, P. Harris, & D. R. Olson (Eds.), *Developing theories of mind* (pp. 387–413). New York: Cambridge University Press.

Chandler, M., Fritz, A. S., & Hala, S. (1989). Small scale deceit: Deception as a marker of 2-, 3-, and 4-year-olds' early theories of mind. *Child Development, 60,* 1263–1277.

Chi, M. T. H., & Ceci, S. J. (1987). Content knowledge and the reorganization of memory. *Advances in Child Development and Behavior, 20,* 1–37.

Christianson, S-Å., & Loftus, E. F. (1987). Memory for traumatic events. *Applied Cognitive Psychology, 1,* 225–239.

Clark, H. H., & Clark, E. V. (1977). *Psychology and language.* New York: Harcourt Brace & Jovanovich.

Clarke-Stewart, A., Thompson, W., & Lepore, S. (1989, May). *Manipulating children's interpretations through interrogation.* Paper presented at the biennial meeting of the Society for Research on Child Development, Kansas City, MO.

Cohen, R. L. (1975). Children's testimony and hearsay evidence. *Law Reform Commission of Canada: Report on evidence.* Ottawa, Ontario, Canada: Information.

Cohen, R. L., & Harnick, M. A. (1980). The susceptibility of child witnesses to suggestion. *Law and Human Behavior, 4,* 201–210.

Cohn, D. S. (1991). Anatomical doll play of preschoolers referred for sexual abuse and those not referred. *Child Abuse and Neglect, 15,* 455–466.

Cole, C. B., & Loftus, E. F. (1987). The memory of children. In S. J. Ceci, M. Toglia, & D. Ross, (Eds.), *Children's eyewitness memory* (pp. 178–208). New York: Springer-Verlag.

Conte, J. R., Sorenson, E., Fogarty, L., & Rosa, J. D. (1991). Evaluating children's reports of sexual abuse: Results from a survey of professionals. *American Journal of Orthopsychiatry, 78,* 428–437.

Cutts, K., & Ceci, S. J. (1988, August). *Memory for cheerios or cheerio memory?* Paper presented at the 96th Annual Convention of the American Psychological Association, Atlanta, GA.

Dale, P. S., Loftus, E. F., & Rathbun, L. (1978). The influence of the form of the question on the eyewitness testimony of preschool children. *Journal of Psycholinguistic Research, 7,* 269–277.

Daro, D., & Mitchel, L. (1990). *Current trends in child abuse reporting and fatalities: The results of the 1989 Annual 50 States Survey.* Washington, DC: National Commission for the Prevention of Child Abuse.

Davidson, D. (1991, April). *Children's recognitions and recall memory for typical and atypical actions in script-based stories.* Paper presented at the biennial meeting of the Society for Research in Child Development, Seattle, WA.

Davies, G. M., Tarrant, A., & Flin, R. (1989). Close encounters of a witness kind: Children's memory for a simulated health inspection. *British Journal of Psychology, 80,* 415–429.

DeAngelis, T. (1990, September). Ruling tracks brief by APA. *APA Monitor,* pp. 1, 16.

Deffenbacher, K. A. (1991). A maturing of research on the behaviour of eyewitnesses. *Applied Cognitive Psychology, 5,* 377–402.

Delamothe, K., & Taplin, E. (1992, November). *The effect of suggestibility on children's recognition memory.* Paper presented at the Annual Meeting of the Psychonomics Society, St. Louis, MO.

Dent, H., & Stephenson, G. M. (1979). An experimental study of the effectiveness of different techniques of questioning child witnesses. *British Journal of Social and Clinical Psychology, 18,* 41–51.

Duncan, E. M., Whitney, P., & Kunen, S. (1982). Integration of visual and verbal information in children's memories. *Child Development, 53,* 1215–1223.

Ervin-Tripp, S. (1978). "Wait for me, Roller Skate!" In S. Ervin-Tripp & C. Mitchell-Kernan (Eds.), *Child discourse* (pp. 165–188). San Diego, CA: Academic Press.

Everson, M., & Boat, B. (1990). Sexualized doll play among young children: Implications for the use of anatomical dolls in sexual abuse evaluations. *Journal of the American Academy of Child and Adolescent Psychiatry, 29,* 736–742.

Farrar, J., & Goodman, G. S. (1990). Developmental differences in the relation between scripts and episodic memory: Do they exist? In R. Fivush & J. Hudson (Eds.), *Knowing and remembering in young children* (pp. 30–64). New York: Cambridge University Press.

Feher, T. (1988). The alleged molestation victim, the rules of evidence, and the Constitution: Should children really be seen and not heard? *American Journal of Criminal Law, 14,* 227.

Fivush, R. (in press). Developmental perspectives on autobiographical recall. In G. S. Goodman & B. Bottoms (Eds.), *Understanding and improving children's testimony.* New York: Guilford Press.

Fivush, R., & Hamond, N. (1990). Autobiographical memory across the preschool years: Toward reconceptualizing childhood amnesia. In R. Fivush & J. Hudson (Eds.), *Knowing and remembering in young children* (pp. 223–248). New York: Cambridge University Press.

Flanagan, O. (1992). Other minds, obligations, and honesty. In S. J. Ceci, M. Leichtman, & M. Putnick (Eds.), *Cognitive and social factors in early deception.* (pp. 111–126). Hillsdale, NJ: Erlbaum.

Flavell, J. H. (1985). *Cognitive development* (2nd ed.). Englewood Cliffs, NJ: Prentice-Hall.

Flavell, J. H., Flavell, E., & Green, F. L. (1987). Young children's knowledge about the apparent-real and pretend-real distinctions. *Developmental Psychology, 23,* 816–822.

Flin, R., Boon, J., Knox, A., & Bull, R. (1992). Children's memories following a five-month delay. *British Journal of Psychology, 83,* 323–336.

Foley, M. A., & Johnson, M. K. (1985). Confusions between memories for performed and imagined actions. *Child Development, 56,* 1145–1155.

Foley, M. A., Johnson, M. K., & Raye, C. L. (1983). Age-related confusion between memories for thoughts and memories for speech. *Child Development, 54,* 51–60.

Foley, M. A., Santini, C., & Sopasakis, M. (in press). Discriminating between memories: Evidence for children's spontaneous elaborations. *Journal of Experimental Child Psychology.*

Freiberg, P. (1990, December). Jurors perceive when children lie about abuse. *APA Monitor,* p. 32.

Freud, S. (1966). New introductory lectures on psychoanalysis. In J. Strachey (Ed. and Trans.), *The standard edition of the complete psychological works of Sigmund Freud* (Vol. 15–16). London: Hogarth Press. (Original work published 1933)

Frye v. the United States, 293 F.1013 (D.C. Cir. 1923).

Garbarino, J., & Stott, F. M. (1989). *What children can tell us.* San Francisco: Jossey-Bass.

Gardner, R. (1989). *Sex abuse hysteria: Salem Witch Trials revisited.* Longwood, NJ: Creative Therapeutics Press.

Garvey, C. (1984). *Children's talk.* Cambridge, MA: Harvard University Press.

Geiselman, R., Saywitz, K., & Bornstein, G. (1990). *Effects of cognitive interviewing, practice, and interview style on children's recall performance.* Unpublished manuscript.

Gelman, R., Meck, E., & Merkin, S. (1986). Young children's numerical competence. *Cognitive Development, 1,* 1–29.

Glaser, D., & Collins, C. (1989). The response of young, non-sexually abused children to anatomically correct dolls. *Journal of Child Psychology and Psychiatry, 30,* 547–560.

Gold, P. (1987). Sweet memories. *American Scientist, 75,* 151–155.

Goodman, G. (1984a). Children's testimony in historical perspective. *Journal of Social Issues, 40,* 9–31.

Goodman, G. (1984b). The child witness: Conclusions and future directions. *Journal of Social Issues, 40,* 157–175.

Goodman, G. S. (1990, August). *Psychology and the media.* In D. Singer (Chair), Symposium conducted at the 98th Annual Convention of the American Psychological Association, Boston.

Goodman, G. S. (1991). Commentary: On stress and accuracy in research on children's testimony. In J. Doris (Ed.), *The suggestibility of children's recollections* (pp. 77–82). Washington, DC: American Psychological Association.

Goodman, G., & Aman, C. (1990). Children's use of anatomically detailed dolls to recount an event. *Child Development, 62,* 1859–1871.

Goodman, G. S., & Clarke-Stewart, A. (1991). Suggestibility in children's testimony: Implications for child sexual abuse investigations. In J. L. Doris (Ed.), *The suggestibility of children's recollections* (pp. 92–105). Washington, DC: American Psychological Association.

Goodman, G. S., Hirschman, J. E., Hepps, D., & Rudy, L. (1991). Children's memory for stressful events. *Merrill Palmer Quarterly, 37,* 109–158.

Goodman, G. S., Levine, M., Melton, G., & Ogden, D. (1991). Child witnesses and the confrontation clause: The American Psychological Association Brief in *Maryland v. Craig. Law and Human Behavior, 15,* 13–30.

Goodman, G. S., & Reed, R. S. (1986). Age differences in eyewitness testimony. *Law and Human Behavior, 10,* 317–332.

Goodman, G. S., Rudy, L., Bottoms, B., & Aman, C. (1990). Children's concerns and memory: Issues of ecological validity in the study of children's eyewitness testimony. In R. Fivush & J. Hudson (Eds.), *Knowing and remembering in young children* (pp. 249–284). New York: Cambridge University Press.

Goodman, G. S., Sharma, A., Golden, M., & Thomas, S. (1991, April). *The effects of mothers' and strangers' interviewing strategies on children's reporting of real-life events.* Paper presented at the biennial meeting of the Society for Research in Child Development, Seattle, WA.

Goodman, G. S., Wilson, M. E., Hazan, C., & Reed, R. S. (1989, April). *Children's testimony nearly four years after an event.* Paper presented at the annual meeting of the Eastern Psychological Association, Boston.

Gordon, B. N., Ornstein, P. A., Clubb, P. A., & Nida, R. E. (1991, November). *Visiting the pediatrician: Long-term retention and forgetting.* Paper presented at the annual meeting of the Psychonomic Society, San Francisco.

Grice, H. P. (1975). Logic and conversation. In P. Cole & J. L. Morgan (Eds.), *Syntax and semantics* (pp. 41–58). San Diego, CA: Academic Press.

Gudjonsson, G. (1986). The relationship between interrogative suggestibility and acquiescence: Empirical findings and theoretical implications. *Personality and Individual Differences, 7,* 195–199.

Harris, P., Brown, E., Marriott, C., Whittall, S., & Harmer, S. (1991). Monsters, ghosts and witches: Testing the limits of the fantasy-reality distinction in young children. *British Journal of Developmental Psychology, 9,* 105–123.

Haugaard, J., & Repucci, N. D. (1992). Children and the truth. In S. J. Ceci, M. Leichtman, & M. Putnick (Eds.), *Social and cognitive factors in early deception.* (pp. 29–46). Hillsdale, NJ: Erlbaum.

Hollingsworth, J. (1986). *Unspeakable acts.* Chicago: Congdon & Weed.

Howe, M. L. (1991). Misleading children's story recall: Forgetting and reminiscence of the facts. *Developmental Psychology, 27,* 746–762.

Hudson, J. (1990). Constructive processes in children's event memories. *Developmental Psychology, 26,* 180–187.

Hudson, J., & Nelson, K. (1986). Repeated encounters of a similar kind: Effects of familiarity on children's autobiographic memory. *Cognitive Development, 1,* 253–271.

Hughes, M., & Grieve, R. (1980). On asking children bizarre questions. *First Language, 1,* 149–160.

Hurlock, E. (1930). Suggestibility in children. *Journal of Genetic Psychology, 37,* 59–74.

Jampole, L., & Weber, M. K. (1987). An assessment of the behavior of sexually abused and nonsexually abused children with anatomically correct dolls. *Child Abuse and Neglect, 11,* 187–192.

Johnson, M. K. (1991). Reality monitoring: Evidence from confabulation in organic brain disease patients. In G. Prigatano & D. Schacter (Eds.), *Awareness of deficit after brain injury* (pp. 124–140). New York: Oxford University Press.

Johnson, M. K., & Raye, C. L. (1981). Reality monitoring. *Psychological Review, 88,* 67–85.

Jones, D., & McGraw, J. M. (1987). Reliable and fictitious accounts of sexual abuse in children. *Journal of Interpersonal Violence, 2,* 27–45.

Jones, D. C., Swift, D. J., & Johnson, M. (1988). Nondeliberate memory for a novelty event among preschoolers. *Developmental Psychology, 24,* 641–645.

Kail, R. V. (1989). *The development of memory in children* (2nd ed.). New York: Freeman.

King, M., & Yuille, J. (1987). Suggestibility and the child witness. In S. J. Ceci, M. Toglia, & D. Ross (Eds.), *Children's eyewitness memory* (pp. 24–35). New York: Springer-Verlag.

Kramer, T., Buckhout, R., Fox, P., Widman, E., & Tusche, B. (1991). Effects of stress on recall. *Applied Cognitive Psychology, 5,* 483–488.

Leekam, S. (1992). Believing and deceiving: Steps to becoming a good liar. In S. J. Ceci, M. Leichtman, & M. Putnick (Eds.), *Social and cognitive factors in early deception* (pp. 47–62). Hillsdale, NJ: Erlbaum.

Leippe, M. R., Romanczyk, A., & Manion, A. P. (1991). Eyewitness memory for a touching experience: Accuracy in eyewitness identification. *Journal of Applied Psychology, 76,* 367–379.

Lewis, M., Stranger, C., & Sullivan, M. (1989). Deception in three-year-olds. *Developmental Psychology, 25,* 439–443.

Lindberg, M. (1980). Is knowledge base development a necessary and sufficient condition for memory development? *Journal of Experimental Child Psychology, 30,* 401–410.

Lindberg, M. (1991). A taxonomy of suggestibility and eyewitness memory: Age, memory process, and focus of analysis. In J. L. Doris (Ed.), *The suggestibility of children's recollections* (pp. 47–55). Washington, DC: American Psychological Association.

Lindsay, D. S. (1990). Misleading suggestions can impair eyewitnesses' ability to remember event details. *Journal of Experimental Psychology: Learning, Memory, and Cognition, 16,* 1077–1083.

Lindsay, D. S., Johnson, M. K., & Kwon, P. (1991). Developmental changes in memory source monitoring. *Journal of Experimental Child Psychology, 52,* 297–318.

Linton, M. (1982). Transformation of memory in everyday life. In U. Neisser (Ed.), *Memory observed: Remembering in natural contexts* (pp. 77–91), New York: W. H. Freeman.

Lipmann, O. (1911). Pedagogical psychology of report. *Journal of Educational Psychology, 2,* 253–261.

Lipscomb, T. J., Bregman, N., & McCallister, H. A. (1984). A developmental inquiry into the effects of postevent information on eyewitness accounts. *Journal of Genetic Psychology, 146,* 551–556.

List, J. A. (1986). Age and schematic differences in the reliability of eyewitness testimony. *Developmental Psychology, 22,* 50–57.

Loftus, E. F. (1979). *Eyewitness testimony.* Cambridge, MA: Harvard University Press.

Loftus, E. F. (1986). Ten years in the life of an expert witness. *Law and Human Behavior, 10,* 241–263.

Loftus, E. F., & Ceci, S. J. (1991). Research findings: What do they mean? In J. L. Doris (Ed.), *The suggestibility of children's recollections* (pp. 129–133). Washington, DC: American Psychological Association.

Loftus, E. F., Miller, D., & Burns, H. (1978). Semantic integration of verbal information into a visual memory. *Journal of Experimental Psychology: Human Learning and Memory, 4,* 19–31.

Loftus, E. F., & Palmer, J. C. (1974). Reconstruction of automobile destruction: An example of the interaction between language and memory. *Journal of Verbal Learning and Verbal Behavior, 13,* 585–589.

Loftus, E. F., & Zanni, G. (1975). Eyewitness testimony: The influence of wording of a question. *Bulletin of the Psychonomic Society, 5,* 86–88.

Loh, W. D. (1981). Psychological research: Past and present. *Michigan Law Review, 79,* 659–707.

Manshel, L. (1990). *Nap time.* New York: Kensington Publishing.

Marin, B. V., Holmes, D. L., Guth, M., & Kovac, P. (1979). The potential of children as eyewitnesses. *Law and Human Behavior, 3,* 295–305.

Martin, C. L., & Halverson, C. F. (1983). The effects of sex-typing schemas on young children's memory. *Child Development, 54* 563–574.

Maryland v. Craig, 110 S. Ct. 3157, 3169 (1990).

Mason, M. A. (1991, Fall-Winter). A judicial dilemma: Expert witness testimony in child sex abuse trials. *Psychiatry & Law,* 185–219.

Masson, J. M. (1984, February). Freud and the seduction theory. *Atlantic Monthly,* pp. 33–60.

McCloskey, M., & Egeth, H. W. (1983). Eyewitness identification: What can a psychologist tell a jury? *American Psychologist, 38,* 550–563.

McCloskey, M., Wible, C., & Cohen, N. J. (1988). Is there a special flashbulb-memory mechanism? *Journal of Experimental Psychology: General, 117,* 171–181.

McCloskey, M., & Zaragoza, M. (1985a). Misleading postevent information and memory for events: Arguments and evidence against the memory impairment hypothesis. *Journal of Experimental Psychology: General, 114,* 1–16.

McCloskey, M., & Zaragoza, M. (1985b). Postevent information and memory: Reply to Loftus, Schooler, and Wagenaar. *Journal of Experimental Psychology: General, 114,* 381–387.

McConnell, T. R. (1963). Suggestibility in children as a function of chronological age. *Journal of Abnormal and Social Psychology, 67,* 286–289.

McGough, L. (in press). *Fragile voices: The child witness in American courts.* New Haven, CT: Yale University Press.

Melton, G. (1992). Children as partners for justice: Next steps for developmentalists. *Monographs of the Society for Research in Child Development, 57,* (5, Serial No. 229).

Melton, G., & Thomson, R. (1987). Getting out of a rut: Detours to less travelled paths in child witness research. In S. J. Ceci, M. Toglia, & D. Ross (Eds.), *Children's eye-witness memory* (pp. 209–229). New York: Springer-Verlag.

Messerschmidt, R. (1933). The suggestibility of boys and girls between the ages of six and sixteen. *Journal of Genetic Psychology, 43*, 422–437.

Mitchell, R. W., & Thompson, N. S. (Eds.) (1986). *Deception: Perspectives on human and non-human deceit.* Albany: State University of New York Press.

Moore, C. (1907). Yellow psychology. *Law Notes, 11*, 125–127.

Moore, C. C. (1908). Psychology in the courts. *Law Notes, 11*, 185–187.

Morison, P., & Gardner, H. (1978). Dragons and dinosaurs: The child's capacity to differentiate fantasy from reality. *Child Development, 49*, 642–648.

Moss, D. C. (1988). "Real" dolls too suggestive: Do anatomically correct dolls lead to false abuse charges? *American Bar Association Journal, 24* (Dec. 1).

Moston, S. (1987). The suggestibility of children in interview studies. *First Language, 7*, 67–78.

Münsternberg, H. (1907a, April). Nothing but the truth. *McClure's Magazine*, pp. 26–29.

Münsternberg, H. (1907b). Yellow psychology: Dr. Münsternberg replies to Mr. Moore. *Law Notes, 11*, 145–146.

Myers, J. B. (1987). *Child witness law and practice.* New York: Wiley.

Myles-Worsley, M., Cromer, C., & Dodd, D. (1986). Children's preschool script construction: Reliance on general knowledge after memory fades. *Developmental Psychology, 22*, 22–30.

Nathan, D. (1993). Revisiting Country Walk. *Issues in Child Abuse Allegations, 5*, 1–11.

Nelson, K., & Gruendel, J. (1979). At morning it's lunchtime: A scriptal view of children's dialogues. *Discourse Processes, 2*, 73–94.

Nurcombe, B. (1986). The child as witness: Competency and credibility. *Journal of the American Academy of Child Psychiatry, 25*, 473–480.

Oates, K., & Shrimpton, S. (1991). Children's memories for stressful and non-stressful events. *Medicine, Science, and the Law, 31*, 4–10.

Ornstein, P. A. (Ed.), (1978). *Memory development in children.* Hillsdale, NJ: Erlbaum.

Ornstein, P. A., Gordon, B. N., & Larus, D. (1992). Children's memory for a personally experienced event: Implications for testimony. *Applied Cognitive Psychology, 6*, 49–60.

Otis, M. (1924). A study of suggestibility in children. *Archives of Psychology, 11*, 5–108.

Perner, J. (1991). *Understanding the representational mind.* Cambridge, MA: MIT Press.

Perris, E. E., Myers, N. A., & Clifton, R. K. (1990). Long term memory for a single infancy experience. *Child Development, 61*, 1796–1807.

Peters, D. P. (1990, March). *Confrontational stress and lying.* Paper presented at the biennial meeting of the American Psychology/Law Society, Williamsburg, VA.

Peters, D. P. (1991a). The influence of stress and arousal on the child witness. In J. L. Doris (Ed.), *The suggestibility of children's recollections* (pp. 60–76). Washington, DC: American Psychological Association.

Peters, D. P. (1991b). Commentary: Response to Goodman. In J. L. Doris (Ed.). *The sug-*

gestibility of children's recollections (pp. 86–91). Washington, DC: American Psychological Association.

Peters, D. P. (1991c, April). *Confrontational stress and children's testimony.* Paper presented at the biennial meeting of the Society for Research in Child Development, Seattle, WA.

Pettit, F., Fegan, M., & Howie, P. (1990, September). *Interviewer effects on children's testimony.* Paper presented at the International Congress on Child Abuse and Neglect, Hamburg, Federal Republic of Germany.

Piaget, J. (1926). *The language and thought of the child.* London: Routledge & Kegan Paul.

Pillemer, D. B. (1990). Clarifying the flashbulb memory concept: Comment on McCloskey, Wible, and Cohen (1988). *Journal of Experimental Psychology: General, 119,* 92–96.

Pillemer, D. B. (in press). Preschool children's memories of personal circumstances: The fire alarm study. In E. Winograd & U. Neisser (Eds.), *Affect and accuracy in recall: The problem of flashbulb memories.* New York: Cambridge University Press.

Pillemer, D. B., Koff, E., Rhinehart, E. D., & Rierdan, J. (1987). Flashbulb memories of menarche and adult menstrual distress. *Journal of Adolescence, 10,* 187–199.

Pipe, M. E., & Goodman, G. S. (in press). Elements of secrecy: Implications for children's testimony. *Behavioral Sciences and the Law.*

Poole, D. A. (in press). Two years later: Effects of question repetition and retention interval on the eyewitness testimony of children and adults. *Developmental Psychology.*

Poole, D. A., & White, L. T. (1991). Effects of question repetition on the eyewitness testimony of children and adults. *Developmental Psychology, 27,* 975–986.

Powers, P., Andriks, J. L., & Loftus, E. F. (1979). Eyewitness accounts of females and males. *Journal of Applied Psychology, 64,* 339–347.

Pratt, C. (1991). On asking children—and adults—bizarre questions. *First Language, 10,* 167–175.

Raskin, D., & Yuille, J. (1989). Problems in evaluating interviews of children in sexual abuse cases. In S. J. Ceci. M. Toglia, & D. F. Ross (Eds.), *Adults' perceptions of children's testimony* (pp. 184–207). New York: Springer-Verlag.

Read, B., & Cherry, L. (1978). Preschool children's productions of directive forms. *Discourse Processes, 1,* 233–245.

Realmuto, G., Jensen, J., & Wescoe, S. (1990). Specificity and sensitivity of sexually anatomically correct dolls in substantiating abuse: A pilot study. *Journal of the American Academy of Child and Adolescent Psychiatry, 29,* 743–746.

Remmers, H., Cutler, M., & Jones, P. (1940). Waking suggestibility in children: General or specific? *Journal of Genetic Psychology, 56,* 87–93.

Romaine, S. (1984). *The language of children and adolescents.* Cambridge, MA: Basil Blackwell.

Rose, S., & Blank, M. (1974). The potency of context in children's cognition: An illustration through conversation. *Child Development, 45,* 499–502.

Ross, D. F., Dunning, D., Toglia, M., & Ceci, S. J. (1990). The child in the eyes of the jury. *Law and Human Behavior, 14,* 5–23.

Rovee-Collier, C., & Borza, M. A. (in press). Infants' eyewitness testimony: Integrating postevent information into a prior memory representation. *Memory & Cognition.*

Rudy, L., & Goodman, G. S. (1991). Effects of participation on children's reports: Implications for children's testimony. *Developmental Psychology, 27,* 527–538.

Saywitz, K. (1987). Children's testimony: Age-related patterns of memory errors. In S. J. Ceci, M. Toglia, & D. Ross (Eds.), *Children's eyewitness memory* (pp. 36–52). New York: Springer-Verlag.

Saywitz, K. (1989). Children's conceptions of the legal system: "Court is a place to play basketball." In S. J. Ceci, M. Toglia, & D. Ross (Eds.), *Perspectives on children's testimony* (pp. 131–157). New York: Springer-Verlag.

Saywitz, K., Geiselman, R., & Bornstein, G. (1992). Effects of cognitive interviewing, practice, and interview style on children's recall performance. *Journal of Applied Psychology, 77,* 744–756.

Saywitz, K., Goodman, G., Nicholas, G., & Moan, S. (1991). Children's memory for genital exam: Implications for child sexual abuse. *Journal of Consulting and Clinical Psychology, 59,* 682–691.

Schneider, W., & Pressley, M. (1989). *Memory development between 2 and 20.* New York: Springer-Verlag.

Schuman, D. C. (1986). False allegations of physical and sexual abuse. *Bulletin of the American Academy of Psychiatry and the Law, 14,* 5–21.

Schwartz-Kenney, B. M., & Goodman, G. S. (1991, April). *Effects of misinformation on children's memory for a real-life event.* Paper presented at the biennial meeting of the Society for Research in Child Development, Seattle, WA.

Sherman, I. (1925). The suggestibility of normal and mentally defective children. *Comparative Psychology Monographs,* No. 2.

Siegal, M., Waters, L., & Dinwiddy, L. (1988). Misleading children: Causal attributions for inconsistency under repeated questioning. *Journal of Experimental Child Psychology, 45,* 438–456.

Sivan, A. B., Schor, D. P., Koeppl, G. K., & Noble, L. D. (1988). Interaction of normal children with anatomical dolls. *Child Abuse and Neglect, 12,* 295–304.

Sodian, B. (1991). The development of deception in young children. *British Journal of Developmental Psychology, 9,* 173–188.

Sonnenschein, S., & Whitehurst, G. (1980). The development of communication: When a bad model makes a good teacher. *Journal of Experimental Child Psychology, 3,* 371–390.

Spencer, J., & Flin, R. (1990). *The evidence of children: The law and the psychology.* London: Blackstone.

Stern, W. (1910). Abstracts of lectures on the psychology of testimony and on the study of individuality. *American Journal of Psychology, 21,* 270–282.

Steward, M. (1989). *The development of a model interview for young child victims of sexual abuse.* (Tech. Rep. No. 90CA1332). Washington, DC: U.S. Department of Health and Human Services.

Stouthamer-Loeber, M. (1987, April). *Mothers' perceptions of children's lying and its rela-*

tionship to behavior problems. Paper presented at the biennial meeting of the Society for Research in Child Development, Baltimore, MD.

Tate, C. S., & Warren-Leubecker, A. R. (1990, March). Can young children lie convincingly if coached by adults? In S. J. Ceci (Chair), *Do children lie? Narrowing the uncertainties.* Symposium conducted at the biennial meeting of the American Psychology/Law Society, Williamsburg, VA.

Tate, C. S., Warren, A. R., & Hess, T. H. (1992). Adults' liability for children's "lie-ability": Can adults coach children to lie successfully? In S. J. Ceci, M. Leichtman, & M. Putnick (Eds.), *Cognitive and social factors in early deception* (pp. 69–88). Hillsdale, NJ: Erlbaum.

Taylor, R., & Howell, M. (1973). The ability of 3-, 4-, and 5-year-olds to distinguish fantasy from reality. *Journal of Genetic Psychology, 122,* 315–318.

Terr, L. (1983). Chowchilla revisited: The effects of psychic trauma four years after a schoolbus kidnapping. *American Journal of Psychiatry, 140,* 1543–1550.

Terr, L. (1988). Anatomically correct dolls: Should they be used as a basis for expert testimony? *Journal of the American Academy of Child and Adolescent Psychiatry, 27,* 254–257.

Terr, L. (1990). *Too scared to cry: Psychic trauma in childhood.* New York: Harper & Row.

Toglia, M. (1991). Commentary: Memory impairment—It is more common than you think. In J. L. Doris (Ed.), *The suggestibility of children's recollections* (pp. 40–46). Washington, DC: American Psychological Association.

Tucker, A., Merton, P., & Luszcz, M. (1990). The effect of repeated interviews on young children's eyewitness memory. *Australian and New Zealand Journal of Criminology, 23,* 117–123.

Tulving, E. E., & Watkins, M. J. (1975). Structure of memory traces. *Psychological Review, 82,* 261–275.

Underwager, R., & Wakefield, H. (1990). *The real world of child interrogations.* Springfield, IL: Charles C Thomas.

Vandermaas, M. (1991, April). *Assessment of young children's anxiety during dental procedures.* Paper presented at the biennial meeting of the Society for Research in Child Development, Seattle, WA.

Varendonck, J. (1911). Les temoignages d'enfants dans un proces retentissant [The testimony of children in a famous trial]. *Archives de Psycholgie, 11,* 129–171.

Vasek, M. E. (1986). Lying as a skill: The development of deception in children. In R. W. Mitchell & N. Thompson (Eds.), *Deception: Perspectives on human and nonhuman deceit* (pp. 144–168). New York: State University of New York: Press.

Walker, A. G. (1988, June). *Questioning young children in court.* Paper presented at the Law and Society annual meeting, Washington, DC.

Warren, A., & Hagood, P. (in press). Effects of timing and type of questioning on eyewitness accuracy and suggestibility. In M. Zaragoza (Ed.), *Memory, suggestibility, and eyewitness testimony in children and adults.* New York: Hemisphere.

Warren, A. R., Hulse-Trotter, K., & Tubbs, E. (1991). Inducing resistance to suggestibility in children. *Law and Human Behavior, 15,* 273–285.

Warren, A. R., & Swartwood, J. N. (in press). Developmental issues in flashbulb memory research: Children recall the *Challenger* event. In E. Winograd & U. Neisser (Eds.), *Affect and accuracy in recall: The problem of flashbulb memories*. New York: Cambridge University Press.

Warren-Leubecker, A. R., Tate, C., Hinton, I., & Ozbek, N. (1989). What do children know about the legal system and when do they know it? First steps down a less travelled path in child witness research. In S. J. Ceci, M. Toglia, & D. Ross (Eds.), *Perspectives on children's testimony* (pp. 158–183). New York: Springer-Verlag.

Whipple, G. M. (1909). The observer as reporter: A survey of the "psychology of testimony." *Psychological Bulletin, 6,* 153–170.

Whipple, G. M. (1911). The psychology of testimony. *Psychological Bulletin, 8,* 307–309.

Whipple, G. M. (1912). Psychology of testimony and report. *Psychological Bulletin, 9,* 264–269.

Whipple, G. M. (1913). Psychology of testimony and report. *Psychological Bulletin, 10,* 264–268.

White, S., Strom, G., Santili, G., & Halpin, B. M. (1986). Interviewing young sexual abuse victims with anatomically correct dolls. *Child Abuse and Neglect, 10,* 519–530.

Whiten, A. (1991). *Natural theories of mind: The evolution, development, and simulation of every day mindreading*. Oxford, England: Basil Blackwell.

Wigmore, J. H. (1909). *Evidence*. Boston: Little, Brown.

Wigmore, J. H. (1935). *Evidence in trials at common law* (Vol. 6). Boston: Little, Brown.

Wilson, J, C., & Pipe, M. E. (1989). The effects of cues on young children's recall of real events. *New Zealand Journal of Psychology, 18,* 65–70.

Winograd, E., & Killinger, W. A., Jr. (1983). Relating age at encoding in early childhood to adult recall: Development of flashbulb memories. *Journal of Experimental Psychology: General, 112,* 413–422.

Wolfner, G., Faust, D., & Dawes, R. (1993). The use of anatomically detailed dolls in sexual abuse evaluations: The state of the science. *Applied and Preventive Psychology, 2,* 1–11.

Yarmey, D., & Jones, J. (1983). Is the psychology of eyewitness identification a matter of common sense? In S. Lloyd & B. Clifford (Eds.), *Evaluating witness evidence* (pp. 13–40). New York: Wiley.

Zacharias, F. (1990). Rethinking confidentiality: II. Is confidentiality constitutional? *Iowa Law Review, 75,* 601.

Zaragoza, M. (1991). Preschool children's susceptibility to memory impairment. In J. L. Doris (Ed.), *The suggestibility of children's recollections* (pp. 27–39). Washington, DC: American Psychological Association.

Zaragoza, M., Dahlgren, D., & Muench, J. (1992). The role of memory impairment in children's suggestibility. In M. L. Howe, C. J. Brainerd, & V. F. Reyna (Eds.), *Development of long term retention.* (pp. 184–216). New York: Springer-Verlag.

9

The Reality of Repressed Memories

Elizabeth F. Loftus

University of Washington, Seattle

Repression is one of the most haunting concepts in psychology. Something shocking happens, and the mind pushes it into some inaccessible corner of the unconscious. Later, the memory may emerge into consciousness. Repression is one of the foundation stones on which the structure of psychoanalysis rests. Recently there has been a rise in reported memories of childhood sexual abuse that were allegedly repressed for many years. With recent changes in legislation, people with recently unearthed memories are suing alleged perpetrators for events that happened 20, 30, even 40 or more years earlier. These new developments give rise to a number of questions: (a) How common is it for memories of child abuse to be repressed? (b) How are jurors and judges likely to react to these repressed memory claims? (c) When the memories surface, what are they like? and (d) How authentic are the memories?

In 1990, a landmark case went to trial in Redwood City, California. The defendant, George Franklin, Sr., 51 years old, stood trial for a murder that had occurred more than 20 years earlier. The victim, 8-year-old Susan Kay Nason, was murdered on September 22, 1969. Franklin's daughter, Eileen, only 8 years old

Reprinted with permission from *American Psychologist*, 1993, Vol. 48, 518–537. Copyright © 1993 by the American Psychological Association, Inc.

Stanley L. Brodsky served as action editor for this article.

This article is an expanded version of an invited address, the Psi Chi/Frederick Howell Lewis Distinguished Lecture, presented at the 100th Annual Convention of the American Psychological Association, Washington DC, August 1992. I thank Geoffrey Loftus, Ilene Bernstein, Lucy Berliner, Robert Koscielny, and Richard Ofshe for very helpful comments on earlier drafts. I thank many others, especially Ellen Bass, Mark Demos, Judie Alpert, Marsha Linehan, and Denise Park for illuminating discussion of the issues. My gratitude for the vast efforts of the members of the Repressed Memory Research Group at the University of Washington is beyond measure. The National Institute of Mental Health and the National Science Foundation have generously supported the underlying research on memory.

herself at the time of the murder, provided the major evidence against her father. What was unusual about the case is that Eileen's memory of witnessing the murder had been repressed for more than 20 years.

Eileen's memory did not come back all at once. She claimed that her first flash-back came one afternoon in January 1989 when she was playing with her two-year-old son, Aaron, and her five-year-old daughter, Jessica. At one moment, Jessica looked up and asked her mother a question like "Isn't that right, Mommy?" A memory of Susan Nason suddenly came back. Eileen recalled the look of betrayal in Susie's eyes just before the murder. Later, more fragments would return, until Eileen had a rich and detailed memory. She remembered her father sexually assaulting Susie in the back of a van. She remembered that Susie was struggling as she said "No don't" and "Stop." She remembered her father saying "Now Susie," and she even mimicked his precise intonation. Next, her memory took the three of them outside the van, where she saw her father with his hands raised above his head with a rock in them. She remembered screaming. She remembered walking back to where Susie lay, covered with blood, the silver ring on her finger smashed.

Eileen's memory report was believed by her therapist, by several members of her family, and by the San Mateo County district attorney's office, which chose to prosecute her father. It was also believed by the jury, which convicted George Franklin, Sr., of murder. The jury began its deliberations on November 29, 1990, and returned a verdict the next day. Impressed by Eileen's detailed and confident memory, they found her father guilty of murder in the first degree.

Eileen's detailed and confident memory impressed a number of people. But is her memory authentic? Did she really witness the murder of her best friend 20 years earlier? The idea of repression of early traumatic memories is a concept that many psychotherapists readily accept (Bruhn, 1990). In fact, it has been said that repression is the foundation on which psychoanalysis rests (Bower, 1990). According to the theory, something happens that is so shocking that the mind grabs hold of the memory and pushes it underground, into some inaccessible cor-ner of the unconscious. There it sleeps for years, or even decades, or even forever—isolated from the rest of mental life. Then, one day, it may rise up and emerge into consciousness. Numerous clinical examples fitting this model can be readily found. Many of these examples involve not memory of murder but rather memory of other sorts of childhood trauma, such as sexual abuse, that allegedly has been repressed for decades until recovered in therapy. Rieker and Carmen (1986) described a woman who entered psychotherapy for sexual dysfunction and recovered memories of incest committed by her father. Schuker (1979) described a woman who entered psychotherapy for chronic insomnia, low self-esteem, and other problems and recovered memories of her father sexually assaulting her. M. Williams (1987) described a man who entered therapy for depression and sleep disturbances and recovered memories of a servant molesting him. These anecdotal reports constitute the clinical evidence that clients do indeed manage later to remember some earlier inaccessible painful experience (Erdelyi, 1985). The reports constitute evidence for the core ideas inherent in the theory of repression. Several respected scholars once made the point that, from a clinical standpoint, "the evidence for repression is overwhelming and obvious" (Erdelyi & Goldberg, 1979, p. 384).

On the other hand, the clinical anecdotes and the loose theory used to explain them remain unconvincing to some psychotherapists and to many laboratory researchers. One psychiatrist who has seen more than 200 severely dissociative patients explicitly referred to such anecdotes as "empirical observations lacking in scientific underpinnings" (Ganaway, 1992, p. 203). One researcher described them as "impressionistic case studies" and claimed that they could not be counted as "anything more than unconfirmed clinical speculations" (Holmes, 1990, p. 97). After reviewing 60 years of research and finding no controlled laboratory support for the concept of repression, Holmes suggested, only half jokingly, that any use of the concept be preceded by a warning: "Warning. The concept of repression has not been validated with experimental research and its use may be hazardous to the accurate interpretation of clinical behavior" (p. 97).

Even if Holmes (1990) was right that there is virtually no scientific evidence to demonstrate the authenticity of repressed memories that return, Eileen's memory could still be authentic. Even if Holmes is proved wrong and there does develop solid scientific evidence to support the authenticity of some repressed memories that return, that would not prove that Eileen's memory is authentic. If Eileen's memory is not authentic, where else might all those details come from? Media reports from 20 years before—December 1969, when the body was found—were filled with some of these same details. The facts that the murdered girl's skull was fractured on the right side and that a silver Indian ring was found on the body were reported prominently on the front page of the *San Francisco Chronicle* ("Susan Nason Body Found," 1969). The fact that she apparently held her hand up to protect herself, inferred from the crushed ring, was also well-known (e.g., *San Jose Mercury*, "Nason Girl Fought," 1969). Most of the details that fill the rich network of her memory, however, are unfalsifiable or uncheckable—such as her memory for the door of the van that her father got out of after he raped Susie. One additional feature of Eileen's memory, worth noting, is that it changed across various tellings. For example, when she gave a statement to the police in November 1989, she told the police that her father was driving her and her sister Janice to school when they first saw Susie and that he made Janice get out of the van when Susie got in. However, months later at the preliminary hearing, she did not report Janice being in the van. In the statement to the police, the trip happened on the way to school in the morning or on the way back from lunch. During the preliminary hearing, after she presumably was reminded that Susie had not been missing until after school was out, she said it was in the late afternoon because the sun was low. Eileen's memory changed over the tellings, and there were alternative possible sources for details that made the memory seem so rich. This proves that at least some portions of these distant memories are wrong, although other parts could, in theory, still be authentic.

When George Franklin, Jr., was convicted on the basis of little more than the return of a repressed memory, *Newsweek* magazine called it an "incredible" story ("Forgetting to Remember," 1991). It was apparently the first time that an American citizen had been tried and convicted of murder on the basis of a freshly unearthed repressed memory.

MORE REPRESSED MEMORIES

Soon after the Franklin case, a string of others involving newly emerged distant memories appeared in the media. People accused by the holders of repressed memories wrote letters asking for help. Lawyers found themselves being asked to represent parties in legal cases involving repressed memories.

Popular Articles

Long-repressed memories that return after decades, often while a person is in therapy, have become highly publicized through popular articles. In 1991, actress Roseanne Barr Arnold's story was on the cover of *People* magazine. Memories of her mother abusing her from the time she was an infant until she was 6 or 7 years old had returned in therapy ("A Star Cries Incest," 1991; Darnton, 1991). Barr Arnold's was not the first such case to capture the cover of *People* magazine that year. Just three months earlier, *People* had also reported a story about former Miss America Marilyn Van Derbur, who had repressed any knowledge of sexual violation by her father until she was 24 years old and told the world about it after her father died ("The Darkest Secret," 1991; Darnton, 1991). Highly publicized cases involving memories that recently sprang into consciousness were told repeatedly in numerous popular articles in such publications as the *Washington Post* (Oldenberg, 1991), the *Los Angeles Times* (Ritter, 1991), *Seventeen* (Dormen, 1991), *Glamour* (Edmiston, 1990), *Newsweek* (Kantrowitz, 1991), and *Time* (Toufexis, 1991).

Letters

Scores of spontaneously written letters from strangers also describe the emergence of memories. I have received letters written by people who had been accused of abuse by their children. A 75-year-old physician from Florida wrote, desperate to understand why his 49-year-old daughter was suddenly claiming that he had abused her during her early childhood and teen years. A woman from Canada wrote about the nightmare of being "falsely accused of sexual abuse by our 30-year-old daughter." A woman from Michigan wrote about her 38-year-old daughter who, "after a year of counseling now accuses us of abuse . . . very much like Roseanne Barr and the former Miss America, Marilyn Van Derbur." A couple from Texas wrote to tell about their youngest son, who had accused them of abusing him long ago. One letter from a mother in California well expresses the pain:

> One week before my husband died after an 8-month battle against lung cancer, our youngest daughter (age 38) confronted me with the accusation that he had molested her and I had not protected her. We know who her "therapist" was: a strange young woman . . . In the weeks, months that followed, the nature of the charges altered, eventually involving the accusation that my husband and I had molested our grandson, for whom we had sometimes cared while our daughter worked at her painting. This has broken my heart; it is so utterly untrue. This daughter has broken off all relationship with her four siblings. She came greatly under the influence of a book, *The Courage to Heal* [by Bass & Davis, 1988].

The letters articulately convey the living nightmares and broken hearts experienced by those accused by their adult children who suddenly remembered past abuse (see also Doe, 1991). The parents vehemently deny the abuse. Who is right and who is wrong? Is the adult child misremembering, or perhaps lying? Are the parents misremembering when they deny abuse, or are they deliberately lying?

Legal Cases

Another development after the Franklin conviction was that lawyers started calling psychologists to obtain assistance with a puzzling new type of legal case. For example, one case involved a 27-year-old San Diego woman (KL) who began to have recollections of molestation by her father (DL), that were repressed but then were later brought out through "counseling and therapeutic intervention" (*Lofft v. Lofft*, 1989). The daughter claimed that her father had routinely and continuously molested and sexually abused her, performing "lewd and lascivious acts, including but not limited to touching and fondling the genital areas, fornication and oral copulation." Her earliest memories were of her father fondling her in the master bedroom when she was three years old. Most of her memories appeared to date back to between the ages of three and eight. She sued her father for damages for emotional and physical distress, medical expenses, and lost earnings. She claimed that because of the trauma of the experience, she had no recollection or knowledge of the sexual abuse until her repression was lifted, shortly before she filed suit.

A few years ago, plaintiffs like KL who claimed to be survivors of childhood sexual abuse would have been barred from suing by statutes of limitations. Statutes of limitations, which force plaintiffs to initiate claims promptly, exist for good reason: They protect people from having to defend themselves against stale claims. They exist in recognition that with the passage of time, memories fade and evidence becomes more difficult to obtain. Succinctly and articulately put, the primary purpose of statutes of limitation is to prevent "surprises through the revival of claims that have been allowed to slumber until evidence has been lost, memories have faded, and witnesses have disappeared" (*Telegraphers v. Railway Express Agency,* 1944, pp. 348–349). When much time has passed, defendants find it hard to mount an effective defense. Although a statute of limitations on child sexual abuse might be suspended until a victim reaches the age of majority or a few years beyond, it previously would not typically have been extended to the age of 27, for example, when KL first recalled her abuse.

In 1989, things changed for plaintiffs in the state of Washington. Legislation went into effect that permitted people to sue for recovery of damages for injury suffered as a result of childhood sexual abuse at any time within three years of the time they *remembered* the abuse (Washington, 1989; see also *Petersen v. Bruen,* 1990). The legislature involved a novel application of the *delayed discovery doctrine,* which essentially says that the statute of limitations does not begin to run until the plaintiff has discovered the facts that are essential to the cause of action. Traditionally, the delayed discovery doctrine has been used in the area of medical malpractice. For example, a patient who discovered during a physical examination that his abdominal discomfort was caused by a surgical instrument left after an appendectomy performed 20 years earlier could sue because he could not have discovered the facts essential to his harm until he had the examination. Analogizing to the surgical instrument that was hidden from the patient until an exam made its presence known, so the memory for abuse was hidden away until it too is discovered and the plaintiff possesses the facts that are essential to the cause of action.

Within three years of enactment of the Washington statute, 18 other states enacted similar legislation allowing for the tolling of the statute of limitations.[1] Many other states introduced bills in the 1991–1992 legislative sessions that would achieve the same result, or they have begun studying similar legislation. As

[1]Alaska, California, Colorado, Connecticut, Florida, Idaho, Illinois, Iowa, Maine, Minnesota, Missouri, Montana, Nevada, New Hampshire (revising an earlier law), Oregon, South Dakota, Vermont, and Virginia (see, for example, Napier, 1990).

a consequence, repressed memories now form the basis for a growing number of civil law suits. As one writer put it, "Such wholesale forgetting—or more precisely, the eventual remembering—is forcing society to grapple in unaccustomed ways with the old problem of child molestation" (Davis, 1991, p. 81). Increasing numbers of women, and also some men, are coming out of therapy with freshly retrieved memories of abuse. They sue for damages rather than file criminal complaints, because criminal charges are often too difficult to prove (Davis, 1991). In a few states (e.g., Wyoming), they can also bring criminal charges, and moves are afoot to change laws in more states to permit criminal prosecutions to go forward. As a consequence, juries are now hearing cases in which plaintiffs are suing their parents, relatives, neighbors, teachers, church members, and others for acts of childhood sexual abuse that allegedly occurred 10, 20, 30, even 40 years earlier. Juries and judges are learning about repression of memory and about newly emerged memories of molestation not only in the United States but also in Canada, Great Britain, and other parts of the world.[2]

Many interesting questions leap to mind about repressed memories. Chief among them are, How common are claims of repressed memory? How do people in general and jurors in particular react to claims of recently unburied repressed memories? What are the memories like? How authentic are they?

HOW COMMON ARE CLAIMS OF REPRESSED MEMORY?

There is little doubt that actual childhood sexual abuse is tragically common. Even those who claim that the statistics are exaggerated still agree that child abuse constitutes a serious social problem (Kutchinsky, 1992). I do not question the commonness of childhood sexual abuse itself but ask here about how the abuse is recalled in the minds of adults. Specifically, how common is it to repress memories of childhood sexual abuse? Claims about the commonness of repressed memories are freely made: It is typical to read estimates such as "most incest survivors have limited recall about their abuse" or "half of all incest survivors do not remember that the abuse occurred" (Blume, 1990, p. 81). One psychotherapist with 18 years of experience has claimed that "millions of people have blocked out frightening episodes of abuse, years of their life, or their entire childhood" (Frederickson, 1992, p. 15). Later, she reported that "sexual abuse is particularly susceptible to memory repression" (p. 23).

Beliefs about the commonness of repressed memories are expressed not only

---

[2]In *Stubbings v. Webb and Another*, 1991, in which a British plaintiff claimed she was raped by her adoptive father and brother while she was a child. She sued 12 years after entering adulthood. The court permitted her suit, even though she knew she had been raped, arguing that she might not have associated the mental impairment that she was experiencing with the past rapes until she gained that knowledge as an adult.

by those in the therapeutic community but also by legal scholars who have used these beliefs to argue for changes in legislation. For example, Lamm (1991) argued in favor of legislation that would ease access to the courts for victims of childhood sexual abuse. She applauded legislation, such as that enacted in California in 1991, that allows victims, no matter how old they are, to sue within three years after discovering their injuries or eight years after reaching majority, whichever date occurs later. As part of her argument that victims should have more time to file claims against their abusers, she expressed a view that "total repression of memories of abuse is common" (p. 2198).

Despite the confidence with which these assertions are made, there are few studies that provide evidence of the extent to which repression occurs. One study (Briere & Conte, in press) sampled 450 adult clinical clients who had reported sexual abuse histories. Therapists approached their individual clients or group clients with this question: "During the period of time between when the first forced sexual experience happened and your 18th birthday was there ever a time when you could not remember the forced sexual experience?" The main result obtained in this largely female (93%) largely White (90%) sample was that 59% said yes. A yes response was more likely in cases involving violent abuse (physical injury, multiple perpetrators, and fears of death if abuse was disclosed) than nonviolent abuse. Reported amnesia was more likely with early molestation onset, longer abuse, and greater current symptomatology. The authors concluded that amnesia for abuse was a common phenomenon (see also Briere, 1992).

Briere and Conte's (in press) result has been taken by others as evidence for the widespread extent of repression. For example, Summit (1992) interpreted the 59% yes rate as evidence that this proportion of people "went through periods of amnesia when they were not aware of their prior abuse" (p. 22). He used the finding to support the commonness of childhood dissociation.

One problem with Briere and Conte's (in press) estimate is that it obviously depends on how the respondent interprets the eliciting question. A yes response to the question could be interpreted in a variety of ways other than "I repressed my memory for abuse." For example, it could mean "Sometimes I found it too unpleasant to remember, so I tried not to"; or "There were times when I could not remember without feeling terrible"; or "There were times I could not bring myself to remember the abuse because I would rather not think about it." Although no question is free of the possibility of multiple interpretations, the great potential for idiosyncratic interpretation by respondents to the particular wording used by Briere and Conte warrants a further examination of the issue with a different eliciting question.

A further problem with Briere and Conte's (in press) study is that the respondents were all in therapy. If some of their clinicians were under the belief that repression of memory is common, they may have communicated this belief to their clients. Clients could readily infer that, if repression of memory is so common, it is likely to have happened to them, thus the answer to the question is probably yes. This would, of course, inflate the estimates of the prevalence of repression.

Other studies have given much lower estimates for the existence of repression. Herman and Schatzow (1987) gathered data from 53 women in therapy groups for incest survivors in the Boston area. Of the 53 cases, 15 (28%) reported severe memory deficits (including women who could recall very little from childhood and women who showed a recently unearthed repressed memory). Severe memory problems were most likely in cases of abuse that began early in childhood and ended before adolescence. Cases of violent or sadistic abuse were most likely to be associated with "massive repression as a defense" (p. 5).[3]

An even lower estimate was obtained in a study of 100 women in outpatient treatment for substance abuse in a New York City hospital (Loftus, Polonsky, & Fullilove, 1993). More than one half of the women in this sample reported memories of childhood sexual abuse. The vast majority of them remembered the abuse their whole lives. Only 18% claimed that they forgot the abuse for a period of time and later regained the memory. Whether the women remembered the abuse their whole lives or forgot it for a period was completely unrelated to the violence of the abuse.

Of course, the data obtained from the New York sample may include an underestimation factor because there could have been many more women in the sample who were sexually abused, repressed the memory, and had not yet regained it. In support of this hypothesis, one could point to the research of L. M. Williams (1992), who interviewed 100 women, mostly African American, known to have been abused 17 years earlier in their lives. Of these, 38% were amnestic for the abuse or chose not to report it. Perhaps there were women in the New York sample who denied sexual abuse but who were still repressing it. Possibly there are women who were actually abused but do not remember it; however, it is misleading to assume that simple failure to remember means that repression has occurred. If an event happened so early in life, before the offset of childhood amnesia, then a woman would not be expected to remember it as an adult, whether it was abuse or something else. This would not imply the mechanism of repression. Moreover, ordinary forgetting of all sorts of events is a fact of life but is not thought to involve some special repression mechanism. For example, studies have shown that people routinely fail to remember significant life events even a year after they have occurred. One study consisted of interviews with 590 persons known to have been

---

[3]One curiosity about this report is that the chief investigator published a landmark book on incest six years before this study (Herman, 1981). In the earlier book, the word *repression* did not even appear in the index. The 40 incest victims interviewed in depth appeared to have persisting, intrusive memories.

in injury-producing motor vehicle accidents during the previous year. Approximately 14% did not remember the accident a year later. Another study consisted of interviews with 1,500 people who had been discharged from a hospital within the previous year. More than one fourth did not remember the hospitalization a year later (U.S. government studies, cited in Loftus, 1982).

How common are repressed memories of childhood abuse? There is no absolute answer available. There are few satisfying ways to discover the answer, because we are in the odd position of asking people about a memory for forgetting a memory. For the moment, figures range from 18% to 59%. The range is disturbingly great, suggesting that serious scholarly exploration is warranted to learn how to interpret claims about the commonness of repression and what abuse characteristics the repression might be related to.

JURORS' REACTIONS TO REPRESSED MEMORY CASES

How do people in general and jurors in particular react to repressed memory cases? Are memories that were once previously repressed as credible as memories that were never repressed? Understanding laypeople's reactions and credibility judgments is important not only for theoretical reasons but for practical ones as well. Theoretically speaking, laypeople's implicit or intuitive theories about repressed memories guide society's thinking on this topic.[4] Such implicit theories can also illuminate how therapists' theories of repression are formed; in part they derive from a therapist's own implicit theories.

On a more practical level, understanding implicit theories of repression is important. Plaintiffs' lawyers who are deciding whether to file repressed memory cases are eager to know their likelihood of a successful outcome. Defense lawyers also care, because such subjective probabilities affect their decisions about whether to proceed to trial or to settle a case early. Perhaps most importantly, the plaintiffs should care. Plaintiffs bring lawsuits for myriad reasons. Some therapists encourage their clients to sue as "hope for emotional justice" (Forward & Buck, 1988). One therapist who had treated more than 1,500 incest victims argued that the lawsuit, although grueling, is "a very important step towards devictimization," "a further source of validation," and that "the personal satisfaction can be significant" (Forward & Buck, p. 159). If the lawsuit is good for a plaintiff's mental health, what happens to mental health if a jury does not find the notion of repressed memories tenable and the plaintiff, consequently, does not prevail?

---

[4]Many cognitive psychologists have argued that implicit theories about any topic (e.g., giftedness) guide a given society's thinking on that topic (e.g., Sternberg, 1992). More generally, intuitive theories are considered constructing working models of the world that people use in the service of understanding their world (Medin & Ross, 1992).

Actual Cases

I start by examining actual cases that have gone to trial in recent years, with a wide range of outcomes. Some trials ended in defense verdicts (e.g., *Lofft v. Lofft,* 1989, in San Diego; *Collier v. Collier,* 1991, in Santa Clara County). Others ended in plaintiff verdicts. For example, a 39-year-old woman sued her father in Los Angeles, and the jury awarded $500,000 (McMillan, 1992). A 33-year-old woman sued her uncle in Akron, Ohio, and the jury awarded $5.15 million ($150,000 in compensatory damages and $5 million in punitive damages; Fields, 1992). Because the laws are new and most cases have settled, there are too few actual trials from which to gather data about reactions to repressed memory claims. Until more cases are tried to verdict, it may be necessary to rely on simulated jury research to gather information on this issue.

Simulations

Several juror simulation studies have explored how people are likely to react to repressed memory cases (Loftus, Weingardt, & Hoffman, 1992). In these studies, mock jurors learned about a legal case that arose out of allegations of sexual assault. Subjects considered the case of a daughter (Roberta) and her father (Jim), a case modeled loosely after an actual case tried in the state of Washington in 1991. Roberta, they learned, accused her father of raping her on several occasions when she was approximately 10 years old. She claimed she repressed all memory for these incidents. At about age 20, Roberta's memory returned while she was in therapy. She filed charges against her father a year after her memory came back. Roberta and her therapist blamed her current problems of depression, anxiety, and sexual dysfunction on the sexual abuse that happened when she was 10. Jim denied the allegations, claiming that Roberta was influenced by her therapist's suggestive questioning and that she was looking for someone or something to blame for her troubles.

How did people react to Roberta's claim? Did their reactions differ from reactions to a case that was identical except for the repression of memory? A different set of subjects reacted to a modified scenario involving a different woman (Nancy) whose memory was not repressed. Nancy's factual situation was identical to Roberta's except, subjects were told, Nancy never told anyone until age 20, when she went into therapy and told her therapist. Who is believed more, Roberta or Nancy? Several consistent findings emerged from these studies. First, people tended to be slightly more skeptical about Roberta's case (the repressed memory) than they were about Nancy's case (the nonrepressed memory). Both male and female subjects reacted this way, with males overall being more skeptical.

When subjects disbelieved the claims, they were more likely to think that the false claims were due to an honest mistake than a deliberate lie. One small difference emerged—repressed and nonrepressed memory cases appear to bring slightly different thoughts to mind. When subjects considered Nancy's case, thoughts of lying were slightly more likely to be evoked than when they considered Roberta's case. One of the clearest results was that, in general, the majority of subjects believed that the claims of both Roberta and Nancy were true and accurate.

WHAT ARE THE MEMORIES LIKE?

The quality of the memories that filter back varies tremendously. They are sometimes detailed and vivid and sometimes very vague. Sometimes they pertain to events that allegedly happened in early childhood and sometimes in adolescence. Sometimes they pertain to events that allegedly happened 5 years ago and sometimes 40 years ago. Sometimes they include fondling, sometimes rape, and sometimes ritualism of an unimaginable sort.

Highly detailed memories have been reported even for events that allegedly happened more than 25 years earlier and during the first year of life. One father–daughter case recently tried in Santa Clara County, California, illustrates this pattern (*Collier v. Collier*, 1991). The daughter, DC, a college graduate who worked as a technical writer, claimed that her father sexually abused her from the time she was six months old until she was 18. She repressed the memories until the age of approximately 26, when she was in individual and group therapy.

Other cases involve richly detailed allegations of a more bizarre, ritualistic type, as in a case reported by Rogers (1992a). The plaintiff, Bonnie, in her late 40s at the time of trial, accused her parents of physically, sexually, and emotionally abusing her from birth to approximately age 25. A sister, Patti, in her mid-30s at the time of trial, said she was abused from infancy to age 15. The allegations involved torture by drugs, electric shock, rape, sodomy, forced oral sex, and ritualistic killing of babies born to or aborted by the daughters. The events were first recalled when the plaintiffs went into therapy in the late 1980s.

In short, reports of memories after years of repression are as varied as they can be. One important way that they differ is in terms of the age at which the events being remembered allegedly happened. In many instances, repressed memory claims refer to events that occurred when the child was one year old or less. This observation invites an examination of the literature on childhood amnesia. It is well known that humans experience a poverty of recollections of their first several years in life. Freud (1905/1953) identified the phenomenon in some of his earliest writings: "What I have in mind is the peculiar amnesia which . . . hides the earliest beginnings of the childhood up to their sixth or eighth year" (p. 174). Contemporary cognitive psychologists place the offset of childhood amnesia at a somewhat earlier age: "past the age of ten, or thereabouts, most of us find it impossible to recall anything that happened before the age of four or five" (Morton, 1990, p. 3). Most empirical studies of childhood amnesia suggest that people's earliest recollection does not date back before the age of about three or four (Kihlstrom & Harackiewicz, 1982; Howe & Courage, 1993; Pillemer & White, 1989). One study showed that few subjects who were younger than three recalled any information about where they were when they heard about the assassination of President Kennedy, although most subjects who were more than eight at the time had some recall (Winograd & Killinger, 1983). Although one recent study suggests that some people might have a memory for a hospitalization or the birth of a sibling that occurred at age two (Usher & Neisser, in press), these data do not completely rule out the possibility that the memories are not true memories but remembrances of things told by others (Loftus, in press). Still, the literature on childhood amnesia ought to figure in some way into our thinking about recollections of child molestation that supposedly occurred in infancy.

ARE THE MEMORIES AUTHENTIC?

Therapists' Beliefs About Authenticity

Many therapists believe in the authenticity of the recovered memories that they hear from their clients. Two empirical studies reveal this high degree of faith. Bottoms, Shaver, and Goodman (1991) conducted a large-scale survey of clinicians who had come across, in their practice, ritualistic and religion-related abuse cases. Satanic ritualistic abuse (SRA) cases involve allegations of highly bizarre and heinous criminal ritual abuse in the context of an alleged vast, covert network of highly organized, transgenerational satanic cults (Braun & Sachs, 1988; Ganaway, 1989, 1991). Clients with SRA memories have reported vividly detailed memories of cannibalistic revels and such experiences as being used by cults during adolescence as serial baby breeders to provide untraceable infants for ritual sacrifices (Ganaway, 1989; Rogers, 1992b). If therapists believe these types of claims, it seems likely that they would be even more likely to believe the less aggravated claims involving ordinary childhood sexual abuse. Bottoms et al.'s (1991) analysis revealed that 30% of responding clinicians had seen at least one case of child sexual abuse. A detailed analysis of 200 clinicians' experiences revealed that a substantial number of cases involved amnesic periods (44% of adult survivor cases). Overall, 93% of clinicians believed the alleged harm was actually done and that the ritualistic aspects were actually experienced by the clients. The conclusion was, in the investigators' own words, "The clinical psychologists in our sample believe their clients' claims" (p. 10).

A different approach to the issue of therapist belief was taken by Loftus and

Herzog (1991). This study involved in-depth interviews with 16 clinicians who had seen at least one repressed memory case. In this small, nonrandom sample, 13 (81%) said they invariably believed their clients. One therapist said, "if a woman said it happened, it happened." Another said, "I have no reason not to believe them." The most common basis for belief was symptomatology (low self-esteem, sexual dysfunction, self-destructive behavior), or body memories (voice frozen at young age, rash on body matching inflicted injury). More than two thirds of the clinicians reacted emotionally to any use of the term *authentic,* feeling that determining what is authentic and what is not authentic is not the job of a therapist. The conclusion from this small study was that therapists believe their clients and often use symptomatology as evidence.

These and other data suggest that therapists believe in their clients' memories. They point to symptomatology as their evidence. They are impressed with the emotional pain that accompanies the expression of the memories. Dawes (1992) has argued that this "epidemic" of belief is based in large part on authority and social consensus (p. 214).

Are the Memories Accurate?

There are those with extreme positions who would like to deny the authenticity of all repressed memories and those who would accept them all as true. As Van Benschoten (1990) has pointed out, these extreme positions will exacerbate our problems: "Denial fosters overdetermination, and overdetermination invites denial" (p. 25).

If we assume, then, that some of the memories might be authentic and some might not be, we can then raise this question: If a memory is recovered that is not authentic, where would it come from? Ganaway (1989) proposed several hypotheses to explain SRA memories, and these same ideas are relevant to memories of a repressed past. If not authentic, the memories could be due to fantasy, illusion, or hallucination-mediated screen memories, internally derived as a defense mechanism. Further paraphrasing Ganaway, the SRA memories combine a mixture of borrowed ideas, characters, myths, and accounts from exogenous sources with idiosyncratic internal beliefs. Once activated, the manufactured memories are indistinguishable from factual memories. Inauthentic memories could also be externally derived as a result of unintentional implantation of suggestion by a therapist or other perceived authority figure with whom the client desires a special relationship, interest, or approval.

The Memories Are Authentic

There is no doubt that childhood sexual abuse is tragically common (Daro, 1988). Surveys reveal a large range in the estimated rates (10%–50%), but as Freyd (1991) has argued, even the most conservative of them are high enough to support the enormity of child abuse. A sizeable number of people who enter therapy were abused as children and have always remembered their abuse. Even when they have severe emotional problems, they can provide rich recollections of abuse, often with many unique, peripheral details (Rogers, 1992a). Occasionally the abuse is corroborated, sometimes with very cogent corroboration, such as pornographic photographs. If confirmed abuse is prevalent, many instances of repressed memory abuse cases also could be authentic. Unfortunately, in the repressed memory cases, particularly when memories do not return for 20 or 30 years, there is little in the way of documented corroboration. This, of course, does not mean that they are false.

Claims of corroborated repressed memories occasionally appear in the published literature. For example, Mack (1980) reported on a 1955 case involving a 27-year-old borderline man who, during therapy, recovered memories of witnessing his mother attempting to kill herself by hanging. The man's father later confirmed that the mother had attempted suicide several times and that the son had witnessed one attempt when he was 3 years old. The father's confirmation apparently led to a relief of symptoms in the son. It is hard to know what to make of examples such as these. Did the son really remember back to age 3, or did he hear discussions of his mother's suicide attempts later in life? The memories could be real, that is, genuine instances of repressed memories that accurately returned much later. If true, this would only prove that some memory reports are authentic but obviously not that all reports are authentic. Analogously, examples of repressed memories that were later retracted, later proved to be false, or later proved to be the result of suggestion would only prove that some memory reports are not authentic but obviously not that all such reports are illusory.

Some who question the authenticity of the memories of abuse do so in part because of the intensity and sincerity of the accused persons who deny the abuse. Many of the thousands of people who have been accused flatly deny the allegations, and the cry of "witch hunt" is often heard (Baker, 1992, p. 48; Gardner, 1991). *Witch hunt* is, of course, a term that has been loosely used by virtually anyone faced by a pack of accusers (Watson, 1992). Analogies have been drawn between the current allegations and the witch craze of the 16th and 17th centuries, when an estimated half million people were convicted of witchcraft and burned to death in Europe alone (Harris, 1974; Trott, 1991b). Although the denials during the witch craze are now seen as authentic in the light of hindsight, the current denials of those accused of sexual abuse are not proof that the allegations are false.

Research with known rapists, pedophiles, and incest offenders has illustrated that they often exhibit a *cognitive distortion*—a tendency to justify, minimize, or rationalize their behavior (Gudjonsson, 1992). Because accused persons are motivated to verbally and even mentally deny an abusive past, simple denials cannot constitute cogent evidence that the victim's memories are not authentic.

The Memories Are Not Authentic

To say that memory might be false does not mean that the person is deliberately lying. Although lying is always possible, even psychotherapists who question the authenticity of reports have been impressed with the honesty and intensity of the terror, rage, guilt, depression, and overall behavioral dysfunction accompanying the awareness of abuse (Ganaway, 1989, p. 211).

There are at least two ways that false memories could come about. Honestly believed, but false, memories could come about, according to Ganaway (1989), because of internal or external sources. The internal drive to manufacture an abuse memory may come about as a way to provide a screen for perhaps more prosaic but, ironically, less tolerable, painful experiences of childhood. Creating a fantasy of abuse with its relatively clear-cut distinction between good and evil may provide the needed logical explanation for confusing experiences and feelings. The core material for the false memories can be borrowed from the accounts of others who are either known personally or encountered in literature, movies, and television.[5]

SOURCES OF DETAILS THAT COULD AFFECT MEMORY

There are at least two important sources that could potentially feed into the construction of false memories. These include popular writings and therapists' suggestions.

Popular Writings

All roads on the search for popular writings inevitably lead to one, *The Courage to Heal* (Bass & Davis, 1988), often referred to as the "bible" of the incest book industry. *The Courage to Heal* advertises itself as a guide for women survivors of child sexual abuse. Although the book is undoubtedly a great comfort to the sex-

---

[5]For those who think it is unlikely that one would ever borrow episodes from movies and popular literature and misremember them as actual events, one only has to examine Lou Cannon's (1991) biography of former President Reagan. A curious journalist who tried to verify Reagan's most famous mismemory of heroism found two that were suspiciously similar—one in the movie *A Wing and a Prayer*, and the other in a *Reader's Digest* story.

ual abuse survivors who have been living with their private and painful memories, one cannot help but wonder about its effects on those who have no such memories. Readers who are wondering whether they might be victims of child sexual abuse are provided with a list of possible activities ranging from the relatively benign (e.g., being held in a way that made them uncomfortable) to the unequivocally abusive (e.g., being raped or otherwise penetrated). Readers are then told "If you are unable to remember any specific instances like the ones mentioned above but still have a feeling that something abusive happened to you, it probably did" (p. 21). On the next page, the reader is told

> You may think you don't have memories, but often as you begin to talk about what you do remember, there emerges a constellation of feelings, reactions and recollections that add up to substantial information. To say, "I was abused," you don't need the kind of recall that would stand up in a court of law. Often the knowledge that you were abused starts with a tiny feeling, an intuition. . . . Assume your feelings are valid. So far, no one we've talked to thought she might have been abused, and then later discovered that she hadn't been. The progression always goes the other way, from suspicion to confirmation. If you think you were abused and your life shows the symptoms, then you were. (p. 22)

What symptoms? The authors list low self-esteem, suicidal or self-destructive thoughts, depression, and sexual dysfunction, among others.[6]

Others have worried about the role played by *The Courage to Heal*. A recent survey of several hundred families accused by derepressed memories revealed that the book was implicated "in almost all cases" (Wakefield & Underwager, 1992, p. 486). Complaints about the book range from its repeated suggestion that abuse probably happened even if one has no memories of it and that demands for corroboration are not reasonable, to its overt encouragement of "revenge, anger, fantasies of murder or castration, and deathbed confrontations" (Wakefield & Underwager, 1992, p. 485). In all fairness, however, it should be mentioned that the book is long (495 pages), and sentences taken out of context may distort their intended meaning. Nonetheless, readers without any abuse memories of their own cannot escape the message that there is a strong likelihood that abuse occurred even in the absence of such memories.

---

[6]Since the publication of *The Courage to Heal*, a number of cases have emerged in which women were led to believe they were abused, and later realized their memories were false (Watters, 1993). Lynn Gondolf is a case in point. During more than a year of therapy she discovered repressed memories of her father raping her. After she stopped therapy, she realized that her therapist had "coerced her and the other members of her group into imagining memories of abuse" (Watters, 1993, p. 26).

The recent incest book industry has published not only stories of abuse but also suggestions to readers that they were likely abused even if there are no memories, that repressed memories of abuse undoubtedly underlie one's troubles, or that benefits derive from uncovering repressed memories and believing them.[7] One popular book about incest is the paperback by E. Sue Blume (1990), the book jacket of which itemizes one of the author's chief credentials as the "Creator of the Incest Survivors' Aftereffects Checklist."[8] Blume, a private practice therapist, tells readers that she has "found that most incest survivors have limited recall about their abuse" (p. 81). She goes on to say that "Indeed, so few incest survivors in my experience have identified themselves as abused in the beginning of therapy that I have concluded that perhaps half of all incest survivors do not remember that the abuse occurred" (p. 81).

Some of the volumes provide exercises to help readers lift the repression. Farmer (1989), for example, tells readers to try one particular exercise "whether or not you have any conscious recollection of the abuse you suffered" (p. 91). The reader is to sit down, relax, and mentally return to childhood. The next step is to choose a particular memory, whether fuzzy or clear, and "bring that memory to your full attention" (p. 91). Details about what to do with the memory are provided, along with an example from the life of "Danielle," who thought about how verbally abusive her father had been, and "Hazel," who remembered anger at her mother's treating her like a rag doll. This exercise allegedly helped to "lift the lid of repression" and unbury the "Hurting Child."

Do these examples lift the lid of repression? Perhaps. But another equally viable hypothesis is that the examples influence the creation of memories or, at the very least, direct the search through memory that the reader will ultimately take.[9]

---

[7]Consider a brief sampling: From Poston and Lison (1990), "Women usually do not make an immediate incest connection. They may not recall for years that the incest occurred: memories have an uncanny way of coming only when the survivor can deal with them" (p. 193); and "Many women do not remember the incest; how are they then to connect adult problems with childhood pain?" (p. 196). From Farmer (1989): "You may have even repressed the memories of the abuse. The more severe the abuse, the more likely you were to repress any conscious recollection of it" (p. 52).

[8]This book proudly displays an endorsement by Gloria Steinem: "This book, like the truth it helps uncover, can set millions free."

[9]Popular writings might also be the source of some questionable lay beliefs about early memories. Bradshaw (1990, 1992), a leading figure in the field of recovery and dysfunctional families, invited readers to consult his "index of suspicion": Do you have trouble knowing what you want? Are you afraid to try new experiences? If someone gives you a suggestion, do you feel you ought to follow it? According to Bradshaw, if you answered even one of these questions "yes," then you "can count on some damage having been done to you . . . between the 9th and 18th months of your life" (1992, p. 49). How many Bradshaw aficionados have struggled through their memories trying to find that childhood trauma?

Therapists' Suggestions

Blume's (1990) observation that so many individuals enter therapy without memories of abuse but acquire memories during therapy naturally makes one wonder about what might be happening in therapy. According to Ganaway (1989), honestly believed but false memories could come about in another way, through unintentional suggestion from therapists. Ganaway noted a growing trend toward the facile acceptance and expressed validation of uncorroborated trauma memories, perhaps in part due to sensitization from years of accusations that the memories are purely fantasy. Herman (1992, p. 180) made a similar point: Whereas an earlier generation of therapists might have been discounting or minimizing their patients' traumatic experiences, the recent rediscovery of psychological trauma has led to errors of the opposite kind. Some contemporary therapists have been known to tell patients, merely on the basis of a suggestive history or symptom profile, that they definitely had a traumatic experience. Even if there is no memory, but merely some vague symptoms, certain therapists will inform a patient after a single session that he or she was very likely the victim of a satanic cult. Once the "diagnosis" is made, the therapist urges the patient to pursue the recalcitrant memories. Although some therapists recommend against persistent, intrusive probing to uncover early traumatic memories (e.g., Bruhn, 1990), others enthusiastically engage in these therapeutic strategies. Evidence for this claim comes in a variety of forms: (a) therapist accounts of what is appropriate to do with clients, (b) client accounts of what happened during therapy, (c) sworn statements of clients and therapists during litigation, and (d) taped interviews of therapy sessions.

Therapist accounts. One therapist, who has treated more than 1,500 incest victims, openly discussed her method of approaching clients (Forward & Buck, 1988). "You know, in my experience, a lot of people who are struggling with many of the same problems you are, have often had some kind of really painful things happen to them as kids—maybe they were beaten or molested. And I wonder if anything like that ever happened to you?" (p. 161). Other clinicians claim to know of therapists who say "Your symptoms sound like you've been abused when you were a child. What can you tell me about that?" (Trott, 1991a, p. 18); or worse, "You sound to me like the sort of person who must have been sexually abused. Tell me what that bastard did to you" (Davis, 1991, p. 82).

At least one clinician advocated "It is crucial . . . that clinicians ask about sexual abuse during every intake" (Frawley, 1990). The rationale for this prescription is that a clinician who asks conveys to the client that the client will be believed and that the clinician will join with the client in working through the memories and emotions linked with childhood sexual abuse. Asking about sexual abuse along with a list of other past life events makes sense given the high instance of actual abuse, but the concern is how the issue is raised and what therapists do when clients initially deny an abusive past.

Evidence exists that some therapists do not take no for an answer. One therapist (who otherwise seemed sensitive to problems of memory tampering) still recommended "When the client does not remember what happened to her, the therapist's encouragement to 'guess' or 'tell a story' will help the survivor regain access to the lost material" (Olio, 1989, p. 6). She went on to provide the example of a client who suspected sexual abuse but had no memories. The client had become extremely anxious at a social gathering in the presence of a three-year-old girl. She had no idea why she was upset except that she wanted the little girl to keep her dress down. When encouraged in therapy to tell a story about what was going to happen to the little girl, the client ultimately related with tears and trembling one of the first memories of her own abuse. She used the story to "bypass her cognitive inhibitions and express the content of the memory" (p. 6). Later she "integrated the awareness that she was indeed the little girl in the story" (p. 6). One cannot help but wonder about these mental fantasy exercises in light of known research showing that the simple act of imagination makes an event subjectively more likely (e.g., Sherman, Cialdini, Schwartzman, & Reynolds, 1985).

Even if the therapist does not encourage the client to guess or tell a story, stories sometimes get told in the form of client dreams. If discussions of incest go on during the day, and day residue gets into the dreams at night, it would not be surprising to see that dreams of incest might result. Poston and Lison (1990) described a woman with "repressed memories" of incest who reported a dream about watching a little girl ice skate on a frozen river. In her dream, the woman tried desperately to warn the child that monsters and snakes were making their way through the ice to devour her. Although frightened, the woman was powerless and could not warn the innocent child. A few days later, the client began remembering incest from her childhood. Knowing she had "a trusted relationship with a therapist and a survivor's group that would understand and accept her" (p. 197), the memories began to flow.

Examples of therapists interpreting dreams as signs of memory of abuse can be found throughout the literature. One clinician described with pride how she communicated to her male patient the basis for her suspicions that he had been abused: "On many occasions, I explained that these dreams had preserved experiences and impressions of an indelible nature" (M. Williams, 1987, p. 152).

Frederickson (1992), who has worked with many incest survivors, has also described in detail her methods of getting patients to remember. She recommended that the therapist guide the patient "to expand on or explore images that have broken through to the conscious mind, allowing related images of the abuse to surface. The process lets the survivor complete the picture of what happened, using a current image or flash as a jumping-off point" (p. 97). She also suggested that the therapist help the patient expand on the images and sensations evoked by dreams "to shed light on or recover our repressed memories" (p. 98). She extolled the virtues of hypnosis to "retrieve buried memories" (p. 98) and recommended that patients "jot down suspected memories of abuse you would like to explore. Include your own felt sense of how you think you were abused" (p. 102).

Even if clinicians are not the first to bring up sexual abuse, they will often reinforce what begins as a mere suspicion. One client developed the idea that she might have been sexually abused, tried hypnosis to help her recover memories, and obsessed for years. Only after her therapist stated that she believed sexual assault was "indeed possible" and cited nightmares, phobia of men, and other symptoms as evidence did the client come up with some specific memories (Schuker, 1979, p. 569).

Before leaving the examples of therapist accounts of what goes on in therapy, it is important to add a word of caution. Sherrill Mulhern, a psychiatric anthropologist, has documented the alarming discrepancies that often exist between therapists' accounts of what they have done in therapy and what is revealed in video- or audiotapes of those same sessions (Mulhern, 1991).

If memories are uncovered—whether after repeated probing, after telling stories, after dreams, or seemingly spontaneously—or even if the memories remain buried, therapists often send their clients to support groups. In one study of clients who had, in the course of therapy, verbalized their victimization through ritualistic abuse, the majority reported that they had participated in these types of groups (Shaffer & Cozolino, 1992). One group, Survivors of Incest Anonymous (SIA), publishes extensive reading materials intended to aid the recovery of incest survivors. (SIA merged with Sexual Abuse Anonymous in 1987.) The criteria for admission make it clear that entry is fine for those with no memories of sexual abuse: "Do you have blocks of your childhood you can't remember? Do you have a sense that 'something happened'?" (SIA, 1985). These and other questions (e.g., Do you have problems with self-confidence and self esteem? Do you feel easily intimidated by authority figures?) are among the set of 20 questions that help a potential survivor decide whether SIA can be of assistance. SIA emphasizes that it is OK not to remember at first, because "Many survivors have 'repressed' actual abuse memories in order to survive." However, the goal is to remember: "Participating in SIA helps us to remember what happened to us so we can stop being controlled by incest" (SIA, 1990, p. 1).

Although support groups are undoubtedly invaluable for genuine survivors of sexual abuse, as they are for other survivors of extreme situations, such as combat and political persecution (Herman, 1992, p. 215), concerns about the incest survivor groups have been expressed. Do these groups foster the development of constructed memories? An investigative journalist attending a four-day workshop watched the construction of memory at work (Nathan, 1992). With members recounting graphic details of SRA abuse, how long will they listen to the person who can only say "I think I was abused, but I don't have any memories." Others have worried in the literature that such groups may induce *proto-extension*—that is, they actually encourage a troubled person to remember details from other survivor stories as having happened to them as well (Ellis, 1992).

Client accounts. Another source for suggestions in therapy can be found in client accounts of what happened to them. Recently, clients have been reporting that a therapist has suggested that childhood abuse was the cause of their current distress. However, these clients have no memories of such abuse. One woman from Oregon entered therapy to deal with depression and anxiety, and within a few months her therapist suggested that the cause could be childhood sexual abuse. She wrote asking for help in remembering:

> Since that time, he has become more and more certain of his diagnosis . . . I have no direct memories of this abuse. . . . The question I can't get past is how something so terrible could have happened to me without me remembering anything. For the past two years I have done little else but try to remember. I've tried self-hypnosis and light trance work with my therapist. And I even travelled to childhood homes . . . in an attempt to trigger memories.

One client revealed the suggestive nature of his therapist's questioning on ABC's *Primetime Live* (ABC News, 1992). Attorney Greg Zimmerman went to a psychotherapist in Boulder, Colorado, to deal with his father's suicide. He told ABC, "I would try to talk to her about the things that were very painful in my life and she kept saying that there was something else" (p. 1). Zimmerman grew more and more depressed as the mystery of that "something else" would not unravel, and then, during a therapy session, his therapist stunned him with her diagnosis: "I don't know how to tell you this, but you display the same kinds of characteristics as some of my patients who are victims of Satanic ritualistic abuse" (p. 1). Zimmerman had said nothing whatsoever to her to provoke this diagnosis, apparently her standard.

It is easy to find published accounts that describe the emergence of memories in therapy and the techniques that therapists have used to uncover those memories (e.g., Bass & Thornton, 1991). One account, written under the pseudonym of Jill Morgan, told of a series of positively horrifying memories of abuse by her father. He raped her when she was 4 years old, again at age 9, once again at age 13, for seven straight days and nights at age 15, and for the final time at age 18. For the next several years, all misery was withheld from conscious memory, and then, at age 29, she was helped to remember in therapy: "Through hypnosis and age regression, a skilled therapist gave me back my memory" (p. 111). The involvement of hypnosis and age regression prompts the natural inquiry into whether these techniques produce authentic memories. Unfortunately, the evidence is discouraging: There is an extensive literature seriously questioning the reliability of hypnotically enhanced memory in general (Smith, 1983), and hypnotic age regression in particular (Nash, 1987). Hypnotic attempts to improve memory increase the confidence in what is recalled more than the accuracy (Bowers, 1992). Even more worrisome is the impossibility of reversing the process; the hypnotically induced memory becomes the person's reality (Orne, 1979). With hypnotic regression, men and women have been known to recall being abducted by aliens aboard exotic spacecraft and other forgotten events (Gordon, 1991).

A more detailed client account is that of Betsy Petersen (1991), as described in an autobiographical account, *Dancing with Daddy*. Petersen, a Harvard graduate and accomplished writer, revealed in her first book that she repressed memory of sexual abuse by her father until she was 45 years old. She now remembers sexual abuse from the time she was 3½ until she was 18. Betsy entered therapy (with "Kris") for problems relating to her children, and almost a year after starting therapy she started worrying, "I'm afraid my father did something to me." She tried hard to recall, putting "together a scenario of what might have happened" (p. 65). When she told her therapist about this, she said "I don't know if I made it up or if it's real." Kris replied, "It feels like a story to you, because when something like that happens, everybody acts like it didn't." Betsy: "You mean it might really have happened!" Kris told her there was a good chance it had happened. Kris told her, in Betsy's words, "It was consistent with what I remembered about my father and my relationship with him, and with the dreams I had been having, and with the difficulties I had being close to my children, and also, she said, with the feelings I had during and after sex with my husband" (p. 65). Betsy worked hard to retrieve incest memories: "I had no memory of what my father had done to me, so I tried to reconstruct it. I put all my skill—as a reporter, novelist, scholar—to work making that reconstruction as accurate and vivid as possible. I used the memories I had to get to the memories I didn't have" (p. 66).[10] If accurate, this account tells us something about one therapist's approach. The therapist convinces the patient with no memories that abuse is likely, and the patient obligingly uses reconstructive strategies to generate memories that would support that conviction. These techniques can be found in numerous autobiographical accounts (see also Smith & Pazder, 1980).

In addition to the first-person accounts, more formal studies of incest survivors provide clues to what might be happening in therapy. One study (Shaffer & Cozolino, 1992) of 20 adults who uncovered ritualistic abuse memories stemming

---

[10]*Dancing with Daddy* was reviewed in the *New York Times* by Culhane (1991). The reviewer called the book "as much a story about our desperate search for one dimensional solutions to multidimensional problems as it is a story about incest and its consequences" (p. 18).

from childhood revealed that the majority sought psychotherapy because of symptoms (e.g., depression and anxiety). The primary focus of their therapy was "the uncovering of memories" (p. 189). The majority participated in 12-step programs (e.g., Incest Survivors Anonymous) as "necessary adjuncts to their psychotherapy" (p. 190). These groups provided substitute families for the clients who had severed ties with their families of origin. Other similar studies of ritualistic abuse rememberers have revealed that most of the victims have no memory of the abuse before therapy (e.g., Driscoll & Wright, 1991) but that techniques such as hypnosis (Driscoll & Wright, 1991) or dreams and artwork (e.g., Young, Sachs, Braun, & Watkins, 1991) were used by therapists to unlock those recalcitrant memories.

Litigation accounts. Information gathered during litigation is another source of knowledge about the emergence of memories in therapy. Take the case of Patti Barton against her father, John Peters, a successful businessman.[11] Depositions taken in the case of *Barton v. Peters* (1990) reveal that Patti Barton began therapy with a Dr. CD, a doctor of divinity, in July 1986. Dr. CD's notes indicate that, during the 32nd session of therapy, Patti expressed "fear her father has sexually tampered with her" (Deposition of CD, April 21, 1991, *Barton v. Peters,* 1990, p. 39). This was the first time that anything like that had come up in any of the sessions. Shortly thereafter, Patti related a dream that a man was after her.[12] Dr. CD apparently then used the technique of visualization wherein Patti would try to visualize her past. He got her to remember eye surgery at the age of 7 months. As for the abuse, one of the earliest acts of abuse he managed to dredge up with this method occurred when Patti was 15 months old. "I visualized that my father stuck his tongue in my mouth."

> After he stuck his tongue in my mouth—Well, it seemed to last for hours and hours even though I know it didn't. But it was awful to me and an event that seemed to last for hours. I started crying, and I

[11]The laws in Washington and other states were changed in part due to the efforts of Kelly Barton and Patti Barton of Seattle. Patti's allegations were described in Seattle newspapers, in *Newsweek* magazine (Darnton, 1991), and on the *Sally Jesse Raphael* show. According to the *Newsweek* account, Patti remembered the alleged abuse when she was in her 30s—too late to sue under the old Washington law. So, with the help of a lawyer, she lobbied to extend the statute of limitations to allow victims to bring suit for up to three years after their memory returns. Patti's father, who denied all charges, moved to Alaska, whereupon Patti turned her efforts on the Alaska legislature and introduced the same legislation there.

[12]In the dream, there was "a fellow who was out to hurt and perhaps rape her. In the dream she could not get rid of him. In her primal, she fought him with words until I nudged her on the shoulder with a batacka (a padded bat), and what I did was, I nudged her on the shoulder and she was there. . . . She came unglued at that. She took the batacka, grabbed it, and began striking out. She worked and worked until she got rid of him at the door. She opened the door of the room and kicked him out and locked the door. The man looked like her manic-depressive brother but had mannerisms like Kelly (her husband)" (p. 43).

crawled over to the wall. And I started banging my head on the wall. And my mother came into the room, and she picked me up. And I tried to tell her in baby talk what had happened. I said "Ma, ma, ma, ma," and I said, "Da, Da, Da, Da" and I said, "Me-e-e-." And that's all that I can remember. (Deposition of PB, May 1991, *Barton v. Peters,* 1990, p. 193)

Later, Patti would remember that her father touched her in her crotch and put his penis in her mouth when she was three years old, and that she stroked his penis over and over at age four. Rape would come later. Patti's father eventually agreed to give his daughter the deed to a piece of land he owned, but he continued to deny the charges. Her brother, a Baptist minister in Alaska, claimed that Satan's wicked spirits planted untruths in Patti's head (Laker, 1992). Did it take 30-some sessions for the therapist to uncover actual memories of abuse, or 30-some sessions for false memories of abuse to begin to be visualized and constructed?

Taped interviews. Often, confidentiality considerations prevent access to interactions between therapists and clients. However, when cases get into litigation, special interviewing is frequently done, and occasionally it is recorded. Recordings were done in a case implicating a man named Paul Ingram from Olympia, Washington (Watters, 1991). Ingram was arrested for child abuse in 1988, amid expressions of shock from his community. At the time he was chair of the county Republican committee and was chief civil deputy in the sheriff's office. He had worked in law enforcement for more than a decade.

The Ingram case began at a time when waves of rumor and media hype over satanic ritualistic abuse were rampant. At first Ingram denied everything, and detectives told him he was in denial. With the help of a psychologist who exerted enormous pressure over endless hours of interrogation, Ingram's memories of abusing his daughter began to appear. Then the psychologist, with the help of a detective, "interviewed" Ingram's son. In that interview, the son reported on his dreams, and the therapist and detective convinced him that the dreams were real.[13]

---

[13]Here is one segment:
Son: "I would have dreams of uh little people . . . short people coming and walking on me . . . walking on my bed."
Psychologist: "What you saw was real."
Son: "Well, this is a different dream . . . everytime a train came by, a whistle would blow and . . . witch would come in my window . . . I would wake up, but I couldn't move. It was like the blankets were tucked under and . . . I couldn't move my arms."
Psychologist: "You were being restrained?"
Son: "Right and there was somebody on top of me."
Psychologist: "[Son's name] these things happened to you. . . . It's real. It's not an hallucination."
Before long, the dreams became the reality: The son soon remembered witches holding him down and joining his father in abuse.

In another case, a father (Mr. K) hired a private investigator after his 26-year-old daughter reported a recently uncovered repressed memory and accused him of incest. The investigator, acting under cover, went to see the daughter's therapist complaining that she had nightmares and had trouble sleeping. On the third visit, the therapist told the undercover agent that she was an incest survivor. According to the investigator's report (Monesi, 1992), the therapist said this to her pseudopatient: "She then told me that she was certain I was experiencing body memory from a trauma, earlier in life, that I could not remember. I could not remember because my brain had blocked the memory that was too painful to deal with." When the patient said she didn't remember any trauma, the therapist told her "that is the case and many people at far later times in their lives go through this when the memory starts to surface." The therapist told her that many people go through this experience, such as "Viet Nam Vets, Earthquake Survivors and Incest Survivors." When the patient said that she had never been in Vietnam or in an earthquake, the therapist nodded her head and said "Yes, I know." The therapist then said she should read *The Courage to Heal,* a book she recommends to all abuse survivors. After that there was the *Courage to Heal Workbook,* which tells survivors how to cope with the fears and memories. She pulled *Secret Survivors* by E. S. Blume (1990) from the shelf, opened the cover, and read the list of symptoms of incest survivors. With two thirds of the symptoms, she would look at the pseudopatient and shake her head yes as if this was confirmation of her diagnosis. She recommended incest survivor groups. In the fourth session, the diagnosis of probable incest victim was confirmed on the basis of the "classic symptoms" of body memory and sleep disorders. When the patient insisted that she had no memory of such events, the therapist assured her this was often the case.

Why Would Therapists Suggest Things to Their Patients?

The core of treatment, it is widely believed, is to help clients reclaim their "traumatic past" (Rieker & Carmen, 1986, p. 369). Therapists routinely dig deliberately into the ugly underbelly of mental life. They dig for memories purposefully because they believe that in order to get well, to become survivors rather than victims, their clients must overcome the protective denial that was used to tolerate the abuse during childhood (Sgroi, 1989, p. 112). Memory blocks can be protective in many ways, but they come at a cost; they cut off the survivors from a significant part of their past histories and leave them without good explanations for their negative self-image, low self-esteem, and other mental problems. These memories must be brought into consciousness, not as an end in itself but only insofar as it helps the survivors acknowledge reality and overcome denial processes that are now dysfunctional (p. 115).

Another reason therapists may be unwittingly suggesting ideas to their clients is that they have fallen prey to a bias that affects all of us, known as the "confirmatory bias" (Baron, Beattie, & Hershey, 1988). People in general, therapists included, have a tendency to search for evidence that confirms their hunches rather than search for evidence that disconfirms. It is not easy to discard long-held or cherished beliefs, in part because we are eager to verify those beliefs and are not inclined to seek evidence that might disprove them.

The notion that the beliefs that individuals hold can create their own social reality is the essence of the self-fulfilling prophecy (Snyder, 1984). How does "reality" get constructed? One way this can happen is through interview strategies. Interviewers are known to choose questions that inquire about behaviors and experiences thought to be characteristic, rather than those thought to be uncharacteristic, of some particular classification. If therapists ask questions that tend to elicit behaviors and experiences thought to be characteristic of someone who had been a victim of childhood trauma, might they too be creating this social reality?

Whatever the good intentions of therapists, the documented examples of rampant suggestion should force us to at least ponder whether some therapists might be suggesting illusory memories to their clients rather than unlocking authentic distant memories. Or, paraphrasing Gardner (1992), what is considered to be present in the client's unconscious mind might actually be present solely in the therapist's conscious mind (p. 689). Ganaway (1989) worried that, once seeded by the therapist, false memories could develop that replace previously unsatisfactory internal explanations for intolerable but more prosaic childhood trauma.

Creation of False Memories.

The hypothesis that false memories could be created invites an inquiry into the important question of what is known about false memories. Since the mid-1970s at least, investigations have been done into the creation of false memories through exposure to misinformation. Now, nearly two decades later, there are hundreds of studies to support a high degree of memory distortion. People have recalled nonexistent broken glass and tape recorders, a cleanshaven man as having a mustache, straight hair as curly, and even something as large and conspicuous as a barn in a bucolic scene that contained no buildings at all (Loftus & Ketcham, 1991). The growing body of research shows that new, postevent information often becomes incorporated into memory, supplementing and altering a person's recollection. The new information invades us, like a Trojan horse, precisely because we do not detect its influence. Understanding how we can become tricked by revised data about our past is central to understanding the hypothesis that suggestions from popular writings and therapy sessions can affect autobiographical recall.

One frequently heard comment about the research on memory distortion is that all changes induced by misinformation are about trivial details (Darnton, 1991;

Franklin & Wright, 1991). There is no evidence, the critics allege, that one can tinker with memories of real traumatic events or that one can inject into the human mind whole events that never happened.

CAN REAL TRAUMATIC MEMORIES BE CHANGED?

There are some who argue that traumatic events leave some sort of indelible fixation in the mind (e.g., "traumatic events create lasting visual images . . . burned-in visual impressions," Terr, 1988, p. 103; "memory imprints are indelible, they do not erase—a therapy that tries to alter them will be uneconomical," Kantor, 1980, p. 163). These assertions fail to recognize known examples and evidence that memory is malleable even for life's most traumatic experiences. If Eileen Franklin's memory of witnessing her father murder her eight-year-old best friend is a real memory, then it too is a memory replete with changes over different tellings. However, there are clearer examples—anecdotal reports in which definite evidence exists that the traumatic event itself was actually experienced and yet the memory radically changed.

In the category of documented anecdotes there is the example of one of the worst public and personal tragedies in the history of baseball (Anderson, 1990; described in Loftus & Kaufman, 1992). Baseball aficionados may recall that Jack Hamilton, then a pitcher with the California Angels, crushed the outfielder, Tony Conigliaro, in the face with a first-pitch fastball. Although Hamilton thought he remembered this horrible event perfectly, he misremembered it as occurring during a day game, when it was actually at night, and misremembered it in other critical ways. Another example will be appreciated by history buffs, particularly those with an interest in the second world war. American Brigadier General Elliot Thorpe recalled the day after the bombing of Pearl Harbor one way in a memoir and completely differently in an oral history taken on his retirement. Both accounts, in fact, were riddled with errors (Weintraub, 1991).

Evidence of a less anecdotal, more experimental nature supports the imperfections of personally experienced traumatic memories. For example, one study examined people's recollections of how they heard the news of the 1986 explosion of the space shuttle *Challenger* (Harsch & Neisser, 1989; Neisser & Harsch, 1992). Subjects were questioned on the morning after the explosion and again nearly three years later. Most described their memories as vivid, but none of them were entirely correct, and more than one third were wildly inaccurate. One subject, for example, was on the telephone having a business discussion when her best friend interrupted the call with the news. Later she would remember that she heard the news in class and at first thought it was a joke, and that she later walked into a TV lounge and saw the news, and then reacted to the disaster.

Another study (Abhold, 1992) demonstrated the malleability of memory for a serious life-and-death situation. The subjects had attended an important high school football game at which a player on the field went into cardiac arrest. Paramedics tried to resuscitate the player and apparently failed. The audience reactions ranged from complete silence, to sobbing, to screaming. (Ultimately, fortunately, the player was revived at the hospital.) Six years later, many of these people were interviewed. Errors of recollection were common. Moreover, when exposed to misleading information about this life-and-death event, many individuals absorbed the misinformation into their recollections. For example, more than one fourth of the subjects were persuaded that they had seen blood on the player's jersey after receiving a false suggestion to this effect.

These anecdotes and experimental examples suggest that even details of genuinely experienced traumatic events are, as Christianson (1992) put it, "by no means, completely accurate" (p. 207).

Can One Inject a Complete Memory for Something That Never Happened?

It is one thing to discover that memory for an actual traumatic event is changed over time but quite another to show that one can inject a whole event into someone's mind for something that never happened. There are numerous anecdotes and experimental studies that show it is indeed possible to lead people to construct entire events.

Piaget's memory. Whole memories can be implanted into a person's real-life autobiography, as is best shown by Piaget's classic childhood memory of an attempted kidnapping (Piaget, 1962; described in Loftus & Ketcham, 1991, p. 19). The false memories were with him for at least a decade. The memory was of an attempted kidnapping that occurred when he was an infant. He found out it was false when his nanny confessed years later that she had made up the entire story and felt guilty about keeping the watch she had received as a reward. In explaining this false memory, Piaget assumed, "I, therefore, must have heard, as a child, the account of this story, which my parents believed, and projected into the past in the form of a visual memory."

Loud noises at night. Although widely disseminated and impressive at first glance, Piaget's false memory is still but a single anecdote and subject to other interpretations. Was this really a memory, or an interesting story? Could it be that the assault actually happened and the nurse, for some inexplicable reason, lied later? For these reasons it would be nice to find stronger evidence that a false memory for a complete event was genuinely implanted.

An apparently genuine 19th-century memory implantation was reported by Laurence and Perry (1983): Bernheim, during hypnosis, suggested to a female subject that she had awakened four times during the previous night to go to the toilet and had fallen on her nose on the fourth occasion. After hypnosis, the woman insisted that the suggested events had actually occurred, despite the hypnotist's insistence that she had dreamed them. Impressed by Bernheim's success, and by explorations by Orne (1979), Laurence and Perry asked 27 highly hypnotizable individuals during hypnosis to choose a night from the previous week and to describe their activities during the half hour before going to sleep. The subjects were then instructed to relive that night, and a suggestion was implanted that they had heard some loud noises and had awakened. Almost one half (13) of the 27 subjects accepted the suggestion and stated *after* hypnosis that the suggested event had actually taken place. Of the 13, 6 were unequivocal in their certainty. The remainder came to the conclusion on basis of reconstruction. Even when told that the hypnotist had actually suggested the noises, these subjects still maintained that the noises had occurred. One said "I'm pretty certain I heard them. As a matter of fact, I'm pretty damned certain. I'm positive I heard these noises" (Laurence & Perry, 1983, p. 524).

The paradigm of inducing pseudomemories of being awakened by loud noises has now been used extensively by other researchers who readily replicate the basic findings. Moreover, the pseudomemories are not limited to hypnotic conditions. Simply inducing subjects to imagine and describe the loud noises resulted in later "memories" for noises that had never occurred (Weekes, Lynn, Green, & Brentar, 1992).

Other false memories. Other evidence shows that people can be tricked into believing that they experienced an event even in the absence of specific hypnotic suggestions. For example, numerous studies have shown that people misremember that they voted in a particular election when they actually had not (Abelson, Loftus, & Greenwald, 1992). One interpretation of these findings is that people fill in the gaps in their memory with socially desirable constructions, thus creating for themselves a false memory of voting.

In other studies, people have been led to believe that they witnessed assaultive behavior when in fact they did not (e.g., Haugaard, Reppucci, Laurd, & Nauful, 1991). In this study, children aged four to seven years were led to believe that they saw a man hit a girl, when he had not, after hearing the girl lie about the assault. Not only did they misrecall the nonexistent hitting, but they added their own details: Of 41 false claims, 39 children said it happened near a pond, 1 said it was at the girl's house, and 1 could not specify exactly where the girl was when the man hit her.

Violent false memories. People can hold completely false memories for something far more traumatic than awakening at night, voting in a particular election, or a simulation involving a man and a girl. Pynoos and Nader (1989) studied children's recollections of a sniper attack at an elementary school playground. Some of the children who were interviewed were not at the school during the shooting, including some who were already on the way home or were on vacation. Yet, even the nonwitnesses had memories:

> One girl initially said that she was at the school gate nearest the sniper when the shooting began. In truth she was not only out of the line of fire, she was half a block away. A boy who had been away on vacation said that he had been on his way to the school, had seen someone lying on the ground, had heard the shots, and then turned back. In actuality, a police barricade prevented anyone from approaching the block around the school. (p. 238)

The memories apparently were created by exposure to the stories of those who truly experienced the trauma.

Memories of being lost. A question arises as to whether one could experimentally implant memories for nonexistent events that, if they had occurred, would have been traumatic. Given the need to protect human subjects, devising a means of accomplishing this was not an easy task. Loftus and Coan (in press), however, developed a paradigm for instilling a specific childhood memory for being lost on a particular occasion at the age of five. They chose getting lost because it is clearly a great fear of both parents and children. Their initial observations show how subjects can be readily induced to believe this kind of false memory. The technique involved a subject and a trusted family member who played a variation of "Remember the time that. . . .?" To appreciate the methodology, consider the implanted memory of 14-year-old Chris. Chris was convinced by his older brother, Jim, that he had been lost in a shopping mall when he was 5 years old. Jim told Chris this story as if it were the truth: "It was 1981 or 1982. I remember that Chris was 5. We had gone shopping at the University City shopping mall in Spokane. After some panic, we found Chris being led down the mall by a tall, oldish man (I think he was wearing a flannel shirt). Chris was crying and holding the man's hand. The man explained that he had found Chris walking around crying his eyes out just a few moments before and was trying to help him find his parents."

Just two days later, Chris recalled his feelings about being lost: "That day I was so scared that I would never see my family again. I knew that I was in trouble." On the third day, he recalled a conversation with his mother: "I remember mom telling me never to do that again." On the fourth day: "I also remember that old man's flannel shirt." On the fifth day, he started remembering the mall itself: "I sort of remember the stores." In his last recollection, he could even remember a conversation with the man who found him: "I remember the man asking me if I was lost."

It would be natural to wonder whether perhaps Chris had really gotten lost that day. Maybe it happened, but his brother forgot. But Chris's mother was subjected to the same procedure and was never able to remember the false event. After five days of trying, she said "I feel very badly about it, but I just cannot remember anything like this ever happening."

A couple of weeks later, Chris described his false memory and he greatly expanded on it.

> I was with you guys for a second and I think I went over to look at the toy store, the Kay-bee toy and uh, we got lost and I was looking around and I thought, "Uh-oh. I'm in trouble now." You know. And then I . . . I thought I was never going to see my family again. I was really scared you know. And then this old man, I think he was wearing a blue flannel, came up to me . . . he was kind of old. He was kind of bald on top . . . he had like a ring of gray hair . . . and he had glasses.

Thus, in two short weeks, Chris now could even remember the balding head and the glasses worn by the man who rescued him. He characterized his memory as reasonably clear and vivid.

Finally, Chris was debriefed. He was told that one of the memories presented to him earlier had been false. When asked to guess, he guessed one of the genuine memories. When told that it was the getting-lost memory, he said, "Really? I thought I remembered being lost . . . and looking around for you guys. I do remember that. And then crying. And mom coming up and saying 'Where were you. Don't you . . . Don't you ever do that again.'"

A false memory of abuse. The lost-in-a-shopping-mall example shows that memory of an entire mildly traumatic event can be created. It is still natural to wonder whether one could go even further and implant a memory of abuse. Ethically, of course, it would not be possible, but anecdotally, as it happens, it was done. It is one of the most dramatic cases of false memory of abuse ever to be documented—the case of Paul Ingram from Olympia, Washington (Ofshe, 1992; Watters, 1991). As described above, Ingram was arrested for child abuse in 1988 at the time he was chair of the county Republican committee. At first Ingram denied everything, and detectives told him he was in denial. After five months of interrogation, suggestions from a psychologist, and continuing pressure from detectives and advisors, Ingram began to confess to rapes, assaults, child sexual abuse, and participation in a Satan-worshipping cult alleged to have murdered 25 babies (Ofshe, 1992). To elicit specific memories, the psychologist or detectives would suggest some act of abuse (e.g., that on one occasion, Ingram and several other men raped his daughter). Ingram would at first not remember these fragments, but after a concerted effort on his part, he would later come up with a detailed memory.

Richard Ofshe, a social psychologist hired by the prosecution to interview Ingram and his family members, decided to test Ingram's credibility. Ofshe had made up a completely fabricated scenario. He told Ingram that two of his children (a daughter and a son) had reported that Ingram had forced them to have sex in front of him. As with the earlier suggestions, Ingram at first could not remember this. But Ofshe urged Ingram to try to think about the scene and try to see it happening, just as the interrogators had done to him earlier. Ingram began to get some visual images. Ingram then followed Ofshe's instructions to "pray on" the scene and try to remember more over the next few hours. Several hours later, Ingram had developed detailed memories and wrote a three-page statement confessing in graphic detail to the scene that Ofshe had invented (Ofshe, 1992; Watters, 1991). Ofshe (1989, 1992) noted that this was not the first time that a vulnerable individual had been made to believe that he had committed a crime for which he originally had no memory and which evidence proved he could not have committed. What is crucial about the Ingram case is that some of the same methods that are used in repressed memory cases were used with Ingram. These include the use of protracted imagining of events and authority figures establishing the authenticity of these events.

These examples provide further insights into the malleable nature of memory. They suggest that memories for personally experienced traumatic events can be altered by new experiences. Moreover, they reveal that entire events that never happened can be injected into memory. The false memories range from the relatively trivial (e.g., remembering voting) to the bizarre (e.g., remembering forcing one's daughter and son to have sex). These false memories, with more or less detail, of course do not prove that repressed memories of abuse that return are false. They do demonstrate a mechanism by which false memories can be created by a small suggestion from a trusted family member, by hearing someone lie, by suggestion from a psychologist, or by incorporation of the experiences of others into one's own autobiography. Of course, the fact that false memories can be planted tells nothing about whether a given memory of child sexual abuse is false or not; nor does it tell how one might distinguish the real cases from the false ones. These findings on the malleability of memory do, however, raise questions about the wisdom of certain recommendations being promoted in self-help workbooks, in handbooks for therapists, and by some therapists themselves. The false memories created in the examples above were accomplished with techniques that are not all that different from what some therapists regularly do—suggesting that the client was probably abused because of some vague symptoms, labeling a client's ambiguous recollections as evidence of abuse, and encouraging mental exercises that involve fantasy merging with reality.

FINAL REMARKS

The 1990s brought a blossoming of reports of awakenings of previously repressed memories of childhood abuse. One reason for the increase may be the widespread statistics on sex abuse percentages that are published almost daily: "By 1980 . . . the government tallied almost 43,000 cases of child sex abuse annually" (Nathan, 1991, p. 154); "One in five women are 'incest victims,'" (p. 155); "6.8 million women nationwide would say they had been raped once, 4.7 million more than once" (Johnston, 1992, p. A9); "In 1972, 610,000 [child abuse cases] were reported nationally, and by 1985 the number had exceeded 1.7 million" (Baker, 1992, p. 37). "If it happens so often, did it happen to me?" is a question many women and some men are asking themselves now more than ever before. The appearance of abuse statistics is one battle in the war waged against an earlier tendency on the part of society to disbelieve the abuse reports of women and children—a tendency that we should all deplore. The repressed memory cases are another outlet for women's rage over sexual violence. Although women's anger is certainly justified in many cases, and may be justified in some repressed memory cases too, it is time to stop and ask whether the net of rage has been cast too widely, creating a new collective nightmare.

Repressed memories of abuse often return in therapy, sometimes after suggestive probing. Today, popular writings have been so fully absorbed by the culture that these too can serve as a source of suggestion that can greatly influence what happens in therapy and outside of it (Guze, 1992). The result is memories that are often detailed and confidently held. Despite lack of corroboration, some of these recollections could be authentic. Others might not be.

Several implications of these observations follow. First, we need a renewed effort at research on the problem of repressed memories. This should encompass, in part, a reexamination of some of the widely cherished beliefs of psychotherapists. Is it true that repression of extremely traumatic experiences is common? Do these experiences invade us despite the fact that "all the good juice of consciousness has drained out" (Dennett, 1991, p. 325). It is common to see analogies drawn between Vietnam War veterans and the incest survivors (e.g., Herman, 1992; Rieker & Carmen, 1986). Do they share in common the use of "massive repression" (Wolf & Alpert, 1991, p. 314) as a mechanism for coping? If so, how do we explain findings obtained with children who witness parental murder and other atrocities? In one study (Malmquist, 1986), not a single child aged 5 to 10 years who had witnessed the murder of a parent repressed the memory. Rather, they were continually flooded with pangs of emotion about the murder and preoccupation with it.

Is it true that repressed material, like radioactive waste, "lies there in leaky canisters, never losing potency, eternally dangerous" (Hornstein, 1992, p. 260) and constantly threatens to erupt into consciousness? Psychotherapists have assumed for years that repressed memories are powerful influences because they are not accessible to consciousness (Bowers, 1992). Is there evidence for this assumption? Is it necessarily true that all people who display symptoms of severe mental distress have had some early childhood trauma (probably abuse) that is responsible for the distress? With cutting-edge research now showing that mental distress involves neuronal and hormonal systems of a much wider scope than previously realized (Chrousos & Gold, 1992; Gershon & Rieder, 1992), should not other potential causes be at least considered?

Questions must also be examined about the well-intentioned treatment strategies of some clinicians. Is it possible that the therapist's interpretation is the cause of the patient's disorder rather than the effect of the disorder, to paraphrase Guze (1992, p. 78)? Is it necessarily true that people who cannot remember an abusive childhood are repressing the memory? Is it necessarily true that people who dream about or visualize abuse are actually getting in touch with true memories? Good scientific research needs to be done to support these assumptions, or they should be challenged. Challenging these core assumptions will not be an easy thing to do, anymore than it was for psychologists of the 1930s to challenge the radical subjectivity of psychoanalysis (Hornstein, 1992), or for psychologists of the 1980s to challenge the reliability of the clinical judgments made by psychologists and psychiatrists (Faust & Ziskin, 1988; Fowler & Matarazzo, 1988).[14] Nonetheless, when we move from the privacy of the therapy session, in which the client's reality may be the only reality that is important, into the courtroom, in which there can be but a single reality, then we as citizens in a democratic society are entitled to more solid evidence.

Until we have better empirical answers, therapists might consider whether it is wise to "suggest" that childhood trauma happened, to probe relentlessly for recalcitrant memories, and then to uncritically accept them as fact. Uncritical acceptance of uncorroborated trauma memories by therapists, social agencies, and law enforcement personnel has been used to promote public accusations by alleged abuse survivors. If the memories are fabricated, this will of course lead to irreparable damage to the reputations of potentially innocent people, according to Ganaway (1989), who discussed the problem in the context of SRA memories.

Uncritical acceptance of uncorroborated trauma memories poses other potentially dangerous problems for society. According to Ganaway (1991), reinforcing the validity of unverifiable memories in the therapeutic setting may lead to diversionary paths in the patient's therapy away from actual childhood trauma. This could lead to interminable therapy and a total draining of the patient's financial

---

[14]British historian, Hugh Trevor-Roper (1967) pointed out that the skeptics during the 16th century witchcraft craze did not make much dent in the frequency of bonfires and burnings until they figured out that they had to challenge the core belief—that is, the belief in Satan.

resources as the therapist and patient collaborate in a mutual deception to pursue a bottomless pit of memories. Worse, the patient's initial wonderings supported by therapist affirmations could then become fixed beliefs, precipitating suicidal thoughts and behaviors based on the new belief system, because the patient would no longer challenge the veracity of the new memories. Like Betsy Ross sewing the first American flag, the abuse becomes a myth that was never true but always will be (E. Frishholz, personal communication, May 1992). Patients who are reinforced into a new belief system could develop newer, larger problems. If actual childhood sexual abuse is associated with numerous negative long-term effects (e.g., severe sexual dysfunction; Ambrosoe-Bienkowski, Stahly, & Wideman, 1991), what might be the consequence of implanted childhood sexual abuse? If the memories are ultimately shown to be false, therapists may then become the targets of future ethics violations and lawsuits. They will be charged with a grave form of mind abuse—charges that have already been initiated in several states.

What should therapists do instead? As a first step, it is worth recognizing that we do not yet have the tools for reliably distinguishing the signal of true repressed memories from the noise of false ones. Until we gain these tools, it seems prudent to consider some combination of Herman's (1992) advice about probing for traumatic memories and Ganaway's (1991) advice about SRA memories. Zealous conviction is a dangerous substitute for an open mind. Psychotherapists, counselors, social service agencies, and law enforcement personnel would be wise to be careful how they probe for horrors on the other side of some presumed amnesic barrier. They need to be circumspect regarding uncorroborated repressed memories that return. Techniques that are less potentially dangerous would involve clarification, compassion, and gentle confrontation along with a demonstration of empathy for the painful struggles these patients must endure as they come to terms with their personal truths.

There is one last tragic risk of suggestive probing and uncritical acceptance of all allegations made by clients, no matter how dubious. These activities are bound to lead to an increased likelihood that society in general will disbelieve the genuine cases of childhood sexual abuse that truly deserve our sustained attention.

REFERENCES

ABC News. (1992, April 2). *Primetime Live* [Transcript]. Washington, DC: American Broadcasting Corporation.

Abelson, R. P., Loftus, E. F., & Greenwald, A. G. (1992). Attempts to improve the accuracy of self-reports of voting. In J. M. Tanur (Ed.), *Questions about survey questions: Meaning, memory, expression, and social interactions in surveys* (pp. 138–153). New York: Russell Sage Foundation.

Abhold, J. (1992). [Unpublished doctoral dissertation data.] University of Arkansas.

Ambroso-Bienkowski, M., Stahly, G. B., & Wideman, K. (1991, August). *Relationship of sexual fantasy and sexual dysfunction to childhood molestation.* Paper presented at the 99th annual Convention of the American Psychological Association, San Francisco.

Anderson, D. (1990, February 27). Handcuffed in history to Tony C. *New York Times,* p. B9.

Baker, R. A. (1992). *Hidden memories.* Buffalo, NY: Prometheus Books.

Baron, J., Beattie, J., & Hershey, J. D. (1988). Heuristics and biases in diagnostic reasoning: Congruence, information, and certainty. *Organizational Behavior and Human Decision Processes. 42,* 88–110.

Barton v. Peters. (1990). Case No 4FA-90-0157, Superior Court for the State of Alaska, 4th Judicial District.

Bass, E., & Davis, L. (1988). *The courage to heal.* New York: Harper & Row.

Bass, E., & Thornton, L. (1991). *I never told anyone: Writings by women survivors of child sexual abuse.* New York: Harper Perennial.

Blume, E. S. (1990). *Secret survivors: Uncovering incest and its aftereffects in women.* New York: Ballantine.

Bottoms, B. L., Shaver, P. R., & Goodman, G. S. (1991, August). *Profile of ritualistic and religion-related abuse allegation reported to clinical psychologists in the United States.* Paper presented at the 99th Annual Convention of the American Psychological Association, San Francisco.

Bower, G. H. (1990). Awareness, the unconscious, and repression: An experimental psychologist's perspective. In J. Singer (Ed.), *Repression and dissociation: Implications for personality, theory, psychopathology, and health* (pp. 209–231). Chicago: University of Chicago Press.

Bowers, K. S. (1992, November 2). *Preconscious processes: How do we distinguish mental representations that correspond to perceived events from those that reflect imaginal processes?* Paper presented at National Institute of Mental Health workshop "Basic behavioral and psychological research: Building a bridge," Rockville, MD.

Bradshaw, J. (1990). *Homecoming.* New York: Bantam Books.

Bradshaw, J. (1992). Discovering what we want. *Lear's, 5,* 49.

Braun, B. G., & Sachs, R. G. (1988, October). *Recognition of possible cult involvement in MPD patients.* Paper presented at the Fifth International Conference on Multiple Personality/Dissociative States, Chicago.

Briere, J. (1992). Studying delayed memories of childhood sexual abuse. *The Advisor* (Publication of the American Professional Society on the Abuse of Children), *5,* 17–18.

Briere, J., & Conte, J. (in press). Self-reported amnesia for abuse in adults molested as children. *Journal of Traumatic Stress.*

Bruhn, A. R. (1990). *Earliest childhood memories: Vol. 1. Theory and application to clinical practice.* New York: Praeger.

Cannon, L. (1991). *President Reagan: The role of a lifetime.* New York: Simon & Schuster.

Christianson, S.-A. (1992). Do flashbulb memories differ from other types of emotional memories? In E. Winograd & U. Neisser (Eds.), *Affect and accuracy in recall: Studies of "flashbulb" memories* (pp. 191–211). New York: Cambridge University Press.

Chrousos, G. P., & Gold, P. W. (1992). The concept of stress and stress system disorders: Overview of physical and behavioral homeostasis. *JAMA: Journal of the American Medical Association, 267,* 1244–1252.

Collier, D. v. Collier, J. (1991, December). Deposition of plaintiff, Case No. 711752, Superior Court, County of Santa Clara, California.

Culhane, D. (1991, August 4). Sins of the father [Peterson, B. Review of *Dancing with Daddy*] *New York Times Book Review,* p. 18.

The darkest secret (1991, June 10) *People,* pp. 88–94.

Daro, D. (1988). *Confronting child abuse.* New York: Free Press.

Darnton, N. (1991, October 7). The pain of the last taboo. *Newsweek.* pp. 70–72.

Davis, L. (1991). Murdered memory. *In Health, 5,* 79–84.

Dawes, R. M. (1992). Why believe that for which there is no good evidence? *Issues in Child Abuse Accusations, 4,* 214–218.

Dennett, D. C. (1991). *Consciousness explained.* Boston: Little, Brown.

Doe, J. (1991). How could this happen? Coping with a false accusation of incest and rape. *Issues in Child Abuse Accusations, 3,* 154–165.

Doe, J. (1991). How could this happen? Coping with a false accusation of incest and rape. *Issues in Child Abuse Accusations, 3,* 154–165.

Dormen, L. (1991, April). A secret life. *Seventeen,* pp. 164–167.

Driscoll, L. N., & Wright, C. (1991). Survivors of childhood ritual abuse: Multigenerational satanic cult involvement. *Treating Abuse Today, 1,* 5–13.

Edmiston, S. (1990, November). Daddy's girl, *Glamour,* pp. 228–231, 280–285.

Ellis, B. (1992). Satanic ritual abuse and legend ostension. *Journal of Psychology and Theology, 20,* 274–277.

Erdelyi, M. H. (1985). *Psychoanalysis: Freud's cognitive psychology.* New York: Freeman.

Erdelyi, M. H., & Goldberg, B. (1979). Let's not sweep repression under the rug: Toward a cognitive psychology of repression. In J. F. Kihlstrom & F. J. Evans (Eds.), *Functional disorders of memory* (pp. 355–402). Hillsdale, NJ: Erlbaum.

Farmer, S. (1989). *Adult children of abusive parents.* New York: Ballantine.

Faust, D., & Ziskin, J. (1988). The expert witness in psychology and psychiatry. *Science, 241,* 31–35.

Fields, R. (1992, August 4). Hood must pay in sex-abuse case. *Beacon Journal* [Akron, OH], p. C5.

Forgetting to remember. (1991, February 11). *Newsweek,* p. 58.

Forward, S., & Buck, C. (1988). *Betrayal of innocence: Incest and its devastation.* New York: Penguin Books.

Fowler, R. D., & Matarazzo, J. D. (1988). Psychologists and psychiatrists as expert witnesses. *Science, 241,* 1143–1144.

Franklin, E., & Wright, W. (1991). *Sins of the father.* New York: Crown.

Frawley, M. G. (1990). From secrecy to self-disclosure: Healing the scars of incest. In G.

Stricker & M. Fisher (Eds.), *Self-disclosure in the therapeutic relationship* (pp. 247–259). New York: Plenum Press.

Frederickson, R. (1992). *Repressed memories: A journey to recovery from sexual abuse.* New York: Simon & Schuster.

Freud, S. (1953). Three essays on the theory of sexuality. In J. Strachey (Ed.), *The standard edition of the complete psychological works of Sigmund Freud* (Vol. 7, pp. 135–243). London: Hogarth Press. (Original work published 1905)

Freyd, J. J. (1991, August 21). *Memory repression, dissociative states, and other cognitive control processes involved in adult sequelae of childhood trauma.* Paper presented at the Second Annual Conference on Psychodynamics–Cognitive Science Interface, University of California, San Francisco.

Ganaway, G. K. (1989). Historical versus narrative truth: Clarifying the role of exogenous trauma in the etiology of MPD and its variants. *Dissociation, 2,* 205–220.

Ganaway, G. K. (1991, August). *Alternative hypotheses regarding satanic ritual abuse memories.* Paper presented at the 99th Annual Convention of the American Psychological Association, San Francisco.

Ganaway, G. K. (1992). Some additional questions. *Journal of Psychology and Theology, 20,* 201–205.

Gardner, R. A. (1991). *Sex abuse hysteria.* Cresskill, NJ: Creative Therapeutics.

Gardner, R. A. (1992). *True and false accusations of child sex abuse.* Cresskill, NJ: Creative Therapeutics.

Gershon, E. S., & Rieder, R. O. (1992). Major disorders of mind and brain. *Scientific American, 267* (3), 127–133.

Gordon, J. S. (1991). The UFO experience. *The Atlantic Monthly, 268,* 82–92.

Gudjonsson, G. (1992). *The psychology of interrogations, confessions and testimony.* Chichester, England: Wiley.

Guze, S. B. (1992). *Why psychiatry is a branch of medicine?* New York: Oxford University Press.

Harris, M. (1974). *Cows, pigs, wars, and witches: The riddles of culture.* NY: Vintage Books.

Harsch, N., & Neisser, U. (1989, November). *Substantial and irreversible errors in flashbulb memories of the Challenger explosion.* Poster presented at the annual meeting of the Psychonomic Society, Atlanta, GA.

Haugaard, J. J., Reppucci, N. D., Laurd, J., & Nauful, T. (1991). Children's definitions of the truth and their competency as witnesses in legal proceedings. *Law and Human Behavior, 15,* 253–272.

Herman, J. L. (1981). *Father–daughter incest.* Cambridge, MA: Harvard University Press.

Herman, J. L. (1992). *Trauma and recovery.* New York: Basic Books.

Herman, J. L., & Schatzow, E. (1987). Recovery and verification of memories of childhood sexual trauma. *Psychoanalytic Psychology, 4,* 1–14.

Holmes, D. (1990). The evidence for repression: An examination of sixty years of research. In J. Singer (Ed.), *Repression and dissociation: Implications for personality, theory, psychopathology, and health* (pp. 85–102). Chicago: University of Chicago Press.

Hornstein, G. A. (1992). The return of the repressed. *American Psychologist, 47,* 254–263.

Howe, M. L., & Courage, M. L. (1993). On resolving the enigma of infantile amnesia. *Psychological Bulletin, 113,* 305–326.

Johnston, D. (1992, April 24). Survey shows number of rapes far higher than official figures. *New York Times,* p. A9.

Kantor, D. (1980). Critical identity image. In J. K. Pearce & L. J. Friedman (Eds.), *Family therapy: Combining psychodynamic and family systems approaches* (pp. 137–167). New York: Grune & Stratton.

Kantrowitz, B. (1991, February 11). Forgetting to remember. *Newsweek,* p. 58.

Kihlstrom, J. F., & Harackiewicz, J. (1982). The earliest recollection: A new survey. *Journal of Personality, 50,* 134–148.

Kutchinsky, B. (1992). The child sexual abuse panic. *Nordisk Sexoligi, 10,* 30–42.

Laker, B. (1992, April 14). A nightmare of memories. *Seattle Post-Intelligencer,* p. C1.

Lamm. J. B. (1991). Easing access to the courts for incest victims: Toward an equitable application of the delayed discovery rule. *The Yale Law Journal, 100,* 2189–2208.

Laurence, J. R., & Perry, C. (1983). Hypnotically created memory among highly hypnotizable subjects. *Science, 222,* 523–524.

Lofft, K. v. Lofft, D. (1989). Complaint for Damages. Case No. 617151, Superior Court of the State of California for County of San Diego.

Loftus, E. F. (1982). Memory and its distortions. In A. G. Kraut (Ed.), *G. Stanley Hall lectures* (pp. 119–154). Washington, DC: American Psychological Association.

Loftus, E. F. (in press). Desperately seeking memories of the first few years of childhood. *Journal of Experimental Psychology: General.*

Loftus, E. F., & Coan, D. (in press). The construction of childhood memories. In D. Peters (Ed.), *The child witness in context: Cognitive, social and legal perspectives.* New York: Kluwer.

Loftus, E. F., & Herzog, C. (1991). Unpublished data. University of Washington.

Loftus, E. F., & Kaufman, L. (1992). Why do traumatic experiences sometimes produce good memory (flashbulbs) and sometimes no memory (repression)? In E. Winograd & U. Neisser (Eds.), *Affect and accuracy in recall: Studies of "flashbulb" memories* (pp. 212–223). New York: Cambridge University Press.

Loftus, E. F., & Ketcham, K. (1991). *Witness for the defense.* New York: St. Martin's Press.

Loftus, E. F., Polonsky, S. & Fullilove, M. T. (1993). *Memories of childhood sexual abuse: Remembering and repressing.* Unpublished manuscript, University of Washington and Columbia University School of Public Health.

Loftus, E. F., Weingardt, K., & Hoffman, H. (1992). *Sleeping memories on trial: Reactions to memories that were previously repressed.* Unpublished manuscript, University of Washington.

Mack, J. E. (1980). Psychoanalysis and biography: Aspects of a developing affinity. *Journal of the American Psychoanalytic Association, 28,* 543–562.

Malmquist, C. P. (1986). Children who witness parental murder: Posttraumatic aspects. *Journal of the American Academy of Child Psychiatry, 25,* 320–325.

McMillan, P. (1992, April 28). Woman, 39, wins $500,000 in incest case. *Los Angeles Times*, p. B3.

Medin, D. L., & Ross, B. H. (1992). *Cognitive psychology*. Ft. Worth, TX: Harcourt Brace Jovanovich.

Monesi, L. (1992). [Reports of a private investigator, Falcon International Inc., Columbus, Ohio.]

Morton, J. (1990). The development of event memory. *The Psychologist, 1*, 3–10.

Mulhern, S. (1991). Satanism and psychotherapy: A rumor in search of an inquisition. In J. T. Richardson, J. Best, & D. Bromley (Eds.), *The satanism scare* (pp. 145–172). New York: Aldine de Gruyter.

Napier, C. W. (1990). Civil incest suits: Getting beyond the statute of limitations. *Washington University Law Quarterly, 68*, 995–1020.

Nash, M. (1987). What, if anything, is regressed about hypnotic age regression? A review of the empirical literature. *Psychological Bulletin, 102*, 42–52.

Nason girl fought. (1969, December 6). *San Jose Mercury*.

Nathan, D. (1991). *Women and other aliens*. El Paso, TX: Cinco Puntos Press.

Nathan, D. (1992, October). Cry incest. *Playboy*, pp. 84–88, 162–164.

Neisser, U., & Harsch, N. (1992). Phantom flashbulbs: False recollections of hearing the news about *Challenger*. In E. Winograd & U. Neisser (Eds.), *Affect and accuracy in recall: Studies of "flashbulb" memories* (pp. 9–31). New York: Cambridge University Press.

Ofshe, R. (1989). Coerced confessions: The logic of seemingly irrational action. *Cultic Studies Journal, 6*, 1–15.

Ofshe, R. J. (1992). Inadvertent hypnosis during interrogation: False confession due to dissociative state, misidentified multiple personality and the satanic cult hypothesis. *International Journal of Clinical and Experimental Hypnosis, 40*, 125–156.

Oldenberg, D. (1991, June 20). Dark memories: Adults confront their childhood abuse. *Washington Post*, p. D1.

Olio, K. A. (1989). Memory retrieval in the treatment of adult survivors of sexual abuse. *Transactional Analysis Journal, 19*, 93–94.

Orne, M. T. (1979). The use and misuse of hypnosis in court. *International Journal of Clinical and Experimental Hypnosis. 27*, 311–341.

Petersen, B. (1991). *Dancing with daddy: A childhood lost and a life regained*. New York: Bantam.

Petersen v. Bruen (1990). 792 P.2d 18 (Nev. 1990).

Piaget, J. (1962). *Plays, dreams and imitation in childhood*. New York: Norton.

Pillemer, D. B., & White, S. H. (1989). Childhood events recalled by children and adults. In *Advances in child development and behavior* (Vol. 21). San Diego, CA: Academic Press.

Poston, C., & Lison, K. (1990). *Reclaiming our lives: Hope for adult survivors of incest*. New York: Bantam.

Pynoos, R. S., & Nader, K. (1989). Children's memory and proximity to violence. *Journal of the American Academy of Child and Adolescent Psychiatry, 28*, 236–241.

Rieker, P. P., & Carmen, E. H. (1986). The victim-to-patient process: The disconfirmation and transformation of abuse. *American Journal of Orthopsychiatry, 56,* 360–370.

Ritter, M. (1991, June 30). Sudden recall of forgotten crimes is a puzzler for juries, experts say. *Los Angeles Times,* p. A10.

Rogers, M. L. (1992a, March). A case of alleged satanic ritualistic abuse. Paper presented at the meeting of the American Psychology–Law Society, San Diego.

Rogers, M. L. (1992b). A call for discernment—natural and spiritual: Introductory editorial to a special issue on SRA. *Journal of Psychology and Theology, 20,* 175–186.

Schuker, E. (1979). Psychodynamics and treatment of sexual assault victims. *Journal of the American Academy of Psychoanalysis, 7,* 553–573.

Sgroi, S. M. (1989). Stages of recovery for adult survivors of child sex abuse. In S. M. Sgroi (Ed.), *Vulnerable populations: Sexual abuse treatment for children, adult survivors, offenders and persons with mental retardation* (Vol. 2, p. 112). Lexington, MA: Lexington Books.

Shaffer, R. E., & Cozolino, L. J. (1992). Adults who report childhood ritualistic abuse. *Journal of Psychology and Theology, 20,* 188–193.

Sherman, S. J., Cialdini, R. B., Schwartzman, D. F., & Reynolds, K. D. (1985). Imagining can heighten or lower the perceived likelihood of contracting a disease. *Personality and Social Psychology Bulletin, 11,* 118–127.

Smith, M. (1983). Hypnotic memory enhancement of witnesses: Does it work? *Psychological Bulletin, 94,* 387–407.

Smith, M., & Pazder, L. (1980). *Michelle remembers.* New York: Congdon & Lattes.

Snyder, M. (1984). When belief creates reality? In L. Berkowitz (Ed.), *Advances in experimental social psychology* (Vol. 18, pp. 247–305). San Diego, CA: Academic Press.

Snyder, M., & Swann, W. (1978). Hypothesis-testing processes in social interaction. *Journal of Personality and Social Psychology, 11,* 1202–1212.

"A star cries incest." (1991, October 7). *People,* pp. 84–88.

Sternberg, R. (1992). *Five-part theory of giftedness.* Paper presented at the Conference on Developmental Approaches to Identifying Exceptional Ability, Lawrence, KS.

Stubbings v. Webb and Another (1991). 3 Weekly Law Reports 383. [Cited in Reports and Developments (1992). *Expert Evidence: The International Digest of Human Behaviour, Science, and Law, 1,* 26.]

Summit, R. (1992). Misplaced attention to delayed memory. *The Advisor* (published by the American Professional Society on the Abuse of Children), *5,* 21–25.

Survivors of Incest Anonymous. (1985). *Is Survivors of Incest Anonymous for you?* Baltimore, MD: Author.

Survivors of Incest Anonymous. (1990). *Questions and answers.* (Distributed at Thursday night San Francisco SIA meeting, October 17).

Susan Nason body found in a dump. (1969, December 3). *San Francisco Chronicle,* p. 1.

Telegraphers v. Railway Express Agency. (1944). 321 U.S. 342, 348–349.

Terr, L. (1988). What happens to early memories of trauma? A study of 20 children under age five at the time of documented traumatic events. *Journal of the American Academy of Child and Adolescent Psychiatry, 27,* 96–104.

Trevor-Roper, H. R. (1967). *Religion, the Reformation, and social change.* London: Macmillan.

Trott, J. (1991a). The grade five syndrome. *Cornerstone, 20,* 16–18.

Trott, J. (1991b). Satanic panic. *Cornerstone, 20,* 9–12.

Toufexis, A. (1991, October 28). When can memories be trusted? *Time,* pp. 86–88.

Usher, J. A., & Neisser, U. (in press). Childhood amnesia and the beginnings of memory for four early life events. *Journal of Experimental Psychology: General.*

Van Benschoten, S. C. (1990). Multiple personality disorder and satanic ritual abuse: The issue of credibility. *Dissociation, 3,* 22–30.

Wakefield, H., & Underwager, R. (1992). Recovered memories of alleged sexual abuse: Lawsuits against parents. *Behavioral Sciences and the Law, 10,* 483–507.

Washington. (1989). Rev. Code Ann. Sec. 4.16.340 (1989 Supp).

Watson, B. (1992). Salem's dark hour: Did the devil make them do it? *Smithsonian, 23,* 117–131.

Watters, E. (1991). The devil in Mr. Ingram. *Mother Jones,* July–August, pp. 30–33, 65–68.

Watters, E. (1993). Doors of memory. *Mother Jones.* January–February, pp. 24–29, 76–77.

Weekes, J. R., Lynn, S. J., Green, J. P., & Brentar, J. T. (1992). Pseudo-memory in hypnotized and task-motivated subjects. *Journal of Abnormal Psychology, 101,* 356–360.

Weintraub, S. (1991, December 4). Three myths about Pearl Harbor. *New York Times,* p. A27.

Williams, L. M. (1992). Adult memories of childhood abuse: Preliminary findings from a longitudinal study. *The Advisor, 5* 19–20.

Williams, M. (1987). Reconstruction of an early seduction and its aftereffects. *Journal of the American Psychoanalytic Association, 15,* 145–163.

Winograd, E., & Killinger, W. A., Jr. (1983). Relating age at encoding in early childhood to adult recall: Development of flashbulb memories. *Journal of Experimental Psychology: General, 112,* 413–422.

Wolf, E. K., & Alpert, J. L. (1991). Psychoanalysis and child sexual abuse: A review of the post-freudian literature. *Psychoanalytic Psychology, 8,* 305–327.

Young, W. C., Sachs, R. G., Braun, B. G., & Watkins, R. T. (1991). Patients reporting ritual abuse in childhood: A clinical syndrome report of 37 cases. *International Journal of Child Abuse and Neglect, 15,* 181–189.

10

Impact of Sexual Abuse on Children: A Review and Synthesis of Recent Empirical Studies

Kathleen A. Kendall-Tackett, Linda Meyer Williams, and David Finkelhor

University of New Hampshire, Durham

A review of 45 studies clearly demonstrated that sexually abused children had more symptoms than nonabused children, with abuse accounting for 15–45% of the variance. Fears, posttraumatic stress disorder, behavior problems, sexualized behaviors, and poor self-esteem occurred most frequently among a long list of symptoms noted, but no one symptom characterized a majority of sexually abused children. Some symptoms were specific to certain ages, and approximately one third of victims had no symptoms. Penetration, the duration and frequency of the abuse, force, the relationship of the perpetrator to the child, and maternal support affected the degree of symptomatology. About two thirds of the victimized children showed recovery during the first 12–18 months. The findings suggest the absence of any specific syndrome in children who have been sexually abused and no single traumatizing process.

Until recently, the literature on the impact of child sexual abuse consisted disproportionately of retrospective studies of adults. For example, the conclusions of

Reprinted with permission from *Psychological Bulletin*, 1993, Vol. 113(1), 164–180. Copyright © 1993 by the American Psychological Association, Inc.

This article is based on a paper presented at the meetings of the American Professional Society on the Abuse of Children, January 1991, San Diego, California. The present research was carried out with funds provided by National Institute of Mental Health Grant T32 MH15161 and National Center for Child Abuse and Neglect Grant 90CA 1406. We thank Elizabeth Royal and Patricia VanWagoner for assistance in preparing the manuscript. We also thank members of the 1991 Family Violence Seminar and the anonymous reviewers for their helpful comments a widely cited review (Browne & Finkelhor, 1986) were based on only 4 studies of children, compared with 23 studies of adults. Not surprisingly, most reviews combined studies of both groups, because research focused on children was rare.

Since 1985, however, there has been an explosion in the number of studies that have concentrated specifically on sexually abused children. Some studies have even focused on specific types of child victims, such as preschoolers, boys, or victims of ritualistic abuse. The studies of child victims have been distinct in several important ways from the research on adults. First, researchers studying children have often used different methodologies, many times relying on parents' or clinicians' reports rather than on children's self-reports. In addition, they have often evaluated specifically child-oriented symptoms, such as regressive behavior. These methodologies and the concentration on child-oriented symptoms make this research more relevant to intervention and treatment with children than the research on the effects of sexual abuse on adults, from which the implications for the treatment of children were difficult to extrapolate.

Research on children has allowed for a developmental perspective and included the first efforts at longitudinal studies of sexual abuse victims. This literature also has important relevance to other theory and research concerning how children process trauma, for example, how trauma expresses itself at various developmental stages, its role in the development of later psychopathology, and the mediating effects of important factors such as familial and community support. Therefore, research on the effect of sexual abuse on children is worthy of its own review.

We undertook such a review to (a) bring together literature from a broad spectrum of fields, including medicine, social work, psychology, and sociology; (b) highlight areas where there is agreement and disagreement in findings; (c) draw conclusions that may be useful for clinicians currently working with child victims and researchers studying this problem; and (d) suggest directions for future research and theory.

DOMAIN

In the present review, we included studies of child victims of sexual abuse,[1] in which all subjects were 18 years of age or younger (see Appendix). In all of these studies, quantitative results of at least one of the following types were reported: a comparison of sexually abused children with nonabused children or norms (clin-

---

[1]Note that when we refer to victims, we mean victims who have come to public attention. The findings from the present review cannot be generalized to unreported victims, for whom impact may be substantially different. In a controversial study of unreported victims from The Netherlands, Sandfort (1982, 1984) claimed that certain (primarily adolescent) boys had relationships with adult pedophiles that they described in positive terms and appeared to have no negative effects. Because these boys were nominated for the research by the pedophiles themselves, who were involved in a pedophile advocacy group, it is difficult to know to what group of children such findings could be generalized.

ical and/or nonclinical) or the age of victims who manifested some symptom. Certain other studies that did not contain these types of data, yet included other relevant data on intervening variables or longitudinal findings, are not listed in the Appendix but are referenced in the appropriate sections. The majority were published within the past 5 years. Because there has been so much research on this topic in the past few years, we also included some unpublished material (most of the manuscripts are currently under review), located through researchers who specialize in research in this area. Although we undoubtedly missed some articles, we are confident that we were able to locate most of them because of the network of researchers we contacted.

Excluded from the present review were nonquantitative or case studies. We also excluded studies in which all subjects manifested a certain behavior (such as teen prostitution or running away) but only some of them had been sexually abused. (In contrast, in the studies we included in the present review, all subjects had been abused.) Finally, we excluded studies that involved both adult and child victims (e.g., ages 15–45) and combined results from these two groups.

The studies used samples from several different sources, but primarily drew from sexual abuse evaluation or treatment programs. Some investigators recruited from specific subgroups of victims, such as day-care victims. Most investigators combined victims of intra- and extrafamilial abuse. The samples also included a wide variety of ages, covering the entire spectrum from preschool to adolescence. The sample sizes ranged from very small ($N = 8$) to large ($N = 369$), with the majority between 25 and 50 children. Approximately half (55%) the studies included comparison groups, and six had both nonabused clinical and nonabused nonclinical controls. This is a major improvement over studies conducted even 10 years ago. The studies used a variety of sources for assessment, including parent report, chart review, clinician report, and children's self-report.

In reviewing these studies, we first looked at the findings with regard to symptoms and then examined the intervening variables that affected these symptoms. We then paid particular attention to the longitudinal studies undertaken thus far. Finally, we drew conclusions for theory and future research.

COMPARISON OF ABUSED AND NONABUSED CHILDREN

A wide range of symptoms have been examined in the studies in which sexually abused children have been compared with nonabused clinical or nonclinical children (or norms). Table 1 groups these symptoms together under major headings. As shown in Column 1, by far the most commonly studied symptom was sexualized behavior, often considered the most characteristic symptom of sexual abuse. Sexualized behavior usually included such things as sexualized play with dolls, putting objects into anuses or vaginas, excessive or public masturbation,

TABLE 1

Sexually Abused (SA) Versus Nonsexually Abused (NSA) Children: Nonclinical and Clinical Comparison Groups

	Nonclinical		Clinical			
Symptom	Total no. studies	SA > NSA[a]/ no. studies	No. studies in which SA > NSA[a]	No. studies in which there was no difference	No. studies in which SA < NSA[b]	Total no. studies
Anxiety	14	5/8	1	2	0	3
Fear	6	5/5	1	0	2	3
Posttraumatic stress disorder						
Nightmares	3	1/1	1	—	—	1
General	5	1/1	1	0	0	1
Depression						
Depressed	17	10/11	1	2	2	5
Withdrawn	14	11/11	—	1	3	5
Suicidal	7	0/1	—	—	—	—
Poor self-esteem	11	3/6	—	—	—	—
Somatic complaints	16	9/11	1	3	3	7
Mental illness						
Neurotic	3	2/2	0	2	2	4
Other	12	6/7	0	4	2	6
Aggression						
Aggressive antisocial	15	10/11	0	1	6	7
Cruel	2	2/2	0	1	0	1
Delinquent	7	6/6	0	1	3	4

Sexualized behavior						
Inappropriate sexual behavior	23	8/8	6	2	0	8
Promiscuity	2	—	0	1	2	3
School/learning problems	13	5/6				
Behavior problems						
Hyperactivity	9	5/7	0	1	4	5
Regression/immaturity	7	2/2	1	0	1	2
Illegal acts	4	—	—	—	—	—
Running away	6	1/1	—	—	—	—
General	5	2/2	—	—	—	—
Self-destructive behavior						
Substance abuse	5	—	—	—	—	—
Self-injurious behavior	4	1/1	—	—	—	—
Composite symptoms						
Internalizing	10	8/8	0	2	1	3
Externalizing	11	7/7	0	1	2	3

Note. The numbers in column 2 do not necessarily add up to the number in column 1 because column 1 includes some studies in which only the percentage of children with symptoms was specified.   [b] SA < NSA = SA children were less symptomatic than NSA children.

[a] SA > NSA = SA children were more symptomatic than NSA children.

seductive behavior, requesting sexual stimulation from adults or other children, and age-inappropriate sexual knowledge (Beitchman, Zucker, Hood, daCosta, & Akman, 1991). Other symptoms that appeared in many studies included anxiety, depression, withdrawn behavior, somatic complaints, aggression, and school problems.

Column 2 shows the number of studies in which sexually abused children were more symptomatic than their nonabused counterparts. The denominator is the number of studies in which this comparison was made. For many symptoms, a difference was found in all of the studies in which such a comparison was made. These symptoms were fear, nightmares, general posttraumatic stress disorder (PTSD),[2] withdrawn behavior, neurotic mental illness, cruelty, delinquency, sexually inappropriate behavior, regressive behavior (including enuresis, encopresis, tantrums, and whining), running away, general behavior problems, self-injurious behavior, internalizing, and externalizing.[3] The symptom with the lowest percentage of studies in which a difference was found (besides suicidal behavior, for which a difference was found in only one study) was poor self-esteem (50%). This may be in part because poor self-esteem is so common and has so many possible causes. It may also be because this symptom was the one most frequently measured by child self-report, a method that may underestimate pathology (see Methodological Issues and Directions for Future Research). Nonetheless, for almost every symptom examined, including self-esteem, in most studies sexually abused children were found to be more symptomatic than their nonabused counterparts.

The comparison between sexually abused children and other clinical, nonabused children (i.e., children in treatment) tells a possibly different story, however (Columns 3–5). For many of the symptoms measured, sexually abused children were actually less symptomatic than these clinical children in the majority of the studies. Sexually abused children showed only two symptoms consistently more often than nonabused clinical children: PTSD (just one study) and sexualized behavior (six of eight studies). Thus, sexually abused children tended to appear less symptomatic than their nonabused clinical counterparts except in regard to sexualized behavior and PTSD. These results must be interpreted very cautiously, especially in the light of two features of the clinical comparison groups with which abused children were often compared. First, most clinical comparison groups of so-called nonabused children probably actually do contain children

---

[2]In this article, we group posttraumatic stress disorder with symptoms even though we realize that it is a cluster of symptoms comprising a diagnostic category.

[3]Internalizing and externalizing are composite symptoms found on the Child Behavior Checklist (Achenbach & Edelbrock, 1984). Internalizing is withdrawn behavior, depression, fearfulness, inhibition, and overcontrol. Externalizing includes aggression and antisocial and undercontrolled behavior.

TABLE 2
Average Effect Sizes for Seven Symptoms of Sexual Abuse

		Effect sizes		
Symptom	No. studies	Range of η^2	Average η	Average η^2
Aggression	4	.37–.71	.66	.43
Anxiety	3	.01–.28	-.39	.15
Depression	6	.06–.68	.59	.35
Externalizing	5	.08–.52	.57	.32
Internalizing	6	.11–.70	.62	.38
Sexualized behavior	5	1.9–.77	.66	.43
Withdrawal	6	.12–.68	.60	.36

whose abuse simply has not been discovered. In this case, the comparison is not a true abused-versus-nonabused comparison. Second, clinical comparison groups generally contain many children who are referred primarily because of their symptomatic behavior. Naturally these children are likely to be more symptomatic than children referred not because of symptoms, but because of something done to them (i.e., abuse). Thus, the lower levels of symptoms in sexually abused children may say more about the clinical comparisons than about the sexually abused children themselves.

For a synthesis of findings such as in Table 1, a comparison of effect sizes would ordinarily be preferable to the so-called simple box score approach we used. Unfortunately, most of the studies we reviewed did not present data in a form amenable to the calculation of effect sizes. We were, however, able to calculate effect sizes (Table 2) for seven symptoms on which enough studies had provided adequate information for a comparison of abused and nonabused nonclinical children (all between-groups comparisons[4]). The symptoms were anxiety, sexualized behavior, depression, withdrawal, aggression, internalizing, and externalizing.

Table 2 shows that sexual abuse status alone accounted for a very large percent-

---

[4]The criteria for including a study in this review were as follows: The authors reported an exact t value or an F value from a univariate analysis of variance, they reported the degrees of freedom, and there was only one degree of freedom in the numerator. Eta allowed us to examine the effects of sexual abuse apart from sample size and therefore provided a standard coefficient by which to compare findings (Rosenthal, 1984). In addition, because eta is comparable to a Pearson r, it provided an index of the strength of the relationship between sexual abuse status and manifestation of a symptom. Eta squared indicated how much of the variance was accounted for by the child's sexual abuse status. One needs to be cautious when interpreting results based on a small number of studies and widely ranging effect sizes. Unfortunately, very few investigators have reported results that are amenable to effect size calculations.

age of the variance for all seven symptoms, with the sexually abused children manifesting significantly more of all these symptoms. The highest effect sizes (etas) were for the acting-out behaviors, such as sexualized behaviors and aggression. Sexual abuse status accounted for 43% of the variance for these two behaviors and 32% of the variance for externalizing. Such a large effect size is less surprising for sexualized behavior than it is for more global symptoms such as aggression and externalizing, which could have a variety of underlying causes.

Sexual abuse status also accounted for a large percentage of the variance (35–38%) for the internalizing behaviors—internalizing, depression, and withdrawal. The smallest percentage of variance accounted for was for anxiety (15%) but even this is a large effect.

Overall, the results of effect size analysis support the conclusion drawn from Table 1 that being sexually abused was strongly related to some symptoms specific to sexual abuse, such as sexualized behavior, as well as a range of more global symptoms such as depression, aggression, and withdrawal. Nonetheless, sexually abused children did not appear to be more symptomatic than were other clinical children, except in the case of PTSD and sexualized behavior.

PERCENTAGES OF VICTIMS WITH SYMPTOMS

Many researchers simply reported whether sexually abused children were more symptomatic than nonabused children. Yet it is also important to know the actual percentage of victims with each symptom. Some symptoms may occur more often in sexually abused than nonabused children but occur so rarely that they are of little concern for the majority of children in treatment. The actual frequency of such symptoms in the population of abused children can be an important guide to clinicians in diagnosis and treatment. Furthermore, this information is helpful for clinicians and researchers who may want to anticipate the consequences of abuse or develop theory about the process of recovery from abuse. In Table 3, we synthesize information about these frequencies.

The range of children with each symptom varied widely from study to study, which is not unusual given the heterogeneity of sources. Therefore, for each symptom we calculated a weighted average across all studies, dividing the total number of children with a symptom by the total number of children in all the studies reporting on that symptom.

Across all studies, the percentage of victims with a particular symptom was mostly between 20% and 30%. It is important to note that, with the exception of PTSD, no symptom was manifested by a majority of victims. However, there have been relatively few studies of PTSD, and half the children included in this calculation were victims of severe ritualistic abuse from Los Angeles-area day-care cases (Kelly, in press-a), thus inflating the percentage. If we exempt these unusu-

TABLE 3
Percentage of Sexually Abused Children With Symptoms

Symptom	% with symptom	Range of %s	No. studies	N
Anxiety	28	14–68	8	688
Fear	33	13–45	5	477
Posttraumatic stress disorder				
Nightmares	31	18–68	5	605
General	53	20–77	4	151
Depression				
Depressed	28	19–52	6	753
Withdrawn	22	4–52	5	660
Suicidal	12	0–45	6	606
Poor self-esteem	35	4–76	5	483
Somatic complaints	14	0–60	6	540
Mental illness				
Neurotic	30	20–38	3	113
Other	6	0–19	3	533
Aggression				
Aggressive/antisocial	21	13–50	7	658
Delinquent	8	8	1	25
Sexualized behavior				
Inappropriate sexual behavior	28	7–90	13	1,353
Promiscuity	38	35–48	2	128
School/learning problems	18	4–32	9	652
Behavior problems				
Hyperactivity	17	4–28	2	133
Regression/immaturity	23	14–44	5	626
Illegal acts	11	8–27	4	570
Running away	15	2–63	6	641
General	37	28–62	2	66
Self-destructive behavior				
Substance abuse	11	2–46	5	786
Self-injurious behavior	15	1–71	3	524
Composite symptoms				
Internalizing	30	4–48	3	295
Externalizing	23	6–38	3	295

ally severely abused children, the average percentage of victims with symptoms of PTSD was 32%, near the level of other frequently occurring symptoms such as poor self-esteem (35%), promiscuity (38%), and general behavior problems (37%). Because the Child Behavior Checklist (CBCL; Achenbach & Edelbrock, 1984) was used in a large number of studies, we also calculated the percentage of children in the clinical range (or with "elevated scores") for internalizing and externalizing symptomatology.

Overall, the percentage of victims with the various symptoms may seem low to those with a clinical perspective. Part of the problem with the analysis of these composite percentages was that many of the symptoms did not occur uniformly across all age groups. We therefore reexamined the weighted percentages presented in Table 3, grouped by the age of the child at assessment. Percentages were calculated for preschool-age (approximately 0–6 years), school-age (approximately 7–12 years), adolescent (approximately 13–18 years), and mixed age (e.g., 3–17 years) groups. The ages reported in different studies varied and overlapped a bit from these guidelines but by and large fell within these ranges. From a developmental standpoint, we should emphasize that these were very crude cuts across large developmental periods. Furthermore, they represented age at the time of report, not at the onset or end of molestation. In addition, there was no control for the context in which the abuse occurred or the variables that mediated the effects of that abuse.

The results of this analysis (Table 4) hint at possible developmental patterns. Differentiating the samples on the basis of major age groups appeared to yield more focused and consistent findings than when age groups were mixed.

For preschoolers, the most common symptoms were anxiety, nightmares, general PTSD, internalizing, externalizing, and inappropriate sexual behavior. For school-age children, the most common symptoms included fear, neurotic and general mental illness, aggression, nightmares, school problems, hyperactivity, and regressive behavior. For adolescents, the most common behaviors were depression; withdrawn, suicidal, or self-injurious behaviors; somatic complaints; illegal acts; running away; and substance abuse. Among the symptoms that appeared prominently for more than one age group were nightmares, depression, withdrawn behavior, neurotic mental illness, aggression, and regressive behavior.

To date, the majority of data on the effects of sexual abuse on children have been collected cross-sectionally, with data obtained only once per child. Nevertheless, from this cross-sectional data it is possible to hypothesize some developmental trajectories of changes in symptomatology. The question remains, however, as to whether these changes in symptomatology occur within a given child at different stages or represent developmental changes in response to sexual abuse at the time of report.

Depression appeared to be a particularly robust symptom across age groups and was also one that appeared frequently in adults molested as children, as two recent reviews have indicated (Beitchman et al., 1992; McGrath, Keita, Strickland, & Russo, 1990). School and learning problems were also fairly prominent in all three age groups, especially school-age children and adolescents. This is a symptom that would not appear in adults but could be parallel to employment difficulties in adults, because both are structured environments to which the person must report every day and both require equivalent types of skills.

Behavior labeled as antisocial in preschool- and school-age children might be labeled as illegal in adolescents. Similarly, the results of our analysis and a recent review by Beitchman et al. (1991) indicate that sexualized behaviors may be prominent for preschool-age children, submerge during latency (or the school-age period), and reemerge during adolescence as promiscuity, prostitution, or sexual

TABLE 4
Percentage of Children With Symptoms by Age Group

Symptom	% of subjects (No. studies/No. subjects)			
	Preschool	School	Adolescent	Mixed
Anxiety	61 (3/149)	23 (2/66)	8 (1/3)	18 (4/470)
Fear	13 (1/30)	45 (1/58)	—	31 (2/389)
Posttraumatic stress disorder				
Nightmares	55 (3/183)	47 (1/17)	0 (1/3)	19 (2/402)
General	77 (1/71)	—	—	32 (3/80)
Depression				
Depressed	33 (3/149)	31 (2/66)	46 (3/129)	18 (2/409)
Withdrawn	10 (1/30)	36 (1/58)	45 (2/126)	15 (3/446)
Suicidal	0 (1/37)	—	41 (3/172)	3 (2/397)
Poor self-esteem	0 (1/25)	6 (1/17)	33 (1/3)	38 (4/438)
Somatic complaints	13 (2/54)	—	34 (1/44)	12 (2/442)
Mental illness				
Neurotic	20 (1/30)	38 (1/58)	24 (1/25)	—
Other	0 (1/37)	19 (1/58)	16 (2/69)	3 (1/369)
Aggression				
Aggressive/antisocial	27 (3/154)	45 (1/58)	—	14 (3/446)
Delinquent	—	—	8 (1/25)	—
Sexualized behavior				
Inappropriate sexual behavior	35 (6/334)	6 (1/17)	0 (1/3)	24 (7/999)
Promiscuity	—	—	38 (2/128)	—
School/learning problems	19 (2/107)	31 (1/58)	23 (2/69)	17 (2/418)
Behavior problems				
Hyperactivity	9 (2/55)	23 (2/75)	0 (1/3)	—
Regression/immaturity	36 (4/159)	39 (2/75)	0 (1/3)	15 (2/389)
Illegal acts	—	—	27 (1/101)	8 (3/469)
Running away	—	—	45 (3/172)	4 (3/469)
General	62 (1/17)	—	—	28 (1/49)
Self-destructive behavior				
Substance abuse	—	—	53 (2/128)	2 (3/658)
Self-injurious behavior	—	—	71 (2/128)	1 (1/369)
Composite symptoms				
Internalizing	48 (1/69)	—	—	24 (2/226)
Externalizing	38 (1/69)	—	—	23 (2/226)

aggression. These same symptoms might manifest themselves as sexual dysfunctions or sex offending in adulthood, although this has yet to be demonstrated empirically.

The results presented in Table 4 suggest that much symptomatology is developmentally specific and the generalizing across large age groups distorts the patterns. Fortunately, this is more a problem of data analysis and presentation of findings than it is of data collection, so future research should be able to address this issue. Developmental theory and suggestions for future research are described in the Discussion section.

PERCENTAGES OF ASYMPTOMATIC VICTIMS

In addition to the percentage of children with specific symptoms, another important statistic is the percentage of children with no symptoms. This figure has important clinical implications for the group of children in whom the impact of abuse may be muted or masked. Unfortunately, few investigators have reported on such asymptomatic children, perhaps out of concern that such figures might be misinterpreted or misused.

Nonetheless, when investigators have made such estimates, they have found a substantial, and perhaps to some surprising, proportion of the victims to be free of the symptoms being measured. For example, Caffaro-Rouget, Lang, and van-Santen (1989) found that 49% were asymptomatic at their assessment during a pediatric examination. Mannarino and Cohen (1986) found that 31% were symptom free, and Tong, Oates, and McDowell (1987) found that 36% were within the normal range on the CBCL. Finally, Conte and Schuerman (1987b) indicated that 21% of their large sample appeared to have had no symptoms at all, even though their assessment included both very specific and broad items such as "fearful of abuse stimuli" and "emotional upset."

There are several possible explanations why so many children appeared to be asymptomatic. The first possibility is that the studies did not include measures of all appropriate symptoms or the researchers were not using sensitive enough instruments. In most individual studies, only a limited range of possible effects were examined. Thus some of the asymptomatic children may have been symptomatic on dimensions that were not being measured.

Another possibility is that asymptomatic children are those who have yet to manifest their symptoms. This could be either because the children are effective at suppressing symptoms or have not yet processed their experiences or because true traumatization occurs at subsequent developmental stages, when the children's victim status comes to have more meaning or consequences for them (Berliner, 1991). We would expect these children to manifest symptoms later on. In one study that supports this interpretation (Gomes-Schwartz, Horowitz,

Cardarelli, & Sauzier, 1990), the asymptomatic children were the ones most likely to worsen by the time of the 18-month follow up: 30% of them developed symptoms. To date, no one has replicated this finding, however.

A final explanation is that perhaps asymptomatic children are truly less affected. Research indeed suggests there is a relationship between the seriousness and duration of the abuse and the amount of impact (see Intervening Variables section, below). The asymptomatic children might be those with the least damaging abuse. They may also be the most resilient children, the ones with the most psychological, social, and treatment resources to cope with the abuse.

In fact, all three explanations may be simultaneously correct. Unfortunately, the issue of asymptomatic children has been peripheral until recently. Too few researchers have even mentioned the issue, and fewer still have looked at the correlates of being symptom free. Future studies need to address this issue more fully, not as a sidebar of unusual findings, but as a central topic in its own right.

INTERVENING VARIABLES

In many studies (25 of the 46 we reviewed), researchers have tried to account for variations in the children's symptomatology by examining characteristics of the abuse experience. The results for variables with consistent findings are listed in Table 5. Variables with contradictory or confusing results are discussed in this section.

Age at the time of assessment has been the most commonly considered intervening variable. The majority of studies indicated that children who were older at the time of assessment appeared to be more symptomatic than those who were younger. However, most of these studies did not control for the effect of duration (those who were older may have had longer molestations), identity of the perpetrator (intrafamilial perpetrators may have been able to continue the abuse for a longer time), or severity of the molestation (older victims may have experienced more severe sexual acts). In three studies, no significant differences related to age at time of assessment were found (Einbender & Friedrich, 1989; Friedrich, Urquiza, & Beilke, 1986; Kolko, Moser, & Weldy, 1988); in one study, younger children were more symptomatic (Wolfe, Gentile, & Wolfe, 1989); and in one study there was a curvilinear relationship between age and symptomatology, with the middle age range being more symptomatic (Gomes-Schwartz, Horowitz, & Sauzier, 1985). Although the data appear to indicate roughly that older children are more negatively affected, these results should be interpreted with caution because of the lack of control over other relevant variables.

Age of onset is another possible intervening variable. However, age of onset was related to symptoms in only one study, which showed that those with early age of onset were more likely to manifest symptoms of pathology (Zivney, Nash,

TABLE 5
Influence of Intervening Variables

Variable	No. studies With significant difference in impact	Total	Direction of findings
Age of child			
At assessment	7	10	Older children were more symptomatic in five studies.
At onset	1	3	Not clear.
Sex of child	5	8	Patterns of symptoms differed for boys and girls.
Penetration/severity	6	10	Oral, anal, or vaginal penetration was related to increased symptoms.
Frequency	4	6	Higher frequency was related to increased symptoms.
Duration	5	7	Longer duration was related to increased symptoms.
Perpetrator	7	9	Symptoms were increased when perpetrator had close relationship with child.
No. perpetrators	1	3	Not clear.
Lack of maternal support	3	3	Lack of support was related to increased symptoms.
Force	5	6	Use of force was related to increased symptoms.
Time elapsed since last abusive incident	1	3	Not clear.
Child's attitudes and coping style	2	2	Negative outlook and coping style were related to increased symptoms.

& Hulsey, 1988). In two other studies no difference was found in level of pathology for early versus late age of onset. By and large, it appears that age of onset must be fit into a total conceptual model of molestation. Research is insufficient to permit any conclusions about whether early versus late age of onset is more likely to lead to greater symptomatology. Age of onset might be related more to other characteristics of the abuse (such as identity of the perpetrator) than to overall number and severity of symptoms. Although the relationship of age of onset to symptomatology in children is not clear at this time, in two recent studies an early age of onset was found to be related to amnesia among adult survivors (Briere & Conte, 1989) and late presentation for treatment (Kendall-Tackett, 1991).

With regard to sex of the subject, consistent differences in the reaction of boys and girls to molestation have been found in only a few studies. The scarcity of these findings is in sharp contrast to the popular belief that boys are likely to manifest externalizing symptoms and girls are more likely to exhibit internalizing symptoms. The absence of consistent gender differences is all the more interesting because girls are more likely to suffer intrafamilial abuse, which has been associated with more severe effects (Finkelhor, Hotaling, Lewis, & Smith, 1990). The lack of more systematic attention to gender differences may be due in part to the small number of male victims in most studies and the possibility that, because of bias in the identification of male victims, only the most symptomatic boys end up in clinical samples. It may also be due to the fact that comparison of boys and girls has produced too few interesting differences to motivate research- ers to place it in center focus. Nevertheless, researchers should address the issue of sex of the victims in future reports.

Penetration (oral, anal, or vaginal) did influence the impact of sexual abuse in the majority of studies, but most researchers differed in their definitions of sever- ity of abuse. To further add to the confusion, some of the investigators added together all the sexual acts that a victim experienced, and therefore their indices of severity included the severity as well as the number of sexual acts. Even with all these variations, it appeared that molestations that contained some form of pen- etration were more likely to produce symptoms than molestations that did not.

The identity of the perpetrator is another factor that has been related to the impact of abuse. The weight of the evidence indicated that a perpetrator who was close to the victim caused more serious effects than one who was less close. To date there does not appear to be a uniform coding scheme for closeness, however. For example, fathers and stepfathers are often coded in the same category. Researchers should try to determine a measure of emotional closeness or degree of caretaking responsibility rather than relying on the kinship label of the perpetrator-victim relationship.

On a similar note, the impact of the number of perpetrators is not clear. The number of perpetrators was positively correlated with number of symptoms in one study, negatively correlated with number of symptoms in another, and not corre- lated with symptoms in another. Future research should address this issue.

Time elapsed since the last abusive incident and assessment is a variable with intuitive appeal, but it has been examined in very few studies. Only 55% of the articles in the present review even mentioned time elapsed, and it varied from a few days to several years. In only three studies was the possible relationship between time elapsed and the impact of abuse examined. In one study (Friedrich et al., 1986), children became less symptomatic over time, whereas in two other studies (McLeer, Deblinger, Atkins, Foa, & Ralphe, 1988; Wolfe et al., 1989) it made no difference. It appears to be too early to decide whether time elapsed is correlated with the number of symptoms. Therefore, we should find out more about this variable before we assume that it makes no difference.

In summary, the findings of the various studies reviewed indicated that moles- tations that included a close perpetrator; a high frequency of sexual contact; a long duration; the use of force; and sexual acts that included oral, anal, or vaginal pen- etration lead to a greater number of symptoms for victims. Similarly, as all the studies that included these variables indicated, the lack of maternal support at the time of disclosure and a victim's negative outlook or coping style also led to increased symptoms. The influence of age at the time of assessment, age at onset, number of perpetrators, and time elapsed between the end of abuse and assessment is still somewhat unclear at the present time and should be examined in future studies on the impact of intervening variables.

It should be kept in mind when interpreting these findings that certain intervening variables are highly correlated. For example, intrafamilial abuse normally occurs over a longer time period and involves more serious sexual activity (i.e., penetration). These natural confounds make it difficult to fully analyze the independent effects of intervening variables. Very few studies have included more than one or two of these variables, and almost no one has statistically controlled for their effects.

LONGITUDINAL STUDIES

Perhaps the most encouraging development in the field has been the appearance of longitudinal studies (Bentovim, vanElberg, & Boston, 1988; Conte, 1991; Everson, Hunter, & Runyan, 1991; Friedrich & Reams, 1987; Gomes-Schwartz et al., 1990; Goodman et al., in press; Hewitt & Friedrich, 1991; Mannarino, Cohen, Smith, & Moore-Motily, 1991; Runyan, Everson, Edelson, Hunter, & Coulter, 1988; Valliere, Bybee, & Mowbray, 1988; Waterman, in press). Most of these studies have followed children for approximately 12–18 months, with a few ranging from 2 to 5 years (Bentovim et al., 1988; Waterman, in press). These studies allow a perspective on two important issues: (a) What is the course of symptomatology over time, and (b) what contributes to recovery?

The picture provided by the longitudinal studies is tentative, but some generalizations are possible. Overall, symptoms seemed to abate with time. The pattern of recovery was different for different symptoms, and some children actually appeared to worsen.

Abatement of Symptoms

Abatement of symptoms has been demonstrated in at least seven longitudinal studies covering all age groups (Bentovim et al., 1988; Conte, 1991; Gomes-Schwartz et al., 1990; Goodman et al., in press; Hewitt & Friedrich, 1991; Mannarino et al., 1991; Runyan et al., 1988). For example, Gomes-Schwartz et al. (1990) noted substantial diminution of emotional distress in 55% of the victims (mixed age group) over 18 months. In Bentovim et al.'s (1988) study, social workers found improvement in the level of symptoms in 61% of the children. Hewitt and Friedrich (1991) noted that 65% of preschool-age children improved over a period of 1 year. About two thirds of even the ritualistically abused pre-schoolers, who were initially in the clinical range on the CBCL (Waterman, in press), had moved back into the normal range on follow-up.

Nonetheless, there was a sizable group—anywhere from 10% to 24%—of children who appeared to get worse (Bentovim et al., 1988 [10%]; Gomes-Schwartz et al., 1990 [24%]; Hewitt & Friedrich, 1991 [18%]; Runyan et al., 1988 [14%]). Some of these were children who had none of the symptoms measured at the time of initial assessment (Gomes-Schwartz et al., 1990).

Some investigators also noted a pattern in which symptoms tended to abate. Gomes-Schwartz et al. (1990) found that signs of anxiety (e.g., sleep problems or fear of the offender) were most likely to disappear, whereas signs of aggressive-ness (e.g., fighting with siblings) tended to persist or worsen. This was consistent with Mannarino et al.'s (1991) finding of a significant reduction over time in the internalizing but not the externalizing scales of the CBCL. Conversely, some symptoms may increase over time. For example, one symptom that may increase over time, at least for the under-12 group, is sexual preoccupations (Friedrich & Reams, 1987; Gomes-Schwartz et al., 1990). It is not entirely clear what this symptom abatement implies. Although some symptoms may be more transient than others, it does not necessarily mean that underlying trauma is resolved, but perhaps only that overt manifestations are more easily masked. Moreover, these changes may have less to do with abatement of trauma than developmental changes in symptomatology, with children at each age manifesting different types of symptoms.

There is a long list of correlates of improvement over time, but few of these findings have been demonstrated in more than one study. Age was not found to be strongly correlated with recovery in any study, although Goodman et al. (in press) found that 6–11-year-olds recovered most quickly in the very short term (3 months after the trial). Neither gender (Gomes-Schwartz et al., 1990; Goodman et al., in press), nor race and socioeconomic status (Gomes-Schwartz et al., 1990) have been factors in recovery. Children who were the most disturbed at the time of first assessment were found to make the most recovery (Gomes-Schwartz et al., 1990), but this may have been an artifact.

Family and Treatment Variables

A key variable in recovery was family support, demonstrated by several studies. Children who had maternal support recovered more quickly (Everson et al., 1991; Goodman et al., in press). Maternal support was demonstrated through believing the child and acting in a protective way toward the child. Waterman (in press) found that the least symptomatic children (5 years after disclosure) were those whose mothers were most supportive and whose families had less strain, enmeshment, and expressions of anger.

Interestingly, the effect of long-term therapy has not been extensively examined. In one study (Gomes-Schwartz et al., 1990), all clients received crisis intervention through the research project. The clients who showed the greatest amount of recovery (15% of subjects) were those who received therapy in the specialized program run by the research team. Those who received therapy in the community at large (20% of subjects) did not appear to recover as well. The authors did not elaborate on the type of long-term therapy that clients received either through the researchers' program or in the community at large, however. In contrast, Goodman et al. (in press) found psychological counseling unrelated to improvement. But again, clients sought therapy in the outside community and there was no control for the type or quality of the therapy they received.

Court Involvement

The impact of court involvement and testimony was also a focus of several of the longitudinal studies because of the intense public policy debate surrounding this issue. In one study (Goodman et al., in press), children involved in court proceedings were slower to recover over both a 7- and an 11-month period than children not involved in court. Recovery was particularly impeded among children who had to testify on multiple occasions, who were afraid of their perpetrators, and who testified in cases in which there was no other corroborating evidence. Whitcomb et al.'s (1991) findings echoed Goodman et al.'s. Whitcomb et al. concluded that there were adverse effects for older children who had to undergo numerous, lengthy, or harshly contested courtroom testimony. The outcome of the trial (conviction or acquittal of the perpetrator), or the number of times that the child was interviewed did not relate to symptomatology (Goodman et al., in press).

Runyan et al. (1988) had more mixed findings with regard to the impact of court involvement. The children who had slower recovery in this study were those who were involved in a criminal case that was still not resolved 5 months after the initial evaluation. However, children whose cases had terminated more quickly with a conviction or plea bargain recovered just as quickly as children who had no court involvement at all. In fact, children who testified in juvenile court proceedings recovered more quickly. However, in a follow-up of adolescents from the same study, Everson et al. (1991) found that having to testify on multiple occasions caused negative effects, concurring with the findings of Goodman et al. (in press).

Although the longitudinal studies showed the risks involved in testimony, at least one cross-sectional study (Williams, 1991) confirmed that testimony in protected court settings can mitigate trauma. In this study of victims abused in day care, children who testified via closed-circuit television or videotaped testimony or in closed courtrooms suffered fewer symptoms of maladjustment than did children who testified in open court.

Overall, this small number of studies suggests that criminal court involvement posed risks to children's recovery, at least in the short run. But the risks were specifically associated with certain aspects of court involvement that can be modified or avoided. For example, negative impact can be lessened by resolving cases quickly, by preventing a child from having to testify on multiple occasions, and by not requiring a frightened child to face a defendant. Thus, although the research urges caution, it cannot be interpreted as a categorical argument against the prosecution of sexual abuse.

Revictimization

Follow-up studies lend an important perspective to the question of whether abuse victims are reabused in the year or two after disclosure. Most of the follow-up studies we reviewed showed the rate of reabuse to be between 6% and 19% (Bentovim et al., 1988 [16%]; Daro, 1988 [19%]; Gomes-Schwartz et al., 1990 [6%]), with follow-up ranging from 18 months to 5 years. Daro (1988) pointed out that the reabuse rate for sexually abused children in her study was still substantially lower than the reabuse rate for victims of neglect or emotional abuse.

Summary

In summary, in the first year or year and a half after disclosure, one half to two thirds of all children became less symptomatic, whereas 10–24% become more so. Six to nineteen percent experienced additional sexual abuse. Fears and somatic symptoms abated the most quickly; aggressiveness and sexual preoccupations were the most likely to remain or increase. Children's recovery was clearly assisted by a supportive family environment, and certain kinds of court experiences delayed recovery.

DISCUSSION

The present review confirms the general impression that the impact of sexual abuse is serious and can manifest itself in a wide variety of symptomatic and pathological behaviors. There is virtually no general domain of symptomatology that has not been associated with a history of sexual abuse. Age and a variety of abuse-related factors can affect both the nature and the severity of symptoms. However, some sexually abused children may also appear to have no apparent symptoms.

Indeed, approximately one third of sexually abused children in the studies we reviewed fell into this category. These findings have a number of important implications for theory development.

Core-Symptom Theories

The first and perhaps most important implication is the apparent lack of evidence for a conspicuous syndrome in children who have been sexually abused. The evidence against such a syndrome includes the variety of symptoms children manifest and the absence of one particular symptom in a large majority of children. Despite the lack of a single symptom that occurs in the majority of victims, both sexualized behavior and symptoms of PTSD occurred with relatively high frequency. These also appeared to be the only two symptoms more common in sexually abused children than in other clinical groups. Even though they do not occur in all victims, some theorists have forwarded PTSD and sexualized behaviors as the core manifestations of sexual abuse trauma (Corwin, 1989; Jampole & Weber, 1987; Wolfe et al., 1989), so the evidence pertaining to these two symptoms is worth reviewing more carefully.

The frequency of sexualized behavior in sexually abused children (including frequent and overt self-stimulation; inappropriate sexual overtures toward other children and adults; and compulsive talk, play, and fantasy with sexual content) is somewhat difficult to determine. Although it is the most regularly studied symptom, its occurrence varies enormously. Across six studies of preschoolers (the children most likely to manifest such symptoms) an average of 35% exhibited sexualized behavior. Friedrich et al. (1992), using an instrument specially designed to measure such behaviors, detected a somewhat higher percentage. But across all sexually abused children it may be only half of all victims. The lowest estimate (7%) was based on a very large study, including many well-functioning and older children (Conte & Schuerman, 1987b). Besides sample and methodological differences, other variations may well arise because the concept itself can be vague (sometimes it is called inappropriate sexual behavior, and other times it is called sexual acting out). Furthermore, some forms of sexualization may be quite minor and transitory (e.g., playing with anatomical dolls), whereas others may be deeply etched, even affecting a child's physiology. Putnam (1990; F. Putnam, personal communication, January 10, 1991) detected elevated hormone levels among some sexually abused girls and evidence that onset of puberty was advanced for these girls by as much as 1 year. Although such physiological changes could be the effect of sexualization or, alternatively, one of its sources, it suggests how profound and pervasive the impact of sexual abuse can be.

Although sexualization is relatively specific to sexual abuse (more so than symptoms such as depression), nonsexually abused children may also be sexualized. For example, Deblinger, McLeer, Atkins, Ralphe, and Foa (1989) found that 17% of physically (but not sexually) abused children exhibited sexually inappropriate behavior. Although sexualized behavior may be the most characteristic symptom of sexual abuse, and the one that best discriminates between abused and nonabused children, as many as half of victims may not be overtly sexualized, and this symptom does not occur only in sexually abused children. From a clinical point of view, this symptom may indicate sexual abuse but is not completely diagnostic because children can apparently appear to be sexualized for other reasons.

The evidence for PTSD as a central effect of sexual abuse is also its relative frequency (particularly in preschool- and school-age victims) and its higher incidence in sexual abuse victims than in other clinical groups. Although PTSD is relatively common in child sexual abuse victims, it is not a universal reaction. In the two most thorough clinical evaluations of PTSD (according to criteria in the revised third edition of the *Diagnostic and Statistical Manual of Mental Disorders;* American Psychiatric Association, 1987). 48% (McLeer et al., 1988) and 21% (Deblinger et al., 1989) of sexually abused children could be diagnosed as having PTSD. Although many other children have related symptoms, such as fears, nightmares, somatic complaints, autonomic arousal, and guilt feelings, it is not clear whether this is evidence for PTSD dynamics or other symptoms. More importantly, PTSD is not specific to sexual abuse in that many nonsexually abused children suffer from PTSD.

PTSD has served as a focal point for the analysis of sexual abuse trauma in part because it is a well-developed, generalized theory of traumatic processes. Finkelhor (1987), however, has raised some questions about how well the model of PTSD accounts for sexual abuse trauma. Theorists describe PTSD as resulting from experiences that are overwhelming, sudden, and dangerous (Figley, 1986; Pynoos & Eth, 1985). Much sexual abuse, however, lacks these components, especially abuse that occurs through manipulation of the child's affections and misrepresentation of social standards. Thus, although many children may suffer symptoms that are explained by the PTSD model, the theory and the empirical findings do not support PTSD symptomatology as universal to sexual abuse or as the most characteristic pattern.

There is at least one other core-symptom theory about the effect of sexual abuse, one that argues that the central damage is to children's self-image (Bagley & Young, 1989; Putnam, 1990). According to this view, it is the damaged self-image, not the sexual abuse per se, that leads to other difficulties. If this theory were true, disturbed self-esteem should be one of the most consistent, pervasive, and long-lasting effects of sexual abuse. Unfortunately, although many victims do have low self-esteem, researchers (e.g., Mannarino et al., 1991) have had considerable difficulty demonstrating this phenomenon. It is not certain whether poor self-esteem, which has been assessed primarily through self-reports, has been effectively measured. But the evidence to date does little to support the theory that self-esteem is the core element of sexual abuse traumatization.

Multifaceted Models of Traumatization

Overall, the absence of one dominant and consistent set of symptoms argues against these core-domain theories. Rather, these data suggest that the impact of sexual abuse is more complicated because it produces multifaceted effects. Several conceptual models are consistent with such a pattern. Finkelhor and Browne's (1985) model suggests that sexual abuse traumatizes children through four distinctive types of mechanisms, which account for the variety of outcomes. The four mechanisms have been termed (a) traumatic sexualization, (b) betrayal, (c) stigmatization, and (d) powerlessness. Traumatic sexualization includes a variety of processes such as the inappropriate conditioning of the child's sexual responsiveness and the socialization of the child into faulty beliefs and assumptions about sexual behavior. Betrayal includes the shattering of the child's confidence that trusted persons are interested in and capable of protecting him or her from harm. Stigmatization covers all the mechanisms that undermine the child's positive self-image: the shame that is instilled, the ostracism the child suffers, and the negative stereotypes that are acquired from the culture and immediate environment. Finally, powerlessness comprises PTSD-type mechanisms (intense fear of death or injury from an uncontrollable event) as well as the repeated frustration of not being able to stop or escape from the noxious experience or elicit help from others. These mechanisms are present to varying degrees and in different forms in different abuse scenarios.

In addition, Finkelhor and Browne (1985) propose that certain symptoms are more closely related to certain dynamics. The sexualization symptoms have an obvious connection to the traumatic sexualization processes, self-esteem is connected to stigmatization, and fears and PTSD are connected to powerlessness. Little research has been carried out to confirm the model in part because of its complexity, the variety of different mechanisms posited, and the difficulty of clearly delineating and measuring them.

Other theorists have also adopted a multiple-dynamics approach to account for the seeming variety of sexual abuse symptoms. Briere (1992) has developed such a model whose dynamics include (a) negative self-evaluation, (b) chronic perception of danger or injustice, (c) powerlessness and preoccupation with control, (d) dissociative control over awareness, (e) impaired self-reference, and (f) reduction of painful internal states.

A different model posits sexual abuse as simply a generalized stressor. Although this model has not been specifically developed, it is another way to understand the impact of sexual abuse. In this model, the child is likely to develop problems in whatever area he or she may have had a prior vulnerability. This model predicts a high degree of similarity between the effects of sexual abuse and the effects of other childhood stressors such as parental divorce. There is some evidence to support this view, particularly our finding in the present review of similarity on some symptoms between sexually abused children and other clinical groups. On the other hand, sexually abused children do tend to exhibit some characteristics (e.g., sexualized behaviors) that are much more common among sexually abused children than they are among other clinical groups. These types of effects argue against sexual abuse as merely a generalized stressor.

A third model posits family dysfunction or a general maltreating environment, not the sexually abusive activities per se, as the root of the trauma in most sexually abused children (Clausen & Crittenden, 1991). This model is supported by apparent similarities in the range and types of problems manifested by all abused children. However, certain evidence from the studies included in the present review argues against such a conceptualization. First, the studies showed that nonabused siblings (i.e., children raised in the same dysfunctional families) displayed fewer symptoms than did their abused siblings (Lipovsky, Saunders, & Murphy, 1989). In addition, the review of the 25 studies in which the influence of intervening variables was examined (Table 5) consistently showed strong relationships between specific characteristics of the sexual abuse and the symptomatology in the children (e.g., Newberger, Gremy, & Waternaux, 1990). All of this argues for traumatic processes inherent in the sexual abuse itself that are independent from a generalized family dysfunction or generalized maltreating environment.

This is not to say that prior vulnerabilities, a maltreating environment, and family dysfunction do not contribute to traumatization as well. Research such as Conte and Schuerman's (1987a, 1987b) demonstrates that both abuse-related factors and family dysfunction contribute to children's trauma. And Conte and Schuerman found that over time, the abuse-related factors were less influential than the continuing family processes, such as the amount of family support for the child. This suggests a grand model of sexual abuse trauma that includes effects that are both more and less specific to sexual abuse and that arise from the abusive acts in particular, which also interact with prior vulnerabilities of the child, the health or toxicity of the family environment, and the social response to the discovery of abuse.

Summary

The research to date points to an array of traumatizing factors in sexual abuse, with sexualization and PTSD as frequent, but not universal, processes. The traumatic impact of the abusive acts themselves (e.g., their frequency and severity) has been established, as well as the likely contribution of other familial and environmental conditions. The role of disturbance to self-esteem and of a child's prior dispositions or vulnerabilities has not been as well substantiated.

This theoretical discussion has implications for clinicians as well as researchers. The range of symptoms, the lack of a single predominant symptom pattern, and the absence of symptoms in so many victims clearly suggest that diagnosis is complex. Because the effects of abuse can manifest themselves in too many ways, symptoms cannot be easily used, without other evidence, to confirm the presence of sexual abuse. Yet the absence of symptoms certainly cannot be used to rule out sexual abuse. There are too many sexually abused children who are apparently asymptomatic. This finding is especially important for those conducting forensic evaluations.

It may be possible, as Corwin (1989) has argued, to find a combination of symptoms that is extremely diagnostic of sexual abuse, especially in certain subgroups of victims (e.g., preschool children with certain kinds of sexualized behavior and posttraumatic play), and research toward such a screening device may be warranted. But the evidence suggests that such a device would identify only a small percentage of victims and that one could conclude nothing at all from the absence of such symptom patterns.

Although conclusions such as these are useful, we also think this discussion highlights a glaring inadequacy in the literature: a nearly universal absence of theoretical underpinnings in the studies being conducted on this subject to date. Researchers evince a great deal of concern about the effects of sexual abuse but disappointingly little concern about why the effects occur. Few studies are undertaken to establish or confirm any theory or explanation about what causes children to be symptomatic. Rather, most researchers simply document and count the existence of symptoms and some of their obvious correlates. This accounts for one of the main reasons that, in spite of numerous studies since Browne and Finkelhor's (1986) review, there have been few theoretical advances.

Future studies need to turn to the development and confirmation of theory. Those who believe that different mechanisms result in different symptoms need to begin to search for such mechanisms. For example, if dissociation is theorized as an acquired strategy for escaping from unpleasant emotions, then researchers need to document the presence of the cognitive, affective, and psychological underpinnings to this mechanism and relate it to the trauma itself. By contrast, those who see sexual abuse as a generalized stressor need to conduct studies that relate the effects of sexual abuse to preexisting vulnerabilities in coping. The dialogue about variables that mediate the effects of abuse needs to be expanded and ideas forwarded about how to study and test their existence. This process of improving research might be assisted when the sexual abuse researchers join forces with those who study related symptomatology in nonabused children. This has already happened in the work generated by the importation of PTSD theory into the field, and it is only by further developing this cross-fertilization that advances can continue.

METHODOLOGICAL ISSUES AND DIRECTIONS FOR FUTURE RESEARCH

Although the studies we reviewed signal an enormous improvement in methodology, they highlight many major areas where current designs could be improved or refined. Some more specific suggestions for improvement are offered in this section.

Improvement in Measures of Impact

The literature on effects has relied extensively on parent-completed checklists of children's symptomatology, particularly the CBCL. However, two sets of findings have raised concern about the validity of these measures. One shows that mothers' judgments about their children's symptoms are highly related to their own level of distress and willingness to believe their children (Everson, Hunter, Runyan, Edelsohn, & Coulter, 1989; Newberger et al., 1990). A second shows a poor association between parents' and children's own reports (Cohen & Mannarino, 1988; Kelly & Ben-Meir, in press).

It does seem plausible that parents might be biased reporters, especially in the context of a family problem like sexual abuse, where parents can experience strong feelings of guilt or ambivalence about a child's disclosure. But other findings suggest that parent reports are nonetheless relatively valid and, in the context of currently used instruments, probably better than their children's reports. For example, although depressed mothers reported more child symptoms than non-depressed mothers on the CBCL, the assessments still differentiated disturbed and nondisturbed children when depression was statistically controlled (Friedlander, Weiss, & Taylor, 1986). Moreover, mothers' ratings tended to be more similar to and correlated better with therapists' and teachers' ratings than with those of their children (Shapiro, Leifer, Martone, & Kassem, 1990; Tong et al., 1987). It appears from several studies (Cohen & Mannarino, 1988; Shapiro et al., 1990) that children's self-reports minimize problems like depression or low self-esteem that are noted by parents and therapists. Why this is so is not clear.

One clear implication from this is that researchers should not rely on children's self-reports alone. Ideally, assessments should be obtained from multiple sources, as Waterman, Kelly, McCord, and Oliveri (in press) recently did. In addition, research needs to be undertaken to improve the validity of parent reports and especially, if possible, children's self-assessments.

A second concern, raised in part by the issue of seemingly asymptomatic children, is whether the instruments currently being used are sensitive enough to measure consistently and accurately the trauma of sexual abuse. Several groups of researchers, recognizing particularly the limitations of the CBCL, have branched out in attempts to develop such sensitive measures. Friedrich et al. (1992) have greatly expanded CBCL symptom items in the domain of sexuality. Lanktree and Briere (1991, 1992) have adapted the Trauma Symptom Checklist, highly successful in differentiating sexually abused adults, for use with children. Wolfe et al. (1989) have developed scales to measure more sensitively PTSD-type symptomatology. Such efforts need to be continued and elaborated.

Greater Differentiation by Age and Gender

Many researchers have studied subjects from very broad age ranges (e.g., 3–18 years) and grouped them together to discuss symptoms. Similarly, they have grouped boys and girls together. As shown in Table 4, this grouping together of all ages can mask particular developmental patterns of the occurrence of some symptoms. At a minimum, future researchers should divide children into preschool, school, and adolescent age ranges when reporting the percentages of victims with symptoms. It would be better to provide even more detail on how age at assessment affects the manifestation of symptoms, by looking at smaller age ranges and tying this information into theory about children's social, emotional, and cognitive development during these difficult developmental periods. A parallel effort is needed with regard to gender.

Expanded Analysis of Intervening Variables

The present review confirms that abuse-related variables are associated with outcome and thus should be regularly included in analyses. However, many other factors probably are influential as well, and more emphasis should be placed on understanding their role. These factors include children's intelligence, coping skills, prior adjustment, and cognitive interpretation of the abuse. It also includes children's family and social environment, as well as the actions taken by professionals in response to their disclosures. Another factor that needs to be regularly taken into account is time elapsed since the end of the abuse. In some samples, several years might have elapsed between the end of the abuse and the assessment of the child, and during this time symptoms may have abated.

Longitudinal Research and Developmental Theory

A developmental perspective is one approach that may encourage more theory-driven research. Researchers using a developmental approach may also respond to some of the methodological issues raised here. Current research has tended to focus on assessments of trauma at a specific age or point in time (a snapshot approach), but it would also be helpful to know more about the course of symptomatology and recovery over time. For example, the symptomatology of a 15-year-old molested at age 4 may be different from that of a 15-year-old molested at age 14. Furthermore, symptoms may tend to recur at different developmental stages and asymptomatic children may later become symptomatic. Studies in which data are collected at more than one time point will encourage this developmental approach for studying sexual abuse and may answer many of our questions (see Baltes, 1987; Starr, MacLean, & Keating, 1991). Even in the absence of funding, any research on outcomes should at least pave the way for possible later follow-up by gaining permission to recontact subjects and by recording data that will facilitate such research in the future.

In addition to studying abuse at multiple time points, developmental research means incorporating the multiple dimensions of children's development. Changes occur in children's behaviors, thoughts, and emotions at every developmental stage. Research on the effects of sexual abuse on children tends to focus predominantly on behavioral and emotional symptoms while ignoring the effects of sexual abuse on cognitive and social development.

A number of research questions can be generated by examining sexual abuse within the multiple dimensions of children's development. For example, cognitive development could influence children's interpretations of sexual abuse and the symptoms they subsequently manifest. Specifically, as children mature, their thinking becomes less egocentric. This issue alone generates several possible research questions. For example, are young children more likely to see themselves as responsible for the abuse ("It happened because I was bad") than are less egocentric older children? Furthermore, are children who see themselves as responsible for the abuse more likely to engage in self-abusive or destructive behavior? How do internal attributions affect children's reactions to prosecution of the perpetrator? Are these attributions more likely to increase the children's sense of guilt when the perpetrator is punished?

Along these same lines, children's cognitive development can influence their emotional and social development and their interpretation of the perpetrators' actions. As thinking becomes decentered, children recognize that people can have both positive and negative traits and that they themselves can have both positive and negative feelings toward others. How does the gradual attainment of decentered thinking affect children's interpretations of the perpetrators' actions, their own behaviors, and the abuse itself? This is especially important to understand when the perpetrator is someone whom the child loves and trusts. Are children who can see conflicting traits in others more likely to report abuse because they see it as only one part of their relationship with the perpetrator ("I love him but I want the abuse to stop")?

These are but a few of the types of research questions that can be generated from examining abuse from a developmental and multidimensional perspective. Future researchers could make specific predictions based on developmental theory and clinical research on related topics (e.g., children's reactions to other types of childhood traumas). This type of framework would also allow researchers to incorporate information about intervening variables such as the timing and duration of the abuse and the identity of the perpetrator.

In summary, studies conducted with a developmental and multidimensional framework could readily incorporate the many intervening variables that modify the effects of abuse. In addition, such a framework offers a richer description of why children and adults manifest certain symptoms at each developmental stage and how people cope with psychic trauma. Developmental psychologists and child clinicians could collaborate to develop models of how children at each developmental stage might be affected by their abuse experience. Researchers studying child sexual abuse have looked in isolation at many of the factors related to the impact of abuse. Now it is time for us to combine them into more realistic models. Research of this type would provide helpful theoretical information about the mechanism and processing of psychological trauma in general. It would also provide guidelines on where clinicians can effectively intervene to aid children in their healing process.

REFERENCES

Achenbach, T. M., & Edelbrock, C. S. (1984). *Child behavior checklist.* Burlington VT: University of Vermont.

Adams-Tucker, C. (1982). Proximate effects of sexual abuse in childhood: A report on 28 children. *American Journal of Psychiatry, 139,* 1252–1256.

American Psychiatric Association. (1987). *Diagnostic and statistical manual of mental disorders* (3rd ed., rev.). Washington, DC: Author.

Bagley, C., & Young, L. (1989). Depression, self-esteem, and suicidal behavior as sequels of sexual abuse in childhood: Research and therapy. In M. Rothery & G. Cameron (Eds.), *Child maltreatment: Expanding our concept of healing* (pp. 183–209). Hillsdale, NJ: Erlbaum.

Baltes, P. B. (1987). Theoretical propositions of live-span developmental psychology: On the dynamics between growth and decline. *Developmental Psychology, 23,* 611–626.

Basta, S. M., & Peterson, R. F. (1990). Perpetrator status and the personality characteristics of molested children. *Child Abuse and Neglect, 14,* 555–566.

Beitchman, J. H., Zucker, K. J., Hood, J. E., daCosta, G. A., & Akman, D. (1991). A review of the short-term effects of child sexual abuse. *Child Abuse and Neglect, 15,* 537–556.

Beitchman, J. H., Zucker, K. J., Hood, J. E., daCosta, G. A., Akman, D., & Cassavia, E. (1992). A review of the long-term effects of child sexual abuse. *Child Abuse and Neglect, 16,* 101–118.

Bentovim, A., vanElberg, A., & Boston, P. (1988). The results of treatment. In A. Bentovim, A Elton, J. Hildebrand, M. Tranter, & E. Vizard (Eds.), *Child sexual abuse within the family: Assessment and treatment* (pp. 252–268). London: Wright.

Berliner, L. (1991). The effects of sexual abuse on children. *Violence Update, 1,* 1–10.

Briere, J. (1992). *Child abuse trauma: Theory and treatment of the lasting effects.* Newbury Park, CA: Sage.

Briere, J., & Conte, J. (1989, August). *Amnesia in adults molested as children: Testing theories of repression.* Paper presented at the 97th Annual Convention of the American Psychological Association, New Orleans, LA.

Browne, A., & Finkelhor, D. (1986). The impact of child sexual abuse: A review of the research. *Psychological Bulletin, 99,* 66–77.

Burgess, A., Hartman, C., McCausland, M., & Powers, P. (1984). Response patterns in children and adolescents exploited through sex rings and pornography. *American Journal of Psychiatry, 141,* 656–662.

Burns, N., Williams, L. M., & Finkelhor, D. (1988). Victim impact. In D. Finkelhor, L. M. Williams, & N. Burns (Eds.) *Nursery crimes: Sexual abuse in daycare* (pp. 114–137). Newbury Park, CA: Sage.

Caffaro-Rouget, A., Lang, R. A., & vanSanten, V. (1989). The impact of child sexual abuse. *Annals of Sex Research, 2,* 29–47.

Clausen, A. H., & Crittenden, P. M. (1991). Physical and psychological maltreatment: Relations among types of maltreatment. *Child Abuse and Neglect, 15,* 5–18.

Cohen, J. A., & Mannarino, A. P. (1988). Psychological symptoms in sexually abused girls. *Child Abuse and Neglect, 12,* 571–577.

Conte, J. R. (1991). *Behavior of sexually abused children at intake/disclosure and 12 months later.* Unpublished manuscript.

Conte, J., & Schuerman, J. (1987a). Factors associated with an increased impact of child sexual abuse. *Child Abuse and Neglect, 11,* 201–211.

Conte, J., & Schuerman, J. (1987b). The effects of sexual abuse on children: A multidimensional view. *Journal of Interpersonal Violence, 2,* 380–390.

Corwin, D. L. (1989). Early diagnosis of child sexual abuse: Diminishing the lasting effects. In G. E. Wyatt & G. J. Powell (Eds.), *Lasting effects of child sexual abuse* (pp. 251–270). Newbury Park, CA: Sage.

Daro, D. (1988). *Confronting child abuse: Research for effective program design.* New York: Free Press.

Deblinger, E., McLeer, S. V., Atkins, M. S., Ralphe, D., & Foa, E. (1989). Post-traumatic stress in sexually abused, physically abused, and nonabused children. *Child Abuse and Neglect, 13,* 403–408.

Einbender, A. J., & Friedrich, W. N. (1989). Psychological functioning and behavior of sexually abused girls. *Journal of Consulting and Clinical Psychology, 57,* 155–157.

Elwell, M. E., & Ephross, P. H. (1987). Initial reactions of sexually abused children. *Social Casework, 68,* 109–116.

Erickson, M. F. (1986, August). *Young sexually abused children: Socioemotional development and family interaction.* Paper presented at the 94th Annual Convention of the American Psychological Association, Washington, DC.

Everson, M. D., Hunter, W. M., & Runyan, D. K. (1991, January). *Adolescent adjustment after incest: Who fares poorly?* Paper presented at the San Diego Conference on Responding to Child Maltreatment, San Diego, CA.

Everson, M. D., Hunter, W. M., Runyan, D. K., Edelsohn, G. A., & Coulter, M. L. (1989). Maternal support following disclosure of incest. *American Journal of Orthopsychiatry, 59,* 197–207.

Feltman, R. I. (1985). *A controlled correlational study of the psychological functioning of female paternal incest victims.* Unpublished doctoral dissertation.

Figley, C. R. (1986). *Trauma and its wake: Vol. II. Traumatic stress theory, research, and intervention.* New York: Brunner/Mazel.

Finkelhor, D. (1987). The trauma of child sexual abuse: Two models. *Journal of Interpersonal Violence, 2,* 348–366.

Finkelhor, D., & Browne, A. (1985). The traumatic impact of child sexual abuse: A conceptualization. *American Journal of Orthopsychiatry, 55,* 530–541.

Finkelhor, D., Hotaling, G., Lewis, I. A., & Smith, C. (1990). Sexual abuse in a national study of adult men and women: Prevalence, characteristics, and risk factors. *Child Abuse and Neglect, 14,* 19–28.

Friedlander, S., Weiss, D. S., & Taylor, J. (1986). Assessing the influence of maternal depression on the validity of the Child Behavior Checklist. *Journal of Abnormal Child Psychology, 14,* 123–133.

Friedrich, W., Beilke, R., & Urquiza, A. (1987). Children from sexually abusive families: A behavioral comparison. *Journal of Interpersonal Violence, 2,* 391–402.

Friedrich, W. N., Beilke, R. L., & Urquiza, A. J. (1988). Behavior problems in young sexually abused boys. *Journal of Interpersonal Violence, 3,* 21–28.

Friedrich, W. N., Grambasch, P., Damon, L., Hewitt, S. K., Koverola, C., Lang, R., & Wolfe, V. (1992). The Child Sexual Behavior Inventory: Normative and clinical comparisons. *Psychological Assessment, 4,* 303–311.

Friedrich, W. N., & Luecke, W. J. (1988). Young school-age sexually aggressive children. *Professional Psychology: Research and Practice, 19,* 155–164.

Friedrich, W. N., & Reams, R. A. (1987). Course of psychological symptoms in sexually abused young children. *Psychotherapy, 24,* 160–170.

Friedrich, W. N., Urquiza, A. J., & Beilke, R. L. (1986). Behavior problems in sexually abused young children. *Journal of Pediatric Psychology, 11,* 47–57.

Gale, J., Thompson, R. J., Moran, T., & Sack, W. H. (1988). Sexual abuse in young children: Its clinical presentation and characteristic patterns. *Child Abuse and Neglect, 12,* 163–170.

Gomes-Schwartz, B., Horowitz, J. M., Cardarelli, A. P., & Sauzier, M. (1990). The aftermath of child sexual abuse: 18 months later. In B. Gomes-Schwartz, J. M. Horowitz, & A. P. Cardarelli (Eds.), *Child sexual abuse: The initial effects.* (pp. 132–152). Newbury Park, CA: Sage.

Gomes-Schwartz, B., Horowitz, J. M., & Sauzier, M. (1985). Severity of emotional distress among sexually abused preschool, school-age, and adolescent children. *Hospital and Community Psychiatry, 36,* 503–508.

Goodman, G. S., Taub, E. P., Jones, D. P. H., England, P., Port, L. K., Rudy, L., & Prado, L. (in press). Emotional effects of criminal court testimony on child sexual assault victims. *Monographs of the Society for Research in Child Development.* Chicago: University of Chicago.

Hewitt, S. K., & Friedrich, W. N. (1991, January). *Preschool children's responses to alleged sexual abuse at intake and one-year follow up.* Paper presented at the meeting of the American Professional Society on the Abuse of Children, San Diego, CA.

Jampole, L., & Weber, M. K. (1987). An assessment of the behavior of sexually abused and nonsexually abused children with anatomically correct dolls. *Child Abuse and Neglect, 11,* 187–192.

Kelley, S. J. (1989). Stress responses of children to sexual abuse and ritualistic abuse in day care centers. *Journal of Interpersonal Violence, 4,* 502–513.

Kelly, R. J. (in press-a). Overall level of distress. In J. Waterman, R. J. Kelly, J. McCord, & M. K. Oliveri (Eds.), *Behind the playground walls: Sexual abuse in preschools.* New York: Guilford Press.

Kelly, R. J. (in press-b). Effects on sexuality. In J. Waterman, R. J. Kelly, J. McCord, & M. K. Oliveri (Eds.), *Behind the playground walls: Sexual abuse in preschools.* New York: Guilford Press.

Kelly, R. J., & Ben-Meir, S. (in press). Emotional effects. In J. Waterman, R. J. Kelly, J. McCord, & M. K. Oliveri (Eds.), *Behind the playground walls: Sexual abuse in preschools.* New York: Guilford Press.

Kendall-Tackett, K. A. (1991). Characteristics of abuse that influence when adults molested as children seek treatment. *Journal of Interpersonal Violence, 6,* 486–493.

Kolko, D. J., Moser, J. T., & Weldy, S. R. (1988). Behavioral/emotional indicators of sexual abuse in child psychiatric inpatients: A controlled comparison with physical abuse. *Child Abuse and Neglect, 12,* 529–541.

Lanktree, C., & Briere, J. (1991, January). *Early data on the Trauma Symptom Checklist for Children (TSC-C).* Paper presented at the meeting of the American Professional Society on the Abuse of Children, San Diego, CA.

Lanktree, C., & Briere, J. (1992, January). *Further data on the Trauma Symptom Checklist for children (TSC-C): Reliability, validity, and sensitivity to treatment.* Paper presented at the San Diego Conference on Responding to Child Maltreatment, San Diego, CA.

Lindberg, F., & Distad, L. (1985). Survival responses to incest: Adolescents in crisis. *Child Abuse and Neglect, 9,* 521–526.

Lipovsky, J. A., Saunders, B. E., & Murphy, S. M. (1989). Depression, anxiety, and behavior problems among victims of father–child sexual assault and nonabused siblings. *Journal of Interpersonal Violence, 4,* 452–468.

Lusk, R. (in press). Cognitive and school-related effects. In J. Waterman, R. J. Kelly, J. McCord, & M. K. Oliveri (Eds.), *Behind the playground walls: Sexual abuse in preschools.* New York: Guilford Press.

Mannarino, A. P., & Cohen, J. A. (1986). A clinical-demographic study of sexually abused children. *Child Abuse and Neglect, 10,* 17–23.

Mannarino, A. P., Cohen, J. A., & Gregor, M. (1989). Emotional and behavioral difficulties in sexually abused girls. *Journal of Interpersonal Violence, 4,* 437–451.

Mannarino, A. P., Cohen, J. A., Smith, J. A., & Moore-Motily, S. (1991). Six and twelve month follow-up of sexually abused girls. *Journal of Interpersonal Violence, 6,* 494–511.

McGrath, E., Keita, G. P., Strickland, B. R., & Russo, N. F. (1990). *Women and depression: Risk factors and treatment issues.* Washington, DC: American Psychological Association.

McLeer, S. V., Deblinger, E., Atkins, M. S., Foa, E. B., & Ralphe, D. L. (1988). Post-traumatic stress disorder in sexually abused children. *Journal of the American Academy of Child and Adolescent Psychiatry, 27,* 650–654.

Mian, M., Wehrspann, W., Klajner-Diamond, H., LeBaron, D., & Winder, C. (1986). Review of 125 children 6 years of age and under who were sexually abused. *Child Abuse and Neglect, 10,* 223–229.

Morrow, K. B., & Sorell, G. T. (1989). Factors affecting self-esteem, depression, and negative behaviors in sexually abused female adolescents. *Journal of Marriage and the Family, 51,* 677–686.

Newberger, C. M., Gremy, I., & Waternaux, C. (1990). *Mothers and children following sexual abuse disclosure: Connections, boundaries, and the expression of symptomatology.* Unpublished manuscript, Children's Hospital, Boston, MA.

Orr, D. P., & Downes, M. D. (1985). Self-concept of adolescent sexual abuse victims. *Journal of Youth and Adolescence, 14,* 401–410.

Putnam, F. W. (1990). Disturbances of "self" in victims of childhood sexual abuse. In R. Kluft (Ed.), *Incest-related syndromes of adult psychopathology* (pp. 113–131). Washington, DC: American Psychiatric Press.

Pynoos, R. S., & Eth, S. (1985). Children traumatized by witnessing acts of personal violence: Homicide, rape, or suicide behavior. In S. Eth & R. S. Pynoos (Eds.), *Post-traumatic stress disorder in children* (pp. 19–43). Washington, DC: American Psychiatric Press.

Rimsza, M. E., Berg, R. A., & Locke, C. (1988). Sexual abuse: Somatic and emotional reactions. *Child Abuse and Neglect, 12,* 201–208.

Rosenthal, R. (1984). *Meta-analytic procedures for social research.* Newbury Park, CA: Sage.

Runyan, D. K., Everson, M. D., Edelsohn, G. A., Hunter, W. M., & Coulter, M. L. (1988). Impact of legal intervention on sexually abused children. *Journal of Pediatrics, 113,* 647–653.

Sandfort, T. (1982). *The sexual aspects of pedophile relations.* Amsterdam: Pan/Spartacus.

Sandfort, T. (1984). Sex in pedophiliac relationships: An empirical investigation among a nonrepresentative group of boys. *Journal of Sex Research, 20,* 123–142.

Shapiro, J. P., Leifer, M., Martone, M. W., & Kassem, L. (1990). Multi-method assessment of depression in sexually abused girls. *Journal of Personality Assessment, 55,* 234–248.

Sirles, E. A., Smith, J. A., & Kusama, H. (1989). Psychiatric status of intrafamilial child sexual abuse victims. *Journal of the American Academy of Child and Adolescent Psychiatry, 28,* 225–229.

Starr, R. H., MacLean, D. J., & Keating, D. P. (1991). Life-span development outcomes of child maltreatment. In R. H. Starr & D. A. Wolfe (Eds.), *The effects of child abuse and neglect: Issues and research* (pp. 1–32). New York: Guilford Press.

Tong, L., Oates, K., & McDowell, M. (1987). Personality development following sexual abuse. *Child Abuse and Neglect, 11,* 371–383.

Valliere, P. M., Bybee, D., & Mowbray, C. T. (1988, April). *Using the Achenbach Child Behavior Checklist in child sexual abuse research: Longitudinal and comparative analysis.* Paper presented at the National Symposium on Child Victimization, Anaheim, CA.

Waterman, J. (in press). Mediators of effects on children;: What enhances optimal functioning and promotes healing? In J. Waterman, R. J. Kelly, J. McCord, & M. K. Oliveri (Eds.), *Behind the playground walls: Sexual abuse in preschools.* New York: Guilford Press.

Waterman, J., Kelly, R. J., McCord, J., & Oliveri, M. K. (in press). *Behind the playground walls: Sexual abuse in preschools.* New York: Guilford Press.

Whitcomb, D., Runyan, D. K., DeVos, E., Hunter, W. M., Cross, T. P., Everson, M. D., Peeler, N. A., Porter, C. A., Toth, P. A., & Cropper, C. (1991). *Child victim as witness research and developmental program* (Final report to the Office of Juvenile Justice and Delinquency Prevention, Office of Justice Programs, U.S. Department of Justice). Washington, DC: U.S. Government Printing Office.

White, S., Halpin, B. M., Strom, G. A., & Santilli, G. (1988). Behavioral comparisons of young sexually abused, neglected, and nonreferred children. *Journal of Clinical Child Psychology, 17,* 53–61.

White, S., Strom, G. A., Santilli, G., & Halpin, B. (1986). Interviewing young sexual abuse victims with anatomically correct dolls *Child Abuse and Neglect, 10,* 519–529.

Williams, L. (1991). *The impact of court testimony on young children: Use of protective strategies in day care cases.* Unpublished manuscript, Family Research Laboratory, University of New Hampshire.

Wolfe, V. V., Gentile, C., & Wolfe, D. A. (1989). The impact of sexual abuse on children: A PTSD formulation. *Behavior Therapy, 20,* 215–228.

Zivney, O. A., Nash, M. R., & Hulsey, T. L. (1988). Sexual abuse in early versus late childhood: Differing patterns of pathology as revealed on the Rorschach. *Psychotherapy, 25,* 99–106.

APPENDIX

Studies of the Effects of Sexual Abuse on Children

Author	Victims			Comparison children		
	Age	N	Source	Age	N	Source
Adams-Tucker (1982)	2–16	28	SAT I/E	—	—	—
Basta & Peterson (1990)	6–10	32	I/E	6–10	16	NA—community
Bentovim & Boston (1988); Bentovim, vanElberg, & Boston (1988)	2–16	411	SAT I/E	2–16	362	NA siblings
Burgess, Hartman, McCausland, & Powers (1984)	6–16	46	SAT E[a]	—	—	—
Burns, Williams, & Finkelhor (1988)	2–5	87	SAT/day care/E	—	—	—
Caffaro-Rouget, Lang, & vanSanten (1989)	1–18	240	SAT I/E	2–18	113	NA—community
Cohen & Mannarino (1988)	6–12	24	SAT I/E	—	—	
Conte & Schuerman (1987a, 1987b)	4–17	369	SAT I/E	4–17	318	NA—community
Deblinger, McLeer, Atkins, Ralphe, & Foa (1989)	3–13	29	Inpatient treatment I/E	3–13 / 3–13	29 / 29	Physically abused—inpatient treatment / NA—inpatient treatment
Einbender & Friedrich (1989)	6–14	46	SAT I/E	6–14	46	NA—community
Elwell & Ephross (1987)	5–12	20	SAT I/E	—	—	—
Erickson (1986)	4–6	11	High-risk infant follow-up	4–6	67	NA—same group
Everson, Hunter, & Runyan (1991)	11–17	44	SAT I/E	—	—	—
Everson, Hunter, Runyan, Edelsohn, & Coulter (1989)	6–17	88	SAT I/E	—	—	—
Feltman (1985)	10–17	31	SAT I	10–17	24	NA—outpatient treatment

Study	Age	N	Measure	Comparison age	Comparison N	Comparison group
Friedrich, Beilke, & Urquiza (1987)	3-12	93	SAT I/E	3-12	64	NA—outpatient treatment
					78	NA—community
Friedrich, Beilke, & Urquiza (1988)	3-8	33	SAT I/E	—	—	—
Friedrich & Luecke (1988)	4-11	22	SAT/ I/E[b]	—	—	—
	5-13	22	SAT I/E[c]			
Friedrich & Reams (1987)	3-7	8	SAT I/E	—	—	—
Friedrich, Urquiza, & Beilke (1986)	3-12	85	SAT I/E	Norms	—	—
Gale, Thompson, Moran, & Sack (1988)	<7	37	SAT I/E	<7	35	NA—outpatient treatment
					13	Physically abused—outpatient treatment
Gomes-Schwartz, Horowitz, & Sauzier (1985); Gomes-Schwartz, Horowitz, Cardarelli, & Sauzier (1990)	4-18	113	SAT I/E	Clinical and nonclinical norms		
Jampole & Weber (1987)	3-8	10	SAT/NR	3-8	10	NA—community
Kelley (1989)	4-11	32	Day care	4-11	67	NA—day care
		35	Ritualistically abused in day care/E			
Kelly (in press-a, in press-b); Kelly & Ben-Meir (in press); Lusk (in press)	4-14; 15	69	Ritualistically abused in day care/SA/E	5-14	32	NA—day care
Kolko, Moser, & Weldy (1988)	5-14	7	SA/inpatient treatment/I/E	5-14	44	NA—inpatient treatment
		22	SA and physically abused	5-14	30	Physically abused—inpatient treatment
Lindberg & Distad (1985)	12-18; M = 12.2	27	Children's home/I	M = 12.5	—	—
Lipovsky, Saunders, & Murphy (1989)		100	SAT I	—	100	NA siblings
Mannarino & Cohen (1986)	3-16	45	SAT I/E	—	—	—
Mannarino, Cohen, & Gregor (1989)	6-12	94	SAT I/E	6-12	89	NA—outpatient treatment
					75	NA—community
McLeer, Deblinger, Atkins, Foa, & Ralphe (1988)	3-16	31	SAT I/E	—	—	—

Continued

Appendix (*cont.*)
Studies of the Effects of Sexual Abuse on Children

Author	Victims			Comparison children		
	Age	N	Source	Age	N	Source
Mian, Wehrspann, Klajner-Diamond, LeBaron, & Winder (1986)	<6	125	Chart review I/E	—	—	—
Morrow & Sorell (1989)	12–18	101	SAT I	—	—	—
Newberger, Gremy, & Waternaux (1990)	6–12	49	SAT I	—	—	—
Orr & Downes (1985)	9–15	20	SAT I/E	9–15	20	NA—emergency room pop
Rimsza, Berg, & Locke (1988)	2–17	72	SAT I/E/chart review	2–17	72	NA—clinic/chart review
Runyan, Everson, Edelsohn, Hunter, & Coulter (1988)	6–17	75	SAT I/E	—	—	—
Shapiro, Leifer, Martone, & Kassem (1990)	5–16	53	SAT I/E	3–16	70	NA—outpatient treatment
Sirles, Smith, & Kusama (1989)	2–17	207	SAT I/E	—	—	—
Tong, Oates, & McDowell (1987)	3–16	49	SAT I/E	3–16	49	NA—community
Valliere, Bybee, & Mowbray (1988)	4–13	34	Day care/E	5–11	136	NA—community Norms
White, Halpin, Strom, & Santilli (1988)	2–6	17	SAT/NR	2–6	23/18	NA—community/neglect
White, Strom, Santilli, & Halpin (1986)	2–6	25	SAT/NR	2–6	25	NA—community
Wolfe, Gentile, & Wolfe (1989)	5–16	71	SAT I/E	—	—	—
Zivney, Nash, & Hulsey (1988)	3–16	80	SAT I/E	3–16	70	NA—outpatient treatment

Note. SAT = sexual abuse treatment or evaluation (outpatient unless indicated), I = intrafamilial abuse, E = extrafamilial abuse, NR = data not reported, SA = sexually abused, pop = population.
[a] Children in sex rings. [b] Sexually aggressive victims. [c] Nonsexually aggressive victims.

Part IV

DEVELOPMENTAL DISORDERS

Although it is generally agreed that the pervasive developmental disorders are neurologically based, knowledge of the mechanisms through which abnormalities of the central nervous system are symptomatically expressed is at best extremely limited. In the first paper in this section, Bishop provides an update of Demasio and Maurer's 1978 hypothesis implicating damage and/or dysfunction of the mesolimbic cortex and associated frontal lobe structures in the etiology of autism. Infant monkeys who sustained bilateral lesions in the amygdala and hippocampus are described as exhibiting a pattern of cognitive and social deficits analogous to those observed in autism. Moreover, neuropsychological studies of executive functions in autistic persons have demonstrated impairments similar to those observed in frontal lobe patients. While executive function tasks measure perseveration and planning ability, theory of mind research explores deficits in social cognition. A considerable body of experimental evidence confirms that autistic persons have particular difficulty appreciating the contents of other people's minds and realizing that these might differ from their own thoughts and beliefs. The body of research summarized in this paper serves to demonstrate that neuropsychological approaches to the exploration of hypothesized frontal and limbic system dysfunction in autism is a potentially powerful tool in clarifying relations within the triad of abnormalities in social relatedness, in communication, and in behavior that is autism.

In the second paper in this section, Tobin, Dykens, Pearson, and Cohen direct attention to a group of children who display a distinctive pattern of disturbance in affect modulation, social relatedness, and thinking, but who fall through the cracks of the DSM-III-R nosology. Clinicians differ in their responses to this diagnostic dilemma; some assign multiple DSM-III-R diagnoses, some apply such "private labels" as borderline or childhood schizophrenia, and some resort to the designation PDD-NOS. The limitations of these solutions are critically discussed and rejected, and criteria for a proposed alternative, Multiple Complex Developmental Disorder (MCDD), are presented. As its name indicates, MCDD is conceptualized as a developmental disorder, and consistent with this conceptualization, children meeting MCDD criteria had an earlier onset of symptoms, poorer social and overall adjustment, longer hospitalizations, and poorer outcomes than did hospitalized children with diagnoses of either conduct disorder or dysthymia. Tobin, Dykens, Pearson, and Cohen emphasize that when affected children are considered from a developmental perspective, treatment efforts shift away from efforts directed towards the eradication of pathological symptoms to a focus on fostering conditions that best support emotional development and educational achievement.

In the final paper in this section on developmental disabilities, Berk and Landau examine the development and functional significance of private speech among children with learning disabilities (LD). As conceptualized by Vygotsky, private speech is externalized thought that serves a self-guiding function and aids children in overcoming obstacles to task success when faced with challenging cognitive problems. With a child's increasing age, audible self-directed utterances are abbreviated and internalized as silent verbal thought. The impetus for the study derived from the observation that learning disabled children are often enrolled in cognitive-behavioral interventions designed to train them in effective use of self-directed or private speech. Despite the face validity of this proposition, Berk and Landau's findings indicate that learning disabled and normally achieving children undergo a similar course of private speech development, and in both groups private speech serves the adaptive function of self-regulation. Learning disabled children, especially those with attentional deficits, use task-relevant private speech actively and freely. However, learning disabled children were delayed in private speech internalization, and this delay was most marked for those learning disabled children who also had an attention deficit hyperactivity disorder (LD/ADHD). Furthermore, partially internalized speech was less successful in modulating task-related behavior than was the audible speech of LD and LD/ADHD children. The authors suggest that cognitive-behavioral interventions that teach children with learning disabilities to talk out loud to themselves while engaged in cognitive tasks may simply be training an already existing skill. Moreover, to expect these children to engage in silent self-communication may be counterproductive. Perhaps learning disabled children would be served best by teachers who, cognizant of the functional significance of private speech, create classroom conditions that permit children to generate audible self-regulatory speech without disturbing classmates.

11

Annotation: Autism, Executive Functions, and Theory of Mind: A Neuropsychological Perspective

D. V. M. Bishop

MRC Applied Psychology Unit, Cambridge, England

It is widely accepted nowadays that some kind of neurological abnormality must be responsible for the symptoms of autism. However, we are still a very long way from understanding how brain damage or dysfunction can cause such a distinctive pattern of symptoms, with impairments in language and social interaction and limitations of the behavioural repertoire. Although some evidence of neurological impairment can be demonstrated in the majority of autistic children if a detailed investigation is undertaken (Steffenburg, 1991) there is considerable variation in etiological factors, which may involve genetic constitution, biochemical disorders and many different types of neurological disease.

Because the majority of autistic children are mentally retarded, it is not surprising to find widespread neuropathology associated with autism. However, although CT and MRI scanning have revealed brain abnormalities in several series of autistic children, there is little agreement from one case to another in the extent and types of impairment found (see reviews by Coleman & Gillberg, 1985; Reichler & Lee, 1987). The unresolved question is why brain dysfunction leads to general mental retardation in some children, and to autistic disorder in others.

This brief paper will not attempt to review the neurobiological or psychological literature on autism, but will rather focus on selected recent studies to show how a neuropsychological approach to autistic

---

Reprinted with permission from the *Journal of Child Psychology and Psychiatry*, 1993, Vol. 34(3), 279–293. Copyright © 1993 by the Association for Child Psychology and Psychiatry.

*symptoms can provide new ways of analysing cognitive deficits in this
syndrome, which may guide the search for neurological correlates of
the disorder using more direct techniques.*

A NEUROLOGICAL MODEL OF AUTISM: DAMASIO AND MAURER

Damasio and Maurer (1978) drew attention to an area of cortex in the mesial
aspect of the frontal and temporal lobes, the *mesolimbic cortex,* that is both
phylogenetically and neurochemically distinct from neighbouring regions (see
Fig. 1). This includes the cingulate gyrus, entorhinal area, perirhinal area,
parahippocampal gyrus, and subicular and presubicular regions of the hippocampal formation. They proposed that impairments of motility, communication, goal-
directed behaviour, attention and perception characteristic of autism could all be
explained in terms of dysfunction of this system and closely related structures in
the frontal lobes and basal ganglia (see Fig. 2).

Their analysis started by considering motor disturbances, which, they pointed
out, are reliably found in autism, but are seldom analysed from the neurological
point of view. Damasio and Maurer argued that many of the motor features of
autism were classical neurological signs indicative of dysfunction in the basal
ganglia, a group of large masses of grey matter that have intimate connections
with mesolimbic cortex. For instance, they found that autistic children show persistent maintenance of a posture by exaggerated muscle tone in both feet and
hands (dystonia of the extremities). Damasio and Maurer further argued that certain repetitive and stereotyped movements produced by autistic children could be
regarded as forms of chorea, athetosis or both. Spasticity, however, was not a
characteristic of autistic children.

Damasio and Maurer went on to consider the language impairments seen in
autism. These do not resemble any of the classical syndromes of acquired aphasia,

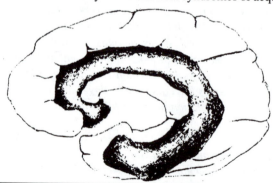

Figure 1. Medial view of the human brain showing neocortex (white) and limbic cortex
(shaded).

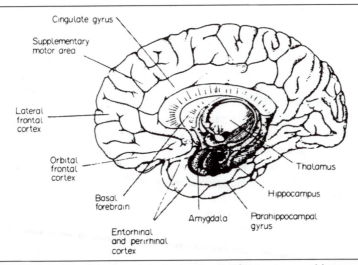

Figure 2. Medial view of the human brain showing limbic structures and interconnected areas in the frontal lobe.

where the deficit is usually specific to verbal communication; in autism nonverbal communication is also impaired. They argued that a much closer parallel could be drawn between the communicative deficits of autism and the syndromes of mutism or speech inhibition that may be seen in the course of recovery from mesial frontal lobe lesions of either hemisphere, particularly those involving the supplementary motor area and cingulate gyrus. These are not aphasias, because basic linguistic capacities to repeat and comprehend language are retained, but there is a failure to initiate conversation spontaneously, which extends to nonverbal as well as verbal interaction. There may be repetitive vocalizations as well as problems in controlling speech volume and pitch.

A third point of similarity between autistic individuals and adults with frontal lesions concerns goal-directed activity. For instance, Ackerly and Benton's (1948) patient with bilateral frontal lobe lesions showed lack of initiative, inability to focus attention, and concreteness in thought and language. Other frontal patients are able to focus attention to a remarkable degree, but do so in a narrow fashion, as if potentially interfering stimuli were completely blocked out (Joseph, 1990). Damasio and Maurer cite animal experiments showing that the mesolimbic system is important in marking the significance of a given stimulus in relation to the goals and emotional state of the organism. Failure to attend to salient stimuli and prolonged interest in less important aspects of the environment could both be caused by an inability to compute the relative significance of different events.

The model proposed by Damasio and Maurer was provocative, but it could be argued that the frontal lobes and limbic system are involved in so many different aspects of behaviour that one could explain almost any pattern of symptoms in terms of dysfunction of this system. As Kolb and Whishaw (1990) have remarked: "There is no cerebral structure in which lesions can produce such a wide variety of symptoms, and thus a more bewildering range of interpretations, than the frontal lobes" (p. 463). In some cases, the parallels drawn by Damasio and Maurer are fragile. For instance, the account of similarities between language disorders in autistic children and those in patients with frontal lesions ignores the fact that comprehension problems are severe in autism, and that when autistic children do speak, their language is characterised by pragmatic abnormalities. Furthermore, one could make a case for localizing certain autistic abnormalities in other parts of the brain. To take just one example, Ornitz (1983) attributed autism to dysfunction of central vestibular control systems in the brainstem and suggested that stereotyped movements were one manifestation of this abnormality. Damasio and Maurer provided a clinical descriptive account of motility disorders similar to those seen in basal ganglia lesions, but they did not specify the characteristics of their patients, the relative frequencies of different impairments or the reliabilities of the observations. It is possible that these neurological signs were correlates of the general retardation that usually accompanies autistic disorder, or even side-effects of antipsychotic medication, rather than being specific to autism.

Overall, then, Damasio and Maurer's model provided a coherent account of a range of autistic features, but the evidence they put forward in its support was circumstantial. Furthermore, at the time they were writing, little emphasis was being placed by researchers on the impairments of social behaviour that are nowadays regarded as a core feature of autistic disorder, and they regarded most of the symptoms of social impairment as secondary to the other deficits seen in this syndrome. However, the passage of time has strengthened their case, with new studies indicating that dysfunction of the mesolimbic system and frontal lobes could provide a plausible neuropsychological account of abnormalities of social behaviour and social cognition, as well as other autistic behaviours.

SOCIAL IMPAIRMENTS AFTER LIMBIC AND ORBITOFRONTAL LESIONS

Studies of both human patients and experimental animals show that destruction of orbital frontal cortex, which has intimate connections with the major limbic nuclei, leads to severe reduction in social and emotional behaviour, whereas with less extensive damage one sees social disinhibition and inappropriate behaviour (see Joseph, 1990, for a review). Changes in social and emotional behaviour after lesions of the limbic system in monkeys have been described by several investigators (e.g. Aggleton & Passingham, 1981). Joseph has argued that one can explain the normal transition from indiscriminate sociability to specific attachments in human infants in terms of the different rates of maturation of the amygdala and septal nuclei of the basal forebrain. Abnormal functioning of the limbic system, therefore, would be entirely compatible with the range of social abnormalities seen in autism.

Until recently, most animal studies looked at the effect of lesions incurred in adulthood. Bachevalier (1991) compared social interactions in infant monkeys who had sustained bilateral lesions of the amygdala and hippocampus with other monkeys with inferotemporal lesions. Lesioned monkeys were observed in a cage with a control monkey of the same age. Those with amygdala-hippocampal lesions had major impairments of social interaction that became more pronounced as they grew older. By 6 months of age these monkeys showed a complete lack of social contact, extreme submissiveness, including active withdrawal, gross motor stereotypies (e.g. twirling in circles and doing somersaults), blank and unexpressive faces, few eye contacts and poor body expression. Animals with lesions in the visual association cortex (inferotemporal cortex) did not show these impairments.

These findings led Bachevalier to propose that autism might be due to early damage to the limbic system and she cited a handful of neuropathological studies that are consistent with this position. An attractive feature of this animal analogue of autism is that it can account for a range of apparently unrelated symptoms; i.e. social and motivational deficits and the motor stereotypies. Bachevalier further argued that the cognitive deficits seen in these animals might have parallels with the puzzling intellectual profile in autism.

Bachevalier's original motivation for carrying out this study was to investigate the functional development of memory. Studies of adults (both human and monkey) have shown that lesions causing conjoint damage to the amygdala and hippocampus lead to severe impairments in the ability to remember, but with preserved ability to learn at least some new skills (see Mishkin & Appenzeller, 1987, for a review). In monkeys, limbic lesions cause substantial impairment in the ability to perform a delayed non-matching to sample task, in which the animal is first rewarded for selecting object A, and then after a delay is presented with a choice between A and B, and is rewarded for selecting B. However, these same animals can learn an object discrimination task, in which they are presented with repeated pairings of objects, A and B, C and D and so on, and must learn which member of each pair is associated with reward (e.g. A but not B, C but not D, etc.). Animals with limbic lesions can not only learn these discriminations but they can also do so when there are prolonged intervals between sessions (24 hours) and when 20 pairs of objects are presented once only in each session. These results have been interpreted as indicating that there are two distinct memory systems: a cognitive memory system (involved in delayed non-matching to sample) and noncognitive habit system (used in discrimination learning). Bachevalier contrasted performance on delayed non-matching to sample and discrimination learning tasks in infant monkeys aged between 3 months and 4 years. Newborn monkeys with damage to the limbic system (amygdala and hippocampus) were severely impaired on the test of cognitive memory but unimpaired in habit formation, and this effect persisted up to 4 years of age. She suggested that the contrast between the intact habit formation system and the severely impaired cognitive memory system might be responsible for the unusual pattern of cognitive strengths and weaknesses observed in autism, where a child may fail to learn basic skills despite having unusually good memory for certain events. There have been relatively few investigations of memory function in autistic children (though see Boucher & Warrington, 1976). Bachevalier's work predicts that if we apply current models of memory derived from work with animals to the study of autistic children we should observe distinctive patterns of strength and weakness (see also Frith & Frith, 1991).

EXECUTIVE FUNCTION DEFICITS AND THE FRONTAL LOBES

Another line of evidence that offers support to Damasio and Maurer's theory comes from recent studies that have used neuropsychological tests sensitive to frontal lobe damage. The frontal lobe is a large and complex structure, with distinct regions varying in cellular composition and interconnection with other brain areas; the consequences of frontal lobe damage will depend on the location and lateralization of the lesion. In his review, Joseph (1990) notes that there are plentiful connections between the frontal lobes and the mesolimbic system; the supplementary motor area has rich interconnections with the cingulate gyrus and basal ganglia, the dorso-lateral area projects to thalamic nuclei, and the orbital frontal lobes receive projections from the inferior temporal lobes, parahippocampal gyrus, and amygdala. Frontal lobe lesions involving the non-motor regions (i.e. dorso-lateral and orbito-frontal cortex) are associated with deficits in executive function, which is defined as the ability to maintain an appropriate problem-solving set for attainment of a future goal (see Duncan, 1986, for a review). Ozonoff, Pennington and Rogers (1991a) noted that some features of autism are reminiscent of executive function deficits. Autistic children are rigid and inflexible and may become distressed at any change to a familiar situation. Their repetitive and stereotyped actions, seen in both spontaneous behaviour and in test situations (e.g. Frith, 1972) may be likened to the response perseveration seen in frontal lobe patients. Autistic individuals do not plan or anticipate long-term consequences and appear not to reflect or self monitor. They frequently appear impulsive and unable to inhibit prepotent but irrelevant responses.

Several investigators have recently attempted to test the hypothesis of frontal lobe dysfunction in autism by administering neuropsychological tests that are designed to assess frontal lobe functions. Prior and Hoffmann (1990) compared 12 autistic individuals of broadly normal nonverbal intelligence (range 76–109) with a control group matched on chronological age and another, slightly younger, control group matched on mental age. Three tests of frontal lobe function were administered. The first was a maze learning task. The subject must learn by trial and error to move a stylus to pick out the correct route through a matrix of metal plates. When an error is made, a click is sounded. Using this task, Milner (1965) found that patients with frontal lesions were not only impaired at learning the route, they also frequently broke the rules of the test by making prohibited diagonal moves or ignoring the need to go back when an error was signalled. Prior and Hoffmann found that autistic subjects took twice as long to complete the task as control children and made three times as many errors. Also, many of the autistic children needed the rules explained repeatedly, suggesting the type of difficulty that typified frontal lobe patients. It was noted that control children often adopted a counting strategy to complete the maze, whereas the autistic children seemed unable to work out how to overcome their difficulties and would persist as if each trial were a new experience.

Prior and Hoffmann also administered the Wisconsin Card Sorting Test (WCST) (Grant & Berg, 1948), which is used to identify perseverative responding in a concept-learning task. The testee is presented with a set of cards that can be sorted by either colour, shape or number, and must deduce the correct sorting rule from the feedback given by the examiner who says whether each classification is right or wrong. In Nelson's (1976) modification of the test, which was used by Prior and Hoffmann, after six correct responses the tester says "The rules have now changed; I want you to find another rule", and starts to adopt a different criterion for feedback. Patients with frontal lesions have been shown to be particularly susceptible to perseveration on this task, persisting in sorting by the original category, despite feedback from the tester (Milner, 1963). Prior and Hoffmann found that on the WCST, children with autism made three times as many errors as controls, and they had more difficulty than control children in naming the categories. Even when aware of making errors, these children seemed unable to change their behaviour to achieve correct responses. However, performance was very variable, and although some autistic children made a substantial number of perseverative errors, others did not.

A final "frontal" task used by Prior and Hoffmann was the Rey–Osterrieth Complex Figure (Rey, 1959), which provides an index of planning and organizational ability. A complex, abstract, two-dimensional figure is copied using different coloured pencils for one minute each until the copy is completed. The testee is then asked to draw the design from memory after a one minute delay. As well as scoring the accuracy of the copy, one can deduce from the colours the order in which different parts of the figure were completed. The usual strategy is to first complete the global outline of the figure, and then add the details. A tendency to draw different sections at random, or to start at one side of the figure indicates a more piecemeal approach to the problem. Prior and Hoffmann found that their three groups did not differ in terms of time or accuracy of the initial copy, but autistic children were significantly poorer than control children in accuracy of recall after a 3 min delay. They commented that the approach to copying was often disorganized and the autistic children would select minor aspects of the model to copy first rather than the overall figure. It was also noted that the poor recall by autistic children could reflect problems with storing material in a coherent way.

Rumsey and Hamburger (1988, 1990) included the WCST and the Rey–Osterrieth Complex Figure in a study comparing the cognitive profiles of 10 autistic men and 15 severely dyslexic men to 25 normal men of similar age and educational level. All subjects had verbal and performance IQs above 80. The autistic subjects showed significant impairments relative to the dyslexic group on the WCST, but were unimpaired on the Rey Complex figure. However, delayed recall of the figure was not tested. The autistic subjects were also impaired on Word Fluency, which is a test sensitive to left frontal lobe injury, and two subtests from the Stanford–Binet Intelligence Test that require the subject to identify the illogical aspect of a story or picture. Rumsey and Hamburger interpreted these results as supporting the involvement of fronto-subcortical systems in autism.

Ozonoff *et al.* (1991a) administered two tests of frontal lobe function to a group of autistic individuals (including some with milder symptoms who were diagnosed as cases of Asperger's syndrome). All subjects had a Full Scale IQ of at least 70. These subjects were compared with a clinical control group, consisting of individuals with diagnoses of dyslexia, hyperactivity or mild mental retardation. Two tests of executive function were included in the assessment battery: the WCST and the Tower of Hanoi, a measure of planning capacities that is sensitive to frontal lobe lesions and requires the ability to inhibit prepotent but irrelevant responses. The autistic group was less efficient than the control group on the Tower of Hanoi task, and made more perseverative errors on the WCST. There were no significant group differences on the WCST number of categories and number of errors, consistent with the idea that the problem is in shifting cognitive set rather than in understanding task demands. Altogether, 96% of the autistic group scored below the control mean on the executive function tasks, and those with Asperger's syndrome were just as impaired as those meeting DSM-III-R diagnostic criteria for autistic disorder (American Psychiatric Association, 1987). These deficits were all the more striking because they occurred in individuals of normal intelligence who were compared with controls matched on age, VIQ, sex, race and SES.

CAN EXECUTIVE FUNCTION DEFICITS EXPLAIN FAILURE ON
THEORY OF MIND TASKS?

Ozonoff *et al.* (1991a) noted that whereas recent neuropsychological studies had emphasised executive function deficits in autism, research by developmental psychologists had focused on other types of impairment. The most influential of these theories has developed from an original study by Baron-Cohen, Leslie and Frith (1985) which set out to test whether autistic children had a "theory of mind", i.e. whether they could appreciate the contents of other people's minds and realise these might differ from their own thoughts and beliefs. In this seminal study, children observed the following scenario. Sally and Anne are together and Sally hides her marble in a basket and leaves the room. Anne moves the marble to a box. Sally returns and the child is asked "Where will Sally look for her marble?" Austistic children tend to respond "in the box", where the marble actually is, rather than "in the basket" where Sally believes the marble to be. This early experiment was followed by an explosion of research on theory of mind in autism, as well as formulation of theoretical accounts of how a selective deficit in understanding the contents of other people's minds might explain the social, behavioural and linguistic deficits that are the core diagnostic features of this disorder (Frith, 1989).

In their study, Ozonoff *et al.* (1991a) explicitly compared performance on tasks of executive function with other measures, including theory of mind tasks. As well as the tasks based on the original study by Baron-Cohen *et al.* ("first order" tasks), they included more difficult "second order" tasks, in which the child had to demonstrate understanding of what one person thought another person believed (Baron-Cohen, 1989a). As noted above, virtually all the autistic subjects scored below the control group mean on the executive function tasks. In contrast, 52% scored below the mean on first order theory of mind tasks and 87% on second order theory of mind tasks. The executive function tasks most clearly separated the two groups, with nearly two standard deviations between the lowest scoring autistic subject and the lowest scoring control. The Tower of Hanoi proved to be the most effective single task at discriminating between groups and was able to correctly classify 80% of subjects in each group. Impairment on this measure was found in both autistic subjects and those with Asperger's syndrome (Ozonoff, Rogers & Pennington, 1991b).

The question arises as to how best to explain these findings of multiple defects on different kinds of tasks. Goodman (1989) has suggested that it may be misguided to look for one primary impairment that can account for all symptoms of autism, and that it is more likely that there are co-existing abnormalities in several neural systems. The classic way to investigate this issue is to consider how far the different symptoms can be dissociated. If the theory of mind impairments and executive function impairments reflected dysfunction of neighbouring brain areas, we might expect to see double dissociations, with some children impaired on one task and not the other. Ozonoff *et al.*, found that whereas the executive function measures were unrelated to theory of mind measures in the control group, there were significant correlations between these measures in the autistic group. Where dissociations were found, they tended to be just in one direction: those with Asperger's syndrome were impaired only on executive function tasks but not on theory of mind tasks (Ozonoff *et al.*, 1991b). This is compatible with an interpretation that treats both deficits as manifestations of the same underlying disorder, which in severe form affects both theory of mind and executive functions, but in milder form affects executive functions only.

On the surface, the theory of mind tasks used by Baron-Cohen and colleagues would seem to have little in common with either the Wisconsin card-sorting task or the Tower of Hanoi. Theory of mind research has emphasised deficits in social cognition. Frontal lobe tasks have been seen as measuring perseveration and a lack of planning ability. The findings of Ozonoff *et al.*, however, raise the intriguing question of whether the co-occurrence of deficits in these different tasks is indicative of any functional relationship in their task requirements.

Ozonoff *et al.* (1991a) proposed that both tests involve the use of stored information to govern behaviour. Impairment in using different types of stored information could affect performance on a wide range of superficially different tasks. To perform well on a theory of mind task, subjects must access internal representations of the mental states of others; to perform executive function tasks, they must generate representations of hypothetical configurations to guide their planning and problem solving. The problem with this explanation is that it is so general that it would be easy to explain almost any deficit on any task in terms of the theory, because most behaviours are governed to some extent by stored information. The particular pattern of strengths and weaknesses seen in autistic children seems to require a more specific explanation.

Consider, for example, the findings from a study by Sodian and Frith (1992), who devised a game where children were encouraged to prevent a bad wolf from obtaining a sweet hidden in a box and to assist a friendly seal to acquire it. If the box were unlocked, the wolf would open it and remove the sweet and eat it. If it was locked, however, he would not bother to try. If the seal was able to open the box to get the sweet, he would reward the child with a sweet, but like the wolf, he would not try to open the box if it were locked. In one condition, the child was given the opportunity to open the box or lock it as a puppet approached. Autistic children were as likely as control children to lock the box if the wolf was advancing, indicating that they knew they should prevent him gaining access to the box. However, if the wolf simply asked the child whether the box was open or locked, autistic children were unable to deceive him and say that the box was locked when it wasn't. Mental-age matched controls, in contrast, quickly learned to tell the wolf that the box was locked even when it was not. This pattern of results cannot be explained by simply arguing autistic children are poor at using stored knowledge to guide behaviour. Both the deception and the sabotage tasks involved predicting a puppet's behaviour, yet it was only in the deception condition, where the child had to tell a lie, that performance was impaired.

An alternative possible point of similarity between frontal lobe patients and autistic children could be that in both cases behaviour is largely driven by external environmental stimulation. Shallice and Burgess (in press) argue that people have available a large but finite set of action and thought schemas that, like computer programs, can be activated if well-learned triggers (either from the environment or from the output of other schemas) are excited. The problem for the organism is how to select the appropriate schema when several are activated at once. According to Shallice and Burgess this process of contention scheduling is controlled by a supervisory system, whose operation depends on the integrity of the frontal lobes. When the supervisory system malfunctions, external stimulation will elicit responses associated with the stimulus, but there will be little evidence of planned behaviour. Impairments of cognitive function will be particularly apparent in situations where the individual is presented with environmental stimuli but required to withold the habitual response to these and to perform some other operation instead. For instance, Baddeley (1986) described a man with an acquired frontal lobe lesion who was given a piece of string, a ruler and scissors and instructed to measure out a piece of string in order to cut it later. He immediately started to cut, and when told not to replied: "Yes, I know I'm not to cut it," while continuing to do so.

Viewed in this light, it is of interest to note that in the theory of mind tasks described so far, the child is required to make a statement that is directly contradictory to the visible evidence. Thus, in the Sally–Anne experiment, children must say that Sally will look for her marble in the basket when in reality they have seen it in the box. In the "deception" condition used by Sodian and Frith, the child had to say that an unlocked box was locked. Russell, Mauthner, Sharpe and Tidswell (1991) suggested that problems in inhibiting a response to a salient object might be the explanation for results on tasks involving false beliefs. They used a strategic game in which the child and adult competed for sweets. Each could open a box and could keep any sweet that was found inside. In one condition, the child but not the adult could see inside the boxes, and the child had to tell the adult where to look. The sensible strategy for the child would be to give false information, so that the adult did not get the reward. Russell *et al.* noted that autistic children were very poor at this task and they did not improve over a series of trials. Hughes and Russell (in press) went on to show that autistic children did poorly on a similar task where they had to point to an empty box to win a sweet, even when there was no opponent and therefore no deception involved. This raises the question as to whether the child actually does have a theory of mind and appreciates false beliefs, but is unable to act on this knowledge because of an inability to inhibit a more prepotent response. This "lack of inhibition" interpretation of theory of mind experiments would be at odds with the conventional account that attributes children's responses to their beliefs rather than to response disinhibition.

However, not all "theory of mind" tasks are easy to account for in these terms. Leslie and Frith (1988) used a "limited knowledge" condition, in which an adult stooge sees a counter hidden in one location and then leaves the room. The child then hides another counter in a new location. The stooge returns and the child must say where she will look for the counter. Note that the correct response does not require the child to describe a nonexistent state of affairs: there *is* a counter hidden in that location. Leslie and Frith showed that autistic children were not appreciably helped by this manipulation, and tended to state that the stooge would look where the child's counter was hidden. This does not completely rule out the possibility that autistic children's responses may be strongly dominated by the immediate environment, because their own placement of a counter could be regarded as a more salient stimulus than their earlier observation of the adult watching a counter being hidden in another place. However, one would expect the "limited knowledge" task to give less striking findings than the "false belief" task. There were no significant differences between the two tasks in Leslie and Frith's study, although the sample was small and the nonsignificant trend was for more children to pass "limited knowledge" than "false belief". Other studies by Baron-Cohen (1989b) have shown difficulties in a range of theory of mind tasks where response disinhibition does not seem a plausible explanation for failure, e.g., autistic children could describe the function of the heart, but were much poorer than mental-age matched controls in describing the function of the brain in mentalistic terms. Baron-Cohen (1991) went on to contrast autistic children's understanding of mental state terms using closely similar methodology in all conditions. In a control task, the child was shown a green brick in a box, the lid was replaced and the child was asked what it was. A yellow brick was then substituted and the child again described the contents of the box. No child had any difficulty in answering the test question "When I first showed you the box, before we opened it, what was inside then?" However, in a closely parallel task that tested understanding of beliefs, the performance of children with autism was very much worse. The child was shown a milk carton and asked: "What do you think is inside this?" All children replied "milk". The box was then opened to reveal that it contained a ball, and all children now agreed that they thought the box contained a ball. The carton was then closed and the subject asked the test question: "When I first asked you, before we opened the carton, what did you think was inside?"

Most normal 4-year-olds, and mentally handicapped young people with a mental age over 4 years, correctly responded "milk". However, the majority of autistic young people of similar mental age failed the task, responding "a ball". This study (which included other conditions testing understanding of pretense and desire) was noteworthy in demonstrating that autistic individuals can give a response that does not describe the current state of affairs (in the control condition) and they do not automatically give the most salient response to the stimulus (in the milk-carton test).

CAN DEFICIENT REPRESENTATIONAL ABILITIES EXPLAIN EXECUTIVE FUNCTION DEFICITS?

Rather than trying to explain away results on theory of mind by proposing an alternative interpretation based on "frontal lobe" hypothesis, it may be more fruitful to turn the question on its head to see how far the executive function impairments might be explicable in terms of the theory that is used to explain the problems with social cognition. In particular, it is of interest to ask whether both theory of mind deficits and executive function impairments could be regarded as manifestations of a common problem: failure to form second order representations.

Leslie (1987) has developed a theoretical account of the development of "theory of mind" in terms of a theory of mental representations. He distinguishes between first order representations, which are based directly on perceptual experience of objects and the customary responses that are made to them, and second order representations, which are "representations of representations". First order representations are used to represent propositions that correspond to things or events in the real world, e.g. "Mary has a ball". Such propositions can be validated or disproved by comparing their content with one's experience, i.e. they are either true or false. Second order representations take a first order representation as an element of a proposition, e.g. "John thinks Mary has a ball". One cannot assess the truth or falsehood of this proposition by considering whether Mary does or does not have a ball. in this case, the proposition "Mary has a ball" has been decoupled from external reality, and is used as a part of another proposition. Leslie used this analysis not just to explain performance on theory of mind tasks but also as an account of development in another area where autistic children are impaired, namely pretend play, which also has the characteristic that one has to decouple a primary representation from reality (e.g. when pretending that a banana is a telephone).

Could a theory of deficient representational abilities be extended to explain frontal lobe functions? Frith and Frith (1991) proposed just such an account, suggesting that "the processing of second-order representations is the job of the frontal cortex and its connections with various posterior structures." Perner (1991) has noted that second order representations must be implicated in thinking about future or hypothetical events. Ability to think about a hypothetical state would seem to be implicated in the process of setting up a list of goals to guide behaviour. In the Tower of Hanoi, for instance, one must imagine future states that do not correspond with the current, observable state of the world. If this analysis of executive function deficits is correct, then frontal lobe patients and people with autism should be able to engage in self-initiated, goal-directed behaviours, provided these do not involve contemplating possible future scenarios. Some of the compulsive and obsessional behaviours seen in autism (e.g. collecting bottle-tops or memorizing bus timetables) would seem to fit this conceptualization.

One can take this line of argument further to explain why autistic children are so poor at the Verbal Comprehension subtest on Wechsler's scales (Bartak, Rutter & Cox, 1975). The items on this subtest involve reasoning rather than demonstrating learned knowledge, and many questions involve hypothetical situations (e.g. "What should you do if you lose a ball that belongs to one of your friends?"). A theory in terms of difficulty in forming second order representations could thus provide an overall account of a wide range of impairments in autism, including nonsocial as well as social deficits. Indeed, it might also be extended to explain the pattern of memory impairment observed by Bachevalier in monkeys with amygdala-hippocampal lesions. Discrimination learning (which the animals could do) involves generating a representation of a previous experience, e.g. [reward = blue square]. Delayed nonmatch to sample (which they could not do) involves forming a representation that incorporates the element [reward = blue square] in a more complex representation (reward now = not [reward past = blue square]).

Attractive although this theory is, recent research has confounded any simple attempt to encompass social and nonsocial cognitive deficits under a single conceptual umbrella. It has been shown autistic children *can* perform a task that is virtually identical to the classic "theory of mind" task in all respects except that it does not have the component of requiring the child to understand another's belief. Leekam and Perner (1991) used a task where the child had to predict what will be shown in a photograph that was taken in one condition (e.g. girl wearing a blue dress) after the situation has been altered (e.g. girl wearing a yellow dress). As with the theory of mind task, the child must give a response (blue dress) that does not correspond to present reality (yellow dress), and that involves deduction without having actually had the specific experience of seeing the photograph. The surprising result was that autistic children *were* able to do this task, which involves working out what a camera has physically represented, but were *not* able to do virtually the same task when they must work out what a person has mentally represented. These findings, which have been replicated and extended (Charman & Baron-Cohen, in press; Leslie & Thaiss, in press) have posed severe problems for any attempt to account for social and nonsocial cognitive impairments in terms of a general impairment of second order representations.*

There is yet another fly in the ointment for those who might wish to propose a common underlying basis for theory of mind and executive function deficits. Welsh, Pennington, Ozonoff, Rouse and McCabe (1990) examined executive function skills in 4-year-old children with early treated phenylketonuria (PKU). Although autism is diagnosed in around 20% of children with untreated PKU (Reiss, Feinstein & Rosenbaum, 1986), it is seldom seen in those who are maintained on a phenylalinine-restricted diet. Welsh *et al.* did not mention whether any of the children in their study were autistic, but this seems unlikely. All were of normal intelligence. Nevertheless, they were significantly impaired on executive function tasks (including the Tower of Hanoi, visual search efficiency, verbal fluency efficiency and motor planning) compared with controls matched on age, IQ and social-economic status. This study suggests, then, that executive function deficits are not sufficient to cause autistic symptoms. The possibility remains, of course, that the executive function deficits in these children might have been milder than those seen in autistic children or that the PKU group might have had some subtle impairments of social cognition. Direct comparison of the two studies is impossible, given the different age ranges of subjects and different tests that were used. It would be of interest to conduct a study that directly compares autistic children with non-autistic children suffering from PKU, to see if similar degrees of executive function impairment could be demonstrated in the two groups.

Attempts to find a common explanation for impairments of social and nonsocial cognition can stimulate new ways of approaching the symptoms of autism, as well as serving the interests of parsimony. However, cases of selective impairment in one area but not another lend support to those who regard these symptoms as indicating underlying dysfunction of adjacent neural systems (cf. Goodman, 1989), rather than as different manifestations of a single primary impairment.

CONCLUSIONS

We are still a very long way from understanding the neurobiological basis of autism, but the work reviewed here suggests that the early proposal of Damasio and Maurer, implicating the mesolimbic system and associated frontal lobe structures, remains a strong contender. Recent studies using neuropsychological tests with autistic individuals draw attention to the similarities between some autistic symptoms and executive function deficits seen in frontal lobe patients. It would,

*It is not possible here to do justice to the theoretical debate that these findings have sparked off. See Perner (1991) and Leslie and Thaiss (in press) for differing approaches to the theory of mental representations.

however, be a gross oversimplification to suppose that frontal lobe lesions will necessarily make children autistic. For a start, the frontal lobe is not a uniform structure (Fuster, 1980): the prediction is that only those areas that are intimately linked with the limbic system would be involved. Furthermore, the lack of conclusive evidence of brain damage from neuroimaging studies suggests that the underlying problem may not be destruction of neural tissue but rather some other process such as depletion of neurotransmitters or developmental cortical malformations. It cannot be emphasized enough that these ideas remain highly speculative. However, as a working hypothesis, the notion of frontal lobe and limbic system dysfunction in autism seems promising, not just in guiding the search for neurobiological correlates of the disorder, but also in suggesting new ways to think about the puzzling range of psychological impairments seen in this condition.

REFERENCES

Ackerly, S. S. & Benton, A. L. (1948). Report of a case of bilateral frontal lobe defect. *Research Publications of the Association for Research in Nervous and Mental Diseases, 27,* 479–504.

Aggelton, J. P. & Passingham, R. E. (1981). Syndrome produced by lesions of the amygdala in monkeys *(Macaca mulatta). Journal of Comparative and Physiological Psychology,* **95,** 961–977.

American Psychiatric Association (1987). *Diagnostic and Statistical Manual* (3rd edn. revised DSM-III-R). Washington, DC: APA.

Bachevalier, J. (1991). An animal model for childhood autism: memory loss and socioemotional disturbances following neonatal damage to the limbic system in monkeys. In C. A. Tamminga & S. C. Schulz (Eds) *Advances in Neuropsychiatry and Psychopharmacology* (Vol. 1, pp. 129–140). New York: Raven Press.

Baddeley, A. (1986). *Working Memory.* Oxford: Clarendon Press.

Baron-Cohen, S. (1989a). The autistic child's theory of mind: a case of specific developmental delay. *Journal of Child Psychology and Psychiatry,* **30,** 285–298.

Baron-Cohen, S. (1989b). Are autistic children "behaviourists"? An examination of their mental–physical and appearance–reality distinctions. *Journal of Autism and Developmental Disorders,* **19,** 579–600.

Baron-Cohen, S. (1991). The development of a theory of mind in autism: deviance or delay? *Psychiatric Clinics of North America,* **14,** 33–51.

Baron-Cohen, S., Leslie, A. M. & Frith, U. (1985). Does the autistic child have a "theory of mind"? *Cognition,* **21,** 37–46.

Bartak, L., Rutter, M. & Cox, A. (1975). A comparative study of infantile autism and specific development receptive language disorder. I. The children. *British Journal of Psychiatry,* **126,** 127–145.

Boucher, J. & Warrington, E. K. (1976). Memory deficits in early infantile autism: some similarities to the amnesic syndrome. *British Journal of Psychology, 67,* 73–87.

Charman, T. & Baron-Cohen, S. (1992). Understanding drawings and beliefs: a further test of the metarepresentation theory of autism. *Journal of Child Psychology and Psychiatry, 33,* 1105–1112.

Coleman, M. & Gillberg, C. (1985). *The Biology of the Autistic Syndromes.* New York: Praeger.

Damasio, A. R. & Maurer, R. G. (1978). A neurological model for childhood autism. *Archives of Neurology, 35,* 777–786.

Duncan, J. (1986). Disorganisation of behaviour after frontal lobe damage. *Cognitive Neuropsychology, 33,* 271–290.

Frith, C. D. & Frith, U. (1991). Elective affinities in schizophrenia and childhood autism. In P. Bebbington (Ed.) *Social Psychiatry: Theory, Methodology and Practice* (pp. 66–88). New Brunswick, NJ: Transactions.

Frith, U. (1972). Cognitive mechanisms in autism: experiments with colour and tone sequence production. *Journal of Autism and Childhood Schizophrenia, 2,* 160–173.

Frith, U. (1989). *Autism: Explaining the Enigma.* Oxford: Blackwell.

Fuster, J. M. (1980). *The Prefrontal Cortex: Anatomy, Physiology and Neuropsychology of the Frontal Lobe.* New York: Raven.

Goodman, R. (1989). Infantile autism: a syndrome of multiple primary deficits? *Journal of Autism and Developmental Disorders, 19,* 409–424.

Grant, D. & Berg, E. (1948). A behavioural analysis of degree of reinforcement and ease of shifting to new responses on a Weigl-type card-sorting problem. *Journal of Experimental Psychology, 38,* 404–411.

Hughes, C. & Russell, J. (in press). Autistic children's difficulty with mental disengagement from an object: its implications for theories of autism. *Developmental Psychology.*

Joseph, R. (1990). *Neuropsychology, Neuropsychiatry, and Behavioral Neurology.* New York: Plenum Press.

Kolb, B. & Whishaw, I. Q. (1990). Fundamentals of Human Neuropsychology (3rd edn). New York: W. H. Freeman.

Leckam, S. R. & Perner, J. (1991). Does the autistic child have a metarepresentational deficit? *Cognition, 40,* 203–218.

Leslie, A. M. (1987). Pretense and representation: The origins of "theory of mind". *Psychological Review, 94,* 412–426.

Leslie, A. M. & Frith, U. (1988). Autistic children's understanding of seeing, knowing and believing. *British Journal of Developmental Psychology, 6,* 315–324.

Leslie, A. M. & Thaiss, L. (1992). Domain specificity in conceptual development: Neuropsychological evidence from autism. *Cognition, 43,* 225–251.

Milner, B. (1963). Effects of different brain lesions on card sorting. *Archives of Neurology, 9,* 90–100.

Milner, B. (1965). Visually-guided maze learning in man: Effects of bilateral hippocampal, bilateral frontal, and unilateral cerebral lesions. *Neuropsychologia, 3,* 317–338.

Mishkin, M. & Appenzeller, T. (1987). The anatomy of memory. *Scientific American,* **256** **(June),** 62–71.

Nelson, H. E. (1976). A modified card sorting test sensitive to frontal lobe deficits. *Cortex,* **12,** 313–325.

Ornitz, E. M. (1983). The functional neuroanatomy of infantile autism. *International Journal of Neuroscience,* **19,** 85–124.

Ozonoff, S., Pennington, B. F. & Rogers, S. J. (1991a). Executive function deficits in high-functioning autistic children: relationship to theory of mind. *Journal of Child Psychology and Psychiatry,* **32,** 1081–1105.

Ozonoff, S., Rogers, S. J. & Pennington, B. F. (1991b). Asperger's syndrome: evidence of an empirical distinction from high-functioning autism. *Journal of Child Psychology and Psychiatry,* **32,** 1107–1122.

Perner, J. (1991). *Understanding the representational mind.* Cambridge, MA: MIT Press.

Prior, M. R. & Hoffmann, W. (1990). Brief report: Neuropsychological testing of autistic children through an exploration with frontal lobe tests. *Journal of Autism and Developmental Disorders,* **20,** 581–590.

Reichler, R. J. & Lee, E. M. C. (1987). Overview of biomedical issues in autism. In Schopler, E. & Mesibov, G. B. (Eds) *Neurobiological Issues in Autism* (pp. 13–41). New York: Plenum Press.

Reiss, A. L., Feinstein, C. & Rosenbaum, K. N. (1986). Autism and genetic disorders. *Schizophrenia Bulletin,* **12,** 724–738.

Rey, A. (1959). *Le Test de Copie de Figure Encomplexe.* Paris: Editions Centre de Psychologie Appliquée.

Rumsey, J. & Hamburger, S. (1988). Neuropsychological findings in high-functioning men with infantile autism, residual state. *Journal of Clinical and Experimental Neuropsychology,* **10,** 201–221.

Rumsey, J. M. & Hamburger, S. (1990). Neuropsychological divergence of high-level autism and severe dyslexia. *Journal of Autism and Developmental Disorders,* **20,** 155–168.

Russell, J., Mauthner, N., Sharpe, S. & Ridswell, T. (1991). The "windows task" as a measure of strategic deception in preschoolers and autistic subjects. *British Journal of Developmental Psychology,* **9,** 331–349.

Shallice, T. & Burgess, P. (in press). Higher-order cognitive impairments and frontal lobe lesions in man. In H. S. Levin, H. M. Eisenberg & A. L. Benton (Eds) *Frontal Lobe Function and Injury* (pp. 125–138). New York: Oxford University Press.

Sodian, B. & Frith, U. (1992). Deception and sabotage in autistic, retarded and normal children. *Journal of Child Psychology and Psychiatry,* **33,** 591–605.

Steffenburg, S. (1991). Neuropsychiatric assessment of children with autism: a population-based study. *Developmental Medicine and Child Neurology,* **33,** 495–511.

Welsh, M. C., Pennington, B. F., Ozonoff, S., Rouse, B. & McCabe, E. R. B. (1990). Neuropsychology of early-treated phenylketonuria: specific executive function deficits. *Child Development,* **61,** 1697–1713.

12

Conceptualizing "Borderline Syndrome of Childhood" and "Childhood Schizophrenia" as a Developmental Disorder

Kenneth E. Towbin, Elisabeth M. Dykens,
Geraldine S. Pearson, and Donald J. Cohen
Yale University School of Medicine, New Haven, Connecticut

Objective: *This is the first attempt to define and validate criteria for an early onset, chronic syndrome of disturbances in affect modulation, social relatedness, and thinking. This study formulates and tests five hypotheses that follow from conceptualizing this syndrome as a developmental disorder. The advantages of viewing this syndrome as a developmental disorder are discussed and compared with alternative formulations such as childhood schizophrenia or borderline syndrome of childhood.* **Method:** *An inpatient cohort (26 boys, 4 girls) was ascertained using specific, defined criteria. Using standardized measures on retrospective chart reviews, these subjects were compared with two different inpatient samples: one diagnosed with dysthymic disorder, the other with conduct disorder.* **Results:** *The criteria readily distinguished between developmentally disordered children and comparison groups. Findings also supported the hypotheses in the predicted directions; index subjects had earlier onset of symptoms, poorer social and overall adjustment, longer hospitalizations, and poorer outcomes.* **Conclusions:** *Findings support the validity of this developmental concept for a multiple complex developmental dis-*

Reprinted with permission from the *Journal of the American Academy of Child and Adolescent Psychiatry*, 1993, Vol. 32(4), 775–782. Copyright © 1993 by the American Academy of Child and Adolescent Psychiatry.

The authors acknowledge the support and encouragement of Drs. Marion Glick and Robert Hodapp in the preparation of this study and manuscript.

order and give preliminary, "first-cut" validity to these specified criteria.

Throughout the past five decades, child psychiatrists have repeatedly described a population of children with a distinctive syndrome characterized by deficits in affect modulation, high levels of anxiety, odd or disturbed relationships, poor social skills, and frequent periods of mild to severe thought disorder. The multiple impairments of this syndrome have their onset from an early age, are enduring, and though persistent, show variable or inconsistent expression. Diagnostically such children pose a dilemma because they possess symptoms that cut across a variety of disorders although they do not typify any specific one. Moreover, this is not a rare phenomenon; children with these symptoms are commonly admitted to residential and hospital services, and they may be among the most chronically impaired patients in outpatient clinics.

Although a large assortment of diagnoses have been awarded to these children (Asarnow and Ben-Meir, 1987; Cohen et al., 1986; Vela et al., 1983; Wenning, 1990), no single *DSM-III-R* diagnosis provides an adequate description. Consequently, some clinicians choose to assign them multiple *DSM-III-R* diagnoses, drawing from combinations of schizotypal personality disorder, attention-deficit hyperactivity disorder (ADHD), overanxious disorder, avoidant disorder, psychotic depression, bipolar disorder, and psychotic disorder-not otherwise specified (NOS).

Alternatively, the diagnostic dilemmas imposed by these problems in affect containment, relatedness, and thinking lead other clinicians to resort to private nosologic labels that are not a part of any *DSM-III*, International Classification of Diseases (ICD), or Research Diagnostic Criteria (RDC) system (Rutter and Gould, 1985; Stengel, 1959). Among those who pursue this route, "childhood schizophrenia" and the "borderline syndrome of childhood" are the most commonly used designations (Petti and Vela, 1990). More recent descriptors of these children include "childhood schizotypal disorder" and "schizoid personality" (Russell, 1991; Wolff and Chick, 1980).

Although these two alternatives, the lengthy lists of diagnoses and private labels, are understandable solutions to a diagnostic enigma, they each fall short of capturing the developmental complexities and severity of disturbance of children affected with this syndrome. On the one hand, the use of multiple diagnoses results in a fragmented, disjointed, potpourri that does not convey what is known of the history, course, prognosis, and symptomatology. On the other hand, the use of private labels of "childhood schizophrenia" and "borderline syndrome of children" is constrained by the absence of agreement on definitions of these terms (Vela and Petti, 1990; Volkmar, 1991). These private labels also allude to continuity with and phenomenological similarity to adult disorders resulting in prognostic and nosologic relationships that may be inaccurate.

CHILDHOOD SCHIZOPHRENIA

The diagnostic ambiguity of the term "childhood schizophrenia" is readily evident in the two different ways this term has been envisioned: the "broad" versus "narrow" conceptualizations. The initial vagueness of criteria offered by Bender (1947) stemmed from her view that children with childhood schizophrenia manifested deficits in the patterning and integration of behavior "at every level" of functioning. "The pathology cannot therefore be thought of as focal in the architecture of the central nervous system, but rather as striking at the substratum of integrative functioning or biologically patterned behavior" (Bender, 1947, p. 40). This broad view, echoed in part by later workers (Cantor et al., 1981; Despert, 1986), was criticized as too vague, and subsequently was countered with the view that the criteria for schizophrenia in children should mirror the more narrow criteria used to diagnose (adult) schizophrenia (Kolvin, 1971; Kolvin et al., 1971; Rutter, 1972). Although this later view has prevailed among most clinicians, considerable confusion remains regarding these two perspectives (Cantor et al., 1982).

The term "childhood schizophrenia" is also misconstrued from the standpoint of the discontinuity between childhood and adult schizophrenia. A variety of studies have established that children presenting with symptoms resembling Bender's "childhood schizophrenia" manifest adult outcomes that are more diverse than schizophrenia using *DSM-III* or other specific criteria (Wolff and Chick, 1980; Zeitlin, 1986). Although these children may be at increased risk for schizophrenia, it is only one of many possible psychiatric outcomes (Eggers, 1978; Zeitlin, 1986). Consequently, both diagnostic ambiguity and the discontinuity with adult schizophrenia suggest that the term "childhood schizophrenia" is an inadequate solution to the diagnostic dilemma imposed by these children.

BORDERLINE SYNDROME OF CHILDHOOD

In a similar vein, the "borderline syndrome of childhood" suffers from a lack of diagnostic specificity and a discontinuity with the adult disorder bearing the same name. Early theorists (Ekstein and Wallerstein, 1954; Freud, 1956; Pine, 1974) depicted "borderline syndrome" cases that seemed to combine features of avoidant and atypical pervasive developmental disorders. Although more recent descriptions of "borderline children" have emphasized severe deficits in object relations (Pine, 1974), others have primarily viewed these children as having disturbances in thinking (Petti and Vela, 1990).

The emphasis on object relations in "borderline syndrome of childhood" mirrors the view of adults with borderline personality disorder, and for several reasons this emphasis creates problems when applied to children. First, deficits in object relations are manifest in a variety of disorders (e.g., autism, chronic post-traumatic stress disorder, and reactive attachment disorder). For this reason it seems that the degree of disturbed object relations should be routinely evaluated in children across various disorders, and extremes of disturbance should not be relegated to a single diagnostic entity.

Second, implying that these children are similar to personality disordered adults is inconsistent with the developmental tenet of personality as existing in a dynamic, unstable state in children. It ordinarily is a term for the functions that give order and congruence in adult functioning (Rutter, 1985). Applying it to disordered children becomes highly confusing. It also understates the pervasive impact of the early onset of these impairments on subsequent development. More than personality is effected; personality impairment does not adequately encompass the severity of disorder in thinking, affect, and relatedness.

Finally, research generally has not supported a continuity between "borderline syndrome of childhood" and adult borderline personality disorder. Some children with this syndrome may emerge as adults with borderline personality disorder, but this association appears "unlikely" (Lofgren et al., 1991). Rather, these children are apt to exhibit a variety of adult psychiatric outcomes that include schizophrenia, affective disorders, and other personality disorders (Greenman et al., 1986; Kestenbaum, 1983; Lofgren et al., 1991; Wenning, 1990; Wolff and Chick, 1980). The term "borderline syndrome of childhood" is thus discontinuous with the adult "borderline" disorder, and suffers also from a lack of commonly used, widely accepted diagnostic criteria. As such, this term generally tends to confuse, rather than clarify, the diagnostic picture of these young children.

MULTIPLE COMPLEX DEVELOPMENTAL DISORDER

Given the limitations of multiple diagnoses and of the terms "childhood schizophrenia" and "borderline syndrome of childhood," many researchers and clinicians have instead placed diagnostic emphases on the early onset and social deficits of these children. These emphases typically result in diagnostic formulations within the constellation of pervasive developmental disorders (PDD) of the nonautistic variety, or pervasive developmental disorder-not otherwise specified (PDD-NOS) in the current *DSM-III-R* nosology. However, as a diagnosis PDD-NOS suffers by this very fact; it is a disorder that lacks specificity. Despite evidence that this "unspecified" PDD group may be more prevalent than its autistic counterpart (Burd et al., 1987; Wing and Gould, 1979), there are no positive criteria for this syndrome. Consequently, the term PDD-NOS lacks an organizational framework and potentially may include a wide spectrum of diverse symptoms and clinical presentations.

In an effort to remedy the lack of specificity for some children in this group of PDD-NOS and to better differentiate PDD, Cohen and coworkers (1986) introduced diagnostic criteria for an early onset developmental disorder characterized by anxiety and deficits in affective states, social relationships, and cognitive processing. These features are inconsistently and variably expressed and were identified in a review of approximately 400 cases of children younger than 6 years with "deviant human relationships and disorganized, bizarre thinking" (Dahl et al., 1986). The term multiple complex developmental disorder (MCDD) was offered by Cohen and coworkers (1986) as means of capturing these young children who seemed to fall between the diagnoses of PDD and the specific developmental disorders. The term MCDD appropriately encompassed the impact of early onset deficits for subsequent development. MCDD also reflected findings that these children showed deficits that were not confined to just a single domain but were instead multiple and complex, with implications for both the fundamental and subtle aspects of experience.

As conceptualized by Cohen et al. (1986), MCDD begins before age 5 years, and is characterized by functional deficits leading to a consistent, enduring pattern of fluctuations in affect regulation, relatedness, and thought. These fluctuations are a great deal wider than those observed in normally developing children and also contrast dramatically to the stability in functioning observed in PDD-autistic individuals. In children with MCDD, regression to highly immature levels of functioning occurs far more readily and frequently than would be expected for the child's mental age. Regressed, immature behavior may last from hours to weeks and is then intermixed with periods of higher functioning that may resemble same age peers. These fluctuations typically endure even when environmental stressors are reduced, and variability in functioning may be more or less dramatic over time and across individual children.

As noted in Table 1, which summarizes the diagnostic criteria for MCDD, these children exhibit affective dysregulation shown by persistent and high levels of anxiety, peculiar anxiety responses, odd phobias or fears, and/or rage reactions that are exaggerated and overwhelming for them. Periods of elevated mood may intrude fleetingly but do not persist beyond hours or days.

The social impairments in MCDD children extend beyond problems in social skills and include fundamental deficits in reciprocity that are qualitatively and quantitatively different from those seen in autistic individuals. Relatedness in MCDD children may be inconsistent, unpredictable, odd, immature, constricted, and lacking understandability. MCDD children may exhibit reciprocal but constrictive and repetitive play, or they may engage in elaborate symbolic and imaginative play that completely ignores the presence of others.

TABLE 1
Diagnostic Criteria Employed for Multiple Complex
Development Disorder

---

1. Regulation of affective state and anxiety is impaired beyond that seen in children of comparable mental age manifested by two of the following:
   (a) intense generalized anxiety, diffuse tension, or irritability;
   (b) unusual fears and phobias that are peculiar in content or in intensity;
   (c) recurrent panic episodes, terror, or flooding with anxiety;
   (d) episodes lasting from minutes to days of behavioral disorganization or regression with the emergence of markedly immature, primitive, and/or self-injurious behaviors;
   (e) significant and wide emotional variability with or without environmental precipitants;
   (f) high frequency of idiosyncratic anxiety reactions such as sustained periods of uncontrollable giggling, giddiness, laughter, or "silly" affect that is inappropriate in the context of the situation.

2. Consistent impairments in social behavior and sensitivity (compared with children of similar mental age) manifest by one of the following:
   (a) social disinterest, detachment, avoidance, or withdrawal in the face of evident competence (at times) of social engagement, particularly with adults. More often attachments may appear friendly and cooperative but very superficial, based primarily on receiving material needs;
   (b) inability to initiate or maintain peer relationships;
   (c) disturbed attachments displaying high degrees of ambivalence to adults, particularly to parents/caregivers, as manifested by clinging, overly controlling, needy behavior, and/or aggressive, oppositional behavior. Splitting affects with shifting love-hate behavior toward parents, teachers, or therapists are common;
   (d) profound limitations in the capacity of empathy or to read or understand others affects accurately.

3. Impaired cognitive processing (thinking disorder) manifested by one of the following:
   (a) thought problems that are well out of proportion with mental age, including irrationality, sudden intrusions on normal thought process, magical thinking, neologisms or nonsense words repeated over and over, desultory thinking, blatantly illogical bizarre ideas;
   (b) confusion between reality and fantasy life;
   (c) perplexity and easy confusability (trouble with understanding ongoing social processes and keeping one thoughts "straight");
   (d) delusions, including fantasies of personal omnipotence, paranoid preoccupations, overengagement with fantasy figures, grandiose fantasies of special powers, and referential ideation;

4. No diagnosis of autism;
5. Duration of symptoms longer than 6 months.

Thought disorder is evident in these children both clinically and on formal projective testing and can include mild slippages and distortions (e.g., inappropriate distance from stimuli, vagueness, clanging, incongruous combinations, tangentiality, perseveration) as well as more severe symptoms (e.g., contaminations, incoherence, neologisms, hallucinations, delusions). Under stress, these deficits may become more severe or frequent, but they also may change without identifiable precipitants. Thought disturbance may be congruent or incongruent with the child's mood, and when frank psychotic symptoms are present, they may be quite syntonic.

Previous work has thus introduced MCDD as a syndrome that is developmentally informed and that may be applicable to many children previously described as "childhood schizophrenic" or "borderline." Despite this rich history, however, research has yet to establish whether MCDD patients can be reliably differentiated from other groups of psychiatrically impaired youngsters. To provide a "first-cut" test of the clinical usefulness of MCDD, the present study compared MCDD children with two groups of psychiatrically impaired children who were hospitalized at the same state facility. It was hypothesized that MCDD patients could be separated from comparison groups on several features that are predicted by the developmental orientation of MCDD. Specifically, it was hypothesized that compared with the contrast groups, MCDD children would (1) have an earlier onset of difficulties, (2) show more severe impairments, (3) be more refractory to treatment, (4) show poorer capacities in peer relations, and (5) have higher rates of serious parental psychopathology.

METHOD

Subjects

Thirty children (26 boys and 4 girls) who reliably met criteria for MCDD were included in the study. These subjects were admitted to a state psychiatric hospital between 1987 and 1990 and ranged in age from 5 to 13 years, with a mean age of 9 years, 7 months (SD = 2.23). MCDD children had a mean IQ of 89 (SD = 15.20), and an IQ range of 50 to 118.

MCDD diagnoses were made using the criteria in Table 1. These criteria were slightly modified from Cohen et al. (1986) and made more specific to reflect clinical information gleaned from the children. All MCDD diagnoses were independently made by raters (K.T., E.D., and G.P.) who were familiar with the cases and completed a checklist of MCDD diagnostic criteria for each child. In this way, only children who met diagnostic criteria for MCDD from all three raters were included in the study. Because the object was to ascertain subjects who unequivocally met criteria for MCDD, each index subject was required to receive the

TABLE 2
Diagnosis before Admission for 30 Multiple Complex
Developmental Disorder Subjects

Diagnosis	N	(%)
ADHD/ADDH	11	(37)
Atypical PDD/PDD-NOS/childhood onset PDD	10	(33)
Conduct disorder	9	(30)
Dysthymia	8	(27)
Schizophrenia/schizophreniform disorder/ "childhood schizophrenia"	7	(23)
Psychotic disorder not otherwise specified	5	(17)
Borderline personality	4	(13)
Oppositional defiant disorder	4	(13)
Developmental language disorder	3	(10)
Specific developmental disorder	3	(10)
Schizotypal personality	2	(7)
No diagnosis	2	(7)

Note: Because multiple diagnoses were possible for patients, the sum of percentages exceeds 100%.

diagnosis by the consensus of all three raters. Frequency counts of diagnoses made before hospitalization on the 30 MCDD patients are reported in Table 2. Inasmuch as multiple diagnoses were possible for any one patient, the sum of percentages exceeds 100.

Two comparison groups were drawn from all patients admitted to the hospital during the same years as MCDD subjects. One group consisted of 30 patients (19 boys, 11 girls) with *DSM-III-R* diagnoses of dysthymia. These 30 subjects did not receive any other psychiatric diagnoses on either Axis I or Axis II. This comparison group ranged in age from 6 to 13 years, with a mean age of 11 years, 5 months (SD = 1.85). Dysthymic subjects had an IQ range of 55 to 126, with a mean IQ of 90 (SD = 14.51).

The second comparison group consisted of 30 patients (24 boys, 6 girls) with *DSM-III-R* diagnoses of conduct disorder. These conduct disordered subjects did not receive any other psychiatric diagnoses. Their mean age was 12 years, 1 month (SD = 1.17), with an age range of 9 to 13 years. Their mean IQ was 92 (SD = 15), with an IQ range of 68 to 123.

The MCDD, dysthymic and conduct disordered groups did not significantly differ in IQ, $F(2, 82) = 0.42$, NS, or in the ratio of boys to girls, $\chi^2 = 4.84$, NS. All subjects shared the low social and economic background that is typical of the state psychiatric facility. The three groups did not differ in racial composition, $\chi^2 = 2.87$, NS, with 60% of the 90 subjects being white, 23% black, 12% Hispanic, and 3% other.

Procedure and Measures

Subjects' medical records were reviewed for age, sex, race, age at first psychiatric contact, age at first psychiatric hospitalization, and length of the target hospitalization. Presence of psychiatric impairments in patients' parents was also noted as determined by diagnoses made directly by hospital clinicians, histories of psychiatric hospitalization, or long-term prescription of antipsychotic medication. Children's Global Assessment Scale (CGAS; Shaffer et al., 1983) ratings of the child's functioning on admission, in the year before hospitalization, and on hospital discharge were also noted from subject's records. Comparison group data were derived from a larger hospital study that included a review of 250 medical records.

In addition to variables directly gleaned from medical records, the Child Behavior Checklist (CBCL; Achenbach and Edelbrock, 1983) was retrospectively completed on each subject. Consistent with the retrospective use of the CBCL, the presence of symptoms was noted using guidelines supplied by Achenbach (1966). CBCL raw scores, based on the presence or absence of symptoms, were calculated for the major factors of internalizing, externalizing, and severity. An item assessing peer relationships from The Premorbid Adjustment Scale (PAS; Cannon-Spoor et al., 1982) was also retrospectively completed on each subject. The PAS is designed for retrospective use based on medical records, and the peer relationship item directly assesses the quality of peer relationships on a 6-point scale ranging from many close friendships to increasingly deviant friendship patterns. In accordance with guidelines supplied by Cicchetti (1984), interrater agreement on CBCL and PAS variables ranged from "good" to "excellent," with intraclass correlations ranging from 0.72 to 0.91.

RESULTS

To assess the first hypothesis, that MCDD patients would have an earlier onset of difficulties than would contrast groups, subjects' ages at first psychiatric contact and ages at first and current psychiatric hospitalizations were compared across groups. As summarized in Table 3, analyses of variance (ANOVAs) revealed that MCDD patients were significantly younger than comparison groups subjects at their first mental health contact and at their first and target psychiatric hospitalizations. Table 3 presents these three mean ages across groups, and F and p values.

To assess the second hypothesis, that MCDD subjects show more severe impairments than do comparison groups subjects, repeated measure ANOVAs compared CBCL scores across groups. As shown in Table 4, MCDD subjects had significantly higher internalizing, externalizing, and severity scores than did their

TABLE 3

Mean Ages in Years, and F and p Values for Early Onset Variables Across Groups

Onset Variables	MCDD[a]	(SD)	Dysthymic	(SD)	Conduct	(SD)	F	(df)
Age at first psychiatric contact	5.89	(2.94)	8.67	(3.36)	8.35	(3.56)	5.54	(2,71)*
Age at first psychiatric hospitalization	8.67	(2.56)	10.87	(2.13)	11.10	(2.32)	9.83	(2,87)*
Age at target psychiatric hospitalization	9.67	(2.23)	11.40	(1.85)	12.07	(1.17)	14.12	(2,87)*

[a]MCDD = Multiple Complex Developmental Disorder.
*$p < 0.001$.

TABLE 4

Mean Symptom Severity Ratings, and F and p Values Across MCDD and Comparison Groups

Domain	MCDD[a]	(SD)	Dysthymic	(SD)	Conduct	(SD)	F	(df)
Child Behavior Checklist								
Internalizing	6.00	(2.62)	2.03	(1.52)	1.33	(1.65)	44.32	(2,82)*
Externalizing	6.84	(3.24)	2.36	(2.21)	4.13	(2.37)	20.83	(2,82)*
Severity	9.38	(3.18)	1.83	(1.39)	1.90	(11.84)	102.84	(2,82)*
Children's Global Assessment Scale								
Year before hospitalization	37.63	(7.69)	46.80	(8.67)	45.72	(9.70)	9.88	(2,86)*
On hospitalization	32.40	(6.37)	38.90	(6.49)	40.14	(8.78)	9.67	(2,86)*

*$p < 0.001$.

TABLE 5

Mean S and F and p Values for Variables Assessing Response to Treatment in MCDD and Comparison Groups

Treatment Variables	MCDD	(SD)	Dysthymic	(SD)	Conduct	(SD)	F	(df)
Length of hospital stay in months	9.53	(6.63)	3.49	(2.51)	4.72	(6.46)	9.08	(2,82)**
CGAS ratings on hospital discharge	40.36	(6.80)	46.37	(8.22)	45.62	(9.91)	3.95	(2,81)*

*$p < 0.05$, **$p < 0.001$.

counterparts. This hypothesis was further tested in a repeated measures ANOVA that evaluated subjects' CGAS scores for the year before admission and on admission across groups. Both these CGAS ratings, also summarized in Table 4, were significantly lower for the MCDD group relative to the contrast groups.

The third hypothesis, that MCDD subjects would be more refractory to treatment than their counterparts, was assessed by hospital length of stay and discharge CGAS ratings. As indicated in Table 5, ANOVAs revealed a longer mean length of hospital stay for MCDD subjects than for comparison group subjects, as well as lower CGAS ratings on hospital discharge.

To assess the hypothesis that MCDD subjects would show poorer peer relating relative to control groups, subjects' peer relating scores on the PAS were assessed across groups in an ANOVA. On the PAS, higher scores indicate greater levels of impairment. This ANOVA proved significant, $F(2, 87) = 10.71, p < 0.001$, with MCDD subjects showing more difficulties relating to peers ($\bar{X} = 4.33$, SD $= 0.51$) than the dysthymic ($\bar{X} = 3.5$, SD $= 1.6$) or conduct disordered groups ($\bar{X} = 3.7$, SD $= 1.0$).

The final hypothesis, that there would be more parental psychopathology in the MCDD group relative to comparison groups, was assessed in separate chi-square analyses for mothers versus fathers. Mothers of MCDD patients had significantly more psychopathology than comparison group mothers, $\chi^2 = 13.99, p < 0.0001$. Sixty-six percent of the mothers in the MCDD group showed psychopathology, although only 40% of the mothers did so in the dysthymic group, and 17% of the mothers showed psychopathology in the conduct disordered group. Although more paternal psychopathology was manifest in the MCDD group (38%) relative to the dysthymic (17%) and conduct disordered groups (15%), the chi-square analysis evaluating these data proved nonsignificant, $\chi^2 = 4.84, p < 0.10$. This nonsignificant finding may be related to missing data; information could not be obtained on 10% of fathers in the sample.

DISCUSSION

The purpose of this study was to propose and begin validation of criteria for a developmental syndrome termed MCDD. Hypotheses derived from a developmental perspective on this disorder were tested by ascertaining a cohort of MCDD patients using specific criteria and comparing it with two other groups of psychiatrically ill children. This "first-cut" test indicated that when compared with children with two other psychiatric diagnoses, those with MCDD possessed criteria-independent features that are consistent with a view of MCDD as a developmental disorder and readily differentiate them from the other groups. All hypotheses were supported in the predicted direction. These findings lend support for the concept of MCDD as a way to both systematically identify children with deficits in affect regulation, relatedness, and thinking and to avoid replication of the problems inherent in other commonly used labels such as "childhood schizophrenia" and "borderline syndrome of childhood."

The findings of this study reveal than on average, MCDD children are likely to make their first mental health contacts at age 6 years; on average this is 3 years earlier than dysthymic or conduct disordered patient. MCDD patients are also hospitalized earlier than are comparison group subjects; in their eighth as opposed to the tenth or eleventh years. Relative to the contrast groups, MCDD subjects also have significantly higher CBCL scores in all three domains of symptoms and lower CGAS ratings of their functioning for the year before and week before hospitalization. The poorer peer relations found in MCDD subjects may be consistent with both their higher rates of symptoms and lower ratings of overall adjustment. Additional support for the severity of disturbance found in MCDD subjects may be found in the increased maternal psychiatric disorder among the MCDD group relative to the comparison groups. It is possible that MCDD subjects may have elevated risk for genetic vulnerabilities of severe symptomatology. Though not specific, this feature may not be as pronounced among other groups of psychiatrically hospitalized patients.

Once hospitalized, MCDD patients are likely to spend two to three times longer in the hospital than their counterparts before they can be transferred to a less structured setting. Despite these longer hospitalizations, however, MCDD children are discharged from the hospital with lower CGAS ratings than comparison group subjects. These findings provide preliminary support for MCDD as an early onset disorder with entrenched features that are quite refractory to treatment. These features of MCDD are prominent even when compared with two other groups of children whose psychiatric impairments and social disadvantage were also severe enough to warrant hospitalization.

This test of criteria for MCDD is consistent with previous and current recommendations for research that seeks to validate psychiatric diagnoses and facilitate the application of these empirical findings to clinical practice (Pincus et al., 1992; Rutter, 1978). More rigorous tests of MCDD diagnostic criteria would be consistent with these recommendations. Research that will test how successfully these definitions distinguish between MCDD children and other groups of developmentally delayed and severely impaired patients is necessary for refining the criteria. In these more rigorous tests, MCDD patients should be compared with children with autism, particularly high-functioning autistic individuals, children with expressive or receptive language delays, with other forms of atypical PDD and with children with the narrowly defined "adult" schizophrenia.

The "first-cut" test is an attempt to corroborate the validity of a developmental perspective on this syndrome. The design of this first-cut test of MCDD employed comparison groups that, by definition, are not prone to the severity or types of symptoms outlined in MCDD diagnostic criteria. By design, patient groups in this study were not directly compared on symptoms but on features that are predicted from the concept that MCDD is a developmental disorder. Therefore, subsequent studies of MCDD need to include direct measurements of the three domains of dysfunction that comprise MCDD diagnostic criteria. To provide the most rigorous test possible, measurements of these three domains should be conducted in various groups of developmentally delayed children. In this way groups of children with different types of developmental delays can be compared on features they are likely to share, to varying degrees, with their MCDD counterparts.

In addition, longitudinal studies to identify the developmental trajectories and diagnostic outcomes of MCDD patients are necessary. The discovery of significant thought disorder in MCDD patients may lead clinicians to predict that these children eventually will develop schizophrenia as adults. Although oddities in relatedness and affective dysregulation are certainly observed in schizophrenia, these two features also are consistently observed in a variety of adult conditions, including chronic affective and personality disorders. MCDD children with these symptoms may be at increased risk for becoming schizophrenic in adolescence or later, but there are too little data available to predict the likelihood of this specific outcome. The ultimate course of this disorder has not been identified, and the risks for particular diagnostic outcomes are unknown.

There are implications of these findings for diagnosis. In children for whom there is a suggestion of thought disorder or extreme affective responses, a complete, careful developmental and symptom history assumes even greater importance. The evaluation should consider the possibility of developmental disorders by pursuing the onset of these symptoms and other evidence of developmental disturbance. Signs of disturbance may be suggested by early oddities, unusual fears, and problems with self-regulation, social relating, and excessive anxiety.

In addition, the diagnosis of a developmental disorder eases the burden of shame from parents who often are blamed for creating or perpetuating their child's disabilities. When parents are relieved of this burden and allowed to grieve, the child may benefit from having their active advocacy for his or her needs.

Advantages offered by understanding this syndrome as a developmental disorder have clinical relevance as well as research implications. When seen as a developmental disorder instead of an acute illness, treatment and educational goals for this syndrome are recast in meaningful ways, and the aims of treatment become clearer. In acute illnesses, the usual goal is to remove pathological symptoms and return the child to his or her premorbid level of function. In developmental disorders, the clinician is required to maintain an awareness of the child's future at all times; interventions should facilitate the child's overall development, educate and strengthen his or her family, and provide support for his or her vulnerabilities. Children with MCDD, like those with other developmental disorders, may be prone to anxiety or become easily undone by changes in their environment or routines and become disorganized and thought disordered. Instead of employing interventions that react to the emergence of thought disorder and disorganization, methods that introduce changes gradually and seek to reduce the child's anxiety may be safer and more effective. Caregivers learn to anticipate that the child will become anxious and plan accordingly. These techniques closely resemble those used with anxious retarded children.

In a similar way, the benefits and side effects of pharmacological treatment must be carefully considered. Physicians experienced in the treatment of developmental disorders weigh the side effects of drugs that hamper a child's development against the impairment caused by symptoms. Prescribing lower doses of neuroleptics or employing other agents that leave mild symptoms requiring occasional behavioral management may keep the child available for learning and relating. This is preferable to the long-term risks, discomfort, sedation, and blunting created by using high doses of neuroleptics that might be necessary to remove all symptoms.

Beyond the advantages conferred clinically and for the study of childhood psychopathology, a developmental perspective on this disorder also is valuable for the science of child development. In autism research, curiosity about the connections between delays in language and socialization has led investigators to propose a core deficit of profound impairment in social reciprocity. Consequently, the study of autistic children has taught us more about normal relatedness and increased our knowledge of the way in which the developing child comes to understand others. In a similar way, investigations with MCDD children can provide opportunities to further this knowledge. Additional study could identify a core deficit that meaningfully links the domains of social relatedness, thinking, and affective regulation. Such a link could explain why these particular impairments are observed in MCDD children. Preliminary suggestions of such a connection have emerged from the concept of "theory of mind" in autism and other pervasive developmental disorders (Baron-Cohen, 1990; Hobson, 1986; Klin et al., 1992; Perner et al., 1989). There are indications that additional study will deepen our appreciation of the psychology and biology of normal social relatedness and the underlying substrates for the capacity to create and maintain durable internal representations (Mayes et al., 1992; Cohen et al., in press).

The present study has provided initial support for MCDD as a developmental disorder that encompasses chronic severe symptoms that do not readily respond to treatment. Dismaying as this current description may be, the findings do offer a fresh viewpoint on the treatment of these children. The aims and objectives of treatment with MCDD children become clearer when their symptoms and disorder are understood as developmental deviance. Instead of moving quickly to remove pathological symptoms, interventions focus on facilitating the child's optimal development in the light of his or her deficits and vulnerabilities. There is an analogy to children with other developmental delays (e.g., autism, mental retardation). When these children experience changes in their routines or environments they may become highly anxious or easily overwhelmed. Treatment and understanding can increase their caregivers' awareness and anticipation of this. It can lead caregivers to introduce changes in less traumatic ways rather than emphasizing the pathological quality of the child's responses. In a similar way, MCDD children can be understood to have critical vulnerabilities to affective and cognitive disorganization. In a developmental perspective, treatment efforts shift away from primarily emphasizing the eradication of chronic oddities or symptoms and give more weight to fostering the conditions that best support the child's emotional development and education. As more about this disorder is learned, more effective and specific treatments may be revealed. Increasing our knowledge holds the possibility of offering better ideas of prognosis, service needs, and treatment approaches to clinicians, their patients, and their patients' families.

REFERENCES

Achenbach, T. M. (1966), The classification for children's psychiatric symptoms: a factor-analytic study. *Psychological Monographs*, 80(7, 615).

Achenbach, T. M. & Edelbrock, C. (1983), *Manual for the Child Behavior Checklist.* Burlington, VT: University Associates in Psychiatry.

Asarnow, J. R. & Ben-Meir, S. (1987), Children with schizophrenia spectrum and depressive disorders: a comparative study of premorbid adjustment, onset pattern and severity of impairment. *J. Child Psychol. Psychiatry,* 29(4):477–488.

Baron-Cohen, S. (1990). Autism: a specific cognitive disorder of "mind blindness." *International Review of Psychiatry,* 2:81–90.

Bender, L. (1947), Childhood schizophrenia. *Am. J. Orthopsychiatry,* 17:40–56.

Burd, L., Fisher, W. & Kerbeshian, J. (1987), A prevalence study of pervasive developmental disorders in North Dakota. *J. Am. Acad. Child Adolesc. Psychiatry,* 26:700–703.

Cannon-Spoor, H. E., Potkin, S. G. & Wyatt, R. J. (1982), Measurement of premorbid adjustment in chronic schizophrenia. *Schizophr. Bull.,* 8:470–484.

Cantor, S., Pearce J., Pezzott-Pearce, T. & Evans, J. (1981), The group of hypotonic schizophrenics. *Schizophr. Bull.,* 7(1):1–11.

Cantor, S., Evans, J., Pearce, J. & Pezzot-Pearce, T. (1982), Childhood schizophrenia: present but not accounted for. *Am. J. Psychol.,* 139(6):758–762.

Cicchetti, D. V. (1984), On a model for assessing the security of infantile attachment: issues of observer reliability and validity. *The Behavioral and Brain Sciences,* 7:149–151.

Cohen, D. J., Paul, R. & Volkmar, F. R. (1986), Issues in the classification of pervasive and other developmental disorders: toward DSM-IV. *J. Am. Acad. Child Psychiatry,* 25(2):213–220.

Cohen, D. J., Towbin, K. E., Mayes, L. & Volkmar, F. (in press), Developmental psycho-pathology of multiplex developmental disorder. In: *Developmental Follow-up: Concepts, Genres, Domains, and Methods,* eds. S. L. Friedman & H. C. Haywood, Orlando, Fla.: Academic Press.

Dahl, E. K., Cohen, D. J. & Provence, S. (1986), Clinical and multivariate approaches to the nosology of pervasive developmental disorders. *J. Am. Acad. Child Psychiatry,* 25(2):170–180.

Despert, L. (1986), *Schizophrenia in Children,* New York: Robert Brunner Inc.

Eggers, C. (1978), Course and prognosis of childhood schizophrenia. *J. Autism and Child. Schizop.,* 8(1):21–36.

Ekstein, R. & Wallerstein, J. (1954), Observations on the psychology of borderline and psychotic children. *Psychoanalytic Study of the Child,* 9:344–369.

Freud, A. (1956), The assessment of borderline cases. In: *The Writings of Anna Freud.* Vol. 5. New York: International Universities Press, pp. 301–314.

Greenman, D. A., Gunderson, J. G., Cane, M. & Saltzman, P. R. (1986), An examination of the borderline diagnosis in children. *Am. J. Psychiatry,* 143:998–1003.

Hobson, R. P. (1986), The autistic child's appraisal of expressions of emotion. *J. Child Psychol. Psychiatry,* 27(3):321–342.

Kestenbaum, C. (1983), The borderline child at risk for major psychiatric disorder in adult life: seven case reports with follow-up. In: *The Borderline Child: Approaches to Etiology, Diagnosis, and Treatment.* ed. K. Robson. New York: McGraw-Hill, 49–81.

Klin, A., Volkmar, F. & Sparrow, S. (1992), Autistic social dysfunction: some limitations of the theory of mind hypothesis in autism. *J. Child Psychol. Psychiatry,* 33:861–876.

Kolvin, I. (1971), Studies in the childhood psychoses: I. Diagnostic criteria and classifi-cation. *Br. J. Psychiatry,* 118:381–384.

Kolvin, I., Ounsted, C., Humphrey, M., & McNay, A. (1971), Studies in the childhood psy-choses: II. The phenomenology of childhood psychoses. *Br. J. Psychiatry,* 118:385–395.

Lofgren, D. P., Bemporad, J., King, J., Lindem, K. & O'Driscoll, G. (1991), A prospec-tive follow-up study of so-called borderline children. *Am. J. Psychiatry,* 148(11):1541–1547.

Mayes, L., Cohen, D. J. & Klin, A. (1991), Experiencing self and others: a psychoanalytic perspective on theory of mind and autism. In: *Understanding Other Minds: Perspectives from Autism.* eds. S. Baron-Cohen, H. Tager-Flusberg & D. J. Cohen. Oxford: Oxford University Press.

Perner, J., Firth, U., Leslie, A. M. & Leekam, S. R. (1989), Exploration of the autistic child's theory of mind: knowledge, belief and communication. *Child Dev.,* 60:689–700.

Petti, T. & Vela, R. (1990), Borderline disorders of childhood. *J. Am. Acad. Child Adolesc. Psychiatry,* 29:327–337.

Pincus, H. A., Frances, A., Davis, W. W., First, M. B. & Widiger, T. A. (1992), *DSM-IV* and new diagnostic categories: holding the line on proliferation. *Am. J. Psychol.,* 149:112–117.

Pine, F. (1974), On the concept "borderline" in children: a clinical essay. *Psychoanalytic Study of the Child,* 29:341–368.

Russell, A. (1991), Schizophrenia. In: *Child Psychopathology: Diagnostic Criteria and Clinical Assessment.* eds. S. Hooper, G. W. Hynd & R. E. Mattison. Hilldale, NJ: Lawrence Earlbaum Associates, pp. 23–65.

Rutter, M. (1972), Childhood schizophrenia reconsidered. *J. Autism Child. Schizophr.,* 2(4):315–337.

Rutter, M. (1978) Diagnostic validity in child psychiatry. *Advances in Biological Psychiatry,* 2(2):2–22.

Rutter. M. (1985), Psychopathology and development: links between childhood and adult life. In: *Child and Adolescent Psychiatry: Modern Approaches.* eds. M. Rutter & L. Hersov. Oxford, U.K.: Blackwell Scientific Publications, pp. 720–739.

Rutter, M. & Gould, M. (1985), Classification. In: *Child and Adolescent Psychiatry: Modern Approaches.* eds. M. Rutter & L. Hersov. Oxford, U.K.: Blackwell Scientific Publications. pp. 304–321.

Shaffer, D., Gould, M. S., Brasic, J., et al. (1983), A children's global assessment scale (CGAS). *Arch. Gen. Psychiatry,* 40:1228–1231.

Stengel, E. (1959), Classification of mental disorders. *Bull. WHO,* 21:21–31.

Vela, R., Gottlieb, E. & Gottlieb, H. (1983), Borderline syndromes in childhood. In: *The Borderline Child: Approaches to Etiology, Diagnosis, and Treatment.* ed. K. Robson. New York: McGraw-Hill, pp. 31–48.

Volkmar, F. (1991), Childhood schizophrenia. In: *Child and Adolescent Psychiatry: A Comprehensive Textbook.* ed. M. Lewis. Baltimore: Williams and Wilkins, pp. 621–629.

Wenning, K. (1990), Borderline children: a closer look at diagnosis and treatment. *Am J. Orthopsychiatry,* 60(2):225–232.

Wing, L. & Gould, J. (1979), Severe impairment of social interaction and associated abnormalities in children: epidemiology and classification. *J. Autism Dev. Disord.,* 9:11–29.

Wolff, S. & Chick, J. (1980), Schizoid personality in childhood. *Psychol. Med.,* 10:85–100.

Zeitlin, H. (1986), *The Natural History of Psychiatric Disorder in Children: A Study of Individuals Known to have Attended Both Child and Adult Psychiatric Departments of the Same Hospital.* Oxford: Oxford University Press.

13

Private Speech of Learning Disabled and Normally Achieving Children in Classroom Academic and Laboratory Contexts

Laura E. Berk and Steven Landau
Illinois State University, Normal

Learning disabled (LD) children are often targets for cognitive-behavioral interventions designed to train them in effective use of a self-directed speech. The purpose of this study was to determine if, indeed, these children display immature private speech in the naturalistic classroom setting. Comparisons were made of the private speech, motor accompaniment to task, and attention of LD and normally achieving classmates during academic seatwork. Setting effects were examined by comparing classroom data with observations during academic seatwork and puzzle solving in the laboratory. Finally, a subgroup of LD children symptomatic of attention-deficit hyperactivity disorder (ADHD) was compared with pure LD and normally achieving controls to determine if the presumed immature private speech is a function of a learning disability or externalizing behavior problems. Results indicated that LD children used more task-relevant private speech than controls, an effect that was especially pronounced for the LD/ADHD subgroup. Use of private speech was setting- and task-specific. Implications for intervention and future research methodology are discussed.

Reprinted with permission from *Child Development,* 1993, Vol. 64, 556–571. Copyright © 1993 by the Society for Research in Child Development, Inc.

Preparation of this article was supported in part by a grant from the Graduate School, Illinois State University. We gratefully acknowledge the assistance of Aimee Callahan, Christine Mitchell, Kristi Moss, Deanna Nagel, Deborah Petrillo, Beth Van Houte, and Cheryl Stein in collecting and compiling the data. We are also grateful to Dr. Sarah Booth, vice principal of Metcalf School, Mr. Larry Daghe, principal of Oakdale School, and Ms. Vicki Freeman, principal of Northpoint School, Normal, IL, for making this study possible, and to the teachers and children for welcoming us into their classrooms.

Private speech is speech spoken out loud that is addressed either to the self or to no particular listener (Zivin, 1979). The dominant perspective on its development and functional significance is that of Vygotsky (1934/1987), who reasoned that private speech is externalized thought, which serves a self-guiding function. Vygotsky hypothesized that private speech aids children in overcoming obstacles to task success when faced with challenging cognitive problems. As private speech gradually gains control over task-related behavior during the late preschool and elementary school years, audible self-directed utterances are abbreviated and internalized as silent verbal thought.

Currently, substantial support for Vygotsky's theoretical assumptions exists (Berk, 1992). Cross-sectional and longitudinal evidence indicates that, in problem-solving contexts, private speech consistently follows a developmental sequence from audible, externalized speech to more internalized, less audible forms (Berk, 1986; Berk & Garvin, 1984; Berk & Potts, 1991; Bivens & Berk, 1990; Frauenglass & Diaz, 1985; Kohlberg, Yaeger, & Hjertholm, 1968). Moreover, the self-guiding function of private speech is supported by two sets of evidence. First, private speech increases under conditions of difficult and demanding tasks (Beaudichon, 1973; Behrend, Rosengren, & Perlmutter, 1989, 1992; Berk & Garvin, 1984; Deutsch & Stein, 1972; Dickie, 1973; Kohlberg et al., 1968), and children are most likely to generate private utterances at points during problem solving in which they fail at particular steps (Goodman, 1981). Second, children's use of private speech predicts self-controlled behavior and eventual task success. In both laboratory and classroom problem-solving contexts, task-relevant private speech is positively associated with concurrent task performance as well as gains in performance over time (Azmitia, 1992; Beaudichon, 1973; Behrend et al., 1992; Bivens & Berk, 1990; Gaskill & Diaz, 1991; Klein, 1964; Murray, 1979; Roberts, 1979). Furthermore, recent longitudinal evidence reveals that progressive internalization of private speech from first to third grade is accompanied by behavioral changes that should facilitate efficient task solution—namely, gains in sustained attention and inhibition of self-stimulating bodily movements while children work at their desks on math seatwork (Bivens & Berk, 1990).

Drawing on the Vygotskian premise that speech is the uniquely human capacity that permits children to master their own actions, cognitive-behavioral investigators have assumed that children with a diverse array of serious learning problems, including impulsivity, hyperactivity, and learning disabilities, suffer from deficits in use of self-guiding private speech (Hughes, 1988). Inducing such speech through a variety of coaching, modeling, and reinforcement procedures is regarded by these theorists as the most efficient and effective means of ameliorating these youngsters' learning difficulties (Camp, Blom, Herbert, & van Doornick, 1977; Harris, 1986; Kendall & Braswell, 1985; Meichenbaum & Goodman, 1971; Palkes, Stewart, & Kahana, 1968; Wong, 1985). However, a careful examination of Vygotsky's theory does not lead inevitably to the conclusion that such children are deficient in verbal self-regulation. If two additional Vygotskian principles are considered—that private speech is a universal human problem-solving tool and that it increases under conditions of cognitive challenge—quite different predictions can be made. First, children with persistent learning problems should follow the same course of private speech development as their normal counterparts. Second, factors that impair cognitive processing and/or ability to sustain attention should act as tenacious obstacles to task success, preventing private speech from gaining efficient mastery over behavior and moving toward internalization. Therefore, children with such deficits should emit greater quantities of externalized, self-guiding speech than their normal agemates and should be delayed in private speech internalization.

Most studies assessing the spontaneous private speech of children with serious learning difficulties have focused on attention-deficit hyperactivity disordered (ADHD) children and the related symptom of impulsive responding. A careful examination of these findings tends to support the second set of predictions specified above (Berk & Potts, 1991; Campbell, 1973; Diaz & Lowe, 1987; Goodman, 1977; Zentall, Gohs, & Culatta, 1983). For example, Berk and Potts (1991) tracked age-related changes in ADHD children's private speech during classroom mathematics seatwork and assessed its relationship to task-related behavior. Movement from externalized self-guiding to internalized speech forms was delayed among ADHD youngsters in comparison to matched controls. Moreover, task-relevant private speech was associated with motor quiescence and attention among only the least distractible ADHD subjects. This finding suggests that only the less symptomatic ADHD children were able to use private speech as a self-regulatory mediational strategy to ameliorate behavioral and attentional difficulties. Although Copeland (1979) reported findings at variance with these studies—namely, less self-guiding and more task-irrelevant utterances among hyperactive youngsters—her results may be an artifact of the conditions under which children were observed. Specifically, Copeland collected private speech data during free play, not while children worked on cognitively demanding tasks.

The current study was designed to extend the body of research summarized above. Its major purpose was to determine if the development and functional significance of private speech among learning disabled (LD) children—both with and without attentional deficits—is similar to that of normal youngsters. As such, this represents the first known investigation to examine LD children's spontaneous use of private speech, in both the naturalistic classroom setting during academic problem solving and in the laboratory. Appraisal of LD children's private speech while engaged in academic work is particularly important, since verbal self-regulatory differences between LD and control children should be most apparent on tasks that tap LD subjects' specific learning disabilities. Furthermore, LD children often have multiple impairments. In particular, a sizable number meet the diagnostic criteria for ADHD (McGee & Share, 1988). If multiple problems place the child at greater risk for delays in private speech internalization, then this trend should be particularly pronounced for LD children who are comorbid with ADHD (i.e., LD/ADHD).

A secondary purpose of this study was to cross-validate naturalistic observations during classroom academic seatwork with laboratory data obtained while children worked on two types of tasks: academic seatwork brought into the lab and puzzle tasks, which have been the most widely used problem-solving context for the study of private speech. In virtually all research that has used puzzle tasks, however, the incidence of private speech has been low. Many children emitted only a few utterances, and in some studies as many as half the sample showed none at all (see review in Berk, 1992). The questionable ecological validity of laboratory puzzle observations is supported by cross-study comparisons indicating that private speech is far more prevalent in classroom than laboratory contexts. For example, when working on academic seatwork, all first through sixth graders observed by Berk and her collaborators used some private speech and most exhibited a great deal. Private speech occurred, on the average, during 60%–80% of 10-sec time-sampling intervals in her series of naturalistic studies (Berk, 1986; Berk & Garvin, 1984; Berk & Potts, 1991; Bivens & Berk, 1990).

Findings by Frauenglass and Diaz (1985), however, suggest that it is not just the laboratory context per se that may depress children's private speech. The type of problem-solving task may be equally or more important. They found that preschoolers displayed more private speech while working on tasks that require verbal mediation (picture ordering and picture sequencing) than during puzzle solving, which depends on visual/spatial strategies. If the lab could serve as a suitable analog for naturalistic data collection, it could represent a more practical and efficient arena for studying the private speech phenomenon. Therefore, we attempted to disentangle the extent to which low rates of private speech in previous studies are due to the laboratory setting, the type of task in which children are engaged, or both factors.

In summary, the specific purposes of this study were to examine the cross-sectional development of LD and normally achieving pupils' private speech during classroom language arts and mathematics seatwork—elementary school tasks that tap LD children's learning deficits and are known to evoke substantial quantities of private speech (Berk, 1986; Berk & Potts, 1991; Bivens & Berk, 1990); to compare the functional significance of private speech in LD and normal children by relating children's self-directed speech to concurrent measures of motor behavior and attention; and to examine setting and task influences on private speech by observing a subset of LD and control subjects in each of three contexts—

classroom academic seatwork, laboratory academic seatwork, and laboratory puzzle tasks.

It was hypothesized that:

1. Both LD and control subjects would show a course of private speech development consistent with Vygotsky's theory and previous research on normal elementary school children, proceeding from task-irrelevant forms to task-relevant externalized private speech to less audible task-relevant speech.

2. Learning-disabled children would display heightened use of task-relevant, self-guiding private speech and diminished use of more internalized, less audible speech forms—a pattern reflecting delays in private speech internalization. This trend would be especially pronounced for a subgroup of LD children also known to present behaviors indicative of ADHD (i.e., LD/ADHD).

3. The private speech of LD children would be less effectively integrated with motor accompaniment to task and attention than that of normal controls.

4. The laboratory context would suppress private speech in both LD and control children, an effect that should be especially pronounced for the puzzle tasks. Moreover, obtained differences between LD and control subjects should be task-specific—that is, apparent during academic tasks that tap LD children's achievement deficits but not evident during laboratory puzzle solving.

METHOD

Subjects

A total of 112 third- through sixth-grade children enrolled in two public schools and a university laboratory school served as subjects. Half the sample was composed of LD children, half of normally achieving controls. Consistent with the demographics of the community, 10% of children were African-American, 2% Hispanic, and 1% Asian. Although SES data were not systematically collected, children in this community represent middle to upper-middle SES groups.

The LD sample met the Illinois state department guidelines for LD placement in special education. As such, each had been referred because of serious academic difficulties, received an individual psychoeducational evaluation that revealed a significant aptitude/achievement discrepancy (at least 1 SD), and had been staffed into learning disabilities special education by the school's multidisciplinary student support team. Each of the LD children was mainstreamed into regular classrooms.

The normal controls were selected by asking regular classroom teachers to nominate a same-sex, average-achieving classmate who was free of externalizing behavior problems to serve as a match for each LD subject. Each group was composed of 13 girls and 43 boys. Mean ages for the LD and control children at each grade were: third grade, 9.6 and 9.0 years ($n = 24$); fourth grade, 10.6 and 10.0 ($n = 32$); fifth grade, 11.2 and 11.0 ($n = 28$); and sixth grade, 12.5 and 11.9 ($n = 28$), respectively. Learning-disabled children were, on the average, 6 months older than their control counterparts. By matching LD with controls on the basis of grade rather than age, the developmental comparison was a conservative one, given the prediction that LD children would be delayed in private speech internalization. The matching procedure also ensured that the behavior of LD and control subjects would be observed under comparable classroom conditions. To have matched on age would have meant that, for a substantial number of the LD subjects, controls would have had to be chosen from a higher-grade classroom.

On the basis of a complete psychoeducational evaluation and the specification of the nature of the learning disability, all LD children included in the sample were identified as impaired in the area of language arts (e.g., reading). To control for verbal ability differences between LD and normal children, all subjects were given the vocabulary subtest of the WISC-R. Consistent with their identified disability, vocabulary scaled scores of LD subjects were significantly lower than those of controls, $M = 9.8$, SD $= 2.8$, and $M = 12.4$, SD $= 1.9$, $t(110) = 5.8$, $p < .01$.

To select a subgroup of LD children who were symptomatic of behaviors suggestive of ADHD, each subject was rated by his or her classroom teacher with the 39-item Conners (1969) Teacher Rating Scale (TRS). As a consequence, the LD sample was divided into pure LD ($n = 47$) and LD/ADHD ($n = 9$) with the use of the Pelham, Milich, Murphy, and Murphy (1989) research diagnostic criteria of 11 or above for third graders and 9 or above for fourth through sixth graders on the Inattention/Overactivity (IO) factor from the Conners TRS (Loney & Milich, 1982). Sixteen percent of the sample met this criterion. The IO factor has been used in previous research to successfully discriminate ADHD children from those with other disorders (Milich & Fitzgerald, 1985; Milich & Landau, 1988) and to validate ADHD diagnosis (Landau, Lorch, & Milich, 1992).

The various LD-control comparisons were organized as follows: First, pure LD children ($n = 47$) and their respective controls ($n = 47$) were compared. Second, to examine the possibility that LD/ADHD subjects differ from both pure LD children and non-LD controls, each LD/ADHD child ($n = 9$) was contrasted with his or her normally achieving control ($n = 9$) as well as a same-sex pure LD subject from his or her classroom ($n = 9$). In instances in which there were more than one possible pure LD match, the child was chosen randomly. The LD/ADHD children and their pure LD matches did not differ significantly in age or vocabulary subtest scores $t(16) = 0.2$, N.S., and $t(16) = 0.6$, N.S., respectively. Furthermore, consistent with the request that teachers designate non-LD controls who were free of externalizing behavior disorders, no control child in the study met the Pelham et al. (1989) Conners TRS research diagnostic criterion for ADHD. Finally, the impact of setting and task on private speech was examined by observing 28 children attending the university laboratory school, half LDs and half matched controls, in both the classroom and the laboratory.

The three schools that LD and control children attended were located in the same small Midwestern city, and each school used similar text and workbook materials. In addition, each LD child worked at a level in language arts and math commensurate with his or her achievement, thereby eliminating the possibility that LD subjects' classroom assignments were overly challenging in comparison to those of their control counterparts.

Procedure

Naturalistic classroom observations. Children's private speech, motor accompaniment to task, and level of attention were recorded by six observers during daily language and math seatwork periods from February through April of the school year. Children were observed only when they worked on assignments requiring individualized written practice in reading and spelling and in arithmetic skills that were part of the school's formal mathematics curriculum.

All observers were blind to the questions under investigation and the group status of subjects. Observations were randomly assigned to observers, and data collection on each child was divided between at least two observers. An adaptation period of several weeks occurred before data collection began (during which time the team of observers received training in the observational system and engaged in practice observations in all three schools). Observers were also instructed to behave as unobtrusively as possible while sitting within hearing distance of each subject to be observed. Children did not know who was being observed on a given occasion, nor were they aware of the phenomena under investigation. Taken together, these precautions reduced the likelihood that either observer bias or subject reactivity influenced the data collected.

Each child was observed for a total of at least 20 min of language and 20 min of math seatwork, distributed across two or more complete seatwork periods in each subject. When the seatwork period began, the observer focused on the target child, sampled the behavior stream for 10 sec, and then recorded events on a code sheet for the next 20 sec. During each observation interval, observers placed codes in subclasses of private speech, motor accompaniment to task, and level of attention.

Previous research has shown that private speech is influenced by classroom contextual factors. For example, when teachers become involved in children's activities or when children move from academic into nonacademic pursuits, the incidence of private speech diminishes substantially (Berk & Garvin, 1984;

Kohlberg et al., 1968). To ensure that the behaviors of interest were recorded under comparable classroom conditions across all subjects, coding procedures similar to those devised by Pechman (1978) and used by Berk and her collaborators (Berk, 1986; Berk & Potts, 1991; Bivens & Berk, 1990) were employed. Private speech and motor accompaniment to task were recorded only when children were at least moderately attentive to language and math seatwork tasks. They were not coded when the child was diverted—that is, engaged in nonacademic activities that were not uniform across children (e.g., conversations with peers, trips to the water fountain, tying shoes, day dreaming). In addition, observers did not code during intervals in which the child sought help with language or math seatwork from the teacher or the teacher offered assistance to the child. Since the adult takes over direction of the task, teacher intervention dramatically lessens children's need for self-guiding private speech (Berk & Garvin, 1984; Diaz, 1992). Consequently, coding during such intervals would have spuriously reduced speech indices for those subjects receiving help from teachers.

Laboratory observations. To examine the impact of setting and task on children's private speech, 28 subjects attending the university laboratory school, half LD and half matched controls, were also videotaped while working on two different kinds of tasks in the laboratory: language seatwork assignments and math seatwork assignments provided by the child's classroom teacher, and a series of four puzzles from the WISC-R object assembly subtest. The object assembly subtest presents different puzzles of graduated difficulty, appropriate for children ages 6-0 to 16-11. As such, it was possible to quantify children's puzzle performance using norms from the WISC-R and relate it to their private speech. According to Sattler (1988), object assembly is an especially good subtest for observing children's thinking and work habits.

Order of administration of the three laboratory tasks was counterbalanced across subjects. Five minutes of observation were obtained for each seatwork assignment. WISC-R administration procedures grant up to 9 min for completion of the object assembly subtest; on the average, children in the subsample took 4.0 min (SD = 2.8). The videotaped records were divided into 10-sec intervals. Both naturalistic and laboratory data were coded using the category system described below.

Observational Categories

Private speech. Private speech was defined as speech that is not clearly and definitely addressed to a listener (Berk & Garvin, 1984). If private speech occurred during an observation interval, it was coded into one of three levels and nine mutually exclusive specific categories devised by Berk (1986), as follows:

1. Level 1: task-irrelevant private speech: (*a*) word play and repetition; (*b*) task-

irrelevant affect expression; (*c*) comments to absent, imaginary, or nonhuman others.

2. Level 2: task-relevant externalized private speech: (*a*) describing one's own activity and self-guiding comments; (*b*) task-relevant, self-answered questions; (*c*) reading aloud and sounding out words; (*d*) task-relevant affect expression (e.g., "I did it!" "This is hard").

3. Level 3: task-relevant external manifestations of inner speech: (*a*) inaudible muttering (remarks involving clear mouthing of words that are not fully audible but that are related to some aspect of the task); (*b*) lip and tongue movement (speech-like lip and tongue movements associated with some aspect of the task; repetitive motor play, such as clicking of the tongue and pursing of the lips, was excluded from this category).

Motor accompaniment to task. These categories were adapted by Berk (1986) from Pechman (1978). All motor accompaniments to task, both self-stimulating and task-facilitating, were included. Since children often exhibited more than one motor behavior, up to two were coded in a given observation interval. Children rarely exhibited more than two motor behaviors at once. In the few instances in which they did, the observer coded the two most salient behaviors—that is, those that represented the largest quantity of motor activity.

1. Self-stimulating behavior: (*a*) self-manipulates (manipulates a part of the body with hands); (*b*) chews (chews on pencil, paper, fingers, gum, comb, or other object); (*c*) rhythmic movement (repeated movement of object, body, or fingers in constant motion); (*d*) body movement (gross movements of the body including stretching and changing positions); (*e*) manipulates object/self-stimulating (manipulates object in a manner unrelated to the task).

2. Task-facilitating behavior: (*a*) manipulates object/task-facilitating (e.g., uses chips to keep track of counting in an arithmetic problem); (*b*) points (uses finger, pencil, or other object to follow a line or read a word); (*c*) gestures (task-related expressive movements with hands, such as counting on fingers); (*d*) watch, look (observes another child, group, or object as an aid to carrying out the task).

3. No movement.

Attention level. The following categories were taken from Pechman (1978) and assess the child's level of attention to the seatwork task:

1. Focused: sustained involvement, resisting interference from outside.

2. Moderate: involvement with the task is momentarily interrupted by another activity, diversion, or input from outside.

3. Diverted: the child is distracted from the task.

Reliability of Observation

For 12% of all observation sessions during data collection, each observer was twice paired with a second observer and scheduled to watch a child simultaneously for an entire language arts or math seatwork period. Kappas (Cohen, 1960) were computed for both the broad and fine categories of private speech, motor accompaniment to task, and attention. Agreements were as follows: private speech broad categories: Level 1 speech, 1.0; Level 2 speech, 1.0; Level 3 speech, .83; motor accompaniment to task broad categories: self-stimulating behavior, .87; task-facilitating behavior, .88; and no movement, .85; and attention to task, .98. In addition, kappas for the 23 fine categories ranged from .67 for manipulates object/self-stimulating to 1.0 for word play/repetition, with a median kappa of .95. These agreement figures are consistent with previous work conducted by this research group (e.g., Berk & Potts, 1991).

RESULTS

Since the number of 10-sec intervals used to complete the classroom seatwork and laboratory puzzle tasks varied across subjects (for classroom language arts seatwork, $M = 141.5$, $SD = 13.8$; for classroom math seatwork, $M = 142.1$, $SD = 13.5$; for puzzles, $M = 24.0$ $SD = 16.8$), percentages of occurrence of the observational variables were entered into the analyses. A preliminary examination of the data revealed no significant sex or sex $\times$ group (LD vs. control) effects on classroom and laboratory private speech indices. Consequently, sex was dropped from the remainder of the analyses. In addition, within-subject comparisons indicated that there were no significant differences between language and math classroom and between language and math laboratory seatwork for any private speech or behavioral variables. Therefore, private speech was combined across language arts and math in each of the two settings for all subsequent analyses.

As in previous research (Berk, 1986; Berk & Potts, 1991; Bivens & Berk, 1990), the overall incidence of private speech during classroom seatwork was extremely high. Some form of private speech occurred, on the average, during 68.3% of the observation intervals ($SD = 17.0$). A total of 31 children (27.7% of the sample) exhibited at least some Level 1 (task-irrelevant) speech, 77 children (68.8%) Level 2 (task-relevant, externalized) speech, and 112 children (100%) Level 3 (task-relevant internalized) speech. An examination of private speech means for all children indicated that the large majority of utterances was of the most mature, Level 3 variety ($M = 61.9$, $SD = 17.6$). Total sample means for Levels 1 and 2 private speech were much lower in occurrence ($M = 1.0$, $SD = 2.6$ and $M = 5.5$, $SD = 6.9$, respectively)—similar to findings of previous investigations that have included older elementary school children (Berk, 1986; Berk & Garvin, 1984; Bivens & Berk, 1990; Kohlberg et al., 1968).

Consistent with earlier studies indicating that internalization of private speech is paced by mental maturity (Berk, 1986; Frauenglass & Diaz, 1985; Kohlberg et al., 1968), WISC-R vocabulary scaled scores were negatively correlated with classroom Level 2 private speech, $r(110) = -.25$, $p < .01$. Consequently, vocabulary was entered as a covariate into analyses comparing the incidence of private speech among LD and control children.

Comparisons of Pure LD and Control Children on Speech and Behavioral Variables in the Classroom

A grade × group (pure LD vs. control) MANCOVA, with the three levels of private speech entered as dependent variables and polynomial trends used to test for grade effects, provided support for Hypothesis 1—that LD children display a pattern of private speech development similar to that of normal controls. As shown in Table 1, grade effects were found for Levels 2 and 3 speech and are consistent with those reported in previous studies of elementary school children (Berk, 1986; Berk & Potts, 1991; Bivens & Berk, 1990). Level 2 speech declined linearly with grade, while Level 3 speech showed a significant quadratic effect—an increase from grade 3 to grade 4 followed by a decline from grade 4 to grade 5, after which it stabilized from grade 5 to grade 6. Absence of significant grade × group interaction effects indicated that these developmental trends characterized both LD and control groups.

A significant main effect for group lent partial support to Hypothesis 2, that LD children would display more externalized self-guiding private speech than their normally achieving classmates. Learning-disabled subjects engaged in more than twice as much task-relevant, Level 2 speech as controls (see Table 2). However, contrary to expectations, the incidence of Level 3 speech did not favor the control subjects; LD children and their normal counterparts showed an equivalently high proportion of the most internalized private speech when observed in

TABLE 1

Relationship of Grade to Private Speech. Expressed in Terms of Percentage of Occurrence

PRIVATE SPEECH	GRADE 3		GRADE 4		GRADE 5		GRADE 6		POLYNOMIAL TREND	$F(1, 85)$
	M	SD	M	SD	M	SD	M	SD		
Level 1	.3	1.0	.7	1.8	.6	1.0	1.3	3.5	. . .	N.S.
Level 2	7.5	9.6	6.1	6.6	3.7	5.5	4.1	4.9	Linear	4.2*
Level 3	57.3	17.6	68.6	19.3	58.4	17.3	60.5	16.3	Quadratic	4.6*

NOTE.—$n = 22$ at grade 3, $n = 28$ at grade 4, $n = 24$ at grade 5, and $n = 20$ at grade 6. Multivariate $F(9, 202)$ = 2.1, $p < .05$.
* $p < .05$.

TABLE 2

Comparisons of Pure LD and Control Children on Classroom Private Speech, Motor Accompaniment to Task, and Attention, Expressed in Terms of Percentages of Occurrence

BEHAVIOR	PURE LD		CONTROLS·		
	M	SD	*M*	SD	*F*(1, 85)
Private speech:					
Level 1	.9	1.6	.6	2.3	.5
Level 2	7.8	7.8	3.0	5.0	8.9**
Level 3	61.4	17.4	61.9	18.9	.1
Motor accompaniment to task:					
Self-stimulating	107.6	20.2	104.3	24.6	.5
Task facilitating	15.4	12.7	9.2	8.2	3.9
No movement	13.8	9.6	19.4	13.0	4.0
Level of attention:					
Focused....................	70.1	13.6	81.0	9.8	14.1**
Moderate	17.8	7.8	12.9	6.7	3.7
Diverted..................	12.7	10.3	6.0	5.7	24.5**

NOTE.—n = 47 for each group. For private speech levels, multivariate $F(3, 83)$ = 2.7, $p <$ .05. For motor accompaniment to task, multivariate $F(3, 83)$ = 2.0, $p < .12$. For level of attention, multivariate $F(3, 83)$ = 8.1, $p < .01$. Since up to two motor behaviors were coded during each observation interval, some motor accompaniment to task means exceed 100%.
* $p < .05$.
** $p < .01$.

the classroom. Also, LD children did not engage in an elevated incidence of task-irrelevant speech. It was low in occurrence for both groups.

A follow-up group × grade MANCOVA was carried out on the Level 2 specific categories to determine which forms were largely responsible for the grade and group differences reported above. Results revealed that LD children's greater use of Level 2 speech was accounted for by the most clearly self-regulatory subtype of describing one's own activity/self-guidance, M's = 4.4 and 1.7, $F(1, 85)$ = 3.9, $p < .05$, and by reading aloud, M's = 2.4 and 0.1, $F(1, 85)$ = 8.0, $p < .01$, a form of private speech previously found to predict successful performance on difficult read-and-answer tasks (Roberts, 1979). These findings lend further credence to Hypothesis 2. Reading aloud was also largely responsible for the linear decline in Level 2 speech with grade, M's = 3.4, 1.0, 1.1, and 0.1, $F(1, 85)$ = 9.3, $p < .01$.

Grade × group (LD vs. control) MANCOVAs, with motor accompaniment to task and attention indices entered as dependent variables and vocabulary as the covariate, revealed that the proportion of time spent in focused attention on classroom seatwork tasks was significantly lower for LD children, and time spent diverted was greater (see Table 2). Although there was a trend for LD children to be less quiescent at their desks and to engage in more task-facilitating motor behavior (e.g., counting on fingers, pointing to follow a line or read a word), the multivariate F for motor accompaniment to task was nonsignificant. No significant grade or grade $\times$ group interaction effects were found for either motor accompaniment to task or attention.

Comparisons of LD/ADHD, Pure LD, and Control Children on Speech and Behavioral Variables in the Classroom

A one-way MANCOVA comparing LD/ADHD subjects with their pure LD and non-LD control classmates offered additional support for Hypothesis 2. As shown in Table 3, LD/ADHD subjects displayed more than three times as much task-relevant, externalized (Level 2) speech as did their pure LD matches and approximately four times as much as controls. In addition, the LD/ADHD subgroup emitted a significantly lower incidence of the most mature, internalized (Level 3) speech forms than did their pure LD and non-LD classmates. These findings suggest that LD/ADHD children are delayed in private speech internalization. As in the LD-control comparison, LD/ADHD children's heightened use of Level 2 speech over their pure LD classmates was accounted for by the subcategories of describing one's own activity/self-guidance, M's = 5.1 and 2.2, $F(1, 15)$ = 4.6, $p < .05$, and reading aloud, M's = 2.4 versus 0.1, $F(1, 15)$ = 5.3, $p < .05$.

The MANCOVAs comparing the three groups on indices of motor accompani-

TABLE 3

Comparisons of LD/ADHD with Pure LD and Control Children on Classroom Private Speech, Motor Accompaniment to Task, and Attention, Expressed in Terms of Percentages of Occurrence

PRIVATE SPEECH	LD/ADHD		PURE LD		CONTROLS		LD/ADHD VS. PURE LD $F(1, 23)$	LD/ADHD VS. CONTROLS $F(1, 23)$
	M	SD	*M*	SD	*M*	SD		
Private speech:								
Level 1	4.0	6.3	.6	1.1	.6	.9	3.7	2.0
Level 2	10.3	7.9	3.1	3.1	2.1	3.6	9.1**	5.2*
Level 3	54.7	17.2	70.6	15.6	67.9	11.3	4.6*	3.9*
Motor accompaniment to task:								
Self-stimulating	121.2	11.2	110.4	17.3	106.8	25.8	2.0	.4
Task facilitating	16.3	9.3	13.4	9.7	9.7	10.4	.4	.9
No movement	9.5	5.2	14.7	8.7	19.5	14.3	1.9	.7
Level of attention:								
Focused....................	67.0	18.3	70.6	11.4	73.0	15.1	.2	.5
Moderate	18.3	6.5	19.4	4.6	17.2	6.4	.1	.2
Diverted....................	14.6	13.0	10.1	8.6	6.5	5.7	.9	2.5

NOTE.—n = 9 for each group. For private speech levels, multivariate $F(6, 42)$ = 2.6, $p < .05$. Since up to two motor behaviors were coded during each observation interval, some motor accompaniment to task means exceed 100%.
  * $p < .05$.
  ** $p < .01$.

ment to task and attention revealed mean differences that would be expected on the basis of diagnostic status—that is, LD/ADHD children were more active and less attentive than their pure LD and control counterparts. However, none of these effects reached significance, perhaps because of the small group sizes (see Table 3).

Relationship of Private Speech to Motor Accompaniment to Task and Attention in the Classroom

To examine the functional relationship of private speech to task-related behavior, correlations of private speech with motor accompaniment to task and attention were computed for the pure LD sample and their normally achieving controls. Grade was partialed out, in view of the earlier reported significant relationship of grade with Level 2 and Level 3 speech. Findings supported Hypothesis 3, that private speech is less effectively integrated with behavior for LD children. As depicted in Table 4, Level 3 speech, the most prevalent form for older elementary school children, was negatively associated with overt behavior—both self-stimulating and task-facilitating—for both pure LD and control youngsters. However, it predicted motor quiescence only for controls and not LD subjects; the difference between these two correlations was marginally significant ($z = 1.96$, $p = .05$). In addition, although Level 3 speech was positively related to focused attention for controls, this relationship did not exist for LD subjects. Again, there was a significant difference between the two correlations ($z = 2.2$, $p < .05$). Finally, correlations of Level 1 and Level 2 speech with behavioral variables resembled findings on previously studied samples of younger normally achieving elementary school pupils (Berk, 1986; Bivens & Berk, 1990). Level 1 (task-irrelevant) speech was negatively related to focused attention and positively related to moderate attention, the former reaching significance for the pure LDs

TABLE 4

Correlations of Classroom Private Speech with Motor Accompaniment to Task and Attention Level for Pure LD and Control Children, Partialing out Grade ($df = 42$)

Behavior	Self-stimulating Behavior	Task-facilitating Behavior	No Movement	Focused Attention	Moderate Attention	Diverted Attention
Pure LD:						
Level 1	.08	−.13	−.06	−.27*	.20	.08
Level 2	.11	.52**	−.38**	−.13	−.07	.15
Level 3	−.56**	−.27	−.03	.04	.00	−.24
Controls:						
Level 1	−.12	−.07	.09	−.26	.33*	.12
Level 2	−.13	.27	.03	−.11	.13	.04
Level 3	−.34*	−.32*	.37*	.48**	.03	.18

NOTE.—$n = 47$ for each group.
* $p < .05$.
** $p < .01$.

and the latter for the controls. Level 2 (task-relevant, externalized) utterances were positively related to task-facilitating motor behavior negatively related to no movement among the LD sample. These relationships were not significant for controls. The Level 2/no movement correlation was significantly greater for LD than control children ($z = 2.1, p < .05$).

Correlations of private speech with task-related behavior, comparing the LD/ADHD subjects with their pure LD and control classmates, indicated that Level 2 speech showed a strong negative association with focused attention, $r(7) = -.74, p < .05$, and a positive relationship with diversion from the task for LD/ADHD children, $r(7) = .72, p < .05$. However, these correlations were nonsignificant for the pure LD subgroup, r's$(7) = -.20$ and $-.04$, and for control classmates, r's$(7) = .19$ and $-.35$. These results resemble findings of Berk and Potts (1991), who reported that ADHD pupils who spent the most time off task emitted the largest proportion of task-relevant externalized utterances. However, because of the low n's, group differences in respective correlations did not reach significance.

Impact of Setting and Task on Private Speech

To examine the first part of Hypothesis 4, that the laboratory context should reduce the incidence of private speech in both LD and control children, three group (LD vs. control) × setting (a two-level, within-subjects factor) MANCOVAs were carried out, comparing private speech indices between classroom and laboratory academic, classroom academic and laboratory puzzle-solving, and laboratory academic and laboratory puzzle-solving contexts. Vocabulary was entered as the covariate. Findings revealed that, in comparison to the classroom, the laboratory academic seatwork setting mildly reduced the incidence of both forms of externalized private speech—Level 1 (task-irrelevant), M's $= 1.3$ and 0.1, $F(1, 22) = 3.9, p < .05$, and Level 2 (task-relevant, externalized), M's $= 5.1$ and 4.7, $F(1, 22) = 8.2, p < .01$. When classroom academic seatwork was compared to the puzzle-solving context, all three forms of private speech were severely reduced—for Level 1, M's $= 1.3$ and 0.0, $F(1, 22) = 4.9$, $p < .03$; for Level 2, M's $= 4.9$ and 0.4, $F(1, 22) = 10.7, p < .01$; and for Level 3, M's $= 52.6$ and 35.6, $F(1, 22) = 5.1, p < .05$. Finally, in comparison to laboratory academic seatwork, the incidence of Level 3 private speech during puzzle solving was significantly curtailed, M's $= 51.8$ and 38.9, $F(1, 22) = 4.1$, $p < .05$. In the above analyses, no group status × setting interaction effects were found, confirming the expectation that private speech was similarly reduced in laboratory contexts for all subjects.

The second part of Hypothesis 4, that behavioral differences between LD and controls would be maintained in the laboratory academic but not in the puzzle-solving context, was explored by conducting several one-way (LD vs. control) MANCOVAs, with laboratory academic and puzzle-solving private speech and behavioral indices entered as dependent variables and vocabulary as the covariate. Findings for private speech showed a trend in the expected direction. In the laboratory academic context, LD children showed a marginally significant tendency to emit more Level 2 speech than controls, M's $= 1.9$ and 0.1, $F(1, 25) = 2.9$, $p < .10$. They also spent significantly more time diverted from the task, M's $= 18.4$ and 8.9, $F(1, 25) = 6.0$, $p < .05$, just as they did during classroom seatwork. In the puzzle context, LD and controls were not significantly different in any of the subtypes of private speech and behavioral variables. Also in support of Hypothesis 4, a t test comparing WISC-R object assembly scaled scores of LD and control subjects revealed no significant differences in puzzle-solving accuracy, M's $= 10.0$ and 12.1, $t(26) = 1.7$, N.S. Moreover, time spent working on puzzles, a measure of persistence, showed no significant differences between LD children and controls, M's $= 4.1$ and 3.1 min, $t(26) = 1.3$, N.S.

Although the private speech analyses reported above reveal that the absolute incidence of private speech is substantially reduced in the laboratory as compared to the natural environment, they do not indicate whether children who score high or low relative to their peers in the natural setting retain their same private speech ranking in the distribution when observed in the laboratory. If they do, then the findings of laboratory research would still be generalizable to classroom environments, with the simple caution that the incidence of private speech is underestimated. To explore this issue, correlations of classroom private speech with private speech in the laboratory academic and puzzle-solving contexts were computed. Level 3 private speech, the most prevalent form in all three contexts, was strongly correlated between classroom and laboratory academic seatwork, $r(26) = .58$, $p < .05$, a finding that held when correlations were computed separately for LD and control children, $r(12) = .67$, $p < .01$, and $r(12) = .60$, $p < .05$, respectively. In contrast, no form of private speech during laboratory puzzle solving was significantly associated with classroom academic private speech. Furthermore, no child emitted any Level 1 (task-irrelevant) private speech during puzzle solving. Consequently, between-setting correlations for this speech form could not be computed.

Relation of Private Speech to Task-related Behavior and Performance in the Laboratory Seatwork and Puzzle Contexts

Secondary analyses were carried out to determine whether private speech during laboratory academic seatwork and puzzle solving predicted motor accompaniment to task and attention in the same way as they did in the classroom academic setting. Correlations between private speech and behavioral variables in the two laboratory contexts revealed no significant relation for either the total sample or for the separate LD and control groups. The lack of association may have been due to the fact that motor activity and distractibility were substantially reduced when children entered the laboratory. As shown in Table 5, group × setting MANOVAS revealed that children exhibited less self-stimulating and task-facilitating motor activity and greater motor quiescence during puzzle solving. They also displayed greater attentional focus and diminished moderate and diverted attention levels in both laboratory academic seatwork and puzzle contexts than they did in the class-room. The absence of significant group × setting interaction effects indicates that these trends characterize both LD and control subjects.

DISCUSSION

The purpose of this investigation was to examine the development and func-tional significance of private speech among children with learning disabilities. This is an important undertaking, since it has been demonstrated that children's use of task-relevant private speech is positively related to self-controlled behav-ior during problem solving and eventual task success (Berk, 1992). If it can be demonstrated that LD children experience a different pattern of private speech development compared to their nondisabled classmates, then the disparity may account, at least in part, for the academic difficulties associated with learning disabilities. In addition, LD children are among those children with learning problems who have been the focus of cognitive-behavioral interventions designed to induce effective use of private speech during problem solving (Hughes, 1988; Wong, 1985). The application of these procedures relies on the

TABLE 5

Within-Subjects Comparisons of Motor Accompaniment to Task and Attention between Classroom and Laboratory Settings, Expressed in Terms of Percentages of Occurrence

	CLASSROOM SEATWORK		LABORATORY SEATWORK		LABORATORY PUZZLES		CLASSROOM VS. LAB SEATWORK	CLASSROOM VS. PUZZLES
BEHAVIOR	M	SD	M	SD	M	SD	$F(1, 26)$	$F(1, 26)$
Motor accompaniment to task:								
Self-stimulating	95.6	24.4	97.2	26.0	47.2	33.1	.1	58.5**
Task facilitating	13.5	10.1	13.3	19.4	1.0	3.5	1.0	39.1**
No movement	20.2	12.8	21.1	15.8	55.0	30.6	.1	43.9**
Attention level:								
Focused	75.4	13.4	90.4	7.8	96.6	6.1	43.4**	75.5**
Moderate	12.1	5.1	7.1	5.7	2.0	4.5	15.4**	66.1**
Diverted	13.6	11.2	2.3	3.9	.1	.8	31.4**	48.7**

NOTE.—For classroom vs. puzzle-solving motor accompaniment to task, multivariate $F(3, 24) = 14.9$, $p < .01$. For classroom vs. lab seatwork attention level, multivariate $F(3, 24) = 40.7$, $p < .01$. For classroom vs. puzzle-solving attention level, multivariate $F(2, 24) = 26.7$, $p < .01$.
** $p < .01$.

assumption that these children are deficient in the production of task-relevant private speech.

The findings of the current study do not support this premise. On laboratory puzzle tasks, pure LD children did not differ from normally achieving classmates in use of any variety of private speech. In academic seatwork contexts, pure LD children used more (not less) task-relevant externalized speech and an equivalent percentage of the most mature, task-relevant internalized variety.

The incidence of the three types of private speech as well as cross-sectional age trends suggest, in agreement with Hypothesis 1, that LD and normally achieving children undergo a similar course of private speech development. Among pure LDs and controls, Level 2 speech showed the Vygotskian-predicted age-related decline repeatedly found in earlier investigations. In addition, Level 3 speech increased between grades 3 and 4, declined between grades 4 and 5, and then stabilized at a high level for both pure LD and control youngsters. The overall high incidence of private speech provides substantial support for Vygotsky's (1934/1987) assumption that private speech is a universal stage of child development in which thought and speech unite to exert control over problem-solving behavior. In addition, the relative balance of private speech subtypes evidenced by these third through sixth graders is congruent with previous research indicating that the three levels of private speech form a developmental sequence that children traverse from the preschool through late elementary school years (Berk, 1986; Berk & Garvin, 1984; Berk & Potts, 1991; Bivens & Berk, 1990; Kohlberg et al., 1968).

The findings also add to the existing literature supporting Vygotsky's belief that private speech serves the adaptive function of self-regulation. The majority of LD and control children's private utterances were task relevant. Moreover, an examination of the Level 2 specific categories revealed that most were clearly self-regulatory in nature—concentrated in subtypes of describing one's own activity/self-guidance and reading aloud. In addition, Level 2 and 3 speech displayed a number of adaptive relationships with task-relevant behavior. Level 2 speech predicted task-facilitating motor activity for LD children, and Level 3 speech predicted motor quiescence and focused attention for normally achieving control children.

The results also supported Hypothesis 2, that LD children would be delayed in private speech internalization. Pure LD children showed heightened use of Level 2 (externalized, task-relevant) speech during academic seatwork, and this trend was particularly pronounced for the LD/ADHD subsample, which also displayed a reduced incidence of Level 3 speech. These findings contribute to the existing literature indicating that investigations of LD children must consider the inadvertent placement of ADHD children in LD research samples. Failure to do so may result in the attribution of a greater than appropriate deficit to LD children. The current results also indicate that LD children's achievement difficulties are not a function of deficits in the production of task-relevant private speech, as some cognitive-behavioral investigators have assumed (e.g., Harris, 1986). Instead, it is more likely that LD children's poor academic performance results from true ability deficits, which act as tenacious obstacles to task success and lead them to produce more externalized speech in an effort to overcome these obstacles. A number of additional findings lend support to this interpretation.

First, even though Level 3 speech of pure LD children was just as well established as that of controls, it was not as effectively integrated with behavior, confirming Hypothesis 3. During classroom academic seatwork, LD children's Level 3 speech showed nonsignificant relations with motor accompaniment to task and attention. The fact that Level 3 speech did not seem to have the same functional relationship with behavior as it did for normal children may explain why LD children relied significantly more often on the externalized, Level 2 forms.

Second, Level 2 speech was used most often by those LD subjects who also felt a need to support their problem solving with task-relevant externalized gestures, such as pointing while reading and counting on fingers while doing arithmetic problems. This association of Level 2 speech with functionally similar forms of motor behavior has been found repeatedly in research on younger, normally achieving children (Berk, 1986; Berk & Potts, 1991; Bivens & Berk, 1990). However, this relationship did not characterize the control children in this study. Instead, normally achieving subjects displayed functionally adaptive relations between the more mature Level 3 speech and behavior. These findings add further credence to the hypothesis that LD youngsters are delayed in private speech internalization.

Third, Level 2 speech was used most often by those LD/ADHD youngsters who spent the greatest amount of time off task. That such speech is itself not task distracting but, rather, is used by these children in an effort to overcome their attentional difficulties is suggested by the fact that the most prevalent Level 2 fine categories involved describing one's own activity/self-guidance and reading aloud. These forms are not only self-regulating in terms of their content but have consistently been found to correlate positively with task success in other populations (Azmitia, 1992; Behrend et al., 1992; Bivens & Berk, 1990; Gaskill & Diaz, 1991; Roberts, 1979).

Findings from this investigation offer strong evidence that children's use of private speech is setting and task specific. As predicted by Hypothesis 4, children's private speech emitted during the laboratory puzzle task was severely reduced and unrelated to utterances during academic seatwork in both the lab and the classroom. Moreover, verbal and behavioral differences between LD and control children in academic contexts did not generalize to puzzle solving. This result underscores the inappropriateness of drawing conclusions about the self-regulatory capacities of LD children based on activities not directly related to their disabilities (see, e.g., Harris, 1986). Specifically, LD children were not significantly different from normally achieving controls in private speech, task persistence, and problem-solving accuracy while working on puzzles. In contrast, LD-control differences in the classroom tended to be maintained in the laboratory setting if children were engaged in academic seatwork, during which the incidence of private speech was only slightly reduced. Furthermore, classroom and laboratory academic private speech were substantially intercorrelated.

These findings suggest that the creation of analog academic settings in the laboratory offers an ecologically valid way to study elementary school children's private speech under conditions of greater experimental control than is possible in everyday classroom environments. However, laboratory research does reduce the opportunity to examine the relation between private speech and certain task-related behaviors. In this study, elimination of naturally occurring distractors led children to display substantially greater focused attention during laboratory than classroom tasks.

Despite the important theoretical and methodological implications of these results, several limitations of the present study suggest that obtained findings should be accepted with caution. First, because learning disabilities are difficult to identify at younger ages, subjects of mid- and late-elementary school years were used, by which time children's use of externalized private speech has diminished. Future investigations need to focus on children with significant achievement difficulties at younger ages, when private speech is still highly audible and can be scrutinized for possible strategic deficits not revealed by this study. Second, the examination of LD subgroups (LD/ADHD vs. pure LD) was limited by a small sample size. Thus, all findings related to this comparison must be considered tentative until replicated in subsequent research. Moreover, the subgroup of LD/ADHD children was selected on the basis of teacher ratings of classroom behavior. Even though the rating scale employed has considerable validity, it is not comparable to referral status for hyperactivity and the resulting clinical diagnosis of ADHD.

The results of this study have implications for use of cognitive-behavioral training procedures with LD and LD/ADHD children. These treatments have been based on the assumption that academic difficulties experienced by such children are due to a failure to generate effective self-regulatory private speech. However, the present findings contradict such an assumption. In spite of the intuitive appeal of these procedures, research on their efficacy indicates disappointing outcomes. Short-term gains in self-control and performance are apparent on experimental tasks on which children are trained, but these gains fail to generalize to behavioral measures and academic achievement in the classroom (Abikoff, 1991; Diaz, Neal, & Amaya-Williams, 1991; Dush, Hirt, & Shroeder, 1989; Hinshaw & Erhardt,

1991; Meador & Ollendick, 1984; Whalen, Henker, & Hinshaw, 1985). The current findings offer a number of explanations as to why these procedures may not be appropriate for ameliorating the academic problems of children with learning and/or attentional deficits.

First, design of these treatments has not been based on systematic information about these youngsters' spontaneous private speech in academic learning situations. Instead, the conventional wisdom presumes that private speech training is indicated because many of these children are impulsive (i.e., "they don't stop, look, and listen") in academic problem solving or interpersonal situations (Douglas, 1972). However, the consensus of current evidence is that such children already use overt, self-guiding speech to a high degree; they are not, as these interventions assume, deficient in their capacity or willingness to produce self-regulating speech. Second, in a typical cognitive-behavioral program, speech is induced through adult coaching, modeling, and reinforcement, after which the child is directed to subvocalize self-directed statements. Yet insistence of treatment programs that children move quickly in the direction of silent self-communication may be counterproductive. The current study indicates that the learning impairments of these subjects rendered their covert speech less successful in modulating task-related behavior. In this study, and in previous research, children with significant learning problems exhibited heightened dependence on *externalized* private speech as a compensatory measure because their impairments exacerbated obstacles to task success.

Results of this investigation show that LD children—especially those who also display attentional deficits—use task-relevant private speech actively and freely. In view of these preliminary findings, cognitive-behavioral interventions that teach children to talk out loud to themselves while engaged in cognitive tasks may simply be training an already existing skill. Instead, interventions that best meet children's needs may be ones that educate teachers about the functional value of private speech and encourage them to arrange classroom conditions, such as special study corners, that allow children to generate audible self-regulatory speech without disturbing nearby classmates.

REFERENCES

Abikoff, H. (1991). Cognitive training in ADHD children: Less to it than meets the eye. *Journal of Learning Disabilities,* **24,** 205–209.

Azmitia, M. (1992). Expertise, private speech, and the development of self-regulation. In R. M. Diaz & L. E. Berk (Eds.), *Private speech: From social interaction to self-regulation* (pp. 101–122). Hillsdale, NJ: Erlbaum.

Beaudichon, J. (1973). Nature and instrumental function of private speech in problem solving situations. *Merrill-Palmer Quarterly,* **19,** 117–135.

Behrend, D. A., Rosengren, K. S., & Perlmutter, M. (1989). A new look at children's private speech: The effects of age, task difficulty, and parental presence. *International Journal of Behavioral Development, 12,* 305–320.

Behrend, D. A., Rosengren, K. S., & Perlmutter, M. (1992). The relation between private speech and parental interactive style. In R. M. Diaz & L. E. Berk (Eds.), *Private speech: From social interaction to self-regulation* (pp. 85–100). Hillsdale, NJ: Erlbaum.

Berk, L. E. (1986). Relationship of elementary school children's private speech to behavioral accompaniment to task, attention, and task performance. *Developmental Psychology, 22,* 671–680.

Berk, L. E. (1992). Children's private speech: An overview of theory and the status of research. In R. M. Diaz & L. E. Berk (Eds.), *Private speech: From social interaction to self-regulation* (pp. 17–53). Hillsdale, NJ: Erlbaum.

Berk, L. E., & Garvin, R. A. (1984). Development of private speech among low-income Appalachian children. *Developmental Psychology, 20,* 271–286.

Berk, L. E., & Potts, M. (1991). Development and functional significance of private speech among attention-deficit hyperactivity disordered and normal boys. *Journal of Abnormal Child Psychology, 19,* 357–377.

Bivens, J. A., & Berk, L. E. (1990). A longitudinal study of the development of elementary school children's private speech. *Merrill-Palmer Quarterly, 36,* 443–463.

Camp, B. W., Blom, G. E., Herbert, F., & van Doornick, W. J. (1977). "Think Aloud": A program for developing self-control in young aggressive boys. *Journal of Abnormal Child Psychology, 7,* 169–177.

Campbell, S. B. (1973). Cognitive styles in reflective, impulsive, and hyperactive boys and their mothers. *Perceptual and Motor Skills, 36,* 747–752.

Cohen, J. (1960). A coefficient of agreement for nominal scales. *Educational and Psychological Measurement, 20,* 37–46.

Conners, C. K. (1969). A teacher rating scale for use in drug studies with children. *American Journal of Psychiatry, 126,* 885–888.

Copeland, A. P. (1979). Types of private speech produced by hyperactive and nonhyperactive boys. *Journal of Abnormal Child Psychology, 7,* 169–177.

Deutsch, F., & Stein, A. H. (1972). The effects of personal responsibility and task interruption on the private speech of preschoolers. *Human Development, 15,* 310–324.

Diaz, R. M. (1992). Methodological concerns in the study of private speech. In R. M. Diaz & L. E. Berk (Eds.), *Private speech: From social interaction to self-regulation* (pp. 55–81). Hillsdale, NJ: Erlbaum.

Diaz, R. M., & Lowe, J. P. (1987). The private speech of young children at risk: A test of three deficit hypotheses. *Each Childhood Research Quarterly, 2,* 181–194.

Diaz, R. M., Neal, C. J., & Amaya-Williams, M. (1991). The social origins of self-regulation. In L. Moll (Ed.), *Vygotsky and education* (pp. 127–154). New York: Cambridge University Press.

Dickie, J. (1973). Private speech: The effect of presence of others, task and interpersonal variables. *Dissertation Abstracts International, 34,* 1292B. (University Microfilms No. 73-20, 329)

Douglas, V. (1972). Stop, look, and listen: The problem of sustained attention and impulse control in hyperactive and normal children. *Canadian Journal of Behavioral Science,* **4,** 159–182.

Dush, D. M., Hirt, M. L., & Shroeder, H. E. (1989). Self-statement modification in the treatment of child behavior disorders: A meta-analysis. *Psychological Bulletin,* **106,** 97–106.

Frauenglass, M. H., & Diaz, R. M. (1985). Self-regulatory functions of children's private speech: A critical analysis of recent challenges to Vygotsky's theory. *Developmental Psychology,* **21,** 357–364.

Gaskill, M. N., & Diaz, R. M. (1991). The relation between private speech and cognitive performance. *Infancia y Aprendisaje,* **53,** 45–58.

Goodman, S. (1977, April). *A sequential functional analysis of preschool children's private speech.* Paper presented at the biennial meeting of the Society for Research in Child Development, New Orleans.

Goodman, S. (1981). The integration of verbal and motor behavior in preschool children. *Child Development,* **52,** 280–289.

Harris, K. R. (1986). Effects of cognitive-behavior modification on private speech and task performance during problem solving among learning-disabled and normally achieving children. *Journal of Abnormal Child Psychology,* **14,** 63–76.

Hinshaw, S. P., & Erhardt, D. (1991). Attention-deficit hyperactivity disorder. In P. C. Kendall (Ed.), *Child and adolescent therapy: Cognitive-behavioral procedures* (pp. 98–128). New York: Guilford.

Hughes, J. N. (1988). *Cognitive behavior therapy with children in schools.* New York: Pergamon.

Kendall, P. C., & Braswell, L. (1985). *Cognitive-behavioral therapy for impulsive children.* New York: Guilford.

Klein, W. L. (1964). An investigation of the spontaneous speech of children during problem solving. *Dissertation Abstracts International,* **25,** 2031. (University Microfilms No. 64-09, 240)

Kohlberg, L., Yaeger, J., & Hjertholm, E. (1968). Private speech: Four studies and a review of theories. *Child Development,* **39,** 691–736.

Landau, S., Lorch, E. P., & Milich, R. (1992). Visual attention to and comprehension of television in attention-deficit hyperactivity disordered and normal boys. *Child Development,* **63,** 928–937.

Loney, J., & Milich, R. (1982). Hyperactivity, inattention, and aggression in clinic practice. In M. Wolraich & D. Routh (Eds.), *Advances in developmental and behavioral pediatrics* (Vol. **3,** pp. 113–147). Greenwich, CT: JAI.

McGee, R., & Share, D. L. (1988). Attention deficit disorder-hyperactivity and academic failure: Which comes first and what should be treated? *Journal of the American Academy of Child and Adolescent Psychiatry,* **27,** 318–325.

Meador, A. E., & Ollendick, T. H. (1984). Cognitive behavior therapy with children: An evaluation of its efficacy and clinical utility. *Child and Family Behavior Therapy,* **6,** 25–44.

Meichenbaum, D. H., & Goodman, J. (1971). Training impulsive children to talk to themselves: A means of developing self-control. *Journal of Personality and Social Psychology,* **34,** 942–950.

Milich, R., & Fitzgerald, G. (1985). A validation of inattention overactivity and aggression rating with classroom observations. *Journal of Consulting and Clinical Psychology,* **53,** 139–140.

Milich, R., & Landau, S. (1988). Teacher ratings of inattention/overactivity and aggression: Cross-validation with classroom observations. *Journal of Clinical Child Psychology,* **17,** 92–97.

Murray, J. D. (1979). Spontaneous private speech and performance on a delayed match-to-sample task. *Journal of Experimental Child Psychology,* **27,** 286–302.

Palkes, H., Stewart, M., & Kahana, B. (1968). Porteus maze performance of hyperactive boys after training in self-directed verbal commands. *Child Development,* **39,** 817–826.

Pechman, E. (1978). Spontaneous verbalization and motor accompaniment to children's task orientation in elementary classrooms. *Dissertation Abstracts International,* **39,** 786A. (University Microfilms No. 78-05, 964)

Pelham, W. E., Milich, R., Murphy, D. A., & Murphy, H. A. (1989). Normative data on the IOWA Conners Teacher Rating Scale. *Journal of Clinical Child Psychology,* **18,** 259–262.

Roberts, R. N. (1979). Private speech in academic problem-solving: A naturalistic perspective. In G. Zivin (Ed.), *The development of self-regulation through private speech* (pp. 295–323). New York: Wiley.

Sattler, J. M. (1988). *Assessment of children's intelligence and spatial abilities* (3d ed.) San Diego: Sattler.

Vygotsky, L. S. (1987). Thinking and speech. In R. W. Rieber & A. S. Carton (Eds.), N. Minick (Trans.), *The collected works of L. S. Vygotsky: Vol. 1. Problems of general psychology* (pp. 37–285). New York: Plenum. (Original work published 1934)

Whalen, C. K., Henker, B., & Hinshaw, S. P. (1985). Cognitive-behavioral therapies for hyperactive children: Premises, problems, and prospects. *Journal of Abnormal Child Psychology,* **13,** 391–410.

Wong, B. Y. L. (1985). Issues in cognitive-behavioral interventions in academic skill areas. *Journal of Abnormal Child Psychology,* **13,** 425–441.

Zentall, S. S., Gohs, D. E., & Culatta, B. (1983). Language and activity of hyperactive and comparison children during listening tasks. *Exceptional Children,* **50,** 255–266.

Zivin, G. (1979). Removing common confusions about egocentric speech, private speech, and self-regulation. In G. Zivin (Ed.), *The development of self-regulation through private speech* (pp. 13–49). New York: Wiley.

Part V
CLINICAL ISSUES

The precursors of adult psychiatric disorder are of interest and concern to child and adolescent and to adult psychiatrists alike. The first paper in this section narrows the focus to the transition between adolescence and young adulthood. Feehan, McGee, and Williams utilize data deriving from the Dunedin Multidisciplinary Health and Development Study to examine the course of psychiatric disorder between 15 and 18 years of age. In this study, which has focused on the assessment of behavioral and emotional problems in a cohort of children followed from birth, the prevalence of DSM-III disorder was determined for 943 subjects at age 15. Of these, prevalence data for DSM-III-R diagnoses were obtained for 890 (94%) at 18 years of age. Psychiatric disorder during adolescence made a significant contribution to psychiatric status during early adulthood. Of the 191 individuals who had a disorder at age 15, 121 (63%) had a DSM-III-R disorder at age 18, compared with 202 (29%) of the 699 without disorder at age 15. Conduct disorders and depression in combination with anxiety were associated with the highest level of risk. Those with "recurrent disorder" (disorder at both ages) were more symptomatic at both 15 and 18 years of age than were those with "transient disorder" (disorder at 15 but not at 18), or those with "new disorder" (disorder at age 18 only). Disadvantage was strongly associated with recurrent disorder. A discussion of the implication of these prospective findings for both clinical practice and public policy concludes with the recommendation that treatment of older adolescents include a focus on social and educational goals. The suggestion that this approach may significantly lessen the risk of later mental illness deserves serious consideration by all who work with this age group.

The approach to diagnosis exemplified by DSM-III/III-R, which encourages the use of multiple diagnostic categories, has served to sharpen concern about the effects of comorbidity. As Angold and Costello note in the second paper in this section, comorbidity may imfluence our understanding of the etiology, course, and treatment of psychiatric disorder. Their review of epidemiological and clinical studies using standardized interviews and DSM-III/III-R diagnoses provides a useful summary of recent work in the area of childhood depression. In summary, there is a high rate of comorbidity in children and adolescents with major depressive disorders or dysthymia. Comorbidity with conduct disorder/oppositional defiant disorder ranged from 21% to 83%; comorbidity with anxiety disorder ranged from 30% to 75%; and comorbidity with attention deficit disorder ranged from 0% to 57.1% in community studies. These rates were similar to rates of depressive comorbidity found in clinical studies. These comorbid disorders, in almost all instances, were more common in depressed children than would be expected by chance. The authors consider several different interpretations of comorbidity with depression during childhood and adolescence, concluding that the mechanisms by which comorbidity occurs are obscure at present. Given the implications for nosology, epidemiology, and treatment, the authors' proposed approaches to future research merit serious consideration.

In the final paper in this section Pennington, Groisser, and Welch provide a different perspective on the problem of comorbidity. Their report illustrates the utility of a neuropsychological approach to clarifying the causal basis of comorbid developmental reading disability (RD) and attention deficit hyperactivity disorder (ADHD). A thorough review of studies of cognitive processing in these two disorders provides a rationale for the selection of measures of phonologic processes and executive functions. A 2 (RD vs. no RD) $\times$ 2 (ADHD vs. no ADHD) $\times$ 2 (domain type) mixed model design was used to test the hypothesis of a double dissociation between reading disability and attention deficit hyperactivity disorder. Specifically, it was predicted that the RD-only group would demonstrate specific impairments on phonologic processes tasks and that the ADHD-only group would be specifically impaired on measures of executive functions. The results confirmed this hypothesis. Moreover, the comorbid group resembled the RD-only group, a finding supportive of the hypothesis that in comorbid ADHD + RD, the ADHD symptoms are secondary to RD. The authors propose an intriguing hypothetical reconstruction of the developmental course of the prototypical ADHD + RD child that may guide future research in the question of how the various comorbid subtypes of ADHD relate to each other.

14

Mental Health Disorders from Age 15 to Age 18 Years

Michael Feehan, Rob McGee, and Sheila M. Williams

University of Otago Medical School, Dunedin, New Zealand

Objective: *To determine the strength of association between mental health disorders in adolescence and disorder in early adulthood.* **Method:** *The study used mental health data from a longitudinal investigation of a New Zealand birth cohort. Of the 943 with prevalence data for DSM-III disorder at age 15, 890 had prevalence data for DSM-III-R disorder when aged 18 years.* **Results:** *Two-thirds of those with disorder at age 15 had disorder at age 18. The residual form of attention deficit disorder, simple phobias, and oppositional disorders (with no other accompanying disorders) were associated with the lowest risk of later disorder and conduct disorder with the highest. With the exception of the overall symptom level, a variety of characteristics examined (e.g., social competence and adversity) could not differentiate between those with transient disorder and those with disorder at both ages. Comparisons of those with recurring disorder and those with new disorder at age 18 showed that in addition to characteristics of the disorder, disadvantage was strongly associated with recurrent disorder.* **Conclusions:** *The risk of later disorder for those with disorder in adolescence was high and differed across type of disorder.*

Reprinted with permission from the *Journal of the American Academy of Child and Adolescent Psychiatry,* 1993, Vol. 32(6), 1118–1126. Copyright © 1993 by the American Academy of Child and Adolescent Psychiatry.

The DMHDRU is supported by the Health Research Council of New Zealand. Collection of the mental health data at ages 15 and 18 was partially supported by grants to Dr. T. E. Moffitt from the Antisocial and Violent Behavior Branch of the U.S. National Institutes of Mental Health (1-23-MH42723, RO1-MH43746, and RO1-MH45070). The authors are indebted to the many people whose contributions continue to make the longitudinal study possible. Thanks are expressed to Dr. P. A. Silva, Ms. S. Nada Raja, and Professor A. Hornblow (Department of Community Health and General Practice, Christchurch School of Medicine) for their comments on earlier versions of this report.

Findings suggest that to reduce the risk of disorder in early adult-hood, clinicians could play a more active role in community interventions with direct social outcomes.

It is increasingly acknowledged that the associations between mental health disorders in adolescence and disorders in early adulthood should be a research priority. Although calls have been made for a greater application of research and clinical resources to child and adolescent mental health services to reduce longer-term distress and disability (Kosky and Hardy, 1992), the "continuities or otherwise [of adult disorder] with adolescence have not been explored" (Hill, 1989).

Researchers have used the term "continuity" to describe a variety of processes and constructs in the development of an individual's social and emotional behavior. Rutter (1984a) has provided a useful definition of continuity suggesting it can be thought of as a "predictable pattern of associations between event and behaviour at an early stage of development and some type of psychological outcome at a later age." Rutter emphasized the elevations of the risk of having later disorder if one experienced certain life events earlier. The experience of mental health disorder in adolescence may not necessarily lead to disorder in adulthood but it may well elevate an individual's risk. Some authors are quite firm in their support for continuity between early and later disorder. Weiner (1982), for example, considered that "adolescents who manifest obvious signs of behavior disorder rarely outgrow them." A more temperate view has been expressed by Sroufe and Rutter (1984) that although the actual degree of continuity may vary, an underlying coherence to the individual's course of development would still remain.

The recent literature appears to accept in principle the notion of continuity. The debate is essentially one of degree, i.e., "to what extent are disorders continuous?" rather than "are they continuous?" Of interest to researchers and clinicians are the relative strengths of association between different types of disorder from adolescence to adulthood. For example, the degree of continuity between adolescent conduct problems and adult antisocial personality disorder is considered high (Rutter, 1984a, Werry, 1992). However, little or nothing is known about the extent of continuity for the affective and anxiety disorders (Kutcher and Marton, 1989; Kovacs, 1989; Rutter, 1984a; Harrington et al., 1990).

Any empirical evidence for continuity in psychopathology between earlier developmental periods and adulthood has largely derived from studies of clinical samples, often using retrospective methods. Inference about the continuity of psychopathology from retrospective studies of adult samples should be made with some caution. In retrospective designs there may be distortions in reporting or effects of illness on recall, and "the few instances" of prospective studies have used highly selected samples where the generalizability of findings may be difficult (Zeitlin, 1986). As Rutter (1984a) pointed out, studies of adults with antisocial personality disorders have shown that the majority were delinquent or antisocial in childhood, yet most antisocial children do not exhibit antisocial personality in adulthood. Recently, support for the notion of continuity between symptomology in adolescence and in late life has come from the Epidemiologic Catchment Area (ECA) studies (Robins and Regier, 1991). Most adult psychiatric disorders had a reported age of onset for symptoms in adolescence (median of 16 years). The disorders with an earlier reported onset tended to follow a more chronic course and were associated with the most subsequent disability during the productive years.

The optimal research strategy to empirically test for continuities in psychopathology is the prospective longitudinal method (Kashani et al., 1989). Given the considerable difficulties in following a large enough sample of children and adolescents into adulthood, such studies are understandably rare (Rutter, 1984b). The Dunedin Multidisciplinary Health and Development Study (DMHDS) is one such study, having followed a cohort of children from birth to early adulthood. The assessment of behavioral and emotional problems has been a focus of the study since its inception, and assessments of psychopathology using structured interviews and recognized diagnostic criteria have been conducted since preadolescence. The prevalence of disorders of childhood and adolescence using *DSM-III* criteria were estimated at ages 11 (Anderson et al., 1987), 13 (Frost et al., 1989), and 15 years (McGee et al., 1990). When the methods used at age 11 and 15 were equated, it was found that of those preadolescents with any disorder, 42% were identified as having disorder in adolescence. However, the majority (81%) of those with disorder at 15 years did not have a history of disorder at age 11 (McGee et al., 1992). At the most recent assessment at age 18, the prevalence of adult disorders in the sample was estimated using *DSM-III-R* criteria (Feehan et al., in press). The overall prevalence of disorder was estimated to be 37%, and the most prevalent disorders were major depressive episode (17%), alcohol dependence (10%), and social phobia (11%). As in earlier assessments of this sample, there was considerable comorbidity among disorders, with 46% having two or more.

The aim of the present paper is to describe the follow-up of the sample from age 15 to 18 years and to examine the degree of continuity of disorder. The paper is structured around three key questions. First, of those persons with disorder in adolescence, what proportion continued to have disorder in early adulthood? Next, given the information about disorder and the characteristics of the presenting adolescent, is it possible to discriminate between those with transient or recurrent disorders? Finally, can those persons with recurrent disorder be differentiated from those who were identified with disorder only at age 18?

METHOD

Sample

The history of the DMHDS, the characteristics of the sample, and its aims have been described by Silva (1990). In summary, the Dunedin study has followed a cohort of children born between April 1, 1972 and March 31, 1973 at Queen Mary Hospital. From the eligible sample of children at age 3, a total of 1,037 were enrolled in the study. Since then the sample has been followed up and assessed biennially to age 15 and again at age 18. At age 15 (1987 and 1988), 976 members of the sample were followed up. At the age 18 assessment (1990 and 1991), 988 provided information about themselves. Among the remainder there had been 10 deaths, 30 members of the sample had refused to participate or were unavailable, four were untraceable, and five had moderate or severe intellectual disabilities.

Procedures

The general assessment procedures were similar at both assessments. Each sample member was invited to attend the Dunedin Multidisciplinary Health and Development Research Unit for a full day of assessments to be conducted as near as possible to their eighteenth birthday. Descriptions of the individual assessments together with a consent form for their signature were mailed out a few weeks before the intended assessment date. At the age-15 assessment, consent for their participation was also gained from the individual's guardian. Consent also was sought to access medical and other personal records. Transport was provided at each assessment for those who resided outside the Dunedin area. The research topics studied were similar at both assessments and included dental, respiratory, and cardiac health; mental health and illegal behavior; injuries; and alcohol and tobacco use. At both assessments, efforts were made to interview those individuals who could not attend the unit, and a staff member traveled to Australia to interview the members living there. In those instances a shortened interview was administrated that included the mental health and illegal behavior questions.

Measures

Assessment of disorder. At the age-15 assessment each member of the sample was interviewed with a modified version of the Diagnostic Interview Schedule for Children (DISC) (Costello et al., 1982). Disorders were identified using the *DSM-III* classification system for children and adolescents. Given the time constraints on the mental health interview, the assessment was restricted to only the more commonly occurring conditions. McGee et al. (1990) described the procedures used to identify mental health disorders at ·that age.

The identification of disorder at age 18 is described by Feehan et al. (in press). To summarize, the prevalence of the more common disorders of adulthood were determined on the basis of *DSM-III-R* criteria using a structured interview developed for adults: the Diagnostic Interview Schedule, version three-revised (DIS-III-R; Robins et al., 1989). The instrument was modified by M.F. and R.M. to meet the requirements of the longitudinal study while retaining as far as possible the actual wording of the questions. The principal modifications involved restricting the onset and recency questions to provide for only a 1-year prevalence estimate, using only those questions that provided for *DSM-III-R* classifications, and adjusting for differences in United States and New Zealand idiom. An additional modification involved assessing depressive symptoms in a fashion comparable with age 15. Major depressive episodes and dysthymia were assessed in two separate sets of questions.

Identification of mental health disorder was based on symptom reports (1) meeting the requisite criteria and (2) being associated with at least some reported impairment in life functioning (on a five-point rating scale), police contact, or help-seeking. This conservative approach to the identification of disorder is in accord with Wakefield's argument (1992) that disorder should be considered as a "harmful dysfunction" and with Bird et al.'s view (1990) that disorder should be related to severity, a need for services, or distress.

The classification of conduct disorder at age 15 was made with items from a 30-item self-report delinquency scale (Moffitt and Silva, 1988) included in the mental health interview. At age 18, the items used to identify conduct disorder came from the Denver Youth Survey Youth Interview Schedule (Huizinga, 1989) administered in a separate interview. At each assessment these items were scored to be compatible with the scoring used in the diagnostic interviews. At the age-18 assessment, the illegal behavior interview had a slightly different response rate than did the mental health interview. Prevalence estimates were only determined for the sample with both sets of data.

At age 15, four symptom scale scores were derived from the diagnostic interview. These comprised an anxiety scale, a depression scale, a conduct disorder scale, and a scale for impulsivity and hyperactivity (Williams et al., 1989). At the age-18 assessment scores for anxiety, depression, conduct disorder, and substance use were derived from the sum of scores of items for each of the major disorder types.

Retest reliability estimates were determined by reinterviewing a group of sample members approximately 2 months after their initial interview. The κ obtained for the diagnostic classifications and the intraclass correlations of the symptom scores indicated the interview had good reliability (Feehan et al., in press). The mental health interviews were completed by five interviewers, all with postgraduate qualifications in psychology. The proportions of the sample identified with disorder for each interviewer were not significantly different. Classifications of disorder were made by the *principal* investigators, blind to the diagnostic status at age 15 years.

Suicidal ideation was assessed at age 15 in the section of the interview pertaining to depressive disorders. Only those members of the sample who responded affirmatively to an initial gate for depressed mood were asked whether they had thought of killing themselves in the last year. Similarly, at the age-18 assessment, this question was asked of those who responded positively to the initial gating questions for depressive disorders. However, it also was asked at the close of the interview of all those who had not completed the depressive assessment, giving the opportunity for all those interviewed to respond.

Significant other report. At the age-15 assessment, parental reports of their children's mental health were obtained with the Revised Behavior Problem Checklist (RBPC) (Quay and Peterson, 1987) together with supplementary questions assessing whether they thought their child had significant behavioral or emotional problems, had police contact, or whether they had sought help or advice for their child. This information was used primarily to "confirm" adolescent self-reports of disorder using criteria described in McGee et al. (1990).

At age 18, reports about each individual's mental health were obtained through a questionnaire mailed to a "significant other" nominated by the 18-year-old. Twelve emotional/behavioral problem items were rated as "no doesn't apply," "yes, applies somewhat," and "yes, applies certainly." For the 930 with complete mental health data, 830 complete questionnaires were returned (89%). Of those, half were completed by a parent and 30% by a close friend. Confirmation of disorder by the significant others is described fully in Feehan et al. (in press). In summary, disorders were confirmed if (1) there was a one-to-one correspondence between an item and a type of disorder, e.g., the sample member was considered to be a major depressive episode and the significant other scored the item "feeling depressed, miserable sad, or unhappy" as "yes, certainly applies;" and (2) the sample member had an internalizing (or externalizing) disorder and he or she scored greater than 1.5 standard deviations above the mean on a scale made up of the internalizing items (or externalizing items) from the problem behavior questionnaire.

Help-seeking. Self-reported seeking-help for behavioral or emotional problems was assessed at age 15 with the item "in the last year, have you sought help or advice from someone other than family or friends? (such as Youthline, school counselor, a doctor, or a teacher)." At age 18 the assessment of help seeking was divided into health-related and other agencies. Respondents were asked if they had "gone to a doctor or other health professional, e.g., general practitioner, psychiatrist, psychologist, or counselor" about mental health problems during the last year. They were similarly asked if they had gone to "anyone else, e.g., a self-help group, minister, telephone counselor, or Department of Social Welfare."

Social competence. Social competence was measured using two comparable indices at ages 15 and 18. At age 15 the index was made up of seven composite scores pertaining to self-perceived strengths (Williams and McGee, 1991), level of recreational activity, part-time work, social support and coping, and attachment to parents, peers, and school. With the exception of part-time work (scored as 0 or 1), each score was coded as 0, 1, or 2 indicating low, medium, and high levels of competence based on each measure's distribution (McGee and Williams, 1991). At age 18 the index did not include part-time work. Also, to shorten administration time, visual analogue scales were used to determine attachment to peers and parents as was done with school attachment at age 15. These scales replaced the shortened form of the Inventory of Parent and Peer Attachment used at age 15 (Armsden and Greenberg, 1987; Nada Raja et al., 1992). The maximum scores were thus 13 and 12, at ages 15 and 18, respectively.

A six-point index of family disadvantage was developed from a parental questionnaire completed at the age-15 assessment. Each item was coded as 0 or 1 based on their distributions, with 1 indicating disadvantage. The items were family socioeconomic status (Elley and Irving, 1976; Irving and Elley, 1977); mother's mental health, principally depression (McGee et al., 1983); family size, parental separations, solo parenting, and family social support, measured with the Family Relations Index derived from subscales of the Family Environment Scale of Holahan and Moos (1983).

At age 18, a five-point index of disadvantage was developed based on the sample member's self-report (Feehan et al., in press). Each of the following was scored as 1 if present: left school with less than 3 years secondary schooling, having no academic qualifications, self-perceived difficulty in supporting themselves financially, the sample member (or their partner) having or expecting a dependent child, and being currently unemployed.

Health ratings. Self-report of health status was obtained at age 15 and at age 18 with a four-point rating scale. The interviewees were asked "how would you rate your overall health?" and could respond with "very good," "good," "not too good" and "poor." Ratings of poor and not too good were used to indicate perceived poor health.

This measure also was included in the retest interviews. Of the 49 persons with retest data, only two reported good health at one interview and poor health at another, indicating excellent reliability ($\chi^2 = 2.0$, 1 *df*, $p > 0.05$) using McNemar's test (Everitt, 1977).

Reading ability. At both ages 15 and 18, reading ability was assessed with the Burt Word Reading Test, 1974 revision (Scottish Council for Research in

Education, 1976). This measure has been administered at each assessment after age 7 (Silva et al., 1987).

Life-stress. Sources of distress at age 15 were assessed with the 20-item "feel bad" scale (Lewis et al., 1984). This scale comprises commonly occurring events such as "not getting along with your teacher," rated on a five-point frequency scale ranging from 0, never, to 4, all the time. Each indicated item is then rated for intensity of distress experienced ("how bad did it make you feel"), on a scale from 0, not bad, to 4, "terrible." Two scores were then obtained: a sum of the number of sources of distress experienced and the total distress reported (McGee and Stanton, 1992). An assessment of life-stress was not conducted at age 18.

RESULTS

Follow-up from Ages 15 to 18 Years

At age 15 years, 943 individuals provided the mental health data from which the prevalence estimates for disorder were made. At age 18, complete data for the identification of disorder were obtained from 930 members of the sample. Of these, 890 (96%) had disorder data at both assessments. This represents 86% of the sample assessed at age 3 years, or 87% of those known to be alive at age 18.

At age 15 years, 207 individuals were judged to have at least one *DSM-III* disorder. At age 18 years, 191 of these were followed up (92%). This was less than the proportion of those without disorder who were followed up (95%), but the difference was not statistically significant. Similarly, the gender ratio of those followed up was not significantly different from the gender ratio of those not seen.

In addition to examining the follow-up rates for males and females and for those with and without disorder to determine if there was a nonresponse bias in the data, those followed up were compared with those missed on symptom scores. The age 15 symptom scale scores (anxiety, depression, conduct disorder, or attention deficit) of the 53 individuals without age 18 disorder data were compared with the scores of those followed up. Student *t*-tests indicated the differences between the means were not significant. Similarly, when the symptom scores at age 18 were compared for those followed up with the 40 individuals without disorder data at age 15, the means for each scale (anxiety, depression, conduct disorder, and substance dependence) were also not significantly different.

What Proportion Continued to Have Disorder in Early Adulthood?

Among the 890 with prevalence data at both ages, those with disorder at age 15 were twice as likely to have a *DSM-III-R* disorder at age 18 than were those without disorder in adolescence ($\chi^2 = 75.5$, 1 *df*, $p < 0.001$). Of the 191 individuals with any *DSM-III* disorder at age 15, 121 (63%) had a *DSM-III-R* disorder at age 18, compared with 202 (29%) of the 699 without disorder at age 15.

To examine differences across types of disorder at age 15, the mutually exclusive *DSM-III* disorder groups identified by McGee et al. (1990) were used. These groups are reproduced in Table 1, along with the proportion of each with a *DSM-III-R* disorder at age 18.

The majority of disorder groups were associated with elevated rates of later disorder compared with the no-disorder group at age 15. However, post hoc chi-square tests indicated that the attention deficit disorder (ADD) residual, simple phobia and oppositional groups were not significantly different from those without disorder at age 15. Within each of the remaining disorder groups at least two-thirds had a disorder at age 18, significantly more than the proportion of those without disorder at age 15 ($\chi^2 > 8.0$, 1 *df*, $p < 0.005$ for each test). The aggressive and nonaggressive conduct disorder groups, along with the depression in combination with anxiety group, were associated with the highest rates of later disorder. Within the group who had only one anxiety disorder in adolescence, the proportions of those with separation anxiety ($n = 31$), overanxious disorder ($n = 8$), or social phobia ($n = 5$) who went on to have later disorder were similar, 68%, 63%, and 60%, respectively.

Examination of Table 1 indicated that the externalizing disorders at age 15 (conduct disorder, oppositional, ADD, and multiple disorders) were associated with both internalizing (depressive and anxiety disorders) and externalizing (conduct disorder and substance dependence) disorder types at age 18 whereas the internalizing disorders showed somewhat more specificity. Those with depression and/or anxiety at age 15 appeared more likely to develop internalizing as opposed to externalizing disorders at age 18.

This became clearer when the age 15 disorder groups were combined into the internalizing, externalizing and multiple disorder groups (those with both internalizing and externalizing disorders). The same procedure was conducted with the disorder types at age 18, with substance-dependence disorders considered as externalizing. As shown in Table 2, although the proportions of each disorder group at 15 who went on to have disorder at 18 were very similar (around two thirds), there were clear differences in the patterns of later disorder. Internalizing disorder at 15 was more likely to be associated with later internalizing disorder.

Different age 18 outcomes for those with internalizing and externalizing disorders at age 15 were also evident when symptom scores (as opposed to classifications) were examined. Figure 1 illustrates the mean anxiety, depression, substance dependence, and conduct disorder symptom scores at age 18, for each principal disorder group at age 15. The scores obtained by the multiple disorder group ($n = 24$) were associated with very large confidence intervals and they were included among those with externalizing disorder.

TABLE 1
Follow-up of Age 15 DSM-III Disorder

DSM-III Disorder at Age 15	N	Depression	Anxiety	Depression + Anxiety	Conduct Disorder	Substance Dependence	Substance Dependence + Conduct Disorder	Multiple Disorder	Total with disorder N	Total with disorder %
Multiple	24	1	0	3	3	0	2	7	16	66.7
CD,[a] aggressive	10	0	1	0	1	0	3	3	8	80.0
CD, nonaggressive	33	4	5	4	1	6	2	1	23	69.7
Oppositional	13	0	1	1	1	1	1	2	7	53.8
ADD,[b] residual	11	0	1	0	1	0	1	1	4	36.4
Depression	13	2	1	2	0	1	0	3	9	69.2
Depression + anxiety	11	3	1	2	0	0	0	2	8	72.7
Multiple anxiety	15	0	3	3	0	0	0	4	10	66.7
Anxiety	44	4	11	6	1	2	1	4	29	65.9
Simple phobia[c]	17	1	2	3	0	0	0	1	7	41.2
No disorder	699	50	56	27	7	27	7	28	202	28.9

*The total number (and percentage) in each age 15 disorder group with DSM-III-R disorder at age 18 are presented along with the numbers with each later disorder type. Total N = 890.
[a]CD = conduct disorder.
[b]ADD = attention deficit disorder.
[c]Social phobia included in the anxiety groups.

TABLE 2
DSM-III Disorders at Age 15 and Percentage with Internalizing, Externalizing, or Multiple DSM-III-R Disorders at Age 18

Disorder at Age 15	N	None %	Internalizing %	Externalizing %	Multiple %
Internalizing	100	37.0	44.0	5.0	14.0
Externalizing	67	37.3	25.4	26.9	10.4
Multiple	24	33.3	16.7	20.1	29.2

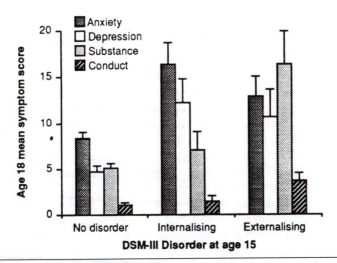

Figure 1. Mean symptom scores at age 18 by disorder status at age 15: no disorder, internalizing disorder, or externalizing disorder. Each mean is presented with its 95% upper confidence interval.

Four analyses of variance (ANOVA) were used to test for significance between the group means on each scale. The main effect for group (no disorder, internalizing and externalizing) was significant for each scale, F *(2,884) > 36.0*, $p < 0.001$, in each analysis. Post hoc Scheffe comparisons indicated that the internalizing group's mean anxiety score was significantly greater than that of the externalizing group ($p < 0.05$), but the mean depression scores did not differ significantly.

For the substance and conduct scales, the significant main group effects were because of elevated scores in the externalizing disorder group. The post hoc comparisons showed the mean substance and conduct scores were not significantly different in the internalizing and no-disorder groups.

Gender had no significant effect on the findings for the depression and anxiety scores, but the group × sex interaction was significant for both the substance and conduct scales ($p < 0.001$ in each analysis). The mean scores obtained by males in the externalizing group (21.5 for substance, 5.7 for conduct) were significantly higher than the mean scores obtained by females (11.3 for substance and 1.6 for conduct).

Is It Possible to Differentiate Between Those with Transient or Recurrent Disorders?

Among those with disorder at age 15, two groups were identified: those who had "recurrent" disorder, i.e., disorder at both ages 15 and 18 ($n = 121$) and those with "transient" disorder who did not go on to have disorder at the later assessment ($n = 70$). When the disorder groups at 15 (Table 1) were examined, 36% of those in the ADD-residual group, 41% of the simple phobia group, and 54% of the oppositional group had recurrent disorder. In the remaining groups the proportion with recurrent disorder ranged from 66% in the anxiety group to 80% in the aggressive conduct disorder group.

It remained possible that although those with transient disorder did not meet criteria for later disorder, they still may have had markedly elevated symptom scores at age 18. To test this hypothesis the mean anxiety, depression, substance, and conduct disorder symptom scores for the four possible disorder groups over the two ages were compared. The mean scores for those with recurrent disorder, transient disorder, no disorder at both ages ($n = 497$) and those with "new disorder" ($n = 202$) are shown in Figure 2. The symptom scores for those with recurrent disorder were clearly the highest, followed by those with new disorder and then by those with transient disorder.

When the mean symptom scores of the transient group were compared with the

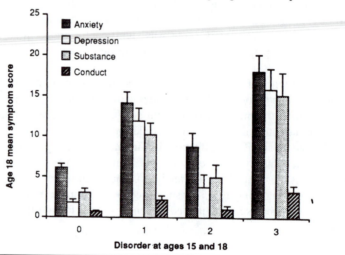

Figure 2. Mean symptom scores at age 18 by disorder groups from age 15 to 18: 0, no disorder at both ages; 1, "new disorder," disorder at age 18 only; 2, "transient," disorder at 15 but not at 18; and 3, "recurrent," disorder at both ages. Each mean is presented with its 95% upper confidence interval.

scores of the 497 without disorder at either age, each of the transient disorder scores were significantly elevated, although, as shown in Figure 2, the differences were small. The total symptom score mean of the transient group was 18.6, and the mean of the no disorder group was 11.7, a statistically significant difference ($t = 5.3$, $df = 565$, $p < 0.001$). However, the difference between the means of 6.9 is less than half a standard deviation unit of the total score and may not be clinically significant.

A series of univariate analyses were conducted using the age-15 assessment data to determine if those with transient disorder could be differentiated from those with recurrent disorder on either disorder or background characteristics. When all four age 15 symptom scales were combined, the mean total score for the recurrent group was significantly greater than the mean for the transient group, 51.1 and 41.3, respectively ($t = 3.4$, $df = 189$, $p < 0.01$) However, the proportions of each group with one, two, or three or more disorders were not significantly different. Other disorder characteristics were also not significantly different between the groups: having an externalizing disorder; having disorder confirmed by a parent; and reporting suicidal ideation.

No significant differences were found between the groups on any of the various background characteristics examined: being male, seeking help for emotional problems, family adversity levels of none, one, or two or more, social competence, poor self-rated health, number of life stress events in the previous year, life stress intensity score, and reading ability.

Are the Disorders Arising in Early Adulthood Different?

As illustrated in Figure 3, those individuals with recurrent disorder had the highest symptom scores at age 15, followed by those with transient disorder. Those with new disorder (i.e., at age 18 only) appeared to have slightly elevated symptom scores compared with the no-disorder group. The mean total score at age 15 for the new disorder group was 22.3 and 15.6 for the no-disorder group. The difference between the means (6.7) was statistically significant ($t = 8.5$, $df = 680$, $p < 0.001$) but was less than half a standard deviation unit of the total score and may not be clinically meaningful.

A series of analyses was conducted to see if those with recurrent disorder could be discriminated from those with new disorder on the age 18 variables. First, the type of disorder at age 18 shown by the two groups was examined. Those with recurrent disorder were more likely to have disorders of the multiple type (i.e., both internalizing and externalizing), and those with new disorder at age 18 were more likely to have internalizing disorder. Of the recurrent disorder group, 23% had multiple disorders, 23% had externalizing disorders only, and 54% had internalizing disorders only. These figures compared with 14%, 20%, and 66%,

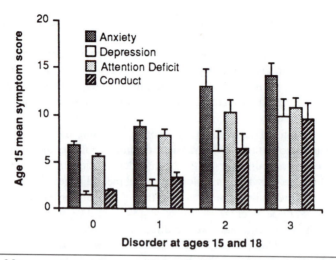

Figure 3. Mean symptom scores at age 15 by disorder groups from age 15 to 18: 0, no disorder at both ages; 1, "new disorder," disorder at age 18 only; 2, "transient," disorder at 15 but not at 18; and 3, "recurrent," disorder at both ages. Each mean is presented with its 95% upper confidence interval.

respectively, in the new disorder groups. These differences almost reached statistical significance ($\chi^2 = 5.9$, 2 *df*, $p = 0.053$).

As seen in Figure 2, those with recurrent disorder had the highest age-18 symptom scale scores. When these scales were combined into a total symptom score, the mean for the recurrent group was significantly greater than the mean score for the new disorder group, 52.4 and 38.4, respectively ($t = 2.9$, *df* = 321, $p < 0.001$). The number of disorders within each group was significantly different with 36% of the recurrent group having three or more compared with 14% of the new disorder group ($\chi^2 = 21.9$, 2 *df*, $p < 0.001$). Those with recurrent disorder were also more likely to have an externalizing disorder, 46% as opposed to 34% in the new disorder group ($\chi^2 = 4.2$, 1 *df*, $p < 0.05$). The proportions of each group who reported suicidal ideation were not significantly different as were the proportions who had made an attempt. Among those with significant other data (176 of the new disorder group and 100 of the recurrent group), the proportion with disorder recognized in the recurrent group was significantly greater than the proportion in the new disorder group, 38% and 22%, respectively ($\chi^2 = 8.6$, 1 *df*, $p < 0.01$).

Differences between the two groups were not significant for gender, seeking help from professionals, seeking help from others, social competence, and reading ability. Those with recurrent disorder were more likely to report poor levels of physical health, 21% compared with 11% ($\chi^2 = 4.4$, 1 *df*, $p < 0.05$) and higher levels of disadvantage ($\chi^2 < 10.5$, 2 *df*, $p < 0.01$). In the recurrent disorder group, 46% had no disadvantage, 30% a level of one, and 24% a level of two or more (compared with 66%, 18%, and 16%, respectively, in the new-disorder group). Although those with recurrent disorder were more likely to report each element of the disadvantage index (including unemployment, less than 3 years secondary schooling, and difficulty supporting self financially), the significant effect for disadvantage was largely owing to have no school qualifications (22% of the recurrent group and 12% of the new-disorder group) or having a dependent child (9% and 4%, respectively).

A logistic regression analysis was carried out to determine whether disadvantage and health status would continue to discriminate between the groups when the effects of disorder were taken into account. The total symptom score was divided into five levels on the basis of quintiles. The unadjusted odds ratio (OR) that those in the upper 20% would have a recurrent disorder was 4.1 [95% confidence interval (CI) 1.6 to 10.7]. The OR for those with three or more disorders was 4.9 (95% CI 2.3 to 10.6), whereas that for an externalizing disorder was 1.7 (95% CI 1.0 to 2.6). The OR associated with poor health was 2.0 (95% CI 1.0 to 3.8), but when this was added to a model that already included the number of disorders, the change in variance was not significant. The OR for any disadvantage was 2.2 (95% CI 1.4 to 3.5). When entered in a model that included the number of disorders, the OR was 1.7 (95% CI 1.1 to 2.9).

A separate logistic regression analysis was conducted for those with significant-other data. In this case the OR of having recurrent disorder if disorder was confirmed by a significant other was 1.5 (95% CI 1.1 to 2.0). This became 1.4 (95% CI 1.1 to 1.9) after adjusting for the number of disorders.

DISCUSSION

Several features of the study give the authors a degree of confidence that the data obtained are adequate to examine the association between adolescent and early adult disorder including the nature of the sample (i.e., an unselected birth cohort), the excellent follow-up rate obtained, the lack of any significant differences for either gender or psychopathology between those followed-up and those not, the use of reliable structured interviews to assess symptomatology, and the cautious approach used to define disorder at each age.

In summary, there was considerable continuity of disorder from age 15 to age 18 years: 63% of the adolescents with *DSM-III* disorder also had *DSM-III-R* disorder at age 18 (14% of the sample). Although a third of those with disorder at age 15 did not have recurrent disorder, they represent only 8% of the sample. The majority of those with disorder at age 18 (also 63%) did not have a history of disorder at age 15 (23% of the sample). The degree of continuity between adolescence and early adulthood appears somewhat greater than between preadolescence and adolescence. In the Dunedin study, 42% of those with disorder at age 11 went on to have disorder at age 15, but 81% of those with disorder at age 15 did not have a history of preadolescent disorder (McGee et al., 1992).

The disorders at age 15 associated most strongly with the presence of disorder at age 18 were the conduct disorders and depression in combination with anxiety. The disorders with the weakest associations with subsequent disorder were simple phobias, oppositional disorder, and the residual form of ADD. It should be noted these are disorders in isolation. The multiple disorder group at age 15 (strongly associated with later disorder) contained several individuals with ADD or ADD-residual in combination with other disorders. There was also a high degree of specificity between disorder types at both ages, with internalizing disorders more likely to be associated with later internalizing disorder and the same for externalizing disorder. This was also evident in the symptom scores. Those with internalizing disorder at age 15 had higher age 18 anxiety scores (although not depression scores) than did those with externalizing disorder at age 15. Similarly, the conduct and substance use scores were higher for those with externalizing disorder than those with internalizing disorder at age 15.

Of particular interest to the practicing clinician may be the findings relating to the differentiation of adolescents with transient or recurrent disorder. Although statistically significant, the age-18 outcome scores of those with transient disorder were not dramatically different from the scores of those without disorder at either age. Their scores were considerably less than those with either recurrent disorder or even those with new disorder at age 18. Given the comparatively good prognosis for the transient group, it may be desirable if clinicians could identify at assessment those most likely to be at less risk. As Robins and Rutter (1990, p. xiv) pointed out, "trying to separate behavior-disordered children into those who will and those who will not recover has proved difficult." In the present study, the only features that discriminated between the two groups were some of the disorder characteristics themselves. The transient group were more likely to have simple phobias, ADD-residual symptoms, or oppositional disorders at age 15, and those with recurrent disorder had higher overall symptom levels. The degree of comorbidity did not discriminate between the groups nor did any of the background characteristics examined. This would imply that when faced with disordered adolescents, the efforts of clinicians may best be directed at the presenting symptoms if the risk of later disorder is to be reduced. However, the findings relating to the discrimination of those with recurrent disorder and new disorder at 18 may be more promising for those interested in prevention.

At age 18, those with recurrent disorder could be clearly differentiated from those with disorder arising at age 18 on a number of variables. The recurrent disorder group had higher presenting symptom scores, were more likely to have externalizing disorders, to have three or more disorders, and to have disorder recognized by a significant other. The major characteristic associated with disorder that could discriminate the two groups was self-reported disadvantage. The effects of disadvantage were evident even when the disorder characteristics were taken into consideration. The measure of disadvantage used in the present study was to some extent based on major life-events that may have occurred in the transition period from age 15 to age 18. These included having a child and leaving school with no formal qualifications. These findings lead to the conclusion that prevention strategies emphasizing social intervention may reduce the likelihood of persistence of disorder from late adolescence to the early adult years. Intervention with enhancing qualifications as the target outcomes may have direct benefits in terms of reduced psychopathology in the community. The same also may be possible for interventions that aim to prevent young motherhood or fatherhood or which are directed to increasing support for young parents.

The findings of the present study suggest two approaches that clinicians interested in reducing the likelihood of mental health disorder in early adulthood might take. First, in the area of secondary prevention, develop effective methods in the identification and treatment of those individuals likely to have disorders with the poorest prognosis in terms of increased risk of later disorder (conduct disorders and multiple internalizing disorders). More attention perhaps could be directed to research investigating the referral pathways and barriers to care (both perceived and actual) for adolescents and to the formulation of screening processes whereby at-risk individuals can be identified and helped into those pathways.

With regard to primary prevention, clinicians should be encouraged to extend their treatment skills beyond those required to deal with single cases or small groups and beyond the amelioration of symptoms as an intervention goal. Cowan (1973) criticized mental health professionals as being "far more concerned with the moment-to-moment effectiveness of their actions than with abstract, removed issues such as the overall good of individually useful but socially limited intervention." Almost two decades later, apparently little has changed: "most mental health personnel do not conceive of their role as including responsibility for influencing social policy" (Swift and Wierich, 1987). Jason (1991) has suggested that even specialist "community psychologists" have devoted more time to descriptive rather than interventive approaches because "the larger social issues appear so overwhelming and intractable." If this is so for those specifically trained to work in the area, one can understand a reluctance of practicing clinicians to address social issues. Nevertheless, psychiatrists and psychologists do have considerable expertise in facilitating individual behavior change. Future research should be directed to the development and evaluation of problem formulations and resultant interventions, whereby the unique skills of mental health professionals are applied directly to social goals (such as the reduction of disadvantage among adolescents). Kosky and Hardy (1992) have called for significant shifts of resources to adolescent mental health services to reduce the toll of later mental illness. Our findings suggest that if existing mental health services broadened their conceptual outlook to include social and educational goals for this age group, resultant interventions may significantly lessen the risk of later mental illness.

REFERENCES

Anderson, J. C., Williams, S., McGee, R. & Silva, P. A. (1987), *DSM-III* disorders in pre-adolescent children: prevalence in a large sample from the general population. *Arch. Gen. Psychiatry,* 44:69–76.

Armsden, G. C. & Greenberg, M. T. (1987), The inventory of parent and peer attachment: individual differences and their relationship to psychological well-being in adolescence. *Journal of Youth and Adolescence,* 16:427–453.

Bird, H. R., Yager, T. J., Staghezza, B., Gould, M. S., Canino, G. & Rubio-Stipec, M. (1990), Impairment in the epidemiological measurement of childhood psychopathology in the community. *J. Am. Acad. Child Adolesc. Psychiatry,* 29:796–803.

Cowen, E. L. (1973), Social and community interventions. *Annu. Rev. of Psychol.,* 24:423–472.

Costello, A., Edelbrock, C., Kalas, R., Kessler, M. & Klaric, S. A. (1982), *Diagnostic Interview Schedule for Children (DISC).* Contract RFP-DB-81-0027. Bethesda, MD: National Institute of Mental Health.

Elley, W. B. & Irving, J. C. (1976), Revised socio-economic index for New Zealand. *New Zealand Journal of Educational Studies,* 11:25–36.

Everitt, B. S. (1977), *The Analysis of Contingency Tables.* London: Chapman and Hall.

Feehan, M., McGee, R., Nada Raja, S. & Williams, S. M. (in press), *DSM-III-R* disorders in New Zealand 18-year-olds. *Aust. N.Z. J. Psychiatry.*

Frost, L. A., Moffitt, T. E. & McGee, R. (1989), Neuropsychological correlates of psychopathology in an unselected cohort of young adolescents. *J. Abnorm. Psychol.,* 98:307–313.

Harrington, R., Fudge, H., Rutter, M., Pickles, A. & Hill, J. (1990), Adult outcomes of childhood and adolescent depression. *Arch. Gen. Psychiatry,* 47:465–473.

Hill, P. (1989). *Adolescent Psychiatry.* Edinburgh: Churchill Livingstone.

Holahan, C. J. & Moos, R. H. (1983). The quality of social support: measures of family and work relationships. *Br. J. Clin. Psychol.,* 22:157–162.

Huizinga, D. (1989), *Denver Youth Survey Youth Interview Schedule.* Boulder, CO: University of Colorado, Institute of Behavioral Science.

Irving, J. C. & Elley, W. B. (1977), A socio-economic Index for the female labour force in New Zealand. *New Zealand Journal of Educational Studies,* 12:154–163.

Jason, L. A. (1991), Participating in social change: a fundamental value for our discipline. *Am. J. Community Psychol.,* 19:1–16.

Kashani, J. D., Orvaschel, H., Rosenberg, T. K. & Reid, J. C. (1989), Psychopathology in a community sample of children and adolescents. *J. Am. Acad. Child Adolesc. Psychiatry,* 28:701–706.

Kosky, R. & Hardy, J. (1992), Mental health: is early intervention the key? *Med. J. Aust,* 156:147–148.

Kovacs, M. (1989), Affective disorders in children and adolescents. *Am. Psychologist,* 44:209–215.

Kutcher, S. P. & Marton, P. (1989), Parameters of adolescent depression. *Psychiatric Clin. North Am.,* 12:895–918.

Lewis, C. E., Siegel, J. M. & Lewis, M. A. (1984), Feeling bad: exploring sources of distress among pre-adolescent children. *Am. J. Public Health,* 74:117–122.

McGee, R., Feehan, M., Williams, S. and Anderson, J. (1992), *DSM-III* disorders from age 11 to age 15 years. *J. Am. Acad. Child Adolesc. Psychiatry,* 31:50–59.

McGee, R., Feehan, M., Williams, S. M., Partridge, F., Silva, P. A. & Kelly, J. (1990), *DSM-III* disorders in a large sample of adolescents. *J. Am. Acad. Child Adolesc. Psychiatry,* 29:611–619.

McGee, R. & Stanton, W. R. (1992), Sources of distress among New Zealand adolescents. *J. Child Psychol. Psychiatry,* 33:999–1010.

McGee, R. & Williams, S. (1991), Social competence in adolescence: preliminary findings from a longitudinal study of New Zealand 15-year-olds. *Psychiatry,* 54:281–291.

McGee, R., Williams, S., Kashani J. H. & Silva, P. A. (1983), Prevalence of self-reported depressive symptoms and associated social factors in mothers in Dunedin. *Br. J. Psychiatry,* 143:473–479.

Moffitt, T. E. & Silva, P. A. (1988), Self-reported delinquency: results from an instrument for New Zealand. *Australian and New Zealand Journal of Criminology,* 21:227–240.

Nada Raja, S., McGee, R. & Stanton, W. R. (1992), Perceived attachments to parents and peers and psychological well-being in adolescence. *Journal of Youth and Adolescence,* 21:471–485.

Quay, H. C. & Peterson, D. R. (1987), *Manual for the Revised Behavior Problem Checklist.* Miami: H. C. Quay & D. R. Peterson.

Robins, L. N., Helzer, J. E., Cottler, L. & Goldring, E. (1989), *NIMH Diagnostic Interview Schedule: Version III Revised.* Written under contract to the NIMH.

Robins, L. N. & Regier, D. A. eds. (1991). *Psychiatric Disorders in America.* New York: The Free Press.

Robins, L. N. & Rutter, M. eds. (1990). *Straight and Devious Pathways from Childhood to Adulthood.* New York: The Free Press.

Rutter, M. (1984a), Continuities and Discontinuities in socioemotional development. In: *Continuities and Discontinuities in Development,* eds: R. N. Emde & R. D. Harmon. New York: Plenum Press.

Rutter, M. (1984b), Psychopathology and development: I. Childhood antecedents of adult psychiatric disorder. *Aust. N.A. J. Psychiatry,* 18:225–234.

Scottish Council for Research in Education. (1976), *The Burt Word Reading Test, 1974 Revision.* London: Hodder and Stoughton.

Silva, P. A. (1990), The Dunedin Multidisciplinary Health and Development Study: A 15-year longitudinal study. *Paediatr. Perinat. Epidemiol.* 4:76–107.

Silva, P. A., Williams, S. & McGee, R. (1987), A longitudinal study of children with developmental language delay at age three: later intelligence, reading and behavior problems. *Dev. Med. Child Neurol.*, 29:630–640.

Sroufe, L. A., & Rutter, M. (1984), The domain of developmental psychopathology. *Child Dev.*, 55:17–29.

Swift, M. & Weirich, T. W. (1987), Prevention planning as social and organizational change. In: *Prevention Planning in Mental Health,* eds: J. Hermalin and J. A. Morell. Beverly Hills, CA: Sage Publications Inc.

Wakefield, J. C. (1992), The concept of mental disorder: on the boundary between biological facts and social values. *Am. Psychol.* 47:373–388.

Weiner, I. B. (1982), *Child and Adolescent Psychopathology.* New York: Wiley.

Werry, J. S. (1992), Child psychiatric disorders: are they classifiable? *Br. J. Psychiatry,* 161:472–480.

Williams, S. & McGee, R. (1991), Adolescents' self-perceptions of their strengths. *Journal of Youth and Adolescence,* 20:325–337.

Williams, S. M., McGee, R., Anderson, J. & Silva, P. A. (1989), The structure and correlates of self-reported symptoms in 11-year-old children. *J. Abnorm. Child Psychol.,* 17:55–71.

Zeitlin, H. (1986), *The National History of Psychiatric Disorder in Children.* Institute of Psychiatry, Maudsley Monographs 29. Oxford: Oxford University Press.

15

Depressive Comorbidity in Children and Adolescents: Empirical, Theoretical, and Methodological Issues

Adrian Angold and Elizabeth J. Costello
Duke University Medical Center, Durham, North Carolina

Objective: *The purpose of the study was to examine comorbidity in the context of child and adolescent depression.* **Method:** *The authors reviewed recent epidemiological studies using standardized interviews and DSM-III or DSM-III-R criteria.* **Results:** *There was a high rate of comorbidity in children and adolescents with major depressive disorders or dysthymia. Comorbidity with conduct disorder/ oppositional defiant disorder ranged from 21% to 83%; comorbidity with anxiety disorder ranged from 30% to 75%; and comorbidity with attention deficit disorder ranged from 0% to 57.1%. Rates of depressive comorbidity found in community studies were similar to the rates found in clinical studies. In almost all cases, the disorders were more common in depressed children than expected by chance, and the rates of other disorders in depressed children were higher than the rates of depression in those with depression.* **Conclusions:** *The mechanisms by which comorbidity occurs are obscure at present. Several possibilities and their implications for nosology, epidemiology, and treatment research are discussed.*

Medicine has long recognized that the simultaneous presence of more than one disorder can complicate both diagnosis and treatment (1). Reasons to be concerned about the effects of comorbidity include the following.

Reprinted with permission from the *American Journal of Psychiatry,* 1993, Vol. 150(12), 1779–1791. Copyright © 1993 by the American Psychiatric Association.

Supported in part by NIMH grant MH-46323, a Leon Lowenstein Foundation grant and a William T. Grant Foundation Faculty Scholar Award to Dr. Angold, and by NIMH grant MH-45244 and a William T. Grant Faculty Scholar Award to Dr. Costello.

1. Etiology. We may identity an etiological factor (for example, family pathology) as a cause of the disorder under study (e.g., childhood depression), when, in fact, it is related causally only to a comorbid condition (e.g., conduct disorder).

2 Course. In the presence of an unmeasured comorbid condition, observed symptoms assumed to be part of the course of the disorder of interest could, in fact, be manifestations of the unmeasured disorder. For example, depressed children referred to an outpatient service might be found to commit more drug-related offenses than those with anxiety disorders. Failure to assess conduct problems in both groups could lead the clinician to believe that depression leads to drug use, whereas the drug use could be related to a higher level of conduct problems in depressed than in anxious children.

3. Treatment. Diagnostic homogeneity is critical for treatment trials, since effects of treatment on the condition of interest may be swamped by differences in outcome related to pretherapeutic comorbidity or may be spuriously inflated because the treatment is actually effective for a comorbid condition rather than the condition of interest. For example, tricyclic antidepressants are known to be effective in the treatment of attention deficit hyperactivity disorder, and the presence of attention deficit hyperactivity disorder in some subjects in a study of antidepressant effects on depression could lead to spurious findings of treatment efficacy for depression. For example, Klee and Garfinkel (2) found that in the treatment of attention deficit disorder, stimulants were more effective in controlling excess motor activity, while tricyclics had a greater effect on dysphoria. It remains to be seen whether tricyclics are most effective in attention deficit disorder when there is comorbid depression.

4. Development. It is important to establish how patterns of comorbidity develop over time as part of the process of defining the natural history of psychiatric disorders.

5. Nosology. Very high levels of comorbidity between two conditions may indicate that current definitions of the individual conditions are inappropriate and that revisions of some of our nosological constructs are needed.

In this paper, we examine comorbidity in the context of child and adolescent depression. First, a review of the research literature defines the extent of depressive comorbidity with three of the more common psychiatric disorders of childhood and adolescence: anxiety disorders, conduct and oppositional disorders, and attention deficit hyperactivity disorders. Next, we examine the history of depressive comorbidity in children and adolescents, reasons for it, both substantive and methodological, and their implications.

DEPRESSIVE COMORBIDITY: THE EVIDENCE

This review of the research data addresses four empirical questions: 1) Is depressive comorbidity more common than expected by chance in studies of child and adolescent psychopathology? 2) Is depression associated with a greater risk of other disorders in general, or do some diagnoses accompany depression more frequently than do others? 3) Are comorbid disorders found more often in children with depression than depression is found in children with other diagnoses? 4) Is comorbidity more common in clinical than in epidemiological studies of depressed children?

To establish rates of comorbidity, and to answer questions 1, 2, and 3, we concentrate on studies that have used samples drawn from the general population, rather than clinical samples. The reason for this is to avoid ascertainment bias: that is, the risk that a depressed child's attendance at a treatment facility is higher if another disorder is also present. This bias could increase the proportion of children with comorbid disorders in a treated sample for reasons unrelated to psychopathology (3). Use of referred samples can also introduce biases in the links observed between causal factors and disease; for example, children with a family history of one or other of the conditions may be more likely than children with no family pathology to be brought for treatment. Of course, this argument does not preclude the use of clinical samples for etiological studies within defined risk groups; it applies only to efforts to establish prevalence or incidence rates or the strength of associations with putative risk factors. However, since the relationship between rates of comorbidity found in clinical and population samples is of interest, we have included a discussion of the rates observed in clinical studies.

As discussed elsewhere (4), research on depression has used that word to mean many different things. In the empirical part of this paper we concentrate on depression defined as a disorder, using the criteria laid down in DSM-III, which was in force when almost all the studies reviewed here were conducted. The reason for using diagnosis as the criterion is that it implies a level of symptom severity equivalent to that seen in clinical settings, which permits the results to be usefully compared to those found in studies using clinical samples. Studies using depression rating scales rather than diagnostic interviews are discussed more briefly. Major depressive disorder and dysthymia are usually combined because of the low prevalence of either in prepubertal children (5) and the high rate of double depression in both clinical and epidemiological studies (6–8).

Samples and Procedure

Samples are all the currently published community studies that permit analyses of comorbidity rates to be made and also meet the following criteria: 1) the sample was reasonably representative of the general population of children in the area from which it was drawn; 2) a standardized psychiatric interview was used to gather data; 3) the child was interviewed, and data were also collected from other informants, using either a standardized interview or questionnaires; 4) decision rules for making diagnoses were specified, and the symptom specifications conformed in general to the DSM-III criteria for that disorder; 5) a diagnosis of depression could be made, either by specific subtypes (e.g., major depressive episode, dysthymia, bipolar disorder) or with subtypes combined; 6) at least one of the following other diagnoses could also be made; attention deficit disorder (with or without hyperactivity), conduct or oppositional disorder, and anxiety disorder. If several subtypes of anxiety diagnosis were made in the study, they are combined into one category. There are too few studies providing rates of depressive comorbidity with any other diagnoses for a detailed review to be possible at this stage. The reason for using an interview with the child as the core of the diagnostic data is the evidence from nearly all epidemiological studies that have addressed the issue that parents report depression in their children less often than children report it in themselves (9).

Six studies met these requirements for one or more comorbid disorders. They are described in several recent reviews (5, 7, 10). Summary information about them is provided in table 1. The Dunedin longitudinal study (11, 12) includes all children born in one New Zealand town's maternity hospital during 1 year. Children have been assessed every 2 years, and at 11 and 15 years they were given a standardized psychiatric interview, with additional information collected by questionnaire from parents and teachers. Repeated measures on children are also available from the survey by Velez et al. (8) of a population living in northern New York state. Three phases of interviews of parent and child have been carried out over a 10-year period; waves 2 and 3 used a structured diagnostic interview. The Puerto Rico survey (13) took a representative sample of 4–17-year-olds on the island, using a two-stage sampling design. Costello and associates' sample (14; unpublished 1993 paper of E.J. Costello et al.) of children aged 7 to 11 was recruited from primary care pediatric clinics and was followed up 5 years later. Although the sample was vulnerable to the risk of ascertainment bias, the fact that 75% of the enrolled children visited their pediatrician during the year of the study, and that on both occasions the prevalence rate of disorder was similar to that found in equal probability population samples, suggests that this is probably not a major concern.

Some other studies provide data that address one or two types of depressive comorbidity. The study of adolescents of Kashani et al. (16) drew a sample from 14–16-year-olds in the public schools of a Midwestern city. No data are available from the sample about comorbidity with attention deficit disorder. Fleming's data (15) come from a random sample of 2,219 children aged 6–16 attending schools

TABLE 1
Community Studies of Depressive Comorbidity

Study	N	Age (years)	Diagnostic System	Diagnostic Rules and Procedures	Informants
New Zealand 1 (11)	786	11	DSM-III	Psychiatrist interviewed child with Diagnostic Interview Schedule for Children; computer algorithms combined symptoms from Diagnostic Interview Schedule for Children and parent and teacher checklist; four levels of diagnosis: 1) independent diagnosis from two or more sources, 2) independent diagnosis from 1 source, confirmed by others, 3) diagnosis based on only one source, 4) diagnosis based on combined data from two or more sources; tables 2–4 based on level 1 or 2 diagnosis	Child (interview); parent (checklist); teacher (checklist)
New Zealand 2 (12)	943	15	DSM-III-R	Children interviewed with 110-item Diagnostic Interview Schedule for Children; parents completed checklist; two levels of diagnosis: 1) diagnosis by Diagnostic Interview Schedule for Children confirmed by parent checklist, 2) Nonconfirmed diagnosis based only on Diagnostic Interview Schedule for Children	Child (interview); parent (checklist)
Puerto Rico (13)[a]	224	4–16	DSM-III	Psychiatrist administered Diagnostic Interview Schedule for Children to both parent and child, then made diagnosis based on own judgment; two levels of diagnosis: 1) based on Diagnostic Interview Schedule for Children interviews, 2) Diagnostic Interview Schedule for Children diagnosis and Children's Global Assessment Scale score <61	Child (interview); parent (interview)

Continued

TABLE 1 (*cont.*)

Community Studies of Depressive Comorbidity

Study	N	Age (years)	Diagnostic System	Diagnostic Rules and Procedures	Informants
New York state 2 (8)	776	9–18	DSM-III-R	Lay interviewers used Diagnostic Interview Schedule for Children with child and parent separately; diagnosis based on algorithms and scale scores from combined symptom set; two levels of diagnosis: 1) Diagnostic Interview Schedule for Children diagnosis and scale score greater than one standard deviation above the mean, 2) Diagnostic Interview Schedule for Children diagnosis and scale score greater than two standard deviations above the mean	Child (interview); parent (interview)
New York state 3 (8)	776	11–20	DSM-III-R	Same as time 2	Child (interview); parent (interview)
Pittsburgh 1 (14)[a]	300	7–11	DSM-III	Lay interviewers used Diagnostic Interview Schedule for Children with parent and child separately; diagnosis based on algorithms used with parent and child data separately	Child (interview); parent (interview)
Pittsburgh 2 (Costello et al., unpublished data, 1993)[a]	278	12–18	DSM-III-R	Same as time 1	Child (interview); parent (interview)
Ontario (15)	3,294	6–17	DSM-III-R	Lay interviewers administered checklist to parent and teacher or parent and child separately; diagnosis present if any scale score above predefined cutoff point	Child[b] (questionnaire); parent (questionnaire); teacher[b] (questionnaire)
Midwest (16)	150	14–16	DSM-III	Clinician interviewers used Diagnostic Interview for Children and Parents with parent and child; diagnosis based on judgment of either interviewer; impairment based on psychiatrist's review of all material; two levels of diagnosis	Child (interview); child (checklist); parent (checklist)

[a]Two-stage study: number shown is the actual number of interviews.

[b]Teacher Report Form used for children aged 6–11; Youth Self-Report used with children aged 12–16.

in Hamilton, Ontario, in 1989. Questionnaires were based on the Child Behavior Checklist, in versions for the parent, child, and teacher, with additional questions on depression. Questionnaire results were validated against psychiatric interviews with a subgroup of the sample. Comorbidity data are available only for anxiety. Other population samples that only partially met the necessary criteria (17–21) are discussed in the text but not included in the tables.

Methodological Issues

Table 1 shows the number of subjects in each study, whether the prevalence rates were based on a single-stage or a two-stage design, and what rules were used to generate diagnoses. Prevalence periods for the studies range from 6 months to 1 year. In the following tables, after listing the prevalence rate of depression and the comorbid disorder under review, we report the number of children with comorbid disorders, the rate of the comorbid condition in depressed children, and the rate of depression in children with the comorbid condition. The prevalence ratio (22), which is approximated by the odds ratio, is a measure of the extent to which the likelihood of the other disorder is increased in the presence of a depressive diagnosis. The probability that the observed association is no different from the association expected by chance, given the base rate of the two disorders, is based on Fisher's exact test. Table 1 shows the studies used in these analyses, with the diagnostic system and sources of information.

RESULTS

Tables 2 through 4 present data on the comorbidity of depression and conduct or oppositional disorder, anxiety disorders, and attention deficit disorder. Conduct/oppositional disorders (table 2) showed a significant association with depression in every study. Rates of conduct/oppositional disorders were between 3.6 and 9.5 times higher in depressed than in nondepressed children.

In the case of anxiety disorders (table 3) a higher prevalence rate was also observed in depressed children in every case; the rate of anxiety disorders was between two and 26 times higher in depressed than in nondepressed children.

In the case of comorbidity with attention deficit disorder (table 4), five studies found a significant association and two did not. The direction of effect, as indicated by the odds ratios, was toward attention deficit disorder being as prevalent or more prevalent in depressed children; in no case was attention deficit disorder less prevalent in the presence of depression. It is particularly noticeable that analyses based on the *same* samples at different times produced different results. In the New Zealand study there was significant comorbidity at age 11 but not at age 15, whereas in the New York study the association was significant in the second

TABLE 2
Studies of Comorbidity of Depression and Conduct/Oppositional Disorders

Study	Prevalence of Disorders				Comorbidity			Prevalence Ratio[a]	p (Fisher's exact test)
	Depression		Conduct/ Oppositional Defiant Disorders			Conduct/ Oppositional Defiant Disorders in Depression (%)	Depression in Conduct/ Oppositional Defiant Disorders (%)		
	N	%	N	%	N				
New Zealand 1 (11)	14	1.8	72	9.2	11	78.6	15.2	42.7	0.001
New Zealand 2 (12)	40	4.2	85	9.0	13	32.5	15.3	5.5	0.001
Puerto Rico (13)[b]	31	8.0	33	10.5	15	55.8	45.4	18.4	0.001
New York 2 (8)	26	3.4	55	7.1	6	23.7	10.9	4.3	0.01
New York 3 (8)	22	2.8	45	5.8	5	22.7	11.1	5.2	0.01
Pittsburgh 1 (14)[b]	8	2.0	33	7.4	3	31.2	8.5	6.0	0.001
Pittsburgh 2 (Costello et al., unpublished data, 1993)[b]	14	3.1	48	12.1	10	65.4	16.8	16.2	0.001
Midwest (16)	12	8.0	22	14.7	10	83.3	45.4	52.5	0.001

[a]Ratio of likelihood of comorbid disorder in the presence of depression to its likelihood in the absence of depression.
[b]For these two-stage studies, figures in the columns labeled "N" are actual numbers based on interviews. Figures in the columns labeled "%," prevalence ratios, and probabilities are based on weighting back to the population sample. Ninety-five percent confidence limits for the estimates can be obtained from Dr. Costello.

TABLE 3
Studies of Comorbidity of Depression and Anxiety Disorders

Study	Prevalence of Disorders				N	Comorbidity		Prevalence Ratio[a]	p (Fisher's exact test)
	Depression		Anxiety			Anxiety in Depression (%)	Depression in Anxiety (%)		
	N	%	N	%					
New Zealand 1 (11)	14	1.8	59	7.5	10	71.5	16.9	36.9	0.001
New Zealand 2 (12)	40	4.2	101	10.7	12	30.0	11.9	3.9	0.001
Puerto Rico (13)[b]	31	8.0	26	6.6	13	38.9	50.0	16.0	0.001
New York 2 (8)	26	3.4	152	19.6	11	42.3	7.2	3.2	0.01
New York 3 (8)	22	2.8	81	10.4	9	40.9	11.1	6.6	0.001
Pittsburgh 1 (14)[b]	8	2.0	58	11.4	3	37.5	6.6	4.9	0.001
Pittsburgh 2 (Costello et al., unpublished data, 1993)[b]	14	3.1	47	13.2	5	47.5	11.2	6.5	0.001
Ontario (15)	86	5.5[c]	261	16.7[c]	50	58.1	19.2	9.7	0.001
Midwest (16)	12	8.0	13	8.7	9	75.0	69.2	100.0	0.001

[a]Ratio of likelihood of comorbid disorder in the presence of depression to its likelihood in the absence of depression.
[b]For these two-stage studies, figures in the columns labeled "N" are actual numbers based on interviews. Figures in the columns labeled "%," prevalence ratios, and probabilities are based on weighting back to the population sample. Ninety-five percent confidence limits for the estimates can be obtained from Dr. Costello.
[c]Based on the sample interviewed.

TABLE 4
Studies of Comorbidity of Depression and Attention Deficit Disorder

Study	Prevalence of Disorders				Comorbidity			Prevalence Ratio[a]	p (Fisher's exact test)
	Depression		Attention Deficit Disorders			Attention Deficit Disorders in Depression (%)	Depression in Attention Deficit Disorders (%)		
	N	%	N	%	N				
New Zealand 1 (11)	14	1.8	53	6.7	8	57.1	15.1	210.0	0.001
New Zealand 2 (12)	40	4.2	20	2.1	0	0.0	0.0		n.s.
Puerto Rico (13)[b]	31	8.0	35	10.0	4	13.0	44.5	37.1	0.01
New York 2 (8)	26	3.4	93	12.0	0	0.0	0.0	12.9	0.0001
New York 3 (8)	22	2.8	59	7.6	5	22.7	8.5	3.8	0.05
Pittsburgh 1 (14)[b]	8	2.0	11	2.2	1	12.5	9.1	11.0	0.05
Pittsburgh 2 (Costello et al., unpublished data, 1993)[b]	14	3.1	48	13.0	4	25.6	6.2	2.4	0.06

[a]Ratio of likelihood of comorbid disorder in the presence of depression to its likelihood in the absence of depression.
[b]For these two-stage studies, figures in the columns labeled "N" are actual numbers based on interviews. Figures in the columns labeled "%," prevalence ratios, and probabilities are based on weighting back to the population sample. Ninety-five percent confidence limits for the estimates can be obtained from Dr. Costello.

wave but only marginal in the third. In the Pittsburgh study, the association was marginal on both occasions.

In summary, the answer to the first question posed is that conduct or oppositional disorder and anxiety disorders are definitely, and attention deficit disorder probably, more common in depressed than nondepressed children and adolescents. As the prevalence ratios show, the presence of depression increases the likelihood of another disorder up to 100-fold; in most cases, the increase is of the order of 20-fold. In answer to question 2, there appears to be some specificity in depressive comorbidity; it is found strongly with conduct or oppositional disorder and anxiety disorders, but the relationship with attention deficit disorder is less strong. The different rates of comorbidity found in various studies may be the result of many different factors (e.g., differences in the age range of subjects, the degrees of reliance on information from parent or child, and the race and socioeconomic class distribution of the subjects). Unfortunately, the samples are too small for the data to be analyzed reliably by subgroups. Results may also be affected by different rates of children with *more* than two disorders (23).

Depression in Children with Other Disorders

Tables 2–4 also present data from the same studies on the increase in rates of depression found in children with conduct/oppositional, anxiety, and attention deficit disorder. In general, these are markedly lower than the rates of other diagnoses carried by depressed children. The only significant exception to this was seen in the Puerto Rican study, where 39% of depressed children were anxious, while 50% of anxious children were depressed. In most other cases, the rate of depression in children with another disorder was less than half the rate of the other disorder in depressed children. This information from tables 2–4 makes it clear that with the possible exception of attention deficit disorder, the likelihood of comorbidity in the presence of depression is considerably higher than is the likelihood of depression in the presence of another disorder.

Other Studies of Depressive Comorbidity

The studies reviewed earlier in this article were selected because they used a similar set of diagnostic criteria, standardized methods of data collection, and multiple informants and provided information about a core set of diagnoses. There are other published studies that do not conform to one or more of these criteria; the findings from those studies are reviewed briefly here.

The Isle of Wight and associated epidemiological studies (19–20), which pioneered the use of structured psychiatric interviews in epidemiological studies of child psychopathology, used a taxonomy that was based on ICD and that differed from DSM-III in several ways. Most important for these analyses is the lack of attention given at that time to depressive disorders in childhood and the use of a specific "mixed disorder" category for children with both conduct disorder and emotional or neurotic disorders. Mixed disorder was the third most common diagnosis in this population when the children were first interviewed at ages 10–11 (24) and also when the children were reinterviewed at ages 14–15. (20) Mixed disorder was diagnosed 14 times more often than would be expected by chance at ages 10–11, given the rates of each disorder individually, and eight times more often at ages 14–15. In a similar study carried out in an inner London borough, all disorders were diagnosed more frequently than on the Isle of Wight, while comorbidity was three times more common than expected by chance. Similar findings were reported from a partial replication of the Isle of Wight study carried out in Mannheim, Germany, on 1,486 children born in 1970. Mixed disorders were nine times more common than expected by chance at age 8, and four times more common at age 13, when they were the third most common diagnosis (25, 26). Vikan (21), using the Isle of Wight interview and the ICD classification with 1,510 Norwegian children, also reported that "mixed" disorders were the third most prevalent diagnosis and were more frequent than the prevalence of either conduct or neurotic disorders alone would predict. None of these studies, however, can be interpreted as referring specifically to depressive comorbidity, since "emotional disorder" was used to include a range of internalizing disorders, of which anxiety disorders are likely to have been the most prevalent.

Another series of epidemiological studies has made use of parent, teacher, and self-report questionnaires, chiefly the Child Behavior Checklist, in recent years. Scales derived from these questionnaires have been used as the basis for prevalence estimates of symptom clusters that approximate diagnoses, including depression (5). Studies that permit estimates of comorbidity tend to mirror the findings of the interview-based studies; thus, Fleming and Offord found that 63.2% of depressed children had one or more other disorders, compared with 11.6% of nondepressed children. The rates of comorbidity were 45% for anxiety disorders, 23% for attention deficit disorder, and 22% for conduct disorder (5). Cole and Carpentieri (17), looking at comorbidity between a child report of depression and a teacher rating of conduct disorder, found that 29% of the depressed children, more than twice the expected number, were also rated as having conduct disorder. The interesting characteristic of this study is that comorbidity was found even when the sources of information about the two disorders were different: children reported on their depressive symptoms, while teachers reported on conduct problems. Levy and Deykin have examined comorbidity with substance abuse in college students aged 18–19 years. Using the Diagnostic Interview Schedule, they found substance abuse in 22% of depressed adolescents, but only in 8.2% of nondepressed adolescents (18).

TABLE 5

Clinical Studies of Comorbidity in Children and Adolescents with Depression

Study and Diagnosis or Group	Number of Depressed Subjects	Percent With Comorbid Disorder	
		Conduct Disorder/ Oppositional Disorder	Anxiety[a]
Hershberg et al. (27)	28	—	39–68
Puig-Antich (28)	43	37	48–59
Kovacs et al. (29)			
Major depressive disorder	46	17	33
Dysthymia	23	22	36
Double depression	16	6	—
Geller et al. (30)			
Prepubertal	36	11	86
Adolescent	23	35	23
Mitchell et al. (31)			
Prepubertal	45	16	11–42
Adolescent	50	14	8–44
Borst et al. (32)	80	33	—
Alessi and Magen (33)	25	40	48
Harrington et al. (34)	80	21	—

[a]A range indicates comorbidity with more than one type of anxiety disorder. For details, see papers cited.

Clinical Studies of Depressive Comorbidity

Table 5 presents an overview of clinical studies, most of them using DSM-III, DSM-III-R, or ICD-9, that report rates of comorbidity in children and adolescents with depressive disorders. In a comparison of these figures with those from community studies reported in tables 2–4, the most notable conclusion to be drawn is that whereas prevalence rates of the various disorders are, of course, higher in clinical settings, comorbidity rates are no higher, and in some cases are lower. Thus, clinical studies have reported rates of comorbidity with conduct disorder that range from 6% (29) to 40% (33), compared with the 22% to 83% reported in table 2. Comorbidity with anxiety disorders ranges from 8% (31) to 86% (30) in clinical studies (table 5); the range for epidemiological studies is 30% to 75% (table 3). Few reports of comorbidity with attention deficit disorder or attention deficit hyperactivity disorder are available in the clinical literature. Kovacs et al. (29) reported that three (13%) of 23 children with dysthymia also had attention deficit disorder; six (24%) of the 25 hospitalized depressed children reported by Alessi and Magen (33) met criteria for attention deficit disorder. Comparable rates from the epidemiological literature are 0% to 57% (table 4).

Clinical studies reporting rates of depressive disorders in children with other diagnoses suggest that these may be similar to the rates of comorbid conditions in depressed patients. For example, 20% of 94 children with anxiety disorders were depressed in a study by Last et al. (35), as were 28% of 106 anxious children in a study by Strauss et al. (36). Last et al. (37) found that depressive comorbidity varied by type of anxiety diagnosis, from 25% in children with obsessive-compulsive disorder to 56% in children with social phobia. Four clinical studies of children with DSM-III attention deficit disorder report depressive comorbidity in 32% to 50% of their subjects (38–41). In several studies, about half of the children with school refusal have been found to have depressive disorders (42–46). Published rates of comorbidity with substance abuse disorders range from 16% (47) to 61% (48). Chiles et al. (49) found that 23% of 13–15-year-olds admitted to a correctional facility were depressed according to Research Diagnostic Criteria. Thus, clinical studies differ from epidemiological surveys in finding that the likelihood of other disorders given depression, and of depression given other disorders, is roughly similar.

PROBLEMS WITH THE AVAILABLE DATA ON COMORBIDITY

The studies reviewed in this article, like most research on comorbidity in children and adolescents, focused on quantifying the coexistence of two or more operationally defined "disorders" at the same time and in the same person. This approach makes strong assumptions about the nature of depression and of comorbidity (23). We will focus our discussion on two of these issues: the definition of child psychiatric disorders and the meaning of comorbidity.

The Definition of Child Psychiatric Disorders

The most vexing problem concerns the definition of "morbid conditions" in childhood and adolescence. In order to determine whether two or more conditions are present, we must be able to define and identify each condition. However, there are no generally accepted, *empirically based* definitions of childhood depression (4, 9, 50, 51). The empirical bases for the comorbid conditions considered here are equally shaky (52). Furthermore, the extent of comorbidity can vary markedly depending on which nosology is used (53). A further problem arises when one considers that the manifestations of individual disorders may change with age. Oppositional and conduct disorder symptoms, for example, are highly age dependent (54). The manifestations of both anxiety and attention deficit hyperactivity disorders are also influenced by age, at least in part (55–58). There is also evidence that patterns of depressive symptoms are age dependent (59). If we cannot precisely define each morbid state, how can we talk of comorbidity?

In fact, a number of approaches are available that will allow us to explore the problem of comorbidity without uncritically adopting any particular diagnostic system. Three of them are considered here.

1. Examine "archetypal" cases of the disorders of interest. Any sample is likely to contain a majority of subjects with relatively mild disorders. When diagnostic categories have fuzzy borders, the inclusion of mild cases will select, among others, individuals whose "depression caseness" is doubtful, or in whom depression does not seem to be the most salient feature of the overall clinical picture. The selection of severe archetypal cases avoids this problem. The problem with this approach is that there are few severely depressed children, even in referred samples. Thus, data collection will be slow, sample sizes will usually be small, and it will be difficult to conduct studies with sufficient power to address the questions of interest. This problem becomes even more acute if "comorbid" status is allowed only when both morbid conditions are archetypal. Diagnostic certainty may only be achieved at the cost of rejecting most of the population of interest and producing findings that apply only to a highly atypical subset of cases.

2. Examine symptom patterns rather than just diagnoses. Another strategy is to shift the focus from diagnostic categories and to examine patterns of association among symptoms themselves. The most extreme version of this strategy is to avoid diagnosis altogether and concentrate on looking at symptom associations by using techniques such as factor analysis, cluster analysis, or grade of membership analysis. This has the advantage of eliminating the comorbidity problem, since individuals are usually not considered to be suffering from one or more distinct disorders but from varying degrees of disturbance or maladaptation (60–64). A lesser degree of diagnostic agnosticism could also be consistent with the use of symptom scales rather than diagnostic categories. For example, it would be quite reasonable to investigate the nature of depression, defined according to adult criteria, in children. The presence or absence of a particular diagnosis could be used to determine group membership for each subject, and then patterns of other symptoms could be examined in the resultant groups. If the depressed children had different conduct symptoms than the nondepressed children, we would have some evidence that depressive conduct disorder is not simply a subcategory of conduct disorder. Furthermore, different diagnostic systems could be employed to determine whether certain types of depression are associated with particular patterns of other symptoms; for instance, whether nonendogenous depression is more frequently associated with conduct or anxiety symptoms than is endogenous depression.

A closer study of symptom patterns could be particularly useful in resolving a major difference between the DSM and ICD nosologies: the use of mixed disorders. ICD-9 and the draft ICD-10 demand that every attempt should be made to allot a single diagnosis to each subject, whereas DSM-III and DSM-III-R permit the more liberal use of multiple diagnostic categories. Thus, when a child manifests a mixture of depressive symptoms and conduct disorder symptoms, the ICD-9 diagnosis would be mixed disorder of conduct and emotions, and ICD-10 offers the diagnosis of depressive conduct disorder; however, separate diagnoses of conduct disorder and one of the depressive disorders would be given according to DSM criteria.

In a sense, the ICD approach arbitrarily solves the problem of comorbidity by doing away with it. There are two major problems with this solution. First, there is a loss of precision in using the ICD-9 and ICD-10 categories. It has been argued that both ICD and DSM suffer from the multiplication of invalid categories (65, 66), but if these categories are good enough for one part of the classification scheme, there is no obvious reason why they should not be relevant throughout. We can ask the question, Do the pure and mixed depressions manifest themselves in the same way?, only if there is a way of subtyping the manifestations of depression. If they are all lumped together, the ability to examine this question at the level of the subtype is lost. Second, it is clear that the comorbidity problem has been translated rather than effectively dealt with. Mixed disorders may actually represent the co-occurrence of quite separate disorders, with different etiologies and requiring different approaches to treatment, in which case their allocation to a separate, combined diagnostic grouping is inappropriate. On the other hand, the ICD system has some conceptual advantages as far as the "archetypal exemplar" approach to comorbidity is concerned, in that it expresses a "heuristic" approach to diagnosis, in which the diagnostician compares the patient's state with the best fitting model diagnosis (67). Thus, the diagnostic task is one of pattern recognition. DSM-III and DSM-III-R, on the other hand, adopt an "algorithmic" approach in which the diagnostician determines the presence or absence of a number of symptoms and then applies a diagnostic algorithm to this information in order to generate a diagnosis. Several of the data sets described in this article permit both ICD and DSM diagnoses to be made, as well as providing detailed symptom data for analysis. It would be a good idea to make use of them to see which diagnostic approach best fits the data—if either does.

3. Examine mixed and pure disorders as defined by different nosologies in relation to their associations with etiological factors, biological markers, and outcome. Some of the problems of diagnostic uncertainty might be resolved by the usual methods of psychiatric syndrome validation (68): testing the validity of a diagnostic category by the strength of its association with putative causes and markers, response to specific treatments, and outcome over time. The extension of these methods to comorbidity involves looking for differential associations between nonphenomenological diagnostic markers in pure and mixed groups. Consider, for instance, the dexamethasone suppression test (DST) as a marker for depression. Work with adults suggests that the DST is quite a good indicator of the presence of endogenous depression in populations containing various subtypes of depression (69). Work on the biophysiology of depression gives little reason to suppose that endogenous depression would cause conduct disorder or vice versa, but we could predict that a child in constant trouble with authority might well be miserable and that pure depressions would more often be associated with abnormal DST results than mixed disorders of conduct and emotions.

The Meaning of Comorbidity

Even supposing that it is possible to define the morbid conditions of interest, one is left with the problem of understanding what their co-occurrence means. It is usually supposed that the presence of two disorders means that two different "disease processes" are in operation in the same individual. By a "disease process" we mean the triad of etiology, pathogenesis, and progression that characterizes the individual disease (70). The usual approach to comorbidity, by addressing just the phenomenological diagnosis according to our rather crude diagnostic criteria, carries an implicit assumption that two or more disease processes are in operation when more than one diagnosis is present. However, because of our shaky nosological foundations, we need to examine a number of other possible meanings. First, we must distinguish between "methodological interpretations" and "substantive interpretations." Methodological interpretations refer to possible explanations of patterns of comorbidity as artifacts of the methods of data collection, data aggregation for diagnostic purposes, or the nosology itself. Substantive interpretations are those intended to reflect an underlying pathogenic process.

Methodological interpretations. Epidemiological studies using structured interview techniques have eliminated from contention the possibility that the observed connection among depression, anxiety, and disruptive behavior disorders is caused by clinician bias (that is, that a clinical interviewer who diagnoses one disorder is more alert to the possibility of others. Parents and teachers, and even children themselves, could be sensitized in a similar way). Respondent-based (highly structured) interviews collect information from parents, teachers, and children in a manner that reduces to a minimum the potential for clinician bias at the information collection level. The use of computer algorithms to generate diagnoses from symptom data further reduces the potential for clinical biases to play a part. Studies that have used a clinician-based "best-estimate" approach to arrive at a final diagnosis provide an opportunity for such a bias to come into play. However, there is no evidence from the existing studies that comorbidity is more likely to occur when best-estimate diagnoses are used. In fact, Bird et al. (71) have reported that the opposite was the case.

On the other hand, some other method-based interpretations cannot be ruled out at present:

1. There is no etiological or pathogenic connection between depression, anxiety, and disruptive behavior disorders, but the individual conditions share some symptoms in common, so that the presence of one disorder reduces the number of symptoms required for the second disorder to reach the threshold for diagnosis. For instance, irritability is allowed to be the basic mood state for the DSM-III-R diagnosis of depression. Irritability may be manifested as temper tantrums, arguments, touchiness, anger and resentment, or fighting, all of which are included as defining criteria for DSM-III-R oppositional defiant disorder or conduct disorder. In effect, the presence of one disorder constitutes a partial fulfillment of the criteria for the second disorder, and thus, in purely operational terms, partially implies the presence of the second disorder. If such an effect were the sole cause of an association between two diagnoses, then the apparent "comorbidity" would be present only in those manifesting the shared symptoms and not in those whose disorders did not involve such symptoms. This hypothesis could be tested with some of the large data bases now available that contain information at the level of individual symptoms from structured psychiatric interviews.

2. There is no etiological or pathogenic connection between depression, anxiety, and disruptive behavior disorders, but the use of multiple informants describing the same phenomena in different terms leads to the spurious appearance of multiple disorders. All of the epidemiological studies and most of the clinical studies of comorbidity have employed some means of combining information from different sources (parents, teachers, children) at either the symptom level or the diagnostic level. In most cases this has meant using a decision rule that if either the parent or the child reports the presence of a symptom, then it is regarded as being present. This approach raises the problem that different individuals may interpret symptoms in different ways. Suppose, for instance, that a child tells his or her mother that he or she is worried about going to school and cries in the process. It is possible that the parent may interpret this as a sign of the child's being depressed and that this may lead to a parental report of depressed mood, while the child's description leads the interviewer to record the presence of anxiety. Using the rule that positive ratings from any informant count toward a diagnosis would result in the same phenomenon being counted twice under different headings that contribute toward two diagnoses and thereby create spurious comorbidity. It is unlikely that such a methodological effect alone is responsible for the entire phenomenon of comorbidity because the finding is so robust across the child studies and in adult data, which rely primarily on self-reports. However, it might help to explain the disparities in the rates of comorbidity seen in the epidemiological studies. A sensitive debriefing of respondents after a structured psychiatric interview might be a way of examining this question.

Substantive interpretations. If methodological explanations are ruled out or controlled through careful design of the research and its analysis, the observed rates of comorbidity can be seen as having some basis in children's symptoms. However, there are several possible substantive explanations that need to be considered.

1. All childhood psychiatric disorders result from the same pathogenic processes. Although a wide range of factors that increase a child's risk of psychiatric disorder have been identified, the degree of specificity of these effects seems to be small (7, 72). For example, it is clear that children with depressed parents suffer from much higher rates of psychopathology than the children of nondepressed parents, but their psychopathology is by no means limited to depression (73–77). A family history of mental illness or criminality, parental marital discord, chronically adverse life circumstances, and acute adverse life events have all been associated with depression, anxiety disorders, and conduct disorder (7). Perhaps the apparently diverse clinical outcomes are products of a single pathogenic process with variable behavioral manifestations; nonspecific responses to a variety of nonspecific insults, so that the supposed "disorders" are nothing more than arbitrary subdivisions unrelated to any useful distinctions between underlying disease processes. Much of the earlier research in child psychiatry (especially epidemiological research) was based on this sort of approach, involving global measures of "maladaptation," rather than measures of specific disorders (78). This also suggests that it might be productive to examine the effects of particular types of insults in producing a range of psychopathological outcomes, rather than investigating the causes of individual types of psychopathology. Recent investigations of the effects of a family history of depression on child psychopathology represent a case in point here.

2. Depressive and anxiety symptoms represent alternative outcomes of the same pathogenic process, but this process is different from that which results in some other disorders (such as conduct disorder). This possibility is similar to the first explanation but less extreme. The broad distinction between the emotional (internalizing) disorders and behavioral (externalizing) disorders has stood the tests of time and repeated investigation. These two broad patterns of disturbance may represent different underlying disease processes, while the diagnostic distinctions within each of the higher order groupings may be arbitrary. If so, some of the observed associations would be the spurious products of the nosology itself, while others would result from real differences in underlying disease processes.

3. Depressive and anxiety symptoms result nonspecifically from a variety of pathogenic mechanisms, which are reflected in other symptoms (such as conduct disorder). This suggestion refers to the possibility that certain supposed disorders represent nonspecific accompaniments of other underlying disease processes. For instance, perhaps what DSM-III-R labels a major depressive episode is the response of the organism to many types of psychosocial problems (e.g., learning difficulties or conduct disorder). Despite the growing evidence that depression in young people is often a chronic or recurring problem (34), it is still possible that such chronic or relapsing depressions are simply accompaniments of other chronic disorders (such as conduct disorder). It remains to be seen whether these affective disorders merit the status of diseases independently of other conditions.

4. Depression directly causes disruptive behavior disorders (or vice versa). This possibility resembles explanation 3 but recognizes that separate disease processes are involved in the production of the two conditions and that one is not simply an epiphenomenon of the other. Thus, one disorder (conduct disorder) may have a variety of causes, of which one is the other disorder (depression).

Possibilities 3 and 4 have been addressed in the distinction between primary and secondary depressions introduced by Woodruff et al. (79). A primary affective disorder is one that occurs in a person who has not had a prior nonaffective psychiatric illness. A secondary affective disorder is one that occurs in a patient who has had a preexisting, diagnosable, nonaffective psychiatric illness. In adults, there seem to be few phenomenological differences between primary and secondary depressions (79–84), although secondary depressions tend to be of earlier onset and may be relatively long lasting. Individuals with secondary depression also tend to be of lower socioeconomic class and to have poorer educational achievement than individuals with primary depression. Secondary depression also seems to be associated with a greater prevalence of alcoholism in relatives. However, these data have necessarily relied upon retrospective recall of the relative onsets of different disorders, with groups of patients who may not always be reliable witnesses (sociopathic patients are an obvious case in point).

A few studies have looked at this distinction in children and adolescents. Carlson and Cantwell (85, 86) found that half of a group of 28 depressed children had another preexisting diagnosis and were felt to constitute subjects with secondary depression. Geller et al. (30) found that in about 80% of their 59 depressed children and adolescents, the onset of separation anxiety postdated that of depression, while the onset of antisocial behavior was later than that of depression in all subjects in whom both disorders were identified. Friedman et al. (87), who studied a group of adolescents and young adults, found that 85% of the adolescents had a primary depression, as did 71% of the adults in the sample. With the two groups combined, it appeared that when their histories were retrospectively reviewed, 59% of the primary group showed only affective disorder (although they were allowed to have additional nonaffective disorders during their major affective episodes). The remaining 41% followed a "complex" course; drug and alcohol abuse figured prominently in their histories. In considering a group of preadolescent boys with major depression who attended a child depression clinic, Puig-Antich (28) found that of the 16 boys with both conduct disorder and depression, the onset of the depression preceded that of the conduct disorder in 14, and the conduct disturbance resolved when the depressive episode responded to treatment in 11 of the 13 who had a full treatment response of the depression. Kovacs et al. (6) reported that the presence of an additional anxiety disorder diagnosis made no difference to the recovery and relapse rates for either major depression or dysthymic disorder, and that in more than half of her cases, recovery from the anxiety disorder accompanied or preceded recovery from depression. Overall, the current evidence seems to point to a preponderance of primary depressions in childhood and adolescence.

However, a problem arises when one considers that the lines of demarcation between certain disorders may be rather arbitrary. Thus, many children with conduct disorder met criteria for oppositional disorder when they were younger, and the age at onset of conduct disorder is to some extent a product of the types of behavior involved in getting the diagnosis (after all, it is difficult to be involved in violent crime as a 6-year-old). The dates of onset of disorders will, therefore, be imperfect markers of the dates of onset of underlying psychopathogenic processes. This situation is common in medicine in general, where the presentation of a disease process through some notable phenomeno-logical marker (such as pain) often occurs late in the development of the disor-der. However, psychiatric diagnosis not only requires the presence of a certain number of symptoms, it also defines the disorder as beginning at the time when the full complement of symptoms is present, rather than when the first key symptom was observed. In this it diverges from most of medicine, which marks the onset of a disease, retrospectively, by the first key symptom. It will be diffi-cult to reach this stage in psychiatry without more reliable ways of recording early symptoms than retrospective recall and a much clearer understanding of the developmental pathways of different disorders. However, this line of work is worth pursuing, especially since developmental analyses can be conducted at the symptom level as well as at the diagnostic level.

5. *The presence of some third factor modulates the relationship of depression with other disorders.* It is possible that the interplay between the various risk and protective factors may affect the diagnostic outcome; for example, a family his-tory of depression might increase the risk of developing depression in the face of risk factors for some other disorder (e.g., conduct disorder). Here again, family genetic studies provide a means of developing a better understanding of the proc-esses involved. However, the need to recruit families with complex patterns of psychiatric comorbidity for comparison with one another greatly complicates both the carrying out and analysis of such studies.

IMPLICATIONS

As Feinstein has pointed out in his discussion of the effects of comorbidity on the course of chronic disease (1), a comorbid condition can affect the time at which a disorder is diagnosed, the outcome to be anticipated with and without treatment, the choice of treatment, and the level of functional impairment to be expected. Assuming that useful treatment is available, comorbidity can be a benefit to the extent that it results in earlier treatment seeking or earlier detection of the child's depression. However, the problems associated with treating depressed children with other disorders have hardly been addressed in clinical research. In addition, longitudinal studies have not yet been done that could clarify the temporal relationships among comorbid conditions and suggest the best approach to early intervention to prevent the development of comorbidity.

Nosology

Diagnostic measures capable of making a wide range of diagnoses are needed for such studies. Furthermore, particular attention should be paid to the definitions of pathological symptom severity in order to minimize some of the problems of clinician bias discussed earlier. Given the differences of approach among the major diagnostic systems, and the lack of evidence that any is clearly superior to the others, it is useful for comparative purposes to make diagnoses according to multiple systems. The ability to detect cases that would attract a particular diagnosis in a number of the available systems would also allow the use of the "archetypal exemplar method" discussed earlier.

It is also clearly advantageous if the diagnostic instruments can provide a measure of overall disturbance, and if their diagnostic scales can be broken down into individual symptom scores, in order that symptom patterns can be investigated both with and without reference to diagnosis. Such an approach also allows for detailed analyses of the relationship between the presence of depression and the severity of comorbid diagnoses, which in turn addresses the possibility that depression is simply an epiphenomenon of the presence of severe problems of other sorts. A further refinement involves looking at the extent to which depression contributes to psychosocial impairment when the level of comorbid symptoms is controlled for. In work of this sort, it is necessary to examine the findings for boys and girls separately, and careful attention needs to be paid to the way the diagnostic process weights data from different informants.

Since none of the present nosological systems can be regarded as having clearly defined a separate depressive syndrome for children, and all are limited in the criteria that they specify as being part of the depressive spectrum, it would be as well not to tie such clinical assessments too rigidly to the symptoms required by the current DSM or ICD definitions. A range of other symptoms that have long been associated with depression, but which are not specifically mentioned in the DSM or ICD glossaries, such as loneliness or social withdrawal, should also be examined. It should also be recognized that a number of other symptoms not usually regarded as specific markers of depression, such as unexplained headaches, abdominal pain, or school refusal, could be defining characteristics of the depressive diathesis in children.

Epidemiological Research

The next generation of epidemiological studies needs to examine the temporal relationships among different disorders and the impact of comorbidity on functioning and treatment seeking. This means that they must be longitudinal studies, following children over the period of risk for both the risk factors of interest and the onset of the disorders. The effect of specific risk factors in relation to a range of disorders is also a topic of central interest. Different patterns of risk and protective factors in relation to individual disorders would support the independent nosological status of those disorders. On the other hand, nonspecificity of risk factors suggests nonspecificity of the disorders with which they are associated. A related strategy that has been little used involves looking at the risk factors for a second disorder given the presence of a particular disorder.

Family genetic studies also have an important place in unravelling these tangled problems. The need here is to simultaneously study the patterns of transmission of multiple disorders. Evidence of the independent transmission of different disorders would strongly suggest their status as separate diseases. Family genetic studies of antisocial personality disorder, alcoholism, and depression in adults have already provided good models of this type of investigation (76, 88). Furthermore, the evidence that early onset is associated with a strong familial loading for both alcoholism and depression indicates that "bottom-up" studies of depression, starting with adolescent or prepubertal probands, offer excellent opportunities for family genetic studies.

Implications for Treatment Research

Treatment outcome studies have particular advantages in the study of depressive comorbidity, since specificity of treatment response has similar implications for nosological status, in our present state of knowledge, as specificity of risk factors. In addition, there are indications in both the adult and child literature that comorbidity affects treatment outcome, so it is now necessary at least to control for potential effects of comorbidity in treatment and outcome studies of depression if group differences are to be interpretable. Of course, if a stratification or statistical control approach is used, the number of subjects required increases, while if stringent study selection criteria are employed, the rate of subject recruitment is slowed. However, there is no alternative to adopting one of these strategies if the treatment and outcome literature is to advance our knowledge.

REFERENCES

1. Feinstein AR: The pre-therapeutic classification of co-morbidity in chronic disease. J Chronic Dis 1970; 23:455–468
2. Klee SH, Garfinkel BD: Identification of depression in children and adolescents: the role of the dexamethasone suppression test. J Am Acad Child Psychiatry 1984; 23:410–415
3. Berkson J: Limitations of the application of fourfold table analysis to hospital data. Biometrics Bull 1946; 2:47–52
4. Angold A: Childhood and adolescent depression, I: epidemiological and aetiological aspects. Br J Psychiatry 1988; 152:601–617
5. Fleming JE, Offord DR: Epidemiology of childhood depressive disorders: a critical review. J Am Acad Child Adolesc Psychiatry 1990; 29:571–580
6. Kovacs M, Gatsonis C, Paulauskas SL, Richards C: Depressive disorders in childhood, IV: a longitudinal study of comorbidity with and risk for anxiety disorders. Arch Gen Psychiatry 1989; 46:776–782
7. Costello EJ: Developments in child psychiatric epidemiology. J Am Acad Child Adolesc Psychiatry 1989; 28:836–841
8. Velez CN, Johnson J, Cohen P: A longitudinal analysis of selected risk factors of childhood psychopathology. J Am Acad Child Adolesc Psychiatry 1989; 28:861–864
9. Angold A: Childhood and adolescent depression, II: research in clinical populations. Br J Psychiatry 1988; 153:476–492
10. Brandenburg NA, Friedman RM, Silver SE: The epidemiology of childhood psychiatric disorders. J Am Acad Child Adolesc Psychiatry 1990; 29:76–83
11. Anderson JC, Williams S, McGee R, Silva PA: DSM-III disorders in preadolescent children: prevalence in a large sample from the general population. Arch Gen Psychiatry 1987; 44:69–77
12. McGee R, Feehan M, Williams S, Partridge F, Silva PA, Kelly J: DSM-III disorders in a large sample of adolescents. J Am Acad Child Adolesc Psychiatry 1990; 29:611–619
13. Bird HR, Canino G, Rubio-Stipec M, Gould MS, Ribera J, Sesman M, Woodbury M, Huertas-Goldman S, Pagan A, Sanchez-Lacay A, Moscoso M: Estimates of the prevalence of childhood maladjustment in a community survey in Puerto Rico: the use of combined measures. Arch Gen Psychiatry 1988; 45:1120–1126
14. Costello EJ, Costello AJ, Edelbrock C, Burns BJ, Dulcan MK, Brent D, Janiszewski S: Psychiatric disorders in pediatric primary care: prevalence and risk factors. Arch Gen Psychiatry 1988; 45:1107–1116
15. Fleming J: The relationship between depressive and anxiety disorders in children and adolescents, in Scientific Proceedings of the Annual Meeting of the American Academy of Child and Adolescent Psychiatry. Washington, DC, AACAP, 1991
16. Kashani JH, Beck NC, Hoeper EW, Fallahi C, Corcoran CM, McAllister JA, Rosenberg TK, Reid JC: Psychiatric disorders in a community sample of adolescents. Am J Psychiatry 1987; 144:584–589; correction, 144:1114

17. Cole DA, Carpentieri S: Social status and the comorbidity of child depression and conduct disorder. J Consult Clin Psychol 1990; 58:748–757

18. Levy JC, Deykin EY: Suicidality, depression, and substance abuse in adolescence. Am J Psychiatry 1989; 146:1462–1467

19. Rutter M, Tizard J, Whitmore K: The selection of children with psychiatric disorder, in Education, Health, and Behaviour. Edited by Rutter M, Whitmore K. London, Longman, 1970

20. Graham P, Rutter M: Psychiatric disorders in the young adolescent: a follow-up study. Proc R Soc Med 1973; 66:1226–1229

21. Vikan A: Psychiatric epidemiology in a sample of 1510 ten-year-old children, I: prevalence. J Child Psychol Psychiatry 1985; 26:55–75

22. Kleinbaum DG, Kupper LL, Morgenstern H: Epidemiologic Research: Principles and Quantitative Methods. New York, Van Nostrand Reinhold, 1982

23. Caron C, Rutter M: Comorbidity in child psychopathology: concepts, issues and research strategies. J Child Psychol Psychiatry 1991; 32:1063–1080

24. Rutter M, Graham P: Psychiatric disorder in 10- and 11-year-old children. Proc R Soc Med 1966; 59:382–387

25. Esser G, Schmidt MH, Woerner W: Epidemiology and course of psychiatric disorders in school-age children—results of a longitudinal study. J Child Psychol Psychiatry 1990; 31:243–263

26. Laucht M, Schmidt MH: Psychiatric disorders at the age of 13: results and problems of a long-term study, in Psychiatric Epidemiology: Progress and Prospects. Edited by Cooper B. London, Croom Helm, 1987

27. Hershberg SG, Carlson G, Cantwell DP, Strober M: Anxiety and depressive disorders in psychiatrically disturbed children. J Clin Psychiatry 1982; 43:358–361

28. Puig-Antich J: Major depression and conduct disorder in prepuberty. J Am Acad Child Psychiatry 1982; 21:118–128

29. Kovacs M, Paulauskas S, Gatsonis C, Richards C: Depressive disorders in childhood, III: a longitudinal study of comorbidity with and risk for conduct disorders. J Affect Disord 1988; 15:205–217

30. Geller B, Chestnut EC, Miller MD, Price DT, Yates E: Preliminary data on DSM-III associated features of major depressive disorder in children and adolescents. Am J Psychiatry 1985; 142:643–644

31. Mitchell J, McCauley E, Burke PM, Moss SJ: Phenomenology of depression in children and adolescents. J Am Acad Child Adolesc Psychiatry 1988; 27:12–20

32. Borst SR, Noam GG, Bartok JA: Adolescent suicidality: a clinical-developmental approach. J Am Acad Child Adolesc Psychiatry 1991; 30:796–802

33. Alessi NE, Magen J: Comorbidity of other psychiatric disturbances in depressed, psychiatrically hospitalized children. Am J Psychiatry 1988; 145:1582–1584

34. Harrington R, Fudge H, Rutter M, Pickles A, Hill J: Adult outcomes of childhood and adolescent depression, II: links with antisocial disorders. J Am Acad Child Adolesc Psychiatry 1991; 30:434–439

35. Last CG, Hersen M, Kazdin A, Orvaschel H, Perrin S: Anxiety disorders in children and their families. Arch Gen Psychiatry 1991; 48:928–934

36. Strauss CC, Last CG, Hersen M, Kazdin AE: Association between anxiety and depression in children and adolescents with anxiety disorders. J Abnorm Child Psychol 1988; 16:57–68

37. Last CG, Perrin S, Hersen M, Kazdin A: DSM-III-R anxiety disorders in children: sociodemographic and clinical characteristics. J Am Acad Child Adolesc Psychiatry 1992; 31:1070–1076

38. Munir K, Biederman J, Knee D: Psychiatric comorbidity in patients with attention deficit disorder: a controlled study. J Am Acad Child Adolesc Psychiatry 1987; 26:844–848

39. Biederman J, Munir K, Knee D, Armentano M, Autor S, Waternaux C, Tsuang M: High rate affective disorders in probands with attention deficit disorder and in their relatives: a controlled family study. Am J Psychiatry 1987; 144:330–333

40. Brown RT, Borden KA, Clingerman SR, Jenkins P: Depression in attention deficit-disordered and normal children and their parents. Child Psychiatry Hum Dev 1988; 18:119–133

41. Biederman J, Faraone SV, Keenan K, Tsuang MT: Evidence of familial association between attention deficit disorder and major affective disorders. Arch Gen Psychiatry 1991; 48:633–642

42. Bernstein GA: Comorbidity and severity of anxiety and depressive disorders in a clinic sample. J Am Acad Child Adolesc Psychiatry 1991; 30:43–50

43. Berney TP, Kolvin I, Bhate SR, Garside RF, Jeans J, Kay B, Scarth L: School phobia: a therapeutic trial with clomipramine and short-term outcome. Br J Psychiatry 1981; 138:110–118

44. Hersov LA: Persistent non-attendance at school. J Child Psychol Psychiatry 1960; 1:130–136

45. Hersov LA: Refusal to go to school. J Child Psychol Psychiatry 1960; 1:137–145

46. Kolvin I, Berney TP, Bhate SR: Classification and diagnosis of depression in school phobia. Br J Psychiatry 1984; 145:347–357

47. Kashani JH: Double depression in adolescent substance users. J Affect Disord 1985; 8:153–157

48. Stowell RJA, Estroff TW: Psychiatric disorders in substance-abusing adolescent inpatients: a pilot study. J Am Acad Child Adolesc Psychiatry 1992; 31:1036–1040

49. Chiles JA, Miller ML, Cox GB: Depression in an adolescent delinquent population. Arch Gen Psychiatry 1980; 37:1177–1184

50. Rutter M: The developmental psychopathology of depression: issues and perspectives, in Depression in Young People: Issues and Perspectives. Edited by Rutter M, Izard C, Read P. New York, Guilford Press, 1986

51. Angold A: The Nosologic Status of Depression in Children and Adolescents, in Sourcebook for DSM-IV. Washington, DC, American Psychiatric Association (in press)

52. Werry JS, Reeves JC, Elkind GS: Attention deficit, conduct, oppositional, and anxiety disorders in children, I: a review of research on differentiating characteristics. J Am Acad Child Adolesc Psychiatry 1987; 26:133–143

53. Angold A, Costello EJ: Comorbidity in children and adolescents with depression. Child and Adolescent Psychiatric Clinics of North America 1992; 1:31–51

54. Loeber R, Green SM, Lahey BB, Christ MAG, Frick PJ: Developmental sequences in the age of onset of disruptive child behaviors. J Child and Family Studies 1992; 1:21–41

55. Werry JS: Diagnosis and assessment, in Anxiety Disorders of Childhood. Edited by Gittelman R. New York, Guilford Press, 1986

56. Loeber R: Development and risk factors of juvenile antisocial behavior and delinquency. Clin Psychol Rev 1989; 9:1–41

57. Klein RG, Mannuzza S: The long-term outcome of the attention deficit disorder/hyperactivity syndrome, in Attention Deficit Disorder and Hyperkinetic Syndrome. Edited by Sagvolden T, Borchgrevink JM, Archers R. Hillsdale, NJ, Lawrence Erlbaum Associates, 1988

58. Marks I: The development of normal fear: a review. J Child Psychol Psychiatry 1987; 28:667–697

59. Angold A, Weissman MM, John K, Wickramaratne P, Prusoff BA: The effects of age and sex on depression ratings in children and adolescents. J Am Acad Child Adolesc Psychiatry 1991; 30:67–72

60. Achenbach TM, Edelbrock CS: The classification of child psychopathology: a review and analysis of empirical efforts. Psychol Rev 1978; 85:1275–1301

61. Edelbrock C, Achenbach TM: A typology of child behavior profile patterns: distribution and correlates for disturbed children aged 6–16. J Abnorm Child Psychol 1980; 8:441–470

62. Verhulst FC, Berden GFMG, Sanders-Woudstra JAR: Mental health in Dutch children, II: the prevalence of psychiatric disorder and relationship between measures. Acta Psychiatr Scand 1985; 72(suppl 324):1–45

63. Verhulst FC, Akkerhuis GW, Althaus M: Mental health in Dutch children, I: a cross-cultural comparison. Acta Psychiatr Scand 1985; 72(suppl 323):1–108

64. Achenbach TM, Conners CK, Quay HC, Verhulst FC, Howell CT: Replication of empirically derived syndromes as a basis for taxonomy of child/adolescent psychopathology. J Abnorm Child Psychol 1989; 17:299–323

65. Gould MS, Shaffer D, Rutter M, Sturge C: UK/WHO study of ICD-9, in Assessment and Diagnosis in Child Psychopathology. Edited by Rutter M, Tuma AH, Lann IS. New York, Guilford Press, 1987

66. Cantwell DP: DSM-III studies. Ibid

67. Achenbach TM: Assessment and Taxonomy of Child and Adolescent Psychopathology. Newbury Park, Calif, Sage Publications, 1985

68. Robins E, Guze SB: Establishment of diagnostic validity in psychiatric illness: its application to schizophrenia. Am J Psychiatry 1970; 126:983–987

69. Carroll BJ: Problems with diagnostic criteria for depression. J Clin Psychiatry 1984; 45:14–18

70. Susser M: Causal Thinking in the Health Sciences: Concepts and Strategies in Epidemiology. New York, Oxford University Press, 1973

71. Bird HR, Gould MS, Staghezza BM: Patterns of diagnostic comorbidity in a commu-

nity sample of children aged 9 through 16 years. J Am Acad Child Adolesc Psychiatry 1993; 32:361–368

72. Williams S, Anderson J, McGee R, Silva PA: Risk factors for behavioral and emotional disorder in preadolescent children. J Am Acad Child Adolesc Psychiatry 1990; 29:413–419

73. Beardslee WR, Keller MB, Lavori PW, Klerman GL, Dorer DJ, Samuelson H: Psychiatric disorder in adolescent offspring of parents with affective disorder in a non-referred sample. J Affect Disord 1988; 15:313–322

74. Weissman MM, Gammon GD, John K, Merikangas KR, Warner V, Prusoff BA, Scholomskas D: Children of depressed parents: increased psychopathology and early onset of major depression. Arch Gen Psychiatry 1987; 44:847–853

75. Orvaschel H, Walsh-Allis G, Ye W, Walsh GT: Psychopathology in children of parents with recurrent depression. J Abnorm Child Psychol 1988; 16:17–28

76. Goodwin DW: Alcoholism and genetics: the sins of the fathers. Arch Gen Psychiatry 1985; 42:171–174

77. Cadoret MD, Troughton E, O'Gorman TW, Heywood E: An adoption study of genetic and environmental factors in drug abuse. Arch Gen Psychiatry 1986; 43:1131–1136

78. Weissman MM, Klerman GL: Epidemiology of mental disorders: emerging trends in the United States. Arch Gen Psychiatry 1978; 35:705–712

79. Woodruff RA, Murphy GE, Herjanic M: The natural history of affective disorders, I: symptoms of 72 patients at the time of index hospital admission. J Psychiatr Res 1967; 5:255–263

80. Guze SB, Woodruff RA, Clayton PJ: Secondary affective disorder: a study of 95 cases. Psychol Med 1971; 1:426–428

81. Weissman MM, Pottenger M, Kleber H, Ruben HL, Williams D, Thompson WD: Symptom patterns in primary and secondary depression: a comparison of primary depressives with depressed opiate addicts, alcoholics, and schizophrenics. Arch Gen Psychiatry 1977; 34:854–862

82. Akiskal HS, McKinney WT: Overview of recent research in depression: integration of ten conceptual models into a comprehensive clinical frame. Arch Gen Psychiatry 1975; 32:285–305

83. Andreasen NC, Winokur G: Secondary depression: familial, clinical and research perspective. Am J Psychiatry 1979; 136:62–66

84. Reveley AM, Reveley MA: The distinction of primary and secondary affective disorders: clinical implications. J Affect Disord 1981; 3:273–279

85. Carlson GA, Cantwell DP: A survey of depressive symptoms in a child and adolescent psychiatric population: interview data. J Am Acad Child Adolesc Psychiatry 1979; 18:587–599

86. Carlson GA, Cantwell DP: Unmasking masked depression in children and adolescents. Am J Psychiatry 1980; 137:445–449; correction, 137:871

87. Friedman RC, Hurt SW, Clarkin JR, Corn R: Primary and secondary affective disorders in adolescents and young adults. Acta Psychiatr Scand 1983; 67:226–235

88. Buydens-Branchey L, Branchey MH, Noumair D: Age of alcoholism onset, I: relationship to psychopathology. Arch Gen Psychiatry 1989; 46:225–230

16

Contrasting Cognitive Deficits in Attention Deficit Hyperactivity Disorder Versus Reading Disability

Bruce F. Pennington, Dena Groisser, and Marilyn C. Welsh
University of Denver

We compared 2 common and sometimes comorbid developmental disorders, reading disability *(RD) and* attention deficit hyperactivity disorder *(ADHD), in 2 cognitive domains, phonological processes (PP) and executive functions (EF). Subjects were 70 boys of early school age, studied by means of a 2 (RD vs. no RD) × 2 (ADHD vs. no ADHD) × 2 (domain type) mixed-model design. The 2 RD groups (RD-only and RD plus ADHD) were significantly impaired compared with both the control and ADHD-only groups on a PP composite score but performed normally on the EF composite score. The ADHD-only group had an opposite profile and was significantly different from both RD groups and from controls on the EF composite score. Thus, there was a double-dissociation between the RD-only and ADHD-only groups. The comorbid group resembled the RD-only group, consistent with the hypothesis that their ADHD symptoms are secondary to RD. These results provide evidence for the separability of PP from EF, as well as one explanation for the comorbidity between RD and ADHD.*

Reprinted with permission from *Developmental Psychology,* 1993, Vol. 29(3), 511–523. Copyright © 1993 by the American Psychological Association, Inc.

Bruce F. Pennington was supported by a National Institute of Mental Health Research Scientist Development Award (MH00419) and MERIT award (MH38870), as well as by grants from the March of Dimes (12-135) and the Orton Dyslexia Society. He was also supported in part by National Institute of Child Health and Human Development Program Project (HD 11681) and Center (HD27802) grants. Marilyn C. Welsh and Dena Groisser were funded by a grant from the Developmental Psychobiology Research Group (159).

One strategy for understanding cognitive development is to see how it is perturbed by different developmental disorders. In this article, we present evidence from two common developmental disorders, *reading disability* (RD) and *attention deficit hyperactivity disorder* (ADHD), which indicate the separability of two different domains of cognitive development, *phonological processes* and *executive functions*. To understand the relations between these two disorders, we had to examine the basis of their frequent overlap or comorbidity.

Comorbidities are a frequently encountered phenomenon in childhood behavioral disorders (Institute of Medicine, 1989), but we know little about their causal bases. Understanding comorbidities is a fundamental issue in the study of developmental psychopathologies, because each different possible explanation has different implications not only for clinical practice but also for developmental theory.

This article addresses the specific problem of the comorbidity of dyslexia (or reading disability, RD) and attention deficit hyperactivity disorder (ADHD) by means of a test for a double dissociation. This methodology addresses the basis of comorbidity (a) by testing whether similar or different domains of cognition are disrupted in the "pure" forms of these two common developmental disorders, and (b) by examining the profile of the comorbid group. We next elaborate on competing hypotheses for the causal basis of a comorbidity, briefly discuss other converging methodologies for testing these hypotheses, and then return to cognitive studies of the relation between RD and ADHD.

There are five competing hypotheses for the causal basis of the development of a comorbidity: (a) Disorder A causes Disorder B; (b) Disorder B causes Disorder A; (c) a third factor causes both disorders in all cases (common etiology); (d) a third factor causes both disorders in an etiologic subtype, but the two disorders are otherwise etiologically independent; or (e) there is no causal basis for the observed association; rather, it is an artifact of some kind. Possibilities a and b can be subdivided. In some cases, the first disorder could produce a complete copy of the second. In other cases, one disorder could produce only the symptoms of the second disorder, not the full syndrome. We call this latter possibility the *phenocopy hypothesis*, because only the symptoms of the secondary disorder would be present but not its deeper characteristics, such as a particular cognitive or brain deficit. This phenocopy hypothesis is particularly germane to the present article (and to the comorbidity of behaviorally defined disorders generally), because it is quite conceivable that RD could produce just the behavioral symptoms of ADHD, or vice versa, without producing the cognitive or brain deficits characteristic of ADHD.

Several methodologies are relevant for evaluating the causal basis of a comorbidity, including epidemiological, longitudinal, behavior genetic, and cognitive studies. For instance, epidemiological studies address whether the observed comorbidity is just an artifact of clinical ascertainment. Because the comorbidity between RD and ADHD is found in both clinic (Cantwell & Baker, 1991; Cantwell & Satterfield, 1978; Dykman & Ackerman, 1991; Holobrow & Berry, 1986; Lambert & Sandoval, 1980) and epidemiologic samples (Gilger, Pennington, & DeFries, 1992; McGee & Share, 1988; Shaywitz & Shaywitz, 1988), it does not appear to be simply an artifact. However, this comorbidity is not always found (Dalby, 1985) and is more likely to be found when the investigator first selects for RD and then looks for ADHD than the reverse (Halperin, Gittelman, Klein, & Rudel, 1984; Shaywitz & Shaywitz, 1988).

Other possible methodologies are longitudinal (McGee, Partridge, Williams, & Silva, 1991) and behavior genetic studies (Gilger et al., 1992; Gillis, Gilger, Pennington, & DeFries, 1992), but these methodologies have been less frequently used than epidemiological or cognitive studies to understand the comorbidity of RD and ADHD. It is noteworthy that our two behavior genetic studies found clear evidence of genetic influence on each disorder considered separately but not significant evidence of genetic overlap (although in both studies there were nonsignificant trends supporting the hypothesis of a small etiological subtype).

In summary, existing epidemiological and behavior genetic evidence clearly reject the artifact and common etiology hypotheses for the basis of the comorbidity between RD and ADHD. The two remaining hypotheses are the phenocopy and etiologic subtype hypotheses. How can cognitive studies help us decide between these two competing explanations?

Evidence for the cognitive separability of two disorders is provided by the finding of a classic double dissociation (Shallice, 1988). In such a double dissociation, the two disorders exhibit opposite profiles on two contrasting cognitive domains, each of which is hypothesized to be central to one disorder and not the other. A priori empirical and theoretical bases are needed for the predicted double dissociation; that is, there must be previous studies supporting different core cognitive deficits in each disorder.

If such a double dissociation is found, then the performance profile of the comorbid group on the two contrasting cognitive domains directly tests the phenocopy hypothesis. The phenocopy hypothesis predicts that the comorbid group's profile will be similar to the profile of one of the pure groups, rather than exhibiting the deficits of both groups. (If the latter pattern were found, either the common etiology or etiologic subtype hypotheses would be supported, because both imply that a single etiology can sometimes produce both full syndromes in the same individual.) Thus, the comorbid group's profile helps to determine which disorder is primary and which is secondary. Finding that the comorbid profile is similar to the pure RD profile would support the interpretation that RD sometimes leads to a secondary phenocopy of ADHD. On the other hand, if the comorbid profile resembles the pure ADHD profile, then the opposite interpretation is supported. It can be seen from this discussion that a cognitive study of four groups based on a 2 (RD vs. no RD) × 2 (ADHD vs. no ADHD) × 2 (domain type) mixed-model design would address both the issues of cognitive separability and the explanation for comorbidity.

We now review previous empirical studies that have used this design (or subsets of it) to examine the relation between RD and ADHD. The results in this area of investigation have been mixed; some studies have found differential deficits, whereas others have not (e.g., Halperin et al., 1984).

One general finding is that ADHD + RD subjects have performed worse than ADHD-only subjects on language measures across several studies (Ackerman, Anhalt, Dykman, & Holcomb, 1986; Ackerman, Dykman, & Gardner, 1990; August & Garfinkel, 1990; Felton & Wood, 1989; Felton, Wood, Brown, Campbell, & Harter, 1987; Halperin et al., 1984; LaBuda, 1988; McGee, Williams, Moffitt, & Anderson, 1989). These results are convergent with other evidence that deficits on certain phonological processing tasks are specific to RD. They also support the phenocopy hypothesis in which primary RD leads to the symptoms of ADHD, because the comorbid group is cognitively distinct from the ADHD-only group but shares cognitive characteristics with RD.

Felton et al.'s (1987) study is noteworthy both for its full 2 × 2 design (RD vs. no RD × ADHD vs. no ADHD) and for the several replication attempts that have followed. Felton et al. tested for main and interaction effects of RD and ADHD on cognitive measures, after covarying out effects of age and of IQ from the Peabody Picture Vocabulary Test—Revised. They found independent main effects of RD on naming tasks, independent main effects of ADHD on verbal memory tasks, and no interaction effects. Both RD and ADHD affected verbal fluency tasks in an additive fashion. These results provide support for ADHD and RD as separate cognitive syndromes. Because there were no interaction effects, we can infer that the comorbid group had the deficits of both pure groups combined, a result consistent with the common etiology or the etiologic subtype hypothesis but not consistent with the phenocopy hypothesis.

These authors (Felton & Wood, 1989) conducted a similar investigation in an unselected sample of first graders. The main effects of RD were found again on naming tasks and were extended to phoneme awareness tasks, both measures of phonological processing. There were also largely separate main effects of ADHD, but these were not a straightforward replication of their earlier results; instead, the effects cut across cognitive domains, including verbal memory, naming phoneme awareness, and visual discrimination. Again, there were no interaction effects.

Two other replications of the original Felton et al. study have failed to find main effects of ADHD. LaBuda (1988), in a study of a twin sample, found independent main effects of RD on measures of verbal memory, fluency, and naming but essentially no independent main effects of ADHD, even though many of her measures overlapped with those used by Felton et al. (1987). Similarly, McGee et al. (1989), using the Dunedin epidemiologic sample, failed to replicate the separate main effects of ADHD on verbal memory. Instead, they found main effects of RD on verbal memory, as well as on verbal IQ. The only deficit specific to ADHD was a slightly lower IQ. Of particular interest here is the fact that the Wisconsin Card Sorting Test, a well-validated measure of prefrontal function in adults, failed to discriminate ADHD from RD children in this study, although ADHD children have performed worse on the Wisconsin test than controls in other studies (e.g., Chelune, Ferguson, Koon, & Dickey, 1986). It may be relevant that McGee et al. used a shortened form of the Wisconsin test.

In summary, across several studies contrasting neuropsychological function in RD versus ADHD samples, verbal deficits specific to RD have been found, but deficits specific to ADHD have been more difficult to pinpoint. Overall, the existing literature provides stronger validation for RD than ADHD as a discrete and specific cognitive syndrome.

An executive function deficit theory of ADHD has been proposed by several ADHD researchers, including Conners and Wells (1986), Douglas (1985), and Stamm and Kreder (1979). Executive functions are those that are involved in the planning, regulation, and verification of activity (Luria, 1966); these functions appear to be mediated by the prefrontal cortices (Shallice, 1988). More research is needed to test this theory, because only a few existing studies of ADHD have used executive function measures.

The present study used the same 2 × 2 design utilized by Felton and colleagues (Felton & Wood, 1989; Felton et al., 1987) but added a within-subjects manipulation of two contrasting neuropsychological domains. Each domain had a priori plausibility as the core area of deficit for one of the disorders: phonological processing for RD and executive functions for ADHD. Multiple measures of each domain were used. Thus, the overall design had three factors: 2(ADHD) × 2(RD) × 2(domain type). The first two factors were between subjects, and the third was within subjects.

The study tested two specific predictions: (a) that a double dissociation between RD and ADHD would be found, with the RD-only group specifically impaired on phonological processing and the ADHD-only group specifically impaired on executive funcitons, and (b) that the comorbid group would resemble the RD-only group. The second prediction derives from the previous evidence, reviewed earlier, supporting the secondary phenocopy hypothesis in which comorbid RD + ADHD is mainly due to RD producing the symptoms of ADHD. In statistical terms, these predictions were that there would be (a) both an RD and an ADHD by domain type, two-way interaction effect and (b) a three-way interaction effect.

METHOD

Subjects

The subjects were 70 boys, 7 to 10 years old. They were recruited from several suburban elementary schools; the Attention Deficit Disorder Advocacy Group, which is a network of parents with ADHD children; and B. F. Pennington's Child Neuropsychology Clinic, which sees many RD children. Although this was not an epidemiological sample, it is likely that the use of three different referral sources helped to reduce the biases associated with any particular referral source. The control group comprised of 20 boys from one of the suburban elementary schools plus 3 others who had been referred to as ADHD or RD but who failed to meet the criteria for either disorder. We used several criteria to screen out children with other serious problems or conditions that would be expected to confound the results. In the initial phone contact, parents were asked whether the child had gross neurological damage, sensorimotor handicap, autism, psychosis, or affective disorder. None of the potential subjects had to be excluded on the basis of these criteria. We examined two other potential exclusionary criteria, IQ and family environment. None of the children had to be excluded for falling below the normal range of intelligence, because all had full-scale IQ (FSIQ) scores greater than 80 on the Wechsler Intelligence Scale for Children—Revised (WISC-R). Nor were any of the children living in a severely chaotic, abusive, or deprived family environment, as far as could be determined from the referral source and the parent questionnaire. This precaution was important, because there is evidence that family factors can produce symptoms similar to those of ADHD or RD.

Diagnostic Criteria

To be classified as ADHD, a child had to meet three criteria (based on Barkley, 1982, and the *Diagnostic and statistical manual of mental disorders* (3rd ed., rev.; *DSM-III-R;* American Psychiatric Association, 1987). The first criterion, severity, was met if the child was rated at least one standard deviation above the mean on the Hyperactive scale of the parent form of the Achenbach Child Behavior Checklist. The second criterion, pervasiveness, was met if the child was rated by the parent as having problems in more than one third of the situations listed in Barkley's (1981) Home Situations Questionnaire. The third criterion, age of onset, was met if the child's problems had started before 6 years old, as reported retrospectively by parents. By these criteria, 32 boys were classified as ADHD and 38 boys were classified as non-ADHD.

To be classified as RD, the child had to meet the criteria outlined in *DSM-III-R* for Specific Developmental Reading Disorder: a significant discrepancy between observed and expected reading levels, taking into account the child's age, general intelligence, and educational experience. This discrepancy was measured with the *reading quotient,* adapted from Finucci, Issacs, Whitehouse, and Childs (1982) and described later. Using a reading quotient of 0.90 as the cutoff, we classified 31 boys as RD and 39 boys as non-RD.

After a child was tested, he was assigned to one of the four groups on the basis of the criteria just described. All subjects were retained, even those who barely missed the cutoff for one (or more) of the clinical groups. For example, if a child missed only one of the three ADHD criteria and missed the reading quotient cutoff for RD by only 0.01, he would be included in the control group. By including all subjects, even borderline cases, we decreased the likelihood of finding significant group differences; however, the generalizability of the results was increased.

The resulting 2 × 2 matrix contained 16 boys in the comorbid cell, 16 in the ADHD-only cell, 15 in the RD-only cell, and 23 who met the criteria for neither diagnosis and constituted the control group.

Procedure

There were 2-hr testing sessions for each child. The measures administered during the first session were the WISC-R, the Spelling subtest from the Wide Range Achievement Test, and the Gray Oral Reading Test. The measures administered at the second session were the Tower of Hanoi disk-transfer task, the Matching Familiar Figures Test, the Wisconsin Card Sorting Test, the Continuous Performance Test, the Pig-Latin Test, and the Woodcock-Johnson Word Attack subtest. If the child was on psychostimulant medication, the parent was asked to withhold medication for 24 hr before the child's participation in the study. Because of the short half-life of psychostimulants, this procedure ensured that there would be minimal medication effects on test performance. The research procedures were administered by D. Groisser and trained research assistants.

Measures

The measures used fall into three broad categories: (a) family background; (b) criterion and related measures; and (c) dependent measures of the two contrasting cognitive domains, phonological processing and executive functions.

Family Background. A questionnaire was used to obtain information on the demographic and socioeconomic characteristics of the family and to obtain parent ratings of the child's behavior. The questionnaire included standard background questions on parents' religion, education, occupation, income, and family composition. A list of major family events and changes that occurred during the past year (e.g., moves, divorce, or death) was elicited to provide a rough measure of familial disruption. Other questions covered the child's past evaluations and diagnoses, remedial classes, therapy, medications, age at which the child's problems were first noticed, family drug/alcohol abuse, and family mental health treatment.

Criterion and related measures. The following parent ratings of child behavior were included in the questionnaire.

The Achenbach *Child Behavior Checklist* (CBCL) was used to assess parents' perceptions of the child's behavior. For this study, we used the behavior problem section of the CBCL, which is composed of a list of 112 problem behaviors. Each behavior is rated on a 3-point scale according to how well it describes the child. The items have been factored into eight subscales, which are in turn grouped into two broadband categories of behavior problems, Internalizing and Externalizing. The CBCL has been found to have good test-retest reliability, interrater agreement, internal consistency, and external validity (Achenbach & Edelbrock, 1983). For this study, scoring at least one standard deviation above the mean (six or above) on the Hyperactive scale was one of the criteria for ADHD.

Barkley's (1981) *Home Situations Questionnaire* lists 16 common home situations (e.g., meals and bedtime) and has the parent rate whether the child's behavior is problematic in each. This measure was used to assess the pervasiveness of the child's behavior problems. Being rated as problematic on more than one third of the items (six or more) was another criterion for ADHD in the present study.

Another measure commonly used to assess ADHD, the *Diagnostic Interview for Children and Adolescents—Parent form* (DICA–P; Herjanic, Campbell, & Reich, 1982), was included. The DICA–P asks the parent to rate the child on 20 common behavioral manifestations of ADHD (e.g., often leaves things unfinished or always on the go).

The *Child Reading Questionnaire,* developed by B. F. Pennington, was included to assess the parent's perception of the child's reading problems. This questionnaire asks the parent to rate the child on 13 common symptoms of RD (e.g., has difficulty sounding out words, makes word substitutions in oral reading).

In addition to these parent rating measures, three psychometric tests were given. The WISC-R was included as a measure of overall intellectual functioning. The child's level of reading and spelling skill was assessed through two tests. The *Gray Oral Reading Test* assesses the child's ability to read aloud passages of increasing difficulty. It yields an age equivalent for reading accuracy (Gray reading age), which is used in the reading quotient formula. The Spelling subtest from the *Wide Range Achievement Test* (WRAT) is a brief written spelling test for young children. It yields an age equivalent for spelling level (WRAT spelling age), which is used in the reading quotient formula.

The reading quotient (adapted from Finucci et al., 1982) was used to determine the degree of reading disability. In the following formula, mental age is obtained by dividing the child's FSIQ by his chronological age. *Age for grade* represents the age equivalent of the child's grade level. For this study, children whose reading quotient was 0.90 or less were classified as RD, and children whose reading quotient was over 0.90 were classified as non-RD.

Reading quotient

$$= \frac{(\text{WRAT spelling age} + \text{Gray reading age})/2}{(\text{Chronological age} + \text{mental age} + \text{age for grade})/3}$$

Cognitive dependent measures. The main dependent measures in the study were drawn from two distinct cognitive domains—phonological processing and executive functions—each plausibly central to RD and ADHD, respectively.

Two measures of phonological processes were used, one involving written language (the Woodcock-Johnson Word Attack subtest) and one involving spoken language (the Pig-Latin test).

1. The Word Attack subtest of the Woodcock-Johnson Psychoeducational Battery was used to measure the child's phonological coding ability, that is, his implicit knowledge of letter-sound correspondences. This test consists of 50 nonsense words that the subject must pronounce.

2. In the Pig-Latin test (Pennington, Van Orden, Smith, Green, & Haith, 1990), the subject must transform words into their Pig-Latin equivalent. This task assesses phonological awareness. The subject is told the rules for transforming words into Pig-Latin (move initial sound to end of word, add long a sound). Half the items are noncluster words (e.g., sat), and half are cluster words (e.g., star). In a cluster word, the initial consonant cluster has to be segmented to produce the correct Pig-Latin (e.g., star becomes tarsay). The subject attempts to produce the Pig-Latin equivalent of 48 words read by the experimenter. Total number correct was used as the response measure.

In the second domain of executive function, we selected measures on the basis of one or more of the following criteria: previous research with normative and ADHD groups, demonstrated sensitivity to prefrontal damage, face validity, and relatively low correlations with IQ. We were also concerned with tapping different aspects of executive function, including planning, set-shifting ability, impulse control, and sustained attention. Three of our executive function tests—the Tower of Hanoi task, the Matching Familiar Figures Test, and the Wisconsin Card Sorting Test—were used in a study of the normative development of executive function in children from 3 to 12 years of age (Welsh, Pennington, & Groisser, 1991). The fourth executive function test—the Continuous Performance Test— was included as a measure of sustained attention.

1. The *Tower of Hanoi* task has been used by cognitive psychologists to assess planning ability (Simon, 1975). The task evaluates the ability to plan and execute a sequence of moves to achieve a designated goal state. Performance on the Tower

of Hanoi has been studied in retarded young adults, who perform worse than mental-age controls (Borys, Spitz, & Dorans, 1982), suggesting executive funcitons may be specifically impaired in some developmental disabilities. Other studies in our laboratory have found deficits on the Tower of Hanoi in comparison with IQ-matched controls in three different, specific developmental disabilities: early-treated phenylketonuria (Welsh, Pennington, Ozonoff, Rouse, & McCabe, 1990); high functioning autism (Ozonoff, Pennington, & Rogers, 1991); and fragile X female adults (Mazzocco, Hagerman, Cronister-Silverman, & Pennington, 1992). Thus, specific impairment on the Tower of Hanoi seems to be a characteristic of several different developmental disabilities in which there is also clinical evidence of problems in behavior regulation. Moreover, performance on a similar measure was impaired in frontally damaged adults (Shallice, 1982) and children (Levin et al., 1991), providing evidence that the Tower of Hanoi is sensitive to prefrontal dysfunction. In addition, young children referred to a clinic for attention problems performed more poorly on the Tower of Hanoi task than did other children referred for language problems (Welsh, Wall, & Towle, 1989).

The version used in this study was developed for the normative study (Welsh et al., 1991). The Tower of Hanoi materials consist of two identical boards, each holding three tapered pegs and three different plastic disks or rings of different sizes (a fourth ring is added for the more difficult problems). The subject is told the rules of the game: A bigger ring may not be put on top of a smaller ring, only one ring may be moved at a time, and a ring always must be moved onto a peg (not put on the table). The rings are placed in a specific configuration on the experimenter's board and in a different configuration on the subject's board. The subject must execute a series of moves that transforms his initial configuration into a duplicate of the experimenter's configuration. A solution is correct if the goal state is achieved in the minimum number of moves. To pass a problem, the child must achieve two consecutive correct solutions in a maximum of six trials. Points are scored according to how many trials are used for each problem. The child progresses through the nine Tower of Hanoi problems, arranged in order of increasing difficulty, until he fails one. Individual problem scores were summed to obtain the total score. The range of possible scores was 0 to 54.

The Tower of Hanoi requires the planning and execution of a strategy in accordance with a set of rules to achieve an externally imposed goal; thus, the subject needs to anticipate the long-range consequences of his actions. For example, sometimes a ring must be moved farther from the goal peg as an intermediate step toward achieving the ultimate goal. The Tower of Hanoi also taps the ability to keep a complex set of rules in working memory and to use these rules to guide behavior. The ADHD-only group was expected to obtain lower total scores on the Tower of Hanoi than the other three groups.

2. The *Matching Familiar Figures Test* has been widely used to assess impul-

sivity of response. The test, devised by Kagan and colleagues (Kagan, Rosman, Day, Albert, & Phillips, 1964), requires the subject to choose from among six pictures the one that is identical to a target picture. Each incorrect picture differs from the target in a single small detail. To do well, the subject must inhibit impulsive responding to give himself time to study the alternatives.

The response measures were total errors (across all problems) and mean response latency (average time to the first response for each problem). The ADHD-only group was expected to show more errors and shorter latencies.

3. The *Wisconsin Card Sorting Test* has been found to discriminate prefrontally damaged adults from adults with other kinds of brain damage (Heaton, 1981). There is some evidence that performance on the Wisconsin test discriminates ADHD children from normal children (Chelune et al., 1986; Gornstein, Mammato, & Sandy, 1989), although research findings are not unanimous (e.g., Loge, Staton, & Beatty, 1990; McGee et al., 1989).

The Wisconsin Card Sorting test requires the ability to generate and implement the correct sorting rule, to shift flexibly to a new sorting rule in response to the experimenter's feedback, and to maintain set while sorting to a reinforced rule. The primary response measure was the number of *perseverative errors,* defined as responses that would have been correct under the previous sorting rule. *Failure to maintain set* was defined as an interruption of the correct sorting strategy after three consecutive responses that were unambiguously correct or any five consecutive correct responses. The number of categories achieved was used to gauge how well the child grasped the concept of sorting to the different categories. The ADHD-only group was expected to have more perseverative errors and failures to maintain set than the other groups but to achieve a similar number of categories.

4. The *Continuous Performance Test* (Rosvold, Mirsky, Sarason, Bransome, & Beck, 1956) can be used to assess vigilance and attention to stimuli over an extended period of time. Previous research with the Continuous Performance Test has found that ADHD children perform worse than control children on contingent-response or delayed-response tasks but not on simple detection tasks (e.g., Anderson, Halcomb, & Doyle, 1973; Cohen & Douglas, 1972; Dykman, Ackerman, Clements, & Peters, 1971). This study used a version of the Continuous Performance Test developed by Garfinkel and Klee (1983). Two 500-letter sequences are administered to the child with different instruction for each sequence. For the first sequence, the child is told to press a specific key whenever a white S flashes on the screen. For the second sequence, the child is told to press the key only when a white S is immediately followed by a blue T. The entire test lasts approximately 15 min. Performance was assessed through the child's correct percentage score for each sequence.

The second sequence of the Continuous Performance Test (Continuous Performance Test–2) which requires the child to inhibit a previously correct response, to conform to an externally impose contingency, and to implement a complex rule over an extended period of time, was considered to tap executive function (and working memory) more than the first sequence, which has no contingency or inhibition demands. The ADHD-only group was expected to perform worse than the other groups on the second sequence only.

RESULTS

We used the Statistical Package for the Social Sciences (SPSS) multivariate analysis of variance (MANOVA) procedure to perform analyses of variance (ANOVAs) and analyses of covariance (ANCOVAs). Post hoc comparisons of pairs of group means (with no covariate) used the Tukey test, which corrects for familywise error. When a covariate was used, we tested contrasts between pairs of group means with the Simple Contrasts subcommand in the MANOVA procedure. Because Simple Contrasts does not correct for the number of comparisons, more stringent significance levels were used when multiple post hoc comparisons were performed (e.g., $p = .013$ for four post hoc contrasts). In other cases, the significance level was set at $p = .050$.

We present the results for the criterion and related measures first, the cognitive dependent measures next, and the family background measures last.

Criterion and Related Measures

Because of the way the groups were defined, it was expected that there would be main effects of ADHD or RD status on the criterion variables but no interaction effects. Indeed, there were highly significant main effects of ADHD status on ADHD measures (Child Behavior Checklist Hyperactivity scale, Barkley's Home Situation Questionnaire, and Diagnostic Interview for Children and Adolescents—Parent form) and of RD status on RD measures (reading quotient and reading questionnaire) but no interaction effects (Table 1). Thus, pairs of groups selected to be high on either clinical dimension were significantly higher than those selected to be low; moreover, post hoc comparisons within such a pair generally revealed no significant differences. In particular, the ADHD + RD group was not significantly different from the ADHD-only group on the three ADHD measures, nor was it significantly different from the RD-only group on the two RD measures. This indicates that comorbidity was not confounded with severity. Likewise, the RD-only group was similar to the control group on ADHD criterion measures, and the ADHD-only group was similar to the control group on the main RD criterion measure (reading quotient), showing that comorbidity was generally restricted to the comorbid group. The sole exception was that the ADHD-only group was significantly higher than the control group (but signifi-

TABLE 1
Sample Description: Mean Scores and Standard Deviations

Variable	ADHD only (n = 16)		RD only (n = 15)		ADHD + RD (n = 16)		Control (n = 23)		F(1, 66)
	M	SD	M	SD	M	SD	M	SD	
Age	8.7	1.0	9.1	0.7	9.1	0.8	8.8	0.9	ns
Education	3.0	1.1	3.3	0.9	3.7	0.8	3.2	1.0	ns
Full-scale IQ	103.3	17.7	106.5	8.5	110.0	10.5	111.7	10.9	4.3**
Verbal IQ	103.1	18.3	103.8	9.6	105.4	12.4	112.7	12.0	ns
Performance IQ	102.4	15.5	109.0	10.4	114.2	8.9	108.4	11.0	4.8[b]*
CBCL Hyperactivity	10.2	2.7	4.0	3.1	9.6	3.3	2.4	2.1	101.6[c]***
Barkley (1981) Home Situation	11.2	2.6	4.3	3.1	10.8	3.6	2.7	2.2	118.0[c]***
DICA–P ADD scale	14.1	4.0	5.3	2.2	13.9	4.0	3.9	4.6	92.1[c]***
Reading quotient	1.09	0.18	0.83	0.05	0.80	0.07	1.06	0.08	102.2[b]***
Reading questionnaire	4.6	2.9	9.4	2.8	10.3	2.2	1.7	2.3	118.3[b]***

Note. Full-scale IQ, verbal IQ, and performance IQ are all from the Wechsler Intelligence Scale for Children—Revised. ADHD = attention deficit hyperactivity disorder; RD = reading disability; CBCL = Childhood Behavior Checklist (Achenbach & Edelbrock, 1983); DICA–P = Diagnostic Interview for Children and Adolescents—Parent form (Herjanic, Campbell, & Reich, 1982). [a] ADHD × RD interactions. [b] RD main effect. [c] ADHD main effect.

* p < .05. ** p < .001.

cantly lower than the two RD groups) on the Child Reading Questionnaire. It seems plausible that some of the symptoms on the Child Reading Questionnaire could be manifestations of inattentiveness or distractibility rather than reading disability (e.g., problems remembering complex instructions or keeping his place on a page), accounting for the higher scores of the ADHD-only group. Whether this symptom-level overlap between ADHD and RD indicates a deeper overlap is addressed by the dependent measures.

The pattern of correlations among these five measures confirmed the potential separability of the ADHD and RD criterion dimensions. The correlation between the Achenbach Child Behavior Checklist Hyperactive score and the Barkley Home Situations score was high, as expected, $r(70) = .75, p < .001$. Scores on the Diagnostic Interview for Children and Adolescents—Parent form were highly correlated with both Achenbach Hyperactivity and Barkley Home Situations scores, $r(67) = .73$ and $r(67) = .76, p < .001$, respectively. Reading quotient was not significantly correlated with the Achenbach Hyperactive, the Home Situations, or the Diagnostic Interview for Children and Adolescents—Parent form scores. Nor was the Child Reading Questionnaire significantly correlated with any of the ADHD criterion measures, whereas scores on the Child Reading Questionnaire and reading quotient were highly correlated, $r(70) = -.74, p < .001$.

Parent ratings of child behavior on Achenbach scales. On both the Internalizing and Externalizing scales of the Achenbach Child Behavior Checklist, there was a significant effect of ADHD such that the high-ADHD groups were rated as having more problems than the low-ADHD groups (Table 2). Within the high-ADHD subjects, there was no difference between the ADHD-only and the ADHD + RD

TABLE 2
Achenbach Child Behavior Checklist Scales: Mean Scores, Standard Deviations, and
ADHD Main Effects

Scale/group	*n*	*M*	*SD*
Internalizing			
ADHD-only	16	22.56	15.50
RD-only	15	11.00	7.01
ADHD + RD	16	23.50	10.16
Control	23	9.17	6.26
Externalizing			
ADHD-only	16	29.38	12.25
RD-only	15	13.00	7.24
ADHD + RD	16	30.88	8.93
Control	23	10.39	8.20

Note. For the Internalizing scale, $F(1, 66) = 28.07, p < .001$; for the Externalizing scale, $F(1, 66) = 67.41, p < .001$. ADHD = Attention-deficit hyperactivity disorder; RD = reading disability.

mean scores. All of the narrower scales that make up the Internalizing and Externalizing scales showed the same significant ADHD main effect, including the Hyperactive scale, as discussed previously. In addition, on the Delinquent scale, pairwise comparisons found that the ADHD + RD group mean ($M = 4.63$, $SD = 2.8$) was significantly higher (indicating more problems) than each of the other three group means (ADHD-only: $M = 2.56$, $SD = 2.1$; RD-only: $M = 1.13$, $SD = 1.1$; and control: $M = 1.39$, $SD = 1.5$), a finding that we highlight in the Discussion.

Age of onset was obtained from the parent's retrospective report of when the child began to demonstrate symptoms of inattentiveness, impulsivity, and high activity. Eight of the control children and 2 of the RD-only children had never shown any of these ADHD symptoms, according to parents, and therefore were not assigned an age of onset. Even without these 10 subjects, the mean age of onset was significantly lower for high-ADHD children than for low-ADHD children (3.09 vs. 4.61 years, respectively), $F(1, 56) = 10.45$, $p = .002$.

Wechsler Intelligence Scale for Children—Revised. For all the children in the study, the range of FSIQ scores was from 81 to 143. The overall mean FSIQ was 108.3 ($SD = 12.5$). As shown in Table 1, the control group had the highest mean FSIQ (111.7), followed by the ADHD + RD group (110.0), the RD-only group (106.5), and the ADHD-only group (103.3). There were no significant main effects of ADHD or RD. The ADHD × RD interaction effect was significant ($p = .043$), but none of the differences between pairs of means was significant according to the Tukey test. It is interesting to note the 7-point difference in FSIQ between the ADHD-only and the ADHD + RD groups, which, although not significant, is the first finding to suggest that these two groups may have divergent cognitive patterns. There were no significant differences among the four groups on verbal IQ, but there was a significant RD main effect on performance IQ; the two groups with RD had higher performance IQs than the two non-RD groups (Table 1).

We also analyzed the three WISC-R factor scores. Parallel to the verbal IQ results, there were no significant differences among the groups for the Verbal Comprehension factor score. Similar to the performance IQ results, the Perceptual Organization factor score was significantly higher for the RD groups than the non-RD groups (ADHD-only: $M = 10.6$, $SD = 2.9$; RD-only: $M = 12.0$, $SD = 2.4$; ADHD + RD: $M = 12.8$, $SD = 2.0$, and controls: $M = 11.5$, $SD = 2.5$; $F(1, 66) = 5.15$, $p = .026$). No pairs of group means differed significantly on Perceptual Organization by the Tukey test.

The overall mean for the Freedom From Distractibility factor was 9.3. The three clinical groups tended to have lower Freedom From Distractibility scores than the control group (ADHD-only: $M = 8.9$, $SD = 3.1$; RD-only: $M = 8.8$, $SD = 2.3$; ADHD + RD: $M = 8.6$, $SD = 1.8$, and controls: $M = 10.5$,

SD = 2.4). However, there were no significant group differences on this variable by ANOVA or by pairwise comparisons. At least for these samples, the so-called "third factor" lacked both diagnostic sensitivity and specificity.

The correlations between FSIQ and the phonological processing and executive function variables were moderate, ranging from $r(69)$ = .22 to $r(69)$ = .43 (Table 3). All except the correlation between FSIQ and the Matching Familiar Figures Test response latency were significant by two-tailed test. Higher FSIQ was associated with better performance on both the phonological processing and executive function measures.

FSIQ as a covariate. Two main factors influenced our decision to use FSIQ as a covariate in the analyses of the phonological processing and the executive function variables. First, FSIQ was related to performance on the executive function and phonological processing measures to a significant degree. Second, the direction of group differences on FSIQ—specifically, the fact that the ADHD-only group had the lowest FSIQ—could have made interpretation of executive function results difficult. Covarying FSIQ in the analyses of phonological processing and executive function variables was considered the best available method of controlling for the differences in FSIQ.

We tested the covariance assumptions of linearity of regression and equal regression slopes for each group. Both were generally satisfied; in particular, there were no significant differences in regression slopes among the four groups. Therefore, it was considered appropriate to use FSIQ as a covariate in the analyses of the phonological processing and executive function variables. We analyzed the data both with and without covariance and compared the two sets of analyses for

TABLE 3

Intercorrelations Between Phonological Processing and Executive Function Variables

Variable	1	2	3	4	5	6	7
1. Word Attack subtest	—	.75**	.13	.09	.01	.14	.39**
		(70)	(69)	(69)	(70)	(43)	(70)
2. Pig-Latin Test		—	.27*	.18	.18	.27	.36**
			(69)	(69)	(70)	(43)	(70)
3. Tower of Hanoi total			—	.38**	.22	.38**	.38**
				(68)	(69)	(.42)	(69)
4. Matching Familiar Figures Test error[a]				—	.27*	.21	.48**
					(69)	(42)	(69)
5. Wisconsin Card Sorting Test, perseverative error[a]					—	.57**	.38**
						(43)	(70)
6. Continuous Performance Test-2, % correct						—	.38*
							(43)
7. Full-scale IQ							—

Note. Values in parentheses are sample sizes.
[a] Recoded so that higher scores correspond to better performance.
* $p < .050$, two-tailed.   ** $p < .012$, two-tailed.

each phonological processing and executive function variable. Comparison of the two sets of analyses showed that, in most cases, the covariance of FSIQ slightly diminished the size of the effects but did not substantially alter the results. The more conservative results, those with FSIQ covaried, are presented. However, tables display unadjusted means.

Cognitive Dependent Measures

The pattern of correlations in Table 3 provided support for the discriminant validity of the two construct domains, and therefore, composite scores were calculated for phonological processing and executive functions. The phonological composite score was the average of the Woodcock-Johnson Word Attack subtest and the Pig-Latin Test z scores. The executive functions composite score was obtained by averaging the z scores for the Tower of Hanoi total score, Matching Familiar Figures Test errors, Wisconsin Card Sorting Test perseverative errors, and Continuous Performance Test-2 correct percentage. The Matching Familiar Figures Test errors and the Wisconsin Card Sorting Test perseverative errors were recoded so that negative scores corresponded to poorer performance.

A 2 (ADHD) $\times$ 2 (RD) $\times$ 2 (domain type) mixed-model ANCOVA with repeated measures on the third factor and covariance of FSIQ was conducted. The main effect of ADHD was significant, $F(1, 65) = 16.92, p < .0001$. The main effects of RD and domain type were nonsignificant. Two of the two-way interactions were significant: ADHD $\times$ Domain Type, $F(1, 66) = 9.26, p < .003$; and RD $\times$ Domain Type, $F(1, 66) = 45.31, p < .0001$. The ADHD $\times$ RD interaction was nonsignificant. Of greatest theoretical importance was the significant three-way interaction, $F(1, 66) = 7.04, p < .01$. That is, the effects of ADHD on performance were dependent on both the cognitive domain measured and the presence or absence of RD.

To illustrate this interaction more clearly, Figure 1 presents the two mean domain scores for each of the four groups. The predicted double dissociation was tested by means of planned pairwise comparisons between the two pure clinical groups within each domain type. With FSIQ covaried, the RD-only group had a significantly lower phonological score than the ADHD-only group, $F(1, 65) = 7.61$, $p = .008$. Conversely, the ADHD-only group had a significantly lower executive function score than the RD-only group, $F(1, 65) = 30.42, p < .001$. Further strengthening this double dissociation conclusion, post hoc comparisons demonstrated that the RD group did not differ significantly from controls on the executive function domain, nor did the ADHD group differ significantly from controls on the phonological domain.

We explored the performance of the comorbid group by means of post hoc comparisons with FSIQ covaried. These analyses indicated that the comorbid

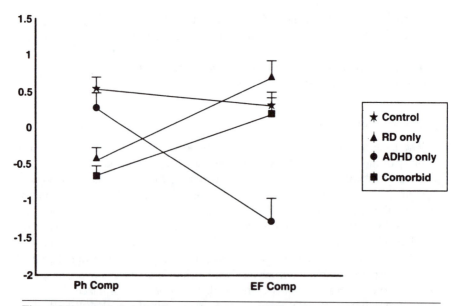

Figure 1 Phonological processing composite score (Ph Comp) and executive function composite score (EF Comp) adjusted *z*-score means (full-scale IQ covaried) for each group. (RD = reading disability; ADHD = attention deficit hyperactivity disorder.)

group did not differ significantly from the RD-only group on either domain score but was significantly different from the ADHD-only group on both the phonological score, $F(1, 65) = 13.35$, $p < .001$, and the executive function score, $F(1, 65) = 18.38$, $p < .001$. As predicted, the comorbid group resembled the RD group, supporting the secondary phenocopy hypotheses in which primary RD sometimes leads to the *symptoms* of ADHD.

Parallel significant effects were found for most of the individual phonological and executive function measures (Table 4), with a few interesting exceptions. For the Pig-Latin Test measure, although there was the expected RD main effect, the ADHD-only group mean fell between that of the RD-only and control groups but did not differ significantly from either on post hoc tests. The ADHD-only mean was significantly ($p < .05$) better than the ADHD + RD group mean. This result, obtained with FSIQ covaried, suggests that ADHD may also affect performance somewhat on this metalinguistic task (perhaps because of the demands it places on working memory), although not as strongly as RD does. For the Matching Familiar Figures Test latency data, the omnibus ANCOVA was only marginally significant ($p = .052$), because of the high variability within groups. Nonetheless, the ADHD-only group was significantly faster (more impulsive) than the RD-only group. High variability

TABLE 4
Individual Phonological and Executive Function Measures Means and Standard Deviations and Results of Analysis of Covariance (Adjusted for Full-Scale IQ)

Measure	ADHD only (n = 16)		RD only (n = 15)		ADHD + RD (n = 16)		Control (n = 23)		F
	M	SD	M	SD	M	SD	M	SD	
Phonological									
Word Attack Subtest	26.4	18.5	12.4	8.0	11.4	8.1	32.2	12.6	43.3**** / 2, 3 < 1, 4
Pig Latin Test	19.0	16.8	14.1	14.0	11.4	12.7	29.5	13.2	13.6**** / 2, 3 < 4 / 3 < 1
Executive Function									
Tower of Hanoi	27.0	9.2	36.4	6.2	37.2	5.7	36.9	6.6	5.78[b]** / 1 < 2, 3, 4
Matching Familiar Figures Test									
Errors	16.6	4.2	10.0	6.1	11.2	4.9	10.2	5.4	8.25[c]*** / 1 > 2, 3, 4
Latency (in s)	11.5	5.8	42.3	52.9	23.9	15.0	26.1	33.2	3.91† / 1 < 2
Wisconsin Card Sorting Test									
Perseverative errors	37.7	23.6	22.2	22.0	23.9	15.0	25.1	18.0	ns
Categories achieved	3.4	2.0	4.7	1.8	4.8	1.8	4.3	2.0	ns
Failure to maintain set	0.9	0.9	1.3	0.9	0.9	0.8	0.9	1.4	ns
Continuous Performance Test									
1st sequence (% correct)	0.66	0.20	0.81	0.9	0.79	0.9	0.82	0.23	ns
2nd sequence (% correct)	0.63	0.17	0.79	0.16	0.76	0.14	0.84	0.08	9.38*** / 1 < 2, 4

Note. ADHD = attention deficit hyperactivity disorder; RD = reading disability.
[a] RD main effect. [b] ADHD × RD interaction effect. [c] ADHD main effect.
* $p < .05$. ** $p < .01$. *** $p < .001$. † $p = .052$.

within groups was also a problem on the Wisconsin Card Sorting Test persever-ative errors, for which the omnibus ANCOVA found no significant differences, although the pattern of means is similar to that of the other executive function tests. As predicted, the groups did not differ appreciably on number of catego-ries attained on the Wisconsin test. Contrary to prediction, they likewise did not differ significantly on failure to maintain set. The Wisconsin test was the least sensitive to deficits in the ADHD-only group of the four executive mea-sures used here.

We next consider the validity of these results by seeing if there are any signif-icant confounds among the family background variables.

Family Background Data

Socioeconomic status. The socioeconomic status variables were occupation and education of the parents. No significant differences among the groups were found for parents' occupational level or father's education, as shown in Table 5. For mother's education, presented in Table 5, there was a significant interaction effect, $F(1, 66) = 14.41, p < .001$. By Tukey test, three significant pairwise dif-ferences were found: RD-only versus controls, RD-only versus ADHD + RD, and ADHD-only versus controls. However, the group differences in maternal edu-cation did not parallel the group differences in IQ, phonological processing, or executive function. Possible implications of the difference in maternal education between the RD-only and ADHD + RD groups are also highlighted in the last part of the Discussion.

Other family characteristics. No significant differences were found across groups for mother's age (overall $M = 36.41$) or father's age (overall $M = 38.79$). All groups were predominantly White (ranging from 81% to 93%), with roughly equal numbers of African-American and Hispanic families making up the bal-ance. Religious affiliation was also quite evenly distributed across the groups. Between 42% and 56% of the families in each group were Protestant, between 25% and 43% were Catholic, and the remainder had other or no religious affil-iation. The chi-squares for ethnicity and religion were not significant. The num-ber of major family events and changes during the past year, as reported on the parent questionnaire, did not differ significantly across the groups.

The families were grouped according to household composition into three groups: *intact* (child living with both biological parents), *mother-only* (child living with mother only), and *other* (child living with mother and stepfather or adoptive parents). The ADHD + RD group had a lower percentage of intact families (56%) and a higher percentage of mother-only households (31%) compared with the three other groups, which ranged from 82% to 88% intact and from 6% to 9% mother-only. Although the chi-square was not significant, this finding raises inter-

TABLE 5
Family and Mental Health Data

Variable	ADHD only (*n* = 16)	RD only (*n* = 15)	ADHD + RD (*n* = 16)	Control (*n* = 23)	*p*
Occupation[a,b]					
M	5.9	6.3	6.5	5.7	*ns*
SD	2.7	2.2	1.7	1.8	
Mother's education (years)[b]					
M	14.8	15.5	13.8	13.2	<.001
SD	1.7	2.3	1.6	1.5	
Father's education (years)[b]					
M	15.6	16.1	14.2	14.7	*ns*
SD	1.8	2.6	2.2	2.1	
Household composition[c]					
Intact	.88	.86	.56	.82	*ns*
Mother-only	.06	.07	.31	.09	*ns*
Other	.06	.07	.13	.09	*ns*
Alcohol/drug use[c]	.19	.20	.50	.04	<.05
Mental health treatment, family[c]	.31	.47	.69	.08	<.01
Therapy for child[c]	.63	.47	.31	.09	<.001
Special classes for child[c]	.31	.53	.75	.13	<.001

Note. ADHD = deficit hyperactivity disorder; RD = reading disability.
[a] Range: 1 = lowest to 9 = highest. [b] Means and standard deviations are given for these three variables. [c] Proportion of total, evaluated by chi-square.

esting possibilities regarding the ADHD + RD group, which are discussed later. According to parent report, the prevalence of drug/alcohol abuse was lowest in the control families, intermediate in the ADHD-only and RD-only families, and highest in the ADHD + RD families (Table 3). The chi-square was significant, $\chi^2(6, N = 70) = 12.84, p = .046$. Similarly, use of mental health services by family members was lowest in the control group, intermediate in the ADHD-only and RD-only groups, and highest in the ADHD + RD group, with the chi-square indicating that the differences were not due to chance, $\chi^2(6, N = 70) = 19.73, p = .003$ (see Table 5).

Child characteristics. The mean age of all the boys in the study was 8.87 years ($SD = 0.85$). Neither omnibus ANOVA tests nor pairwise comparisons found any significant age differences among the groups (see Table 1). Average grade level of the entire sample was 3.26, with no significant group differences.

The highest use of therapeutic services for the child (including speech, vision, and psychological therapy) occurred in the ADHD-only group, as shown in Table 5. However, the ADHD + RD group had the highest percentage attending special classes at school, for which there were significant group differences by chi-square, $\chi^2(6, N = 70) = 16.75, p = .001$. One child in the control group and 2 children in each of the other groups had repeated a grade at school.

In summary, examination of the family data and child characteristics did not reveal significant confounds. There were interesting differences between the ADHD + RD group and the RD-only group, which we discuss later.

DISCUSSION

We examined the comorbidity of RD and ADHD by means of 2 (RD) × 2 (ADHD) × 2 (domain type) mixed-model design, in which the first two factors operated between groups and the last, within. The within-subjects manipulation examined two contrasting cognitive domains: phonological processes and executive funcitons. Based on previous research, we made two predictions: (a) that there would be a double dissociation between the RD-only and ADHD-only groups, and (b) that the comorbid group would resemble the RD-only group, supporting the secondary phenocopy hypothesis.

Consistent with our first prediction, there were significant two-way interactions between domain type and both the RD and the ADHD group factors. In other words, we found a classical double dissociation between the ADHD-only group and the RD-only group on measures of executive function and phonological processing. Planned pairwise comparisons with FSIQ covaried revealed that the ADHD-only group showed a significant impairment in executive function (compared with both controls and the RD-only group) but no impairment in phonological processing, whereas the RD-only group showed an impairment in phonological processing (compared with both controls and the ADHD-only group) but no impairment in executive function (see Figure 1).

Two implications of these results are (a) that the ADHD-only and the RD-only groups represent two distinct clinical syndromes and (b) that separate cognitive processes underlie ADHD and RD. Although we did not study brain mechanisms directly, our results are consistent with the view that the cognitive deficits of ADHD and RD are mediated by separate brain systems, a view that is consistent with recent explorations of brain structure and blood flow in these two groups (Hynd, Semrud-Clikeman, Lorys, Novey, & Eliopulos, 1990; Zametkin et al., 1990).

The distinctive performance of the ADHD-only group in contrast to the other three groups (see Figure 1) provides evidence for the validity of pure ADHD (without accompanying RD) as a distinct diagnostic category. Our results suggest that ADHD is characterized by an underlying executive function impairment, a result that supports the executive function model of ADHD, at least for a subgroup of pure ADHD children. Our results ar consistent with those of a recent study (Grodzinsky & Diamond, 1992), which found deficits in ADHD boys across a broad range of tests sensitive to frontal damage in adults. Furthermore, the intact executive function skills of the ADHD + RD and RD-only groups provide evidence that executive function impairment is specific to pure ADHD and is not simply a corollary of inattentiveness or clinical status per se.

Consistent with our second prediction, we found a significant three-way interaction, indicating that the effects of the ADHD factor on performance were dependent on both the cognitive domain measured and the presence or absence of RD. The comorbid group did not differ significantly from the RD-only group on either domain score but was significantly different from the ADHD-only group on both scores. Thus, the comorbid group's profile was statistically indistinguishable from that of the RD-only group's and was also doubly dissociable from the profile of the ADHD-only group. These findings support the phenocopy hypothesis in which the presence of a primary reading disability leads to secondary symptoms of ADHD.

Why did our study demonstrate a double dissociation between ADHD and RD, when previous studies have failed to find deficits specific to ADHD apart from RD? Why did our study find nonadditive deficits in the comorbid group, when previous studies have found additive or overlapping deficits in the comorbid subgroup? Unlike previous studies, we had clear a priori hypotheses about the two contrasting cognitive domains affected in the two disorders. Other studies using the 2 × 2 design have not separated the cognitive variables into two domains and thus could not test for a double dissociation. Ascertainment bias is another consideration. Several studies contrasting ADHD-only with ADHD + RD have drawn their entire sample from a mental health clinic sample of ADHD children (e.g., August & Garfinkel, 1990; Halperin et al., 1984). As Epstein, Shaywitz, Shaywitz, and Woolston (1991) have demonstrated, ADHD children in such settings tend to have more severe symptomatology. They are also more likely to have comorbid diagnoses. If there is in fact a small comorbid subtype of ADHD + RD with a common etiology, that subtype would likely be overrepresented in such clinic samples. For all these reasons, additive deficits in the comorbid group would be expected, as would less clear differentiation between ADHD-only and ADHD + RD. In contrast, our study used a different ascertainment procedure and included milder cases.

One of the most potentially important aspects of this study is the performance of the ADHD + RD group. Our results are consistent with the phenocopy hypothesis that primary RD can lead to secondary ADHD symptomatology. For this claim to be plausible, we need a way to understand why some children with primary RD develop ADHD behavioral symptoms and some (the RD-only group) do not. There are at least two possibilities here.

One artifactual possibility is simply that parent differences in the comorbid group (such as maternal education and higher rates on nonintact, mother-only households) may have led to different parent perceptions of their son's behavior, since the ADHD diagnosis in this study was based on parent reports. We cannot completely exclude this possibility, but it is important to point out that parent perceptions in both ADHD groups were corroborated by professional diagnoses and prescribed medication treatment. For instance, 14 of 16 boys in the ADHD-only group and 13 of the 16 boys in the ADHD + RD groups had been previously diagnosed as ADHD by a pediatrician or child psychiatrist. In the ADHD-only group, 13 of 16 boys had received prescribed psychostimulant medication, as had 10 of 16 boys in the ADHD + RD group. Thus, the rates of this kind of external validation of parental perceptions were similar in both ADHD groups.

The second, speculative possibility is that family environment differences in the comorbid group could have predisposed the children in that group to the development of the secondary diagnosis. How might this have occurred? Throughout the Results section, we highlighted differences between the ADHD + RD group and the RD-only group that might be relevant to their different developmental courses. In summary, the differences are as follows: The ADHD + RD group, compared with the RD-only group, had (a) lower maternal educational level, (b) more mother-only households, (c) more family members with drug/alcohol abuse and mental health treatment, (d) fewer children receiving therapy, (e) more children in special classes at school, and (f) higher Delinquent scale scores.

We now present a hypothetical reconstruction of the development of the prototypical ADHD + RD child. The child has a congenital mild language disability, with noticeable problems in aspects of early language development, such as articulation and productive syntax (Scarborough, 1990). The child's mother is stressed by the demands of being a single parent and finds it difficult to devote as much time and energy to the child as she would like. Alcohol or drug abuse and other problems requiring mental health treatment are present in the extended family. The child's early language difficulties interact with his environment, which, although adequate, does not provide consistent structure and support. The child begins to show ADHD symptoms, such as not listening to adults and short attention span, possibly as early as 3–4 years old. In kindergarten, demands begin for prereading skills, such as learning letter names and letter–sound correspondences. As reading demands grow over the years, the child experiences increasing frustration, leading to more ADHD symptoms, including fidgeting, not following instructions, and speaking out of turn. His problems in both reading and behavior become evident to the school, and he is placed in special classes. His mother, pressed by the demands of being a single parent, does not recognize the need for intervention or does not have the time or money for therapy. Therefore, the child does not get the therapeutic services that he needs. The child begins to see himself as a troublemaker and begins to seek out other children with antisocial tendencies. Increasingly, his behavior brings him into conflict with rules and expectations. By the age of 9, he has the full-blown behavioral symptomatology of ADHD, according to both parent report and professional diagnosis. In cognitive testing, he demonstrates impaired phonological processing skills, but he performs well on tests of executive function skills, because his ADHD symptoms are not caused by a primary executive function deficit.

Clearly, empirical testing of this explanation is needed. For example, one could conduct longitudinal studies beginning in preschool (or earlier) of children at high risk for each disorder.

It is also known that ADHD is comorbid with conduct disorder and that in this comorbid group, academic problems and poor long-term outcome are commonly found (Moffitt & Henry, 1989). Likewise, it is known that ADHD is comorbid with other disorders, such as depression and anxiety (Biederman, Neucorn, & Sprich, 1991). Much more work is needed on the broader question of how the various comorbid subtypes of ADHD relate to each other; the converging methodologies discussed in the introduction provide a way to begin to tackle this complex problem.

More research is also needed to test competing models of ADHD + RD comorbidity. Additional studies comparing comorbid groups with pure groups on the contrasting cognitive domains studied here will be informative, as will behavior genetic studies. We are currently combining both approaches by examining these two cognitive domains within an RD and control twin sample. This approach will permit both a replication test of the current results and further tests of the genetic relation between the two cognitive domains. There is no reason to assume that all ADHD + RD children must fit the same model of comorbidity; our ADHD + RD sample may represent only a subgroup of the ADHD + RD population. As noted earlier, there may also be a small etiologic subtype of RD + ADHD, in which both disorders are fully present. Further research will help to determine whether other groups of ADHD + RD children are better described by a different comorbid hypothesis or whether the phenocopy hypothesis supported here is prevalent across the ADHD + RD population.

REFERENCES

Achenbach, T. M., & Edelbrock, C. (1983). *Manual for the Child Behavior Checklist and Revised Child Behavior Profile.* Burlington, VT: University of Vermont Press.

Ackerman, P. T., Anhalt, J. M., Dykman, R. A., & Holcomb, P. (1986). Inferential word decoding weakness in RD children. *Learning Disability Quarterly, 9,* 315–324.

Ackerman, P. T., Dykman, R. A., & Gardner, M. Y. (1990). ADD students with and without dyslexia differ in sensitivity to rhyme and alliteration. *Journal of Learning Disabilities, 23,* 279–283.

American Psychiatric Association. (1987). *Diagnostic and statistical manual of mental disorders* (3rd ed., rev.). New York: Author.

Anderson, R. P., Halcomb, C. G., & Doyle, R. B. (1973). The measurement of attentional deficits. *Journal of Learning Disabilities, 6,* 534–539.

August, G., & Garfinkel, B. D. (1990). Comorbidity of ADHD and reading disability among clinic-referred children. *Journal of Abnormal Child Psychology, 18,* 29–45.

Barkley, R. A. (1981). *Hyperactive children: A handbook for diagnosis and treatment.* New York: Guilford Press.

Barkley, R. (1982). Guidelines for defining hyperactivity in children: Attention deficit disorder with hyperactivity. In B. E. Lahey & A. B. Kazdin (Eds.), *Advances in clinical psychology* (pp. 137–180). New York: Plenum Press.

Biederman, J., Newcorn, J., & Sprich, S. (1991). Comorbidity of attention deficit hyperactivity disorder with conduct, depressive, anxiety, and other disorders. *American Journal of Psychiatry, 148,* 564–577.

Borys, S. V., Spitz, H. H., & Dorans, B. A. (1982). Tower of Hanoi performance of retarded young adults and nonretarded children as a function of solution length and goal state. *Journal of Experimental Child Psychology, 33,* 87–110.

Cantwell, D. P., & Baker, L. (1991). Association between attention deficit-hyperactivity disorder and learning disorders. *Journal of Learning Disabilities, 24,* 88–95.

Cantwell, D. P., & Satterfield, J. H. (1978). Prevalence of academic achievement in hyperactive children. *Journal of Pediatric Psychology, 3,* 168–171.

Chelune, G. L., Ferguson, W., Koon, R., & Dickey, T. O. (1986). Frontal lobe disinhibition in attention deficit disorder. *Child Psychiatry and Human Development, 16,* 221–234.

Cohen, N. J., & Douglas, V. I. (1972). Characteristics of the orienting response in hyperactive and normal children. *Psychophysiology, 9,* 238–245.

Conners, C. K., & Wells, K. C. (1986). *Hyperkinetic children: A neuropsychosocial approach.* Beverly Hills, CA: Sage.

Dalby, J. T. (1985). Taxonomic separation of attention deficit disorders and developmental reading disorders. *Contemporary Educational Psychology, 10,* 228–234.

Douglas, V. I. (1985, April). *Attention deficit disorder.* Invited address at the annual meeting of the Society for Research in Child Development, Toronto, Ontario, Canada.

Dykman, R. A., & Ackerman, P. T. (1991). Attention deficit disorder and specific reading disability: Separate but often overlapping disorders. *Journal of Learning Disabilities, 24,* 96–103.

Dykman, R. A., Ackerman, P. T., Clements, S. D., & Peters, J. E. (1971). Specific learning disabilities: An attentional deficit syndrome. In H. R. Myklebust (Ed.), *Progress in learning disorders* (pp. 56–98). New York: Grune & Stratton.

Epstein, M. A., Shaywitz, S. E., Shaywitz, B. A., & Woolston, J. L. (1991). The boundaries of attention deficit disorder. *Journal of Learning Disabilities, 2,* 78–86.

Felton, R. H., & Wood, F. B. (1989). Cognitive deficits in reading disability and attention deficit disorder. *Journal of Learning Disabilities, 22,* 3–22.

Felton, R. H., Wood, F. B., Brown, I. B., Campbell, S. K., & Harter, M. R. (1987). Separate verbal memory and naming deficits in attention deficit disorder and reading disability. *Brain and Language, 31,* 171–184.

Finucci, J. M., Isaacs, S. D., Whitehouse, C. C., & Childs, B. (1982). Empirical validation of reading and spelling quotients. *Developmental Medicine in Child Neurology, 24,* 733–744.

Garfinkel, B. G., & Klee, S. H. (1983). A computerized assessment battery for attention deficits. *Psychiatric Hospital, 14,* 163–166.

Gilger, J. W., Pennington, B. F., & DeFries, J. C. (1992). A twin study of the etiology of comorbidity: Attention deficit-hyperactivity disorder and dyslexia. *Journal of American Academy of Child and Adolescent Psychiatry, 31,* 343–348.

Gillis, J. J., Gilger, J. W., Pennington, B. F., & DeFries, J. C. (1992). Attention deficit hyperactivity disorder in reading disabled twins: Evidence for a genetic etiology. *Journal of Abnormal Child Psychology, 20,* 303–315.

Gornstein, E. E., Mammato, C. A., & Sandy, J. M. (1989). Performance of inattentive–overactive children on selected measures of prefrontal-type function. *Journal of Clinical Psychology, 45,* 619–632.

Grodzinsky, G. M., & Diamond, R. (1992). Frontal lobe functioning in boys with attention-deficit hyperactivity disorder. *Developmental Neuropsychology, 8,* 427–445.

Halperin, J., Gittelman, R., Klein, D., & Rudel, R. (1984). Reading disabled hyperactive children: A distinct subgroup of attention deficit disorder with hyperactivity? *Journal of Abnormal Child Psychology, 12,* 1–14.

Heaton, R. K. (1981). *Wisconsin Card Sorting Test Manual.* Odessa, FL: Psychological Assessment Resources.

Herjanic, B., Campbell, J., & Reich, W. (1982). Development of a structured psychiatric interview for children: Agreement between child and parent on individual symptoms. *Journal of Abnormal Child Psychology, 10,* 307–324.

Holobrow, P. L., & Berry, P. S. (1986). Hyperactivity and learning disabilities. *Journal of Learning Disabilities, 19,* 426–431.

Hynd, G. W., Semrud-Clikeman, M., Lorys, A. R., Novey, E. S., & Eliopulos, D. (1990). Brain morphology in developmental dyslexia and attention deficit disorder/hyperactivity. *Archives of Neurology, 3,* 345–362.

Institute of Medicine. (1989). *Research on children and adolescents with mental, behavioral, and developmental disorders.* Washington, DC: National Academy Press.

Kagan, J., Rosman, B. L., Day, L., Albert, J., & Phillips, W. (1964). Information processing in the child: Significance of analytic and reflective attitudes. *Psychological Monographs, 78* (No. 578).

LaBuda, M. (1988). *Reliability and validity of subgroups of reading-disabled twins within the Colorado reading project.* Unpublished doctoral dissertation, University of Colorado.

Lambert, N. M., & Sandoval, J. (1980). The prevalence of learning disabilities in a sample of children considered hyperactive. *Journal of Learning Disabilities, 19,* 426–431.

Levin, H. S., Culhane, K., Mendelsohn, D., Chapman, S., Harward, H., Hartmann, J., Bruce, D., Fletcher, J., & Ewing-Cobbs, L. (1991, February). *Effects of frontal versus extrafrontal lesions on planning ability in head-injured children.* Paper presented at the annual meeting of the International Neuropsychological Society, San Antonio, TX.

Loge, D. V., Staton, R. D., & Beatty, W. W. (1990). Performance of children with ADHD on tests sensitive to frontal lobe dysfunction. *Journal of the American Academy of Child and Adolescent Psychiatry, 29,* 540–545.

Luria, A. (1966). *Higher cortical functions in man.* New York: Basic Books.

Mazzocco, M. M. M., Hagerman, R. J., Cronister-Silverman, A., & Pennington, B. F. (1992). Specific frontal lobe deficits among women with the fragile X gene. *Journal of the American Academy of Child and Adolescent Psychiatry, 31,* 1141–1148.

McGee, R., Partridge. F., Williams, S., & Silva, P. A. (1991). A twelve-year follow-up of preschool hyperactive children. *Journal of the American Academy of Child and Adolescent Psychiatry, 30,* 224–232.

McGee, R., & Share, D. L. (1988). Attention deficit-hyperactivity and academic failure: Which comes first and what should be treated? *Journal of the American Academy of Child and Adolescent Psychiatry, 27,* 318–325.

McGee, R., Williams, S., Moffitt, T., & Anderson, J. (1989). A comparison of 13-year-old boys with attention deficit and/or reading disorder on neuropsychological measures. *Journal of Abnormal Child Psychology, 17,* 37–53.

Moffitt, T. E., & Henry, B. (1989). Neuropsychological assessment of executive functions in self-reported delinquents. *Development and Psychopathology, 1,* 105–118.

Ozonoff, S., Pennington, B. F., & Rogers, S. J. (1991). Executive function deficits in high-functioning autistic individuals: Relationship to theory of mind. *Journal of Child Psychology and Psychiatry, 32,* 1081–1105.

Pennington, B. F., Van Orden, G. C., Smith, S. D., Green, P. A., & Haith, M. M. (1990). Phonological processing skills and deficits in adult dyslexics. *Child Development, 61,* 1753–1778.

Rosvold, H., Mirsky, A., Sarason, I., Bransome, E., & Beck, I. (1956). A continuous performance test of brain damage. *Journal of Consulting Psychology, 20,* 343–350.

Scarborough, H. (1990). Very early language deficits in dyslexic children. *Child Development, 61,* 1728–1743.

Shallice, T. (1982). Specific impairments of planning. *Philosophical Transactions of the Royal Society of London B, 298,* 199–209.

Shallice, T. (1988). *From neuropsychology to mental structure.* Cambridge, England: Cambridge University Press.

Shaywitz, S. E., & Shaywitz, B. A. (1988). Attention deficit disorder: Current perspectives. In J. F. Kavanagh & T. J. Truss (Eds.), *Learning disabilities: Proceedings of the national conference* (pp. 369–523). Parkton, MD: York Press.

Simon, H. A. (1975). The functional equivalence of problem solving skills. *Cognitive Psychology, 7,* 268–288.

Stamm, J. S., & Kreder, S. V. (1979). Minimal brain dysfunction: Psychological and neuropsychological disorders in hyperkinetic children. In M. S. Gazzaniga (Ed.), *Handbook of behavioral neurology: Vol. 2. Neuropsychology.* New York: Plenum Press.

Welsh, M., Pennington, B. F., & Groisser, D. B. (1991). A normative-developmental study of executive function: A window on prefrontal function in children? *Developmental Neuropsychology, 7,* 131–149.

Welsh, M. C., Pennington, B. F., Ozonoff, S., Rouse, B., & McCabe, E. R. B. (1990). Neuropsychology of early-treated phenylketonuria: Specific executive function deficits. *Child Development, 61,* 1697–1713.

Welsh, M. C., Wall, B. M., & Towle, P. O. (1989), April). *Executive function in children with attention deficit: Implications for a prefrontal hypothesis.* Paper presented at the biennial meeting of the Society for Research in Child Development, Kansas City, MO.

Zametkin, A. J., Nordahl, T. E., Gross, M., King, A. C., Sample, W. E., Rumsey, J., Hamburger, S., & Cohen, R. M. (1990). Cerebral glucose metabolism in adults with hyperactivity of childhood onset. *The New England Journal of Medicine, 323,* 1361–1366.

Part VI
SPECIAL ISSUES

The papers in this section address a variety of issues of importance in the lives of children and those who have the responsibility for their care. Although the world has been free from global conflict for almost 50 years, these have not been peaceful years. As episodic conflicts have come to involve civilian populations to an increasingly greater extent, there has been a concurrent expansion of concern for the effects of war on children. In the first paper in this section, Jensen and Shaw direct attention to the psychological consequences of war and armed conflict on children and adolescents. Current knowledge regarding the stressors of war, its relation to psychopathology, its impact on values and attitudes, and the effects of war-related parental separation, loss, and absence are systematically reviewed. Jensen and Shaw conclude that the multiple adversities of war significantly interfere with the emotional, social, and intellectual development of exposed children. Massive exposure to war-time trauma is likely to overwhelm the defenses of a very great many children. Nevertheless, cognitive immaturity, plasticity, and innate adaptive capacities may well serve to mitigate the effects of exposure to war-time situations of lower intensity resulting in the emergence of adaptive styles that permit effective functioning to continue after acclimatization. Although much of the evidence derives from studies beset by significant methodologic limitations, including a confounding of stressors, a reliance on clinical samples, and an absence of controls, Jensen and Shaw's review provides a valuable reminder of the victimization of children during war-time.

Although the importance of AIDS education before the initiation of high-risk behaviors is well recognized, those who seek to develop developmentally appropriate health education programs for children in the primary and elementary grades have had little to guide them. In the second paper in this section Schonfeld, Johnson, Perrin, O'Hare, and Cicchetti address this gap in the course of examining the level of understanding of the concepts of causality, treatment, and prevention of AIDS in healthy, elementary school children. A new, developmentally based, semistructured interview protocol (ASK, AIDS Survey for KIDS) was administered to 361 children in kindergarten through sixth grade. Responses to questions about causality, treatment, and prevention were scored for each of three illnesses—AIDS, colds, and cancer. Children's understanding of AIDS was found to follow the same systematic developmental sequence of increasing conceptual sophistication with increasing grade level as did their understanding of colds and cancer. Understanding was not affected by race, gender, or socioeconomic status. However, comparisons across illnesses showed that children's conceptual understanding of causal processes is significantly less advanced for both cancer and AIDS than for colds. This disparity is interpreted as suggesting that elementary school children do have the conceptual ability to achieve a more sophisticated understanding of AIDS given appropriate educational intervention. Knowledge of children's understanding of causality, treatment, and prevention of disease in general and AIDS in particular makes an important contribution to the development of AIDS education curricula.

In the third paper in this section Pfefferbaum and Hagberg examine the use of analgesics and psychopharmacological adjuvants in children experiencing pain. The specific contributions of peripheral analgesics, narcotics, major tranquilizers, minor tranquilizers, tricyclic antidepressants, stimulants, and benzodiazepines are discussed against the background of a review of general management principles. The authors stress that pain is a complicated subjective experience and that its treatment should be initiated only after careful assessment and monitored frequently. The importance of establishing a trusting relationship with the child, beginning with believing the complaint and encouraging participation in the definition of treatment goals and the assessment of effectiveness is underscored. Knowledge of drug profiles allows for selection of an appropriate agent, dose, and route for essentially any pain situation, but there may be great variation in response. When associated emotional or behavioral symptoms complicate the picture, adjuvant pharmacological and nonpharmacological treatment methods may be necessary. Child psychiatrists, who are consulted regarding children suffering from pain, whether as a consequence of trauma, burns, cancer, or procedural and surgical treatments, will find this thoughtful and thorough review invaluable.

The results of the nine-year followup of children enrolled in the Vermont Intervention Program for Low Birthweight Infants reported by Achenbach, Howell, Aoki, and Rauh in the final paper in this section raise important questions regarding the effectiveness of psychosocial interventions to compensate for biologic risk. Twenty-four low birth weight children who had received an experimental intervention (LBWE) during the neonatal period, 31 control children who had received no treatment (LBWC) and 36 normal birth weight (NBW) children were compared. The intervention was designed to optimize caretaking interactions by assisting the mother in appreciating her baby's specific behavioral and temperamental characteristics, sensitizing her to the baby's cues and teaching her how to respond appropriately. A neonatal intensive care nurse worked with the mother and baby in seven daily sessions during the week prior to the baby's discharge from the hospital plus four home sessions at 3, 14, 30, and 90 days after discharge. Although no significant differences were found between the LBWE and LBWC groups at six or at 12 months, when both groups lagged significantly behind the NBW group, the two LBW groups had begun to diverge at age three.

By nine years of age, the LBWE children obtained significantly more favorable scores than the LBWC children on cognitive and achievement tests, as well as on standardized parent and teacher ratings of school functioning. Also, at age nine LBWE children were not significantly inferior to normal birth weight children on any measure. The progression—so clearly shown by the data of this study—from no significant LBWE vs. LBWC differences in early cognitive and achievement scores to significant differences in an array of measures of school-related functioning underscores the need for long-term followup to assess the effectiveness of early intervention. What is particularly exciting about these findings is that a relatively inexpensive intervention appears to have produced important long-term effects. While additional long-term outcome studies are needed to test the robustness of the findings, the simplicity of the intervention, which can be provided by the existing staff of neonatal intensive care units at very little additional costs, suggests that the introduction of programs to help mothers of LBW infants adapt to their babies need not await replication studies.

17

Children as Victims of War: Current Knowledge and Future Research Needs

Peter S. Jensen

National Institute of Mental Health, Rockville, Maryland

John Shaw

University of Miami School of Medicine

Recent international events have drawn attention to the effects of war-related events and processes on children and their families. This review of the literature concerning the existence, frequency, and type of social, emotional, and behavioral problems in children exposed to war indicates significant methodological problems in previous research. Available evidence suggests that massive exposure to wartime trauma seems likely to overwhelm most children's defenses; however, children's cognitive immaturity, plasticity, and innate adaptive capacities may mitigate war's effects in low-to-moderately intense wartime settings, resulting in self-protective, adaptive, cognitive styles that allow effective functioning after acclimatization. Promising recent research has shifted from the focus on psychopathology to social awareness, values, and attitudes. More research will be needed to determine how age, developmental, family, and community factors may mediate the strength and nature of wartime effects, and to determine which interventions are most effective in a variety of settings and cultural contexts.

Reprinted with permission from the *Journal of the American Academy of Child and Adolescent Psychiatry,* 1993, vol. 32(4), 697–708. Copyright © 1993 by the American Academy of Child and Adolescent Psychiatry.

The opinions and assertions contained in this paper are the views of the authors and are not to be construed as official or as reflecting the views of the Department of Health and Human Services, the National Institute of Mental Health, or the University of Miami School of Medicine.

The authors wish to acknowledge the careful, critical review and useful suggestions by John Richters, Ph.D.

There is increasing awareness of the effects of stressful and traumatic events on children and adolescents. Although most research has focused on natural disasters or discrete man-initiated acts of violence such as rape, kidnapping, sniper shooting, etc., the recent events in Operation Desert Shield and Desert Storm have heightened awareness and concerns about the effects of war on this youthful population. This paper will specifically address the effects of war-related stressors on children and adolescents. War-related stressors include both direct effects when there is clear, unequivocal exposure to life threatening situations, violent injury, and death (as seen in conditions of acute and chronic war settings), as well as indirect effects of war, such as the effects of parental separation, loss, and absence. Of particular concern in the recent conflict in Iraq was the number of American families where both parents were military members and were sent overseas, leaving their children with no familiar primary caregiver.

SCOPE OF CONCERNS

Armed conflicts around the world increasingly have been characterized by low intensity and episodic conflict with the employment of guerrilla armies, and there has been an accelerating victimization of civilian population. Concurrently, there has been an increasing awareness and sensitivity to the plight of "children in a warring world" (Escalona, 1975). In his monograph, *Children of War,* Rosenblatt (1983) states, "There are places in the world like Northern Ireland, Israel, Lebanon, Cambodia, and Vietnam that have been at war for the past twenty years or more . . . the children living in these places have known nothing but war in their experiences. The elements of war, explosions, destructions, dismemberments, eruptions, noises, fire, death, separation, torture, grief, which ought to be extraordinary and temporary for any life are for those children normal and constant."

As might be expected, the level and intensity of the effects of war on children and adolescents engender strong reactions from many concerned persons, including clinicians, researchers, educators, and policy makers. These concerns have spanned many decades and have been described by spokespersons from all over the world. Although a moral-philosophical discussion of war is beyond the scope of this review, it is the authors' position that war must be regarded with abhorrence in terms of its terrible human toll in human suffering, especially on its most innocent bystanders—children and adolescents. [In the authors' view, circumstances may arise in which war is a necessary, unavoidable evil and the only possible recourse to aggression or oppression. Nonetheless, the consequences to children, families, and society cannot be viewed dispassionately or removed from a larger, moral context.] However, such ardent, albeit widely shared concerns, may tend to shape clinical approaches, educational practices, national policy, and even research strategies in ways that may not be grounded in empirically established information. For this reason, a review of the empirical and clinical literature is warranted.

What are the psychological consequences of war and armed conflict on children and adolescents? How do children experience the exposure to death and injury of loved ones, bodily and life threats, the loss of family, community, and the sense of danger and uncertainty that suddenly pervades their lives? The context of war, given its broad scope, imposes an enormous diversity of stressors, not only on its active participants but also its more passive bystanders, such as children and families. The exposure to war with its multiple stressors may constitute a significant interference with children's development. Yet their cognitive immaturity, plasticity, and adaptive capacities often have veiled the effects of war in a certain obscurity. Garmezy and Rutter (1985) noted that frequently children's response to stress is such that their "behavior disturbances appear to be less intense than might have been anticipated." For these reasons, there is a conflicting and controversial literature debating the existence, frequency, and configuration of psychological and psychiatric morbidity in children exposed to war.

STRESSORS IN WAR

There are relatively few studies of the effects of military action per se on children, and most relevant reports have been limited to clinical-descriptive approaches. Nonetheless, one might reasonably assume that children who have been exposed to war may be similar to other victims of overwhelming, disastrous life events. For example, studies from the post-traumatic stress disorder (PTSD) literature indicate that children can and do manifest post-traumatic stress symptomatology, such as intrusive recollections of thoughts and sensory images, and various behavioral reenactments expressed in traumatic play, dreams, story telling, music, and other behaviors. Alternatively, they may manifest avoidance behaviors such as emotional constriction, reduced interests, and estrangement from others. The PTSD literature suggests that the particular configuration of stress response symptomatology is likely mediated by biological and psychosocial risk factors, parental responsivity, developmental effects, and the proximity and the degree of exposure to the stressors. Particular characteristics of the stressors are most likely important mediators, and include the stressors' particular intensity and duration, the degree of injury or life threats, the losses of family members, and the disruption of the continuity of community, school and family (Bloch, 1956; Breslau et al., 1991; Erikson, 1976; McFarlane, 1987; Newman, 1976; Pynoos et al. 1987).

Applying PTSD constructs to children of war-torn settings, a number of authors have described the children of war as manifesting regressive behaviors, episodic aggression, psychophysiological disturbances, guilt, grief reactions, changes in school performance, personality changes, and various depressive and anxiety symptoms (Arroyo and Eth, 1985; Baker, 1990; Chimienti et al., 1989; Dyregrov et al., 1987; Kinzie et al., 1986; Shaw and Harris, 1989).

However, although war is undoubtably "stressful" for children, the concept of PTSD (as usually employed) may have limited applicability to the full understanding of the effects of war on children. War usually represents a chronic, enduring condition, in which the entire context and social fabric may be dramatically altered. Entire nations and cultures may be disrupted, whereas most events leading to PTSD occur under much more limited circumstances. The dramatic contextual changes of war may result in conditions in which the stressful events and circumstances seem normal, with the possibility that the child may become somewhat acclimated to these new surroundings. Thus, for many children, the context and climate of war may be the only environment they have experienced. In this sense, war may be a chronic form of privation, and there may be little opportunity for the child to feel "deprived" per se. Furthermore, the meanings of war's stressful events and processes often are embedded in a larger national context that is bound up with patriotism, heroism (e.g., Desert Storm for the children of Multinational Forces personnel who were mobilized), or even stigma (e.g., the Vietnam war for U.S. personnel, or the Afghanistan occupation for former Soviet Union military personnel). Such considerations likely have less relevance for the construct of PTSD.

In a review of the childhood traumas, Terr (1991) noted the important role of psychic trauma as a crucial etiological factor in the development of a number of serious disorders of childhood and adulthood. She has described two basic types of traumatic experiences in children: type I (event stressor) refers to childhood trauma usually characterized by a single, sudden, and unexpected exposure to an overwhelming stressor, whereas type II (process stressor) traumas result from prolonged and sustained exposure to repeated stressors, as often occur in child physical or sexual abuse. Type I traumas may become type II traumas. One might see this type II pattern in children who have been exposed in an ongoing manner to the enduring stressors of war, but the careful application of this model to these settings awaits empirical study.

When dealing with the effects of war on children, consideration should be given to the careful examination of the nature of the stressors themselves, including actual damage to body or property, loss of family and friends (or threats of such losses), and the geographic and psychological proximity of the war-related stressors. In addition, careful scrutiny of the intrinsic adaptive capacities of the child and the social and community resources he or she has at hand to deal with the stressful circumstances are necessary to disentangle the effects of war from those of other adverse or detrimental conditions.

PROXIMITY OF EFFECTS OF WAR EVENTS AND PROCESSES

Stoltz (1951) hypothesized that the effects of war on children are likely a function of the psychological and geographic proximity of the stressful and traumatic events to the child. Whereas this tenet seems fairly well established in the PTSD literature (Pynoos et al., 1987), studies of the relationship between proximity and the effects of war on children are more contradictory.

For example, Dunsdon (1941) reported that children who remained under bombing attacks in Bristol, England, were eight times more likely to demonstrate psychological distress compared with those who were evacuated to the countryside. Bodman (1941) observed that only 4% of school children exposed to air bombings in the general vicinity demonstrated psychological distress, although 61% of those children in a hospital hit by bombs showed signs of distress several weeks after the incident. Chimienti et al. (1989) noted that children in Lebanon exposed to war conditions of shelling, destruction of home, death, and forced displacement were 1.7 times more likely to manifest regression, depression, and aggressive behaviors. Saigh (1991) has demonstrated that 24 of 72 Lebanese adolescents exposed to major war-related stressors met diagnostic criteria for PTSD.

In contrast, other accounts have suggested that little if any psychological morbidity is associated with proximity, suggesting that other variables are important. Gillespie (1942) described the remarkably low incidence of child psychiatric casualties on the English "home front," compared with the number anticipated. More recently, reports from Israel contradict the notion of the effects of shelling on children and adolescents. A study of the dreams and sleep habits of Israeli youth in a border town subject to terrorist activities indicated they slept longer and had fewer bad dreams, compared with nonexposed children (Rofe and Lewin, 1982). Similarly, these exposed children had fewer daydreams about violent themes, the enemy, and other wartime themes. The authors suggested that those with a certain degree of wartime exposure develop a repressive style with a better attendant adjustment and better school performance, compared with nonexposed children who remain more sensitive and aware about the potential threat of their circumstances. Likewise, Ziv and Israeli (1973) using measurements of anxiety discovered that children from frequently shelled kibbutzim were no different from nonshelled kibbutzim.

Given the potentially adaptive nature of low-to-moderate degrees of exposure to war-related stressors, geographic and psychological distance from the war events may not always serve adaptation if the child is then suddenly faced with a potential trauma. Raviv and Klingman (1983) reported an incident where 86 Israeli children were held hostage by terrorists for 16 hours. During the storming of the building by Israeli forces, 22 children were killed and 60 wounded. In a follow-up study of these children, three-quarters of the children had continuing problems with insomnia, nightmares, and psychosomatic problems, but only a small percentage had significant behavioral problems or personality problems. The author noted the importance of "subjective psychological distance," and concluded that for the child who is in the "rear" (away from the front lines where one could become acclimated to the threat of war-related events) and who is attacked by terrorists in a relatively calm setting, the attack may seem to be quite personally directed. In a related vein, Ayalon (1983) has drawn important distinctions between "face-to-face" experiences with terrorism and "remote-control" situations (e.g., missile attacks, bombings, etc.). In "remote control" experiences, the danger is immediate, finite, and impersonal, compared with the psychological dissonance one might experience in face-to-face interactions with a terrorist.

Although little research has directly investigated the effects of physical war trauma on children, Ayalon (1983) noted that within groups of children who are exposed to a terrorist attack, those who suffer only mild wounds seemed to fare best. In contrast, uninjured children seem to suffer from a great deal of guilt, and those with more significant wounds suffer from both the direct physical and psychological trauma, as well as later disability and disfigurement. These assumptions seem plausible, but unfortunately we have been unable to obtain further evidence documenting the nature and severity of children's responses to these types of traumatic events. Given their acute, intense nature, they likely share many of the characteristics of acute PTSD-like experiences.

Thus, whereas massive exposure to wartime trauma seems likely to overwhelm many children's defenses, more moderate degrees of exposure may result in self-protective, adaptive, cognitive styles that allow effective functioning. Minimal degrees of threat may not invoke these protective mechanisms for some children. Although these hypotheses may be plausible, more research will be needed to determine how age, developmental, family, and community factors may mediate the strength and nature of these effects.

WAR AND PSYCHOPATHOLOGY

A common concern raised by researchers since World War II until the present has been the potentially specific effects of wartime conditions on the emergence of child and adolescent antisocial behavior and delinquency. For example, Cook (1941) warned of an alarming increase in juvenile delinquency during World War II and likened this growing problem to the situation of "the child wolves of post-revolutionary Russia." Similarly, Alcock (1941) concluded that those children exposed to major wartime stresses responded with "unruly behavior," and those whose major stress was separation from the home were likely to exhibit psychosomatic and neurotic symptoms. In Northern Ireland, Lyons (1979) studied 217 patients (including children) seen in the general medical practice. Based on his assessment of the types of symptoms with which children presented in this setting, the author concluded that these youth had become "conditioned to violence." Undue reliance on clinically referred samples is problematic, however, and such studies are suspect.

Fee (1980) studied 6,604 children from Belfast primary schools and compared these findings with those from similar studies in London and the Isle of Wight by Rutter and colleagues (1970, 1975). The author reported that Belfast school children scored much higher in levels of antisocial behavior than did either of the other two groups. However, the London children appeared to have twice the levels of neurotic disturbance. Overall levels of disturbance were higher in the Northern Ireland sample than in the Isle of Wight studies but lower than levels seen in inner London.

Although the evidence from Fee (1980) seems to support the notion of the effects of chronic warlike conditions on children's development of antisocial behavior, several caveats deserve consideration: as a number of commentators have noted (Heskin, 1980; McWhirter, 1983), despite the social unrest in Northern Ireland, the number of indictable offenses in that area is only two thirds the number in England and Wales. Furthermore, politically motivated offenses constitute only a very small part of the total Northern Ireland official crime statistics, and many more children die of motor vehicle accidents in Northern Ireland than owing to violence (McWhirter and Trew, 1981). The vast majority of juvenile crimes in this area are not political terrorism or violence but theft (McWhirter, 1983).

Other lines of evidence do not provide support for the notion of profound effects of Northern Ireland's sectarian violence on development of aggression and violence in children. McWhirter (1983) studied 200 3- to 16-year-old Belfast children and asked them about their perceptions of causes of death in their society. Children's perceptions indicated they attribute death more to sickness and old age than to violence; these perceptions paralleled official death statistics. Because of evidence that children may become acclimated to these chronic, low to moderate levels of violence, and because of evidence that children's responses to such difficulties tend to be short-lived, more recent research has shifted from the focus on psychopathology to social awareness, values, and attitudes.

VALUES AND ATTITUDES

Growing evidence indicates that wartime stresses, particularly at the low to moderate levels experienced by most children in a major or global conflict, have more important effects in shaping children's attitudes and perceptions than any direct expressions of psychopathology. For example, Ziv et al. (1974) compared 144 children who had been exposed to wartime stress with 54 children without such exposure. Children's peer relationships, levels of aggression, and attitudes toward war, peace, and terrorists were contrasted. Findings indicated that those children who had been exposed to shelling in the immediate vicinity placed increased value on courage in their peers, compared with nonshelled children. There were no differences between the two groups in overt aggression toward terrorists, although there was some evidence of increased covert aggressive attitudes and increased patriotism among shelled children. Both groups equally valued peace. Contrary to popular notions, shelled children showed no more increased positive attitudes toward war than did nonshelled children. Exposed children appeared to demonstrate a stronger identification with the community, however. In another Israeli study Ziv and Nebenhaus (1973) assessed 659 children to determine their wishes and thoughts about peace during different periods of war intensity. Only one child expressed any hostile wishes toward the perceived aggressor, suggesting that the phenomenon of "identification with the aggressor" was quite infrequent.

Exposure to wartime conditions may result in other subtle, but perhaps more important, shifts in interactions in relationships within families. Cohen and Dotan (1976) studied the war and postwar communication patterns of a stratified random sample of 118 married Israeli women with 6- to 18-year-old children. Their findings indicated that wartime stress resulted in increased mother-child conversations and time spent together watching television. These effects were greater for families of a higher socioeconomic background. Surprisingly, the husband's draft status did not affect the findings.

Thus, the literature concerning the type and frequency of psychiatric morbidity in children exposed to war is somewhat conflicting. Few would disagree that the exposure to war with its multiple adversities constitutes a significant interference with the child's emotional, social, and intellectual development, but the native adaptive capacities of children and adolescents may mute more pronounced effects of the exposure to war. As Garmezy and Rutter (1985) have noted, children's response to stressful conditions appears to be less intense than might have been anticipated. Because the preponderance of evidence suggests that many children exposed to stressful wartime conditions show no important increases in significant psychopathology (at least under conditions of low to moderate wartime stress), increased attention should be focused on factors that may mediate or buffer the effects of wartime conditions on children.

PARENTAL SEPARATION, LOSS, AND ABSENCE

Wartime Evacuation of Children from Parents

Some of the first lines of evidence about the effects of war-related parental separations on children came from the fairly common World War II British policy of evacuating children to the safer countryside away from the bomb-stricken cities. These children were separated from parents and frequently placed abruptly in unknown surroundings with unfamiliar caregivers. Straker and Thouless (1940) described the "Cambridge Evacuation Survey," where 6,700 children were evacuated from their homes in September 1939. Fully half returned to their homes in the first month, due to dissatisfaction with the foster care arrangements, finances, or homesickness. Burt (1940) studied changes in children's symptoms before and after evacuation and noted a marked increase in anxiety after evacuation, especially among girls. He concluded there was an increase in "mild conditions" owing to evacuation but not in "serious conditions." Likewise, Henshaw and Howarth (1941) concluded that the air raids themselves caused less disturbance than did evacuation.

Although most World War II British child care workers, scientists, and policy makers concluded that the evacuation policy probably was harmful to children, not all workers in this area agreed. To compare evacuated and nonevacuated children, Boyd (1941) surveyed school teachers after the children returned to their homes and concluded that evacuated children did better in the areas of "speech and discipline" than those who had not been evacuated. Nonetheless, rigorous scientific evidence on this point was not forthcoming from the World War II studies, and carefully controlled studies may have been unethical. Some tentative conclusions are possible, however. As Rutter (1974) has indicated, the reason and circumstances surrounding a given separation may be more relevant to the question of untoward effects on the child than the simple separation itself: thus, in the case of separations in the midst of great sense of danger, fears for the child's, family's, or parents' safety, and/or lack of adequate preparation of the child, the effects may be quite different than instances where separations occurred under more ideal circumstances.

Prisoner of War Studies

A few studies available have examined the effects of parental separation in families of male prisoners of war (POWs). As one would expect, the POW's family fares poorly during his absence. Understandably, the determination of effects of prolonged husband-father absence per se in this select population is difficult, inasmuch as many other changes occur to these families in addition to the POW's imprisonment (e.g., the family's ever-present fears for his safety and their reasonable doubts about his eventual return). Using standardized interview schedules, McCubbin and Dahl (1976) investigated 100 Army, Navy, and Marine Corps POW families before the POWs' return and found that 12% of 204 POW children had been in treatment and an additional 20% needed psychiatric treatment. In a follow-up study of a subset of these families, McCubbin and Dahl (1976) studied 43 American Navy POW families 1 year after reunion and found that the children scored significantly lower on the California Test of Personality major subscales

(Total Personal Adjustment and Total Social Adjustment) as well as the overall scale (Total Adjustment), compared with standardized norms. Fathers' increasing length of absence was associated with better child adaptation, suggesting that with increasing lengths of father absence, children (and possibly wives) were able to develop partially compensatory adaptive strategies to cope with the father's POW separation and absence.

"Routine" Father Absence

Previous studies of U.S. military families suggest that "routine" (non-POW) wartime father absence does not necessarily produce uniform, adverse effects on children. Hill (1949) and Boulding (1950) studied 135 randomly selected Iowa veterans and their families with extensive interviews at the war's end and found that good marital adjustment and the degree of family affection before separation predicted good reunion adjustment. Families that only partially "closed ranks" (i.e., kept the absent father's role and importance central to the family emotional environment, yet got on with the business at hand) suffered more during his absence but did better at reunion than those families that "closed ranks" completely at the time of father separation, as if to shut out the reality of the father's absence. Individual instances occurred in which a family did not have a stable situation before the father's departure but was nonetheless poised for a developmental spurt. Some families used the period of father absence as one of significant growth and development.

Thus, effects of parental absence during wartime may be variable and may not always be deleterious. Several studies during the Vietnam War documented significant effects (both positive and negative) of father absence on children, particularly boys. Hillenbrand (1976) studied 73 boys and 53 girls in a sixth grade classroom in a school for military children and demonstrated that cumulative father absence (defined as the total amount of time separated from the child and family to that point in the child's life) was associated with higher IQ scores in first-born boys. But for younger boys with older siblings, "early-beginning" father absence (not defined by the authors) was related to increased aggression and dependency as well as greater verbal than math scores. Nice (1978) studied the personal adjustment of 53 children 1 to 4 months before the wartime deployment of their fathers aboard a U.S. Navy aircraft carrier and again 1 to 3 months after their fathers' return. During the course of the absence, children demonstrated significant gains on standardized personality tests. Although such findings were not hypothesized a priori, similar findings have been described by other researchers who have noted the "steeling" effect of certain life challenges can facilitate growth and adaptation (e.g., Garmezy, 1974).

Overall findings from the military father-absence literature indicate that relatively brief parental absences during wartime situations are associated with modest, temporary behavioral and emotional symptoms in family members, particularly in wives and sons. The reintegration and reunion process is critical to the resolution of these difficulties. Absence of greater length, frequency, or under combat or wartime conditions may exert more persistent effects. The data at hand suggest that absence effects are mediated by preexisting father-family relationships, the age, gender, and birth order of siblings, meaning of the absence to the family, extent of danger to which the father is exposed, and how the mother copes with the father's absence. Under some circumstances, father absence may be associated with adaptive outcomes and enhanced personality development.

The relatively recent increase in families with two military parents as well as increase in female active-duty parents are important phenomena and deserve further study. Unfortunately, we have been unable to locate any systematic literature on the effects of female military parent absence on children.

Bereavement Issues

There are a few systematic studies of the effects of parental loss and bereavement on children and adolescents during times of war. Unfortunately, there is a similar absence of systematic research concerning the effects of bereavement on children under normal, nonwartime conditions, although recent evidence suggests that more than one third of grieving children meet criteria for major depression (Weller et al., 1991). Nonetheless, because of the overall lack of systematic studies of bereavement in children, comparisons between wartime and nonwartime situations are difficult. It is reasonable to expect that the effects of parental loss and the process of bereavement may be similar to that of children who lose their parents during peacetime conditions, but the context and meaning of the loss may have unique significance. For example, to the grieving child, the lost parent (usually father) may be regarded as a hero, or the child may feel that the father's death was due to some kind of failure on the father's part. Circumstances in which the larger national community also shares the grief and respect of the lost one may result in different consequences for bereaved children. Nonetheless, a continuing study of 25 Israeli children who lost their fathers to military action when they were 2 to 10 years old indicates the sustained effect of parental death on the psychological health of these children. Fifty percent of these children continued to have significant behavioral and emotional problems 3½ years after the father's death (Elizur and Kaffman, 1982, 1983). Unfortunately, these studies were uncontrolled, rendering it difficult to compare the effects of parental loss owing to military action with parental loss and bereavement under other circumstances, as well as with children who did not lose their parents.

MEDIATORS OF THE EFFECTS OF WAR

A variety of factors must be considered to understand why some children do not appear to be as susceptible to the effects of war as others. These mediators may be divided into child factors, family factors, and social cultural factors.

Child Specific Factors

Variables intrinsic to the individual child likely to affect ultimate outcomes in children exposed to wartime conditions include such factors as age, inborn coping style and capacity, cognitive level and other developmental factors, guilt, preexisting psychopathology, and temperament. Some evidence suggests that a substantial proportion of children are able to call on intrinsic coping capabilities during wartime crises and generate new levels of adaptation and coping. For example, during the 1967 Arab-Israeli War, de Shalit (1970) reported that many children responded in a remarkable manner, often displaying high levels of self-sacrifice and desire to help the community. In this situation, children's fears often seemed less than one might have expected. One child said to his mother (a child psychiatrist), "At a time like this, each of us has a job to do. Mine is to go to school and be with my friends. We must not try to get out of our obligations." When war affects the home front, children (like adults) may prefer active roles (filling sandbags, etc.) to passive roles (sitting in shelters).

The opportunity to play an active role and to exert some control over one's individual responses to war stressors may have important eventual consequences on children's outcomes. For example, Brander (1941) noted that those who were evacuated to the countryside under voluntary conditions fared better than those who remained in the city. He theorized that evacuation was not harmful when it was voluntary and unhurried, in agreement with the findings of Dunsdon (1941). Brander concluded that the separation of children from parents was more harmful than the evacuation itself, especially when evacuation was conducted en masse and without consideration of individual needs.

Recent evidence provides additional support of the importance of the opportunity to exercise personal control in one's response to war stressors. Baker (1990) studied self-esteem, locus of control, and behavioral symptoms in 796 Gaza and West Bank children and found evidence of higher levels of positive self-esteem and locus of control since the Intifada, which allowed the children to more actively respond to the stresses of the Israeli occupation of that territory by the local residents.

The ability to exert and develop an internal locus of control may be more characteristic of older children, and it may be the adaptive result of a response to stressors. Lifschitz (1975) found that adolescents who had lost fathers during the

Six Day War or the Yom Kippur War tended to exercise a more internal locus of control and assert responsibility for their lives, as compared with controls.

A child's ability to invoke a variety of cognitive defense mechanisms may enhance adaptive outcomes. For example, Rofe and Lewin (1982) noted that adolescents exposed to moderate levels of bombing stress seemed to develop a repressive cognitive style; for example they have fewer sleep difficulties during war periods than nonexposed children. Bodman (1941) noted that among 44 children who had experienced severe bombing of a hospital in which they were being treated, older children tended to describe the event in retrospect as "an adventure." Among the oldest children, reactions were remarkably slight, and adaptive outcomes seem related to these children's sense of responsibility to care for the younger children.

Age and developmental factors may set important limits on children's and adolescents' capacity to respond adaptively to war crises. The young child lacks the cognitive capacities available to the adult. His/her theories of causality are egocentric, and he or she may be unable to talk about frightening experiences. Unable to transform internal conflicts and feelings into words, the child may express such feelings in action, play, or aggressive behaviors or activities. In contrast, the older child and adolescent may have a wider repertoire of adaptive responses and coping capabilities.

A number of authors have noted that older children and adolescents who have suffered pronounced effects of war often demonstrate remarkable resiliency. Whereas some evidence suggests that such youths may be at risk for the eventual development of anxiety and depressive symptoms, some of these youths also may identify with the "helping professions" (medicine, law, etc.) and prepare themselves for future positions in a society without war or violence (Dyregrov et al., 1987; Shaw, 1987). However, such findings cannot be understood without long-term studies, inasmuch as such early responses to war stress could eventually become dysfunctional. The importance of longitudinal follow-up study is indicated in the studies of Kinzie and colleagues (1986), who noted that 50% of Cambodian war refugee children who were traumatized while between 6 and 12 years of age had a diagnosis of PTSD in young adulthood. Follow-up of Cambodian refugees 3 years after fleeing Cambodia indicated that nearly half continued to exhibit PTSD (Kinzie et al., 1989).

Possibly, younger children may be at increased risk for later consequences of war stress, because of their increased preponderance of idiosyncratic and egocentric thought. Thus, a young child whose father is killed during wartime may wonder why the father was killed and whether the father failed somehow. Young children's tendency to attribute blame associated with their inner feelings is well described among clinical populations and may be an important contributing factor for some adverse outcomes. Freud and Burlingham (1943) suggested that very young children must be protected from war and violence, not because the horrors are strange and traumatic, but because the outer violent circumstances may parallel the children's inner experiences. Under such conditions, the normal processes of sublimation and repression are made much more difficult.

When considering the role of war stressors on children and adolescents, it should be known that the war traumas may unmask latent psychopathology or, perhaps more commonly, may serve as a framing construct for more normal developmental fears. Thus, the child who at a given age may be quite normally afraid of certain animals or strangers may just as well become afraid of that country's enemies, e.g., the "Russians" for the U.S. child, the "Israelis" for the Palestinian child. In this sense, the war events may serve as metaphors or vehicles for the child to express normal developmental anxieties.

Parental and Family Responses

Understandably, the preschool child living within the security of a constantly available and supporting family often mirrors the parental response to wartime stressors. When there is parental physical injury, significant parental emotional responses, premorbid parental psychopathology, or excessive intolerance of the child's tendency to regress behaviorally, an emotional contagion may occur that passes like a "ripple effect" on the child (Bloch et al., 1956; McFarlane, 1987; Newman, 1976; Pynoos et al., 1987). Although these concepts are grounded in a substantial clinical and developmental literature, the actual extent to which parent-child emotional contagion occurs is unclear, and inferences about such factors often are drawn from selected clinical cases. This is problematic, inasmuch as equally dramatic instances of adaptive outcomes have been seen in other selected case vignettes (e.g., Epstein, 1979), which describe how children whose parents were in concentration camps coped with the traumatic experiences of their parents. Parent-child interactions obviously were importantly shaped by the parent's history of trauma, outcomes were most commonly quite adaptive, and adverse outcomes were not necessarily reflected in the traditional domains of psychopathology.

Unfortunately, case studies of clinical populations and samples have popularized the notion of common mental health problems among children of concentration camp survivors (Bergman and Jucovy, 1982; Sigal and Rakoff, 1971). In a much more carefully controlled and conducted study, Leon and colleagues (1981) examined a community based sample of concentration camp survivors and their children, and compared them with matched control families who were European immigrants. Findings indicated neither increases in psychopathology nor survivor guilt among children of concentration camp survivors. Likewise, additional evidence from Israeli studies suggests that although parents must cope with certain anxieties about the safety and welfare of their children under wartime conditions, most parents do not become unnecessarily overprotective or anxious; in fact, they seem to facilitate adaptive responses in their offspring (de Shalit, 1970).

Highly individualized, specific aspects of the child-parent relationship may be more explanatory of adverse outcomes than are generic war events and processes. For example, Lifschitz and colleagues (Lifschitz, 1975; Lifschitz et al., 1977) noted that among children who had lost their fathers during the Yom Kippur War, children with an affectionate relationship with the mother were better adjusted. This finding was particularly related to adaptation in boys whom the mothers regarded as similar in characteristics to the deceased father. Nonetheless, these findings are not surprising, and are quite consistent with findings one would expect for children who have lost parents under nonwartime conditions.

Although parental responses are likely to mediate important adaptive and maladaptive outcomes in children, no evidence supports the notion that many adverse outcomes are explained by this phenomenon, particularly in view of the relatively remarkable outcomes in most children exposed to war events and processes. Likely, most parents respond quite appropriately during wartime conditions on behalf of their children. Inferences from clinical samples cannot be applied to the broader populations exposed to these stressors.

Acclimatization

A fair degree of evidence suggests that under slight to moderate levels of war stress, children and their parents may acclimate to these situations. For example, Ziv et al. (1974) compared 144 children who had been exposed to wartime shelling with 54 children without such exposure with regard to their peer relationships, aggression, and attitudes toward war, peace, and terrorists. Findings indicated that stressed children did not have significantly worse outcomes. Similarly, Ziv and Israeli (1973) studied anxiety levels of 103 children whose neighborhoods were shelled during the Six Day War and compared them with 90 children who were never shelled during the same time period. Findings indicated no differences between the two groups in anxiety levels, contrary to a priori hypotheses. These authors concluded that shelling may become a somewhat routine part of life, since no significant, specific trauma directly impacted on the children's lives. Similar findings have been reported by Milgram (1982), who found that anxiety levels in 50 11-year-old children living along the Jordanian border were no different from levels of children living in the middle of the country where terrorist attacks were very uncommon. Surprisingly, the group most exposed to wartime stresses along the border showed higher levels of autonomy and self-confidence than did the nonexposed group.

Not all investigators have reported no effects of wartime stress on children.

Kristal (1978) compared 66 shelled children ages 10 to 12 with 71 nonexposed peers and found a higher prevalence of bruxism among exposed children. Although the groups did not differ in neutral situations, exposed children reported higher anxiety levels after watching a film of a terrorist attack. Thus, a provocative stimulus was required to demonstrate the differences between exposed and nonexposed children. In a less carefully controlled, but nonetheless interesting study, Milgram and Milgram (1975) longitudinally studied 85 fourth and fifth grade students using a variety of questionnaires and psychological tests; their findings demonstrated a twofold increase in anxiety in these children from the beginning to the end of the Yom Kippur War. However, socioeconomic changes and the effects of mobilization and other uncontrolled variables may have mediated children's response rather than the threat of war per se.

Findings are not conclusive, but the weight of the evidence concerning the effects of war-related stresses on children and adolescents indicates that children may acclimate to relatively low or moderate levels of war-related stressors, particularly when such stressors do not involve direct physical trauma to the child or immediate family. The proximity of the threat and stressor is apparently a critical determining variable in mediating outcomes, and the child's potential acclimatization may be a function of the war stresses to which he or she must respond, including their level, intensity, and his or her history of exposure to the stresses, as well as the context in which they are presented. However, more research is needed to answer this question with certainty.

Social and Community Contexts

Beyond the role that child and family characteristics may play in shaping children's reactions to war, the social context of specific war-related events is likely also an important mediator of eventual outcomes. For example, researchers who have studied the effects of the chronic political and social unrest in Northern Ireland have noted that the reported differences in children's behavior in comparative studies between Ireland and England cannot be adequately understood without considering the broader socioeconomic conditions in these two comparisons. For example, unemployment has tended to be much higher in Ireland than in England (e.g., 15.4% versus 6.6%) (Heskin, 1980). Furthermore, housing conditions are much worse, neonatal mortality is higher, and more families are on welfare (Heskin, 1980). Thus, even if the data were to suggest (which they do not) that the Northern Ireland political unrest leads to adverse long-term effects on these children, such concerns must be tempered by the fact most Northern Ireland children would continue to be "under stress" long after the political unrest ceased.

Another social contextual factor is the meaning of the war-related tensions within the community. For example, Ziv and Israeli (1973) suggest that Israeli children who have been exposed to bombings may have been protected by their "hero" status, inasmuch as their situation was well known and met with great sympathy throughout the country. Conceivably, war-related stresses occurring during an unpopular war (such as Vietnam) could have quite different consequences than similar events occurring during a war that was widely regarded as justified and "moral."

Other researchers of the effects of war on children in Israel have concluded that the presence of strong social and community supports may buffer the effects of adverse experiences on children and adolescents. Lifschitz and colleagues (Lifschitz, 1975; Lifschitz et al., 1977) noted that children who had lost their fathers during the war fared better when they lived in kibbutzim than in less cohesive supportive settings (e.g., the moshav or traditional environments). Authors have noted that among children living in the 150 kibbutzim in Israel the incidence of psychological disturbance after the Yom Kippur War was no higher than during the 2 years before the outbreak of the war (Milgram, 1982). Such positive outcomes may be the result of specific steps taken within the kibbutzim to ameliorate or prevent stressful responses in children during these war tensions, but concerns have been raised that such optimistic assessments of outcomes may be partly related to political motivations (Milgram, 1982). Nonetheless, similar findings have been noted for adults, indicating that under high levels of stress, a higher degree of social supports may buffer the effects of stressful events (Zuckerman-Bareli, 1979). Additional support for the stress-buffering hypothesis has been found in studies of Palestinian women (Punamaki, 1986).

Ayalon (1983) has identified three community variables that may mediate child and family responses to terrorist and war-induced stresses. First, the historical and cultural characteristics of the community, as well as its previous experience with such trauma, may shape its reactions to subsequent traumas. Second, community features such as leadership, community cohesion, and communication can play an important role, particularly during and after the stressful situations. Third, the community's specific anticipatory responses to the possibility of the occurrence of such traumatic events likely shape responses during and after the traumas.

In addition to these factors, it seems plausible that the community's specific responses after the traumatic situation may further shape eventual outcomes. For example, Ayalon (1983) noted that after one terrorist attack on a school in which many children were significantly injured, traumatized children were treated insensitively by the school system, which tended to regard the children's later concentration difficulties as "taking advantage of the situation." In some instances, responses were punitive: girls were expelled who violated the dress codes by wearing slacks to school to cover disfigurement and scarring to their legs.

INTERVENTIONS

In the consideration and development of interventions for children who have been affected by war events and processes, attention to three possible levels of intervention is indicated. One may intervene directly with the child, with his or her family, or at community/social structure level.

Child Specific Interventions

It is not totally clear what constitutes an ideal intervention for children who have been affected by terrorist or war-related acts. Some authors (Ayalon, 1983) have described a series of interventions including ventilation, abreaction, channeling of aggression, gradual in vivo exposure to feared situations, and cognitive reappraisal. Shaw and Harris (1989) have proposed a transitional psychosocial program to facilitate war-traumatized children's reorganization of their lives to enable them to again meet normal developmental expectations and participate in family and community. This program, consisting of an intensive residential program with high levels of staff involvement, group activities, psychodrama, and psychiatric consultation, is being implemented in Mozambique (Shaw and Harris, 1991). However, such interventions may be most useful for children whose traumatic experiences have entailed the separation and massive disruption of family and social ties and would not apply to children under most circumstances.

Child-focused interventions in clinical settings often entail: (1) identifying and understanding the pattern of symptoms and dysfunction, (2) facilitating the child's expression of emotions, fears, and anxieties embedded in the symptom complex, and ultimately (3) enabling the child's interpretation and understanding of the traumatic situation. Younger children with behavioral or emotional symptoms may be given an opportunity to draw or play out their traumatic experiences, thus providing a forum for discussion. Older children and adolescents can be more directly encouraged to express and verbalize feelings, questions, and concerns, so they will not feel overwhelmed with feelings of guilt, shame, grief, and helplessness. Avenues must be made available for the expression of affects, conflicting feelings, confusing and muddled impressions, and perceptions, which otherwise are all too often quickly distorted in a search for egocentric explanations of causality. Although there are a number of therapeutic avenues by which one can address traumatized children and adolescents, a critical component employed in most settings is a psychosocial treatment designed to facilitate the child's assimilation and integration of the reality and meaning of the traumatic situation, such that he or she is able to progress with developmental tasks.

Using less traditional clinical approaches, Lifschitz and colleagues (Lifschitz,

1975; Lifschitz et al., 1977) noted that children who have lost their fathers benefit from identification with and pairing with "big brothers" or "big sisters." Other observers (Eloul, 1982; Morawetz, 1982) have noted that many children do not seem to be able or willing to cope directly or verbally with loss but do like to be with other children who have experienced similar losses. Parents should know that such difficulties do not constitute a lack of love for the lost one or shallowness on the child's part but are relatively common responses.

Group intervention with child victims of war is a promising technique, with its provision of opportunities for clarification of cognitive distortions, normalization of the recovery process and further assessment of psychiatric and psychological comorbidity. However, one must be aware that children may suffer from a spectrum of emotional and behavioral problems that require individualized, targeted interventions. When children manifest symptoms of noradrenergic hyperarousal and continuing failure of modulation, consideration may be given to using psychopharmacological interventions, e.g., propranolol, clonidine, and the tricyclics (Famularo et al., 1988; Friedman, 1991). Nonetheless, because there are many different contexts and great variations in children's responses to war situations, great care must be given to develop interventions that consider the child's and family's ecological and cultural context.

Family Interventions

At the level of family interventions, traditional individually focused mental health concepts and approaches may need further restructuring. During crises, how does one treat families without disrupting the social structure? If children's responses to such traumas will be partly mediated through the effects on the broader family structure, interventions designed to assist the larger family group may be most effective. For families where a parent is away owing to war (either as a POW or more routine military combat duty), Frank, Shanfield, and Evans (1981) recommended that the absent parent's place be kept "open" during the time of separation, to facilitate that parent's eventual reintegration into the family on return. Although we are unaware of systematic research evidence documenting the actual usefulness of such strategies, many workers in the field recommend the use of frequent letters and tapes from the absent parent whenever possible, as well as the provision of ongoing support structures for the remaining parent (e.g., through the use of support groups, etc.).

Dreman and Cohen (1982) have recommended specific family therapy approaches as a strategy for dealing with children and adolescents who have been victimized by terrorist and war-related events. With this approach they deemphasize the importance of individual psychopathology and concentrate instead on promoting family strengths, cohesion, and coping.

Community Interventions

Given the broad and far-reaching impact of war-related events and processes on children and families, it seems likely that conventional mental health practices at the individual or even family level may not be possible during wartime due to the lack of available resources. In addition, it is possible that such individual- or family-specific interventions may be wasteful, ineffective, or even harmful. Traditional mental health concepts often are derived from Western thought and culture and may not be useful in other cultural contexts. As one method of choosing among treatment approaches, Benyamini (1976) has recommended the consideration of community level interventions for broad and potentially mild problems (e.g., school interventions), group level interventions for more severe problems (e.g., therapeutic approaches) family or group, and individual level interventions (e.g., child and family therapeutic approaches) for the most severe war-related difficulties.

Community level interventions draw on the premise that the breakdown of social structure may be a critical factor in determining the overall impact of war traumas on children and families. Because the social structure provides the norms and context for interpreting and understanding traumatic events and circumstances, interventions at the level of these community structures may provide a highly relevant, potentially effective vehicle for intervention. Benyamini (1976) has described a school psychological emergency intervention after a terrorist attack. Similarly, at the community and school level Koubovi (1982) has advocated the use of "therapeutic teaching" of literature during the war-related events and their aftermath. This approach involves selecting books with war-related themes and conducting classroom discussion. Koubovi suggests that such an approach promotes intellectualization, cognitive reappraisal, and reassurance of the likelihood of positive outcomes, while avoiding the unstructured and potentially harmful ventilation of feelings. At the group and community level other authors have suggested the use of art (Pergamenter, 1982; Schwarcz, 1982).

In Israel, some communities have prepared for the threat of war and terrorist attacks by systematic training and development. Such approaches are characterized by attack drills, allocation of roles and responsibilities to individual members, and the development and use of communications structures (Ayalon, 1983). These approaches seem plausible, but Ayalon (1983) has cautioned that an actual terrorist attack or war may be so traumatic that no amount of preparation through cognitive approaches can prepare one for the actual assault. Furthermore, it is possible that such rehearsals may increase children's anxieties and phobic responses and reinforce children's stereotyping of others as "the enemy." Nonetheless, promising systematic approaches have been developed to orient a community and its children to respond to emergency situations (e.g., COPE,

Community Oriented Preparation for Emergency, developed at the University of Haifa), but studies of the effectiveness of such interventions are needed.

Although a variety of child, family, and social system level approaches have been developed, there is no research evidence documenting the superiority of one intervention over the other. Benyamini's (1976) recommendations for interventions at three system levels (based on the severity and breadth of the problem) are sensible but may not be possible under widespread or severe war-related conditions. Studies of combat stress reactions in the United States and Israeli military suggest that group- and social-level interventions may be more effective than individually focused interventions. In adult soldiers, traditional, individual, psychopathology oriented psychotherapeutic interventions may lead to prolonged morbidity (Wise, 1988). These adverse outcomes may be partly because of secondary gain resulting from ongoing morbidity in military soldiers, but caution is warranted in the use of individual approaches without careful consideration of the broader context in which the traumas occurred and the systems and cultures in which people must adapt after the resolution of the traumas.

Ethical and Political Issues

Although additional research is needed to better understand the effects of war events and processes on children, one must question whether it is ethical to expend valuable resources during wartime situations in conducting research. Hopes of eventually developing more effective preventive and intervention programs are not unwarranted, but the stressful situations and difficulties under which such research can be conducted may limit the likelihood that effective, well-designed research can be adequately carried out in most wartime situations.

Under some circumstances, political and economic considerations may impede the development and implementation of effective research, including adequate needs assessment of the affected communities. Government agencies or structures responsible for the funding of services may become concerned that the well-defined description of needs and problems within a traumatized community may place great burdens on funding resources to provide such services. In war-torn and refugee situations, concerns may be raised that if the needs are adequately met, refugee camps and other temporary by-products of war may become too attractive, thereby delaying the reintegration of displaced persons and communities back into their home settings.

The recent events of Desert Shield and Desert Storm have galvanized concerns among advocacy and professional groups that during times of national mobilization and preparations for war, all efforts should be made to prevent the separation of mothers from their children. Interestingly, the same recommendation and concern was raised 40 years ago by Stoltz (1951), who noted that mothers should be the last source of manpower during wartime. Such recommendations deserve careful consideration, and may warrant a special panel of scientists, lawmakers, and military leaders to consider the scientific evidence for and against such a step as well as to assess the potential impact of such a decision on military families and national security.

METHODOLOGICAL AND RESEARCH CONSIDERATIONS

Most earlier studies of the effects of war on children (particularly those from World War II) suffered from significant methodological limitations, including the lack of systematic standardized assessments, absence of controls or specification of replicable methods, the absence of longer term follow-ups, and the apparent confounding of many interrelated stressful conditions apart from the war experience itself (e.g., bombings and evacuation being considered simultaneously, without separating the effects of one from the other). Although more recent studies also have suffered (albeit to a lesser extent) from many of these same methodological limitations, the quality of research has improved. Nonetheless, a commonly recurring difficulty has been the heavy use and reliance on clinical samples, from which inferences have been drawn to the larger population.

An important limitation affecting almost all of the reported studies has been the difficulty in establishing adequate controls. Some success in this regard has been achieved in a few of the Israeli studies, but these studies constitute the exception rather than the rule. Even in the better controlled studies, attempts to directly assess child and adolescent psychopathology as a result of war stresses may be hampered by several factors. First, reliance on single informants (e.g., parents or teachers) may unduly shape outcome assessments. Second, findings are most commonly retrospective and unblinded, increasing the likelihood that responses are shaped by children's or adult wishes to potentially "look good" or "look bad" and Hawthorne effects. [Hawthorne effects are defined as effects based upon the actual conduct of a study and subjects' knowledge that they are being tested, rather than from any other experimental variable.] Last, self-report and parent-report checklists have been commonly used for the better controlled studies, but it is unclear whether such instruments are adequately sensitive to what may be significant changes in self-perceptions, values, attitudes as well as subtle forms of psychopathology. Exclusive attempts to focus on assessment of psychopathology may constitute misplaced precision: effects may be most seen in the domains of the children's value systems, later attitudes toward child-rearing, etc. These variables may have only distal relationships to psychopathology that may eventually emerge in later years (or generations).

In addition to these considerations, others have questioned the usefulness of adult-derived models and measures in assessing children's responses to wartime stresses, given the fact that children's responses may be quite different. For example, investigators have noted that children are less likely to demonstrate amnesia, flashbacks, and psychic numbness in response to trauma than they are to exhibit traumatic play or other behavioral reenactments and cognitive distortions (Terr, 1981).

Whereas the effects of direct massive exposure to war trauma may be undisputed, the effects of more "normative" war events and processes often are so confounded with other ongoing events, that it is difficult to tease out the war factors from other potential events (loss of parents, change in social structure, etc.). It is likely that in many instances, the effects of the more "normative" war events and processes will pale in the face of the magnitude and immediacy of other events that often accompany the wartime experience.

Our review suggests that additional attention must be paid to the adequate assessment of children and families who have been affected by war. Although the traditional domain of psychopathology as a potential outcome remains relevant for research, additional studies assessing the impact of wartime conditions on the values and attitudes of children and families are of critical importance. A better understanding of why some children seem to acclimate to low-to-moderate levels of stress, while others remain anxious or become dysfunctional is needed. Greater clarification of the optimal level of intervention for traumatized children and communities is necessary.

The notion of psychological and geographic proximity of the wartime stressors has provided useful clues to comprehending the magnitude of war-related effects under some circumstances, but increased understanding and development of a typology of environments is necessary for us to better understand how similar events with similar psychological and geographic proximity exert dissimilar effects in some persons and some communities, compared with others. Hopes have been raised for a "new world order," but the long and continuing history of international disorder indicates that these research issues deserve ongoing highest priority.

REFERENCES

Alcock, A. T. (1941). War strain on children. *Br. Med. J.,* 1:124.

Arroyo, W. & Eth, S. (1985), Children traumatized by Central American Warfare. In: *Post-Traumatic Stress Disorder in Children,* eds. S. Eth & R. Pynoos. Washington, DC: American Psychiatric Press.

Ayalon, A. (1983), Coping with terrorism. In: *Stress Reduction and Prevention,* eds., D. Meichenbaum & M. Jaremko. New York: Plenum Press, pp. 293–339.

Baker, A. M. (1990), The psychological impact of the Intifada on Palestinian children in the occupied West Bank and Gaza: an exploratory study. *Am. J. Orthopsychiatry,* 60:496–505.

Benyamini, K. (1976), School psychological emergency intervention: proposals for guidelines based on recent Israeli experience. *Ment. Health Soc.,* 3:22–32.

Bergman, M. S. & Jucovy, N. E. (1982), *Generations of the Holocaust,* New York: Basic Books.

Bloch, D., Silber, E. & Perry, S. (1956), Some factors in the emotional reaction of children to disaster. *Am. J. Psychiatry,* 113:416–422.

Bodman, F. (1941), War conditions and the mental health of the child. *Br. Med. J.,* 2:486–488.

Boulding, E. (1950, Family adjustments to war separation and reunion, *Am. Acad. Polit. Soc. Sci. Ann.,* 272:59–67.

Boyd, W. (1941), The effects of evacuation on the children. *Br. J. Educ. Psychol.,* 11:120–126.

Brander, T. (1941), Kinderpsychiatrische Beobachtungen waehrend des Krieges in Finnland, 1939–1940. *Z. Kinderpsychiatr.,* 7:177–187.

Breslau, N., Davis, G. C., Andreski, M. A. & Peterson, E. (1991), Traumatic events and posttraumatic stress disorder in an urban population of young adults. *Arch. Gen. Psychiatry,* 48:216–222.

Burt, C. (1940), The incidence of neurotic symptoms among evacuated school children. *Br. J. Educ. Psychol.,* 10:8–15.

Chimienti, G., Nasr, J. A. & Khalifeh, I. (1989), Children's reactions to war-related stress: affective symptoms and behavior problems. *Soc. Psychol. Psychiatry Epidemiol.,* 24:282–287.

Cohen, A. A. & Dotan, J. (1976), Communication in the family as a function of stress during war and peace. *J. Marriage Family,* 38:141–148.

Cook, P. H. (1941), Evacuation problems in Britain. *Trans. Kans. Acad. Sci.,* 44:343–345.

Dahl, B. B., McCubbin, H. I. & Lester, G. R. (1976), War-induced father absence: comparing the adjustment of children in reunited, non-reunited, and reconstituted families. *Int. J. Sociol. Family,* 6:99–108.

de Shalit, N. (1970), Children in war. In: *Children and Families in Israel: Some Mental Health Perspectives,* eds. A. Jarus, J. Marcus, J. Oren & C. Rapoport. New York: Gordon and Breach.

Dremen, S. & Cohen, E. C. (1982), Children of victims of terrorist activities: a family approach to dealing with tragedy. *Am. J. Family Therapy,* 10:39–47.

Dunsdon, M. I. (1941), Juvenile delinquency in war time, report from the British Child Guidance Clinic. *Lancet,* 2:572–574.

Dyregrov, A., Raundalen, M., Lwanga, J. & Mugisha, C., (1987), Children and War. Paper presented to the Annual Meeting of the Society for Traumatic Stress Studies, October, Baltimore, MD.

Elizur, E. & Kaffman, M., (1982) Children's reaction following the death of the father: the first four years. *J. Am. Acad. Adolesc. Child Psychiatry,* 21:474–480.

Elizur, E. & Kaffman, M., (1983) Factors influencing the severity of childhood bereavement reactions. *Am. J. Orthopsychiatry,* 53:668–676.

Eloul, J. (1982), A description of group work with war widows. In: *Stress and Anxiety,* Vol. 8, eds. C. D. Spielberger, I. G. Sarason & A. Milgram, Washington. DC: Hemisphere.

Epstein, H. (1979), *Children of the Holocaust.* New York, NY: G. P. Putnam's Sons.

Erikson, K. (1976), Loss of community at Buffalo Creek. *Am. J. Psychiatry,* 133:302–395.

Escalona, S. K. (1975), Children in a warring world. *Am. J. Orthopsychiatry,* 45:765–772.

Famularo, R., Kinscherff, R. & Fento, T. (1988), Propranolol treatment for childhood post-traumatic stress disorder, acute type: a pilot study. *Am. J. Dis. Child.,* 142:1244–1247.

Fee, F. (1980), Responses to a behavioural questionnaire of a group of Belfast children. In: *A Society Under Stress: Children and Young People in Northern Ireland,* eds. J. Harbison & J. Harbison. Somerset, England: Open Books, pp. 31–42.

Frank, M., Shanfield, S. B. & Evans, H. E. (1981), The in-and-out parent: strategies for managing reentry stress. *Milit. Med.,* 146:846–849.

Freud, A. & Burlingham, D. T. (1943), *War and Children,* New York: Medical War Books, Ernst Willard.

Friedman, A. (1991) Biological approaches to the diagnosis and treatment of post-traumatic stress disorder. *J. Traumatic Stress,* 4:67–91.

Garmezy, N. (1974), Children at risk: the search for antecedents of schizophrenia. Part II: Ongoing research programs, issues, and intervention. *Schizophr. Bull.,* 9:55–125.

Garmezy, N. & Rutter, M., (1985) Acute reactions to stress. In: *Child and Adolescent Psychiatry: Modern Approaches,* 2nd edition, eds. M. Rutter & L. Hersov. Oxford, Blackwell, pp. 152–176.

Gillespie, R. D. (1942), *Psychological effects of war on citizen and soldier.* New York: W. A. Norton.

Henshaw, E. M. & Howarth, H. E. (1941), Observed effects of wartime conditions on children. *Mental Health,* 2:93–101.

Heskin, K. (1980), *Northern Ireland: A Psychological Analysis.* New York, N.Y.: Columbia University Press.

Hill, R. (1949), *Families Under Stress: Adjustment to the Crises of War Separation and Reunion.* Westport: Greenwood Press.

Hillenbrand, E. D. (1976), Father absence in military families. *Family Coordinator,* 25:451–458.

Kinzie, J. D., Sack, W., Angell, R., Clarke, G. & Ben, R. (1989), A three-year follow-up of Cambodian young people traumatized as children. *J. Am. Acad. Child Adolesc. Psychiatry,* 28:501–504.

Koubovi, D. (1982), Therapeutic teaching of literature during the war and its aftermath. In: *Stress and Anxiety,* Vol. 8, eds. C. D. Spielberger, I. G. Sarason & N. A. Milgram. Washington, DC: Hemisphere.

Kristal, L. (1978), Bruxism: an anxiety response to environmental stress. In: *Stress and Anxiety,* Vol. 5, eds. C. D. Spielberger, I. G. Sarason & N. A. Milgram. Washington, DC: Hemisphere, pp. 45–59.

Leon, G. R., Butcher, J. N., Kleinman, M., Goldberg, A. & Almagor, M. (1981),

Survivors of the Holocaust and their children: current status and adjustment. *J. Pers. Soc. Psychol.,* 41:503–516.

Lifschitz, M. (1975), Long-range effects of father's loss: the cognitive complexity of bereaved children and their school adjustment. *Br. J. Med. Psychol.,* 49:187–197.

Lifschitz, M., Berman, D., Galili, A., & Gilad, D. (1977), Bereaved children: the effects of mother's perception and social system organization on their short range adjustment. *J. Child Psychiatry,* 16:272–284.

Lyons, H. A. (1979), Civil violence—the psychological aspects. *J. Psychosom. Res.,* 23:373–393.

McFarlane, A. C. (1987), Posttraumatic phenomena in a longitudinal study of children following a natural disaster. *J. Am. Acad. Child Adolesc. Psychiatry,* 25:764–769.

McWhirter, L. (1983), Northern Ireland: Growing up with the "troubles." In: *Aggression in Global Perspective,* eds. A. P. Goldstein & M. H. Segall. New York: Pergamon Press, pp. 367–400.

McWhirter, L. & Trew, K. (1981), Social awareness in Northern Ireland children. *Bull. Brit. Psychological Soc.,* 34:308–311.

Milgram, N. A. (1982), War related stress in Israeli children and youth. In: *Handbook of Stress: Theoretical and Clinical Aspects,* eds. L. Goldberger & S. Breznitz. New York: Free Press, pp. 656–676.

Milgram, R. & Milgram, N. (1975), The effects of the Yom Kippur war on anxiety level in Israeli children. *J. Psychology,* 94:107–113.

Morawetz, A. (1982), The impact on adolescents of the death in war of an older sibling. In: *Stress and Anxiety:* Vol. 8, eds. C. D. Spielberger, I. G. Sarason & N. A. Milgram. Washington, DC: Hemisphere.

Newman, J. (1976), Children of disaster: clinical observations at Buffalo Creek. *Amer. J. Psychiatry,* 133:306–312.

Nice, D. S. (1978), The androgynous wife and the military child. In: *Children of Military Families: A Part and Yet Apart,* eds. E. J. Hunter & D. S. Nice. Washington, DC: U.S. Government Printing Office, pp. 25–37.

Pergamenter, R. (1982), Crisis intervention with child-care personnel in an Israeli border kibbutz. In: *Stress and Anxiety,* Vol. 8, eds. C. D. Spielberger, I. G. Sarason & N. A. Milgram. Washington, DC: Hemisphere.

Punamaki, R. (1986), Stress among women under military occupation: women's appraisal of stressors, their coping modes, and their mental health. *Int. J. Psychol.,* 21:445–462.

Pynoos, R., Frederick, C., Nader, K. et al., (1987), Life threat and post-traumatic stress in school age children. *Arch. Gen. Psychiatry,* 44:1057–1063.

Raviv, A. & Klingman, A. (1983), Children under stress. In: *Stress in Israel,* eds. S. Breznitz. New York: Van Nostrand Reinhold Company, pp. 138–162.

Rofe, Y. & Lewin, I. (1983), The effect of war environment on dreams and sleep habits. In: *Stress and Anxiety,* Vol. 8, eds. C. D. Spielberger, I. G. Sarason & N. A. Milgram. Washington, DC: Hemisphere, pp. 59–75.

Rosenblatt, R. (1983), *Children of War.* Garden City, New York: Anchor Press/Doubleday.

Rutter, M. (1974), Parent-child separation: Psychological effects on the children. *J. Child Psychol. Psychiatry,* 12:233–260.

Rutter, M., Tizard, J. & Whitmore, K. (1970), *Education, Health, and Behavior.* London: Longman.

Rutter, M., Cox, A., Tupling, C., Berger, M. & Yule, W. (1975), Attainment and adjustment in two geographical areas: I. The prevalence of psychiatric disorder. *Br. J. Psychiatry,* 126:520–533.

Sack, W. H., Angell, R. H., Kinzie, J. D., Ben, R. (1986), The psychiatric effects of massive trauma on Cambodian children: II. The family, the home, and the school. *J. Am. Acad. Child Psychiatry,* 25:377–383.

Saigh, P. (1991), Affective and behavioral parameters of traumatized and nontraumatized adolescents, presented to the Annual Meeting of the Society for Traumatic Stress Studies, October, Washington, D.C.

Schwarcz, J. H. (1982), Guiding children's creative expression in the stress of war. In: *Stress and Anxiety,* Vol. 8, eds. C. D. Spielberger, I. G. Sarason & N. A. Milgram. Washington, DC: Hemisphere.

Shaw, J. (1987), Unmasking the illusion of safety: psychiatric trauma in war. *Bull. Menninger,* 51:49–63.

Shaw, J. & Harris, J. (1989), A prevention-intervention program for children of war in Mozambique, presented to the annual meeting of the American Academy of Child and Adolescent Psychiatry, October, New York.

Shaw, J. & Harris. J. (1991), Child victims of terrorism in Mozambique. In: *Human Response to Trauma and Disaster,* eds. R. J. Ursano et al. England: Cambridge Press.

Sigal, J. J. & Rakoff, V. (1971). Concentration camp survival: a pilot study of the effects on the second generation. *Canad. Psychiatry Assoc. J.,* 6:393–397.

Stoltz, L. (1951), The effect of mobilization and war on children. *Social Casework,* 32:143–149.

Straker, A. & Thouless, R. H. (1940), Preliminary results of Cambridge survey of evacuated children. *Br. J. Educ. Psychol.,* 10:97–113.

Terr, L., (1981), Psychic trauma in children: observations following the Chowchilla schoolbus kidnapping. *Am. J. Psychiatry,* 138:14–19.

Terr, L. (1991), Childhood traumas: an outline and overview, *Am. J. Psychiatry,* 148:10–19.

Weller, R. A., Weller, E. B., Fristad, M. A. & Bowes, J. M. (1991), Depression in recently bereaved children. *Am. J. Psychiatry,* 148:1536–1540.

Wise, M. G. (1988), Adjustment disorders and impulse disorders not otherwise classified. In: *Textbook of Psychiatry,* eds. J. A. Talbott, R. G. Hales & S. C. Yudofsky. Washington, DC: American Psychiatric Press, pp. 605–620.

Ziv, A. & Israeli, R. (1973), Effects of bombardment on the manifest anxiety level of children living in kibbutzim. *J. Consult. Clin. Psychol.,* 40:287–291.

Ziv, A., Kruglanski, A. W. & Shulman, S. (1974), Children's psychological reactions to wartime stress. *J. Pers. Soc. Psychol.,* 30:24–30.

Ziv, A. & Nevenhaus, S. (1973), Frequency of wishes for peace of children during different periods of war intensity. *Israeli J. Behav. Sci.,* 19:423–427.

Zuckerman-Bareli, C. (1979), Effects of border tension on residents of an Israeli town. *J. Human Stress,* 5:29–40.

18

Understanding of Acquired Immunodeficiency Syndrome by Elementary School Children—A Developmental Survey

David J. Schonfeld
Yale University School of Medicine, New Haven, Connecticut

Susan R. Johnson
University of California, San Francisco

Ellen C. Perrin
University of Massachusetts, Worchester

Linda L. O'Hare
Yale University School of Medicine, New Haven

Domenic V. Cicchetti
Yale University School of Medicine, West Haven
VA Medical Center, New Haven

Objectives. *The developmental process by which young children acquire an understanding of the concepts of causality, treatment, and prevention of illness as related to acquired immunodeficiency syndrome (AIDS) is poorly understood. Previous studies have focused on adolescent populations and have measured the* facts *that children seem to know rather than their* understanding *of relevant concepts. Such approaches are likely to overestimate the child's true level of understanding and obscure significant misconceptions. The aims of*

Reprinted with permission from *Pediatrics*, 1993, Vol. 92(3), 389–395. Copyright © 1993 by the American Academy of Pediatrics.

Presented in part at the 32nd annual meeting of the Ambulatory Pediatric Association, Baltimore, MD, May 6, 1992, and the VI International Conference on AIDS Education, Washington, DC, August 17, 1992.

this project are to measure directly the level of understanding of the concepts of causality, treatment, and prevention of AIDS in healthy, elementary school children and to assess the sociodemographic variables associated with their conceptual understanding.

Methods. *Using a new, developmentally based, semistructured interview protocol (ASK, AIDS Survey for Kids), 361 children (57% black, 24% Hispanic, 19% white) in kindergarten through sixth grade at four public schools in New Haven, CT were interviewed. Responses to questions about causality, treatment, and prevention were scored for each of three illnesses (AIDS, and for comparison, colds and cancer) based on the level of conceptual sophistication of the response, irrespective of its factual accuracy.*

Results. *Scores for each of the concepts were highly intercorrelated and were correlated most strongly with grade level (R = .31 to .50, P < .0001 for each of these correlations, with the exception of the treatment of AIDS). Gender, race, and socioeconomic status did not contribute significantly to the variance observed for any of the concept scores in a linear regression model. Overall, children's level of understanding of causality was significantly less sophisticated for AIDS than for colds (P < .0001); their level of conceptual understanding for the causality of AIDS was not significantly different from that of cancer (P = .9).*

Conclusions. *Children's understanding of causality, treatment, and prevention of AIDS, as measured by the ASK, follows the same developmental sequence reported for children's understanding of general physical illness. Sociodemographic variables, such as race, gender, and socioeconomic status do not affect children's level of sophistication of these developmental concepts. These results have implications for the creation of developmentally appropriate and effective AIDS education curricula for primary and elementary grades. They also offer guidance to health care providers in their efforts to educate parents and young children about this important topic.*

Early and effective education currently is the most viable means of confronting the acquired immunodeficiency syndrome (AIDS) crisis.[1,2] In general, health education seems to be more effective in preventing the initiation of undesired behaviors than in modifying behavior already present.[3,4] AIDS education therefore needs to begin at a young age,[5] before the initiation of high-risk behaviors. Young children have a right and a need to know about the nature of the AIDS epidemic and how to avoid behaviors associated with transmission of human immunodeficiency virus (HIV) infection. Many studies have documented adolescents' factual knowledge about AIDS,[6-22] but minimal data are available about the knowledge of younger children,[3,4,23-26] and virtually nothing is known about the conceptual process by which children acquire an understanding of the concepts of illness (eg, causality, treatment, and prevention) related to AIDS.[3] There is little information to offer guidance in the creation of effective, developmentally appropriate health education programs for children in the primary and elementary grades, or to guide health care providers and parents in their efforts to educate young children on this topic.

The developmental sequence of the acquisition of concepts about physical illness in general, especially those related to causality and treatment, has been well studied.[27-31] With increasing age and cognitive maturity, a child's understanding of both the cause and treatment of illness increases in a predictable manner,[32] through a series of discrete stages that are characterized by qualitatively different cognitive structures.[28] This developmental progression is not influenced much by gender[28,29,33] or socioeconomic status.[28,33] This model of cognitive development, based on the theories of Piaget, has been utilized as a guiding framework for research in multiple areas of health-related conceptual development, including sexuality, death, and physical illness—three areas that are directly relevant to AIDS education.[29]

Less is known about the development of children's understanding about AIDS in particular. Most previous studies have focused on adolescent populations.[6-22] Through written questionnaires[7-21] these studies catalogued the facts that children can report at different ages, but failed to assess directly their understanding of relevant concepts. Questionnaires that measure only the content of the response (eg, "You get AIDS from sex") without exploring the underlying conceptual understanding (eg, how it is transmitted via sexual relations), do not provide insight into how children learn this information or how it can be taught. Furthermore, this approach is likely to overestimate children's level of understanding and fail to identify their misconceptions (eg, what is meant by sex or sexual relations).

The aims of this project are to measure directly the level of conceptual understanding about AIDS in healthy, elementary school children and to assess the sociodemographic variables associated with children's understanding of these concepts. A semistructured interview was designed to elicit responses from which children's conceptual understanding, in addition to factual knowledge, about AIDS could be quantified. For comparison, the same questions were also asked about colds and cancer. The interview was administered to a cross-sectional sample of kindergarten through sixth grade children in New Haven Public Schools (New Haven, CT); a parallel research project utilizing a comparable interview in an urban public school system in northern California is described in a separate report.[34]

METHODS

Sample

Two elementary schools and their affiliated middle schools, which are representative of the entire school district, were selected by New Haven Public Schools. Children who attend regular education classes in kindergarten through sixth grade in these four schools were invited to participate; full-time special education classes and bilingual classes were excluded. Letters that described the project and consent forms were sent to parents of all eligible children. To minimize any discomfort to the child from the interview, the letter recommended that parents who were concerned about their child's or a family member's HIV status (ie, those with suspected or confirmed AIDS/HIV infection) should not participate. Only those children who agreed to participate and whose parents provided written consent were enrolled. Children who did not return a completed consent form were given additional copies; one phone call was made to the parents to verify that they had received the information sent home with their children and to answer any of their questions about the study.

Signed informed consent was obtained from the parents of 44% of the children who were invited to participate (9% of the parents refused to participate and 48% did not respond), so that 361 children, about equally distributed from grades kindergarten through sixth, were interviewed (see Table 1). The racial distribution of the sample (57% black, 24% Hispanic, 19% white) is highly representative of all students enrolled in elementary schools (kindergarten through fifth grade) in New Haven Public Schools (56% black, 22% Hispanic, 20% white). The socioeconomic status of the sample, as measured by the students' school lunch status (55% free, 9% reduced, 36% full-pay), and gender distribution (52% female, 48% male) were highly representative of all students enrolled in the two elementary schools used in the study (55% free, 7% reduced, 38% full-pay; 47% female, 53% male).

At the time of the study, formal AIDS education was beginning in the sixth grade in one of the participating schools, potentially involving 9% of the study subjects; no formal instruction was provided in the other grade levels. During the interview, children were asked about sources of information about AIDS; 46% reported that they had heard about AIDS from a teacher. In a questionnaire completed by the parents of children participating in the study, 44% of the parents stated that their children had learned about AIDS in school.

Research Instruments and Procedures

ASK (AIDS SURVEY FOR KIDS). The ASK is a semistructured interview lasting approximately 30 to 40 minutes; it is based on the interview protocol described

TABLE 1
Characteristics of the Study Sample (N = 361)

Characteristics	N	%
Grade		
Kindergarten	40	11
1st grade	50	14
2nd grade	51	14
3rd grade	57	16
4th grade	51	14
5th grade	51	14
6th grade	61	17
Total	361	100
Gender		
Female		52
Male		48
Race		
Black		57
Hispanic		24
White		19
School Lunch status		
Free		55
Reduced		9
Full-pay		36

by Perrin and Gerrity[28,33] that examines the child's understanding of the concepts related to physical illness. The ASK includes a series of open-ended questions, listed in Table 2, about the causality, treatment, and prevention of AIDS, and, for comparison, of colds and cancer. The ASK also includes open-ended questions exploring conceptual understanding in other domains (ie, transmission, vulnerability, irreversibility, and symptoms) and additional forced choice questions regarding AIDS (ie, specific mechanisms of casual transmission, fears of having or catching the disease, sources of information, and desire for further education) that are not included in this report.

Responses are probed by the interviewer in a standardized manner until children indicate that their highest level of conceptualization has been reached either by explicitly stating they have no further information or by providing circular or redundant responses. Interviews were conducted by one research assistant and were recorded and transcribed verbatim for later blinded scoring.

The coding scale is organized hierarchically, and it is based on the conceptual sophistication of the response, independent of its accuracy. The answers are scored on a scale from 1 to 6 (with a higher score indicating a more advanced level of conceptual understanding) for each of the three concepts (causality, treatment,

TABLE 2
Questions on the AIDS Survey for Kids Related to Causality, Treatment, and Prevention

Causality
How does someone get AIDS* (a cold, cancer)?
How does a child get AIDS (a cold, cancer)?
How do you get AIDS (a cold, cancer)?

Treatment
When someone has AIDS (a cold, cancer), can that
person get better again?
    Probes
        (If child responds yes) How does someone get
        better?
        (If child responds no) Why not?

Prevention
How can someone keep from getting AIDS (a cold,
cancer)?
    Probes
        What can people do so that they don't get AIDS
        (a cold, cancer)?
        How can a child keep from getting AIDS (a cold,
        cancer)?
        How can you keep from getting AIDS (a cold,
        cancer)?
        What can you do so you don't get AIDS (a cold,
        cancer)?

* AIDS, acquired immunodeficiency syndrome.

and prevention) for each of the three illnesses (AIDS, colds, and cancer), yielding a total of nine concept scores for each child. Scoring criteria are parallel across the three concepts and do not differ by illness. A brief overview of the scoring criteria for the concept of causality is shown in Table 3.

All interviews were scored by one research assistant (L. L. O.) using a detailed scoring guidebook. A random sample of 50 interviews were scored independently by another member of the research team (D. J. S.) as well, to quantify interrater reliability. Observed agreement ranged from 92% to 99% for each concept and illness, using a linear weighting system for partial agreement. In this linear weighting system[35] a score of 1.0 represented perfect agreement between the two scorers. Disagreements that were one category apart (eg, (1,2), (2,1), (2,3), (3,2), etc.) received a score of 0.8; similarly, disagreements that were 2, 3, 4, or 5 categories apart were given respective scores of 0.6, 0.4, 0.2 and 0. Weighted κ, which controls for expected agreement, ranged from 0.63 to 0.97, representing very good to excellent interrater reliability across all concepts and illnesses.[35-37] *Other data.* The Peabody Picture Vocabulary Test-Revised (PPVT-R)[38] was administered to all children just before the administration of the ASK. The

TABLE 3
Sample Scoring Criteria for the Concept of Causality

1 = "I don't know" or off-subject response (eg, "I never had AIDS, but I once had chicken-pox.")
2 = Circular (eg, "You get AIDS by getting sick.") or phenomenistic response, wherein the child refers to a phenomenon associated with having the illness, such as a symptom, as if it were the cause (eg, "You get AIDS by having a fever.")
3 = Concrete, specific causal agents or actions are named (eg, "From a virus.")
4 = Internalization is indicated (eg, "When you have sex, the virus gets inside of you.")
5 = Specific effect of the illness-causing agent is stated (eg, "The virus gets into your body and kills your white blood cells.")
6 = Causal mechanism or process is elaborated (eg, "When your white blood cells don't work you can't fight off other sicknesses and you get real sick.")

PPVT-R is an individually administered, norm-referenced, wide-range, power test of receptive vocabulary designed for administration to persons 2½ through 40 years of age and was used in this study as a measure of verbal fluency and as a proxy estimate of cognitive abilities. Demographic information available from school records included date of birth, gender, race, grade, and school lunch status (free lunch, reduced-pay lunch, full-pay lunch), which was used as a measure of socioeconomic status.

Analyses. Intercorrelations among the nine concept scores were computed by Pearsonian R. Correlations between each concept score and grade level were determined by both Pearsonian R and Stuart's Tau-C (τ). (When measuring the correlation between ordinal variables that do not have the same number of scale points, Stuart's Tau-C is the preferred statistic[39]). Scores for each concept were dichotomized and analyzed by the Jonckheere test of ordinal trend[40,41] to assess whether there is a linear association between grade level and the proportion of children with a more sophisticated level of conceptual understanding. To compare the children's level of understanding of the concept of causality between pairs of illnesses, the score for the concept of causality for one illness was subtracted from the score for the concept of causality for the second illness. The differences in the scores were then analyzed by two-tailed paired t-tests. For each concept and illness, a linear regression model was constructed, with concept score as the dependent variable. Correlation coefficients (Pearsonian R) were determined for any independent variables that contributed significantly to the variance observed in the concept score within the linear regression models. Analyses were conducted using SAS/STAT System for Personal Computers (Release 6.04) proprietary software.[42]

RESULTS

As expected, scores for each of the three concepts (causality, treatment and prevention) for the same illness were moderately correlated (Pearsonian R ranged from .38 to .49, $P < .0001$). Similarly, scores for each illness (AIDS, colds, and cancer) for the same concept were moderately correlated (Pearsonian R ranged from .32 to .46, $P < .0001$).

Grade level (or age) was the single variable most strongly correlated with each of the three concept scores for each of the three illnesses, with a medium to large effect [Pearsonian R[43] ranged from .31 to .50 (corresponding Stuart's Tau-C values ranged from 0.20 to 0.40); $P < 0.0001$] with the exception of treatment for AIDS, for which Pearsonian $R = .14$ ($P = .05$). The most likely reason for the small correlation between grade level and children's level of conceptual understanding of the treatment of AIDS was that 50% of the children stated that AIDS was not treatable, so their responses could not be scored for this concept. Older children were more likely to state that AIDS could not be treated than were younger children [66% (107/163) of children in grades 4 through 6 vs 36% (72/198) of children in grades kindergarten through 3; χ^2 corrected (1 $df = 30.66$; $P < .0001$]. If the response that AIDS is not treatable is rescored as the highest level response for treatment, then a moderate correlation between grade level and level of conceptual understanding of treatment of AIDS is achieved (Pearsonian $R = .30$; $P < .0001$).

To assess further the nature of the relationship between grade level and concept scores, scores for each concept were dichotomized into two levels: low (scores 1 to 3) and high (scores 4 to 6). There was a consistent increase in the percent of children with high concept scores as grade level increased, for each concept and illness ($P < .001$ except for treatment of AIDS: Jonckheere test of ordinal trend[40,41]).

In the Figure, the mean score and standard error of the mean (SEM) for the concept of causality for each illness is shown for each grade, demonstrating that (1) the mean concept score for causality for each of the three illnesses increased consistently as grade level increased, and (2) the children's level of conceptual understanding was less sophisticated for the causality of AIDS than for the causality of colds. This difference was statistically significant for all grade levels combined ($P < .0001$), and for each grade level separately ($P < .01$) except for 4th and 6th. In contrast, the children's level of conceptual understanding of the causality of AIDS was not significantly different from that of cancer ($P = .9$ for all grade levels combined; $P \geq .2$ for each grade).

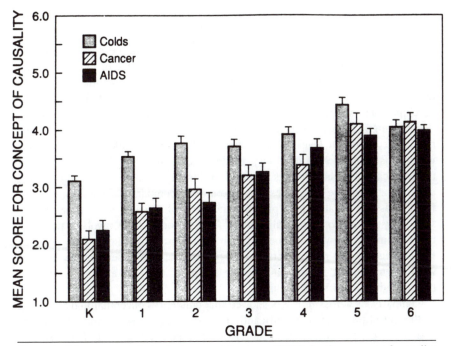

Figure 1. Mean score and standard error of the mean (SEM) for the concept of causality for each of three illnesses (colds, cancer, and acquired immunodeficiency syndrome [AIDS]) as a function of grade level.

For each concept and illness, a linear regression model was constructed, with concept score as the dependent variable. Only grade level contributed significantly ($P \leq .05$) to the variance observed for each concept score and illness. The score on the PPVT-R also contributed significantly to the variance observed for causality for all three illnesses and for treatment and prevention of colds. The overall correlation (Pearsonian R) between PPVT-R score and concept score ranged from .17 to .34 ($P \leq .001$) for each concept and illness, except for the treatment ($R = .06, P = .4$) and prevention of AIDS ($R = .11, P = .03$). The lack of a significant correlation between PPVT-R score and concept score for the treatment of AIDS probably resulted from the large percent of older children who stated that AIDS could not be treated and therefore did not receive a score for the concept of the treatment of AIDS, as discussed previously. Gender, race, and school lunch status did not contribute significantly to the variance observed in the concept score within the linear regression models.

DISCUSSION

Children's understanding of the causality, treatment, and prevention of general physical illness follows a systematic developmental sequence of increasing conceptual sophistication with increasing age (and grade level). This study has shown that children's understanding of AIDS, as measured by the ASK, follows the same developmental sequence, as does their understanding of colds and cancer. Sociodemographic variables such as race, gender, and socioeconomic status did not affect children's level of sophistication for these developmental concepts within this population of inner-city, predominantly minority children. A concurrent replication of the findings reported in this paper was obtained through the administration of the same questions, as part of a comparable interview, to a different cross-sectional sample of elementary school students in an urban public school system in northern California.[34] These studies both involved predominantly minority, lower income children in inner-city public school systems. Further studies with more diverse populations are needed to determine what role, if any, demographic factors have on the timing of the progression of children's understanding of these concepts.

Comparisons across illnesses showed that children's conceptual understanding of the causal processes is significantly less advanced for both cancer and AIDS than for colds, even when the accuracy of the response is ignored. This disparity suggests that, with appropriate educational intervention, children have at least the conceptual ability to achieve a more sophisticated understanding of AIDS. It is unlikely that this discrepancy results from the relative ease of comprehension of the causal processes of colds as opposed to those of AIDS. Both illnesses are caused by viruses that must be internalized. Although the signs and symptoms of a cold (eg, rhinorrhea, nasal congestion, pharyngeal irritation, cough, sneezing, fever, etc) may be more familiar to young children, the direct effects of the virus on the human body and their underlying causal mechanisms are difficult to explain. The mechanism by which HIV impairs the immune system does not appear to be more difficult to explain to children than *how* a rhinovirus causes rhinorrhea or how a "cold" (that many children think is caused by going out in cold weather) makes your body hot. Children's less advanced conceptual understanding of the causal processes of AIDS, as compared with colds, more likely reflects the relative absence of developmentally appropriate explanations about the cause of AIDS and their lesser familiarity with the disease, than it indicates that one illness is inherently more difficult to understand.

Unlike most previous reports of children's understanding of AIDS, this study has concentrated on the level of conceptual sophistication of children's responses and not on the actual content or accuracy of the responses. In other words, the emphasis is placed not on *what* children know, but on *how well* they understand

TABLE 4
Drugs as a Cause of Acquired Immunodeficiency Syndrome (AIDS)

Response	No. of Responses	No. of Children
Drugs, not specified		
Intravenous implied	30	
Intravenous not implied	52	
Total	82	82*
Drugs, specified		
Cigarettes	15	
Alcohol	14	
Cocaine		
Inhaled/smoked	4	
Intravenous	2	
Eaten	1	
Marijuana	2	
Total specific drugs	38	27
Any drug response	120	96

* Thirteen children gave responses that were classified under both drugs, not specified and drug(s), specified, (eg, if the child responded that one can get AIDS from nonspecified "drugs" and also from cigarettes).

it. Superficial analyses of the content of children's responses often overestimate their true understanding and fail to identify major misconceptions. As an illustration, a description of a further analysis of the 120 responses (by 96 children) indicating drugs as one of the means of acquiring AIDS is presented in Table 4.

Overall, 96 children mentioned drugs as a cause of AIDS. Most of these children (82) referred to "drugs" but did not identify a particular drug, although 30 did allude to intravenous drugs (eg, "you get AIDS from drug needles"). Only 27 children were able to indicate a particular drug: 15 listed cigarettes, 14 alcohol, 4 cocaine inhaled or smoked, 2 intravenous cocaine, 1 crack that is eaten, and 2 marijuana. The inaccurate responses, such as cigarettes and alcohol, were equally distributed across grades. Approximately one-fourth of the study sample mentioned drugs as a cause of AIDS. However, of these children, more than two-thirds had a very limited underlying comprehension and did not imply in any way in their response, even after probing, that intravenously administered drugs were involved. This example illustrates the common phenomenon that children are often able to parrot back what appear to be appropriate "facts," but lack an underlying conceptual understanding. Serious misconceptions may develop, as one second grader's response to the question "How does someone get AIDS?" illustrates:

Well, by doing drugs and something like that . . . By going by a drug dealer who has AIDS. (How would you get AIDS by doing drugs?) Well, you go by a person who's a drug dealer and you might catch the AIDS from 'em . . . By standing near 'em.

Similar misconceptions (despite superficially "correct" responses) were also noted regarding sexual transmission. Misconceptions such as these may heighten the child's anxiety about the disease and interfere with efforts to promote appropriate behavioral change. It is therefore inappropriate to rely simply on the *content* of children's answers to estimate the level of their comprehension about AIDS; the use of fact-based multiple choice or true/false questions may be misleading. A developmentally based, semistructured interview, such as the ASK, is a useful tool for the empirical study of children's understanding of this illness.

This study involved elementary school-age children, but misconceptions persist into adolescence and even adulthood. One of the authors (D. J. S.), in addressing classes of high school students, has been asked on more than one occasion whether someone can catch AIDS through anal intercourse even if neither partner is infected with the virus. Similarly, Skurnick et al[11] reported that despite an overall high level of knowledge about AIDS in their survey of New Jersey high school students, 19% believed that AIDS can be spread by sex between two uninfected persons. It appears that these adolescents may memorize the "fact" that (anal) intercourse is a means of AIDS transmission but, lacking a well-developed conceptual framework for a germ theory, may conclude incorrectly that the sexual act itself causes the illness. This apparent paradox of appearing to know a fact, while failing to comprehend truly its meaning, may explain a consistent but puzzling finding in virtually all recent studies of adolescents' understanding of AIDS. Although nearly all adolescents report that AIDS is transmitted through blood and intravenous drug use, an alarming 30% to 60% of the same adolescents will include donating blood as one of the mechanisms of acquiring the illness.[6,11,13,14,16,18,19,21,22] It appears that these adolescents may have memorized the "fact" that HIV may be transmitted via blood, without truly understanding the underlying mechanism; failing to understand that (infected) blood merely serves as a vehicle for the transmission of the viral agent, they may incorrectly conclude that blood transmission, per se, causes the illness. These observations are strong evidence of the need for educational programs that stress conceptual understanding and not simply the memorization of lists of risky and nonrisky behaviors.

An AIDS education curriculum for children in the elementary grades should present in simple but accurate terms how the AIDS virus is transmitted, with an emphasis on correcting misconceptions that may lead to unnecessary anxiety about the disease. Because many children, even at the lower grade levels, have heard about sex and drugs as a cause of AIDS, these means of transmission should be presented without unnecessary elaboration. Instruction should focus on how AIDS is *not* transmitted through drugs, such as alcohol and cigarettes, that do not involve the transfer of blood, and that common means of expressing affection that involve casual contact, such as hugging or holding hands, are not ways of transmitting HIV through "sex." Children need help understanding that drugs do not *cause* AIDS, but that the infected blood that resides within shared drug needles is a means of transmitting HIV.

Children tend to generalize from a familiar condition to a related condition for which they have little information. This study has illustrated that children's understanding of AIDS is less advanced than their understanding of more familiar illnesses, such as the common cold. It should be anticipated that children will overgeneralize from their understanding of the cause of colds to assume that such common actions as coughing, sneezing, or sharing cups or utensils are means of transmitting AIDS. A curriculum developed by one of the authors (D. J. S.) therefore begins each lesson by reminding the children that there are many different types of illnesses. Different illnesses have different causes, different symptoms, different treatments, and different outcomes. And while there are some general lessons we can learn about illnesses, we must also know something about each illness itself. The lessons then proceed to introduce the children to accurate information about the unique characteristics of the causes, treatment, and prevention of AIDS.

IMPLICATIONS

When the AIDS epidemic first became recognized, educators and health care providers quickly attempted to identify the facts that children and adults needed to know to prevent further transmission of this disease. We suggest that further educational efforts for children, by both teachers and health care providers, must be based on an appreciation of the developmental sequence of children's understanding of concepts relevant to this illness.

The information learned from this cross-sectional survey of elementary school children has been used to design developmentally based curricula for AIDS education for children in the primary and elementary grades. One of the authors (D. J. S.) is currently completing a randomized, controlled trial of a multifaceted educational intervention program with these curricula, utilizing the ASK as the outcome measure. Findings from this project will provide information about the efficacy of empirically derived and developmentally based AIDS education curricula.

ACKNOWLEDGMENTS

This research was supported in part by a FIRST Award from the National Institute of Mental Health (5 R29 MH47251) awarded to D. J. S. and a VA Merit Review Grant (MRIS 1416) awarded to D. V. C.

The authors wish to thank Eugene D. Shapiro, MD for critical review of the manuscript, and to acknowledge the continuing support and assistance of New Haven Public Schools—the administrators, teachers, staff, parents, and above all the students, whose efforts allowed this project to be conducted.

REFERENCES

1. Centers for Disease Control. Guidelines for effective school health education to prevent the spread of AIDS. *MMWR.* 1988;37(suppl 2):1–14
2. Brown L, Fritz G. AIDS education in the schools: a literature review as a guide for curriculum planning. *Clin Pediatr.* 1988;27:311–316
3. Brown L, Reynolds L, Brenman A. Out of focus: children's conceptions of AIDS. *J Health Educ.* In press
4. Sly D, Eberstein I, Quadagno D, Kistner J. Young children's awareness, knowledge, and beliefs about AIDS: observations from a pretest. *AIDS Educ Prev.* 1992;4:227–239
5. Quackenbush M, Villarreal S. *Does AIDS Hurt?": Educating Young Children About AIDS.* 2nd ed. Santa Cruz, CA: ETR Associates; 1992
6. Strunin L, Hingson R. Acquired immunodeficiency syndrome and adolescents: knowledge, beliefs, attitudes and behaviors. *Pediatrics.* 1987;79:825–828
7. Price J, Desmond S, Kukulka G. High school students' perceptions and misperceptions of AIDS. *J Sch Health.* 1985;55:107–109
8. DiClemente R, Zorn J, Temoshok L. Adolescents and AIDS: a survey of knowledge, attitudes and beliefs about AIDS in San FRancisco. *Am J Public Health,* 1986;76:1443–1445
9. Helgerson S, Petersen L, The AIDS Education Study Group. Acquired immunodeficiency syndrome and secondary school students: their knowledge is limited and they want to learn more. *Pediatrics.* 1988;81:350–355
10. Brown L, Fritz G. Children's knowledge and attitudes about AIDS. *J Am Acad Child Adolesc Psychiatry,* 1988;27:504–508
11. Skurnick J, Johnson R, Quinones M. Foster J, Louria D. New Jersey high school students' knowledge, attitudes, and behavior regarding AIDS, *Aids Educ Prev.* 1991;3:21–30
12. Huszti H, Clopton J, Mason P. Acquired immunodeficiency syndrome educational program: effects on adolescents' knowledge and attitudes. *Pediatrics.* 1989;84:986–994
13. Goodman E, Cohall A. Acquired immunodeficiency syndrome and adolescents: knowledge, attitudes, beliefs, and behaviors in a New York City adolescent minority population. *Pediatrics.* 1989;84:36–42

14. Steiner J, Sorokin G, Schiedermayer D, Van Susteren T. Are adolescents getting smarter about acquired immunodeficiency syndrome? Changes in knowledge and attitude over the past 5 years. *AJDC*. 1990;144:302–306

15. Nagy S, Hunt B, Adcock A. A comparison of AIDS and STD knowledge between sexually active alcohol consumers and abstainers. *J Sch Health*. 1990;60:276–279

16. Centers for Disease Control. HIV-related knowledge and behaviors among high school students—selected U. S. sites, 1989. *MMWR*. 1990:39:385–397

17. Ross M, Caudle C, Taylor J. Relationship of AIDS education and knowledge to AIDS-related social skills in adolescents. *J Sch Health*. 1991;61:351–354

18. Kann L, Anderson J, Holtzman D, et al. HIV-related knowledge, beliefs, and behaviors among high school students in the United States: Results from a national survey. *J Sch Health*. 1991;61:397–401

19. Siegel D, Lazarus N, Krasnovsky F, Durbin M, Chesney M. AIDS knowledge, attitudes, and behavior among inner city, junior high school students. *J Sch Health*. 1991;61:160–165

20. Shafer M. Boyer C. Psychosocial and behavioral factors associated with risk of sexually transmitted diseases, including human immunodeficiency virus infection, among urban high school students. *J Pediatr*. 1991;119:826–833

21. DuRant R, Ashworth C, Newman C, Gaillard G. High school students' knowledge of HIV/AIDS and perceived risk of currently having AIDS. *J Sch Health*. 1992;62:59–63

22. Hingson R, Strunin L, Berlin B. Acquired immunodeficiency syndrome transmission: changes in knowledge and behaviors among teenagers, Massachusetts statewide surveys, 1986 to 1988. *Pediatrics*. 1990;85:24–29

23. Fassler D, McQueen K, Duncan P, Copeland L. Children's perceptions of AIDS. *J Am Acad Child Adolesc Psychiatry*, 1990;29:459–462

24. Brown L, Nassau J, Barone V. Differences in AIDS knowledge and attitudes by grade level. *J Sch Health*. 1990;60:270–275

25. Montauk S, Scoggin D. AIDS: Questions from fifth and sixth grade students. *J Sch Health*. 1989;59:291–295

26. Walsh M, Bibace R. Children's conceptions of AIDS: a developmental analysis. *J Pediatr Psychol*. 1991;16:273–285

27. Bibace R. Walsh M. Development of children's concepts of illness. *Pediatrics*. 1980;66:912–917

28. Perrin E, Gerrity S. There's a demon in your belly: children's understanding of illness. *Pediatrics*. 1981;67:841–849

29. Burbach D. Peterson L. Children's concepts of physical illness: a review and critique of the cognitive-developmental literature. *Health Psychol*. 1986;5:307–325

30. Pidgeon V. Children's concepts of illness: implications for health teaching. *Matern Child Nurs J*. 1985;14:23–35

31. Potter P, Roberts M. Children's perceptions of chronic illness: the roles of disease symptoms, cognitive development, and information. *J Pediatr Psychol*. 1984;9:13–27

32. Schonfeld D. The child's cognitive understanding of illness. In: Lewis M, ed. *Child*

and Adolescent Psychiatry: A Comprehensive Textbook. Baltimore, MD: Williams & Wilkins; 1991:949–953

33. Perrin E, Sayer A, Willett J. Sticks and stones may break my bones . . . Reasoning about illness causality and body functioning in children who have a chronic illness. *Pediatrics.* 1991;88:608–619

34. Johnson S, Schonfeld D, Boyce T, et al. Urban elementary students' conceptual understanding of causality in AIDS, colds, and obesity. *J Dev Behav Pediatr.* 1992;13:306

35. Cicchetti D, Sparrow S. Developing criteria for establishing interrater reliability of specific items: applications to assessment of adaptive behavior. *Am J Ment Deficiency.* 1981;86:127–137

36. Cohen J. Weighted kappa: nominal scale agreement with provision for scaled disagreement or partial credit. *Psychol Bull.* 1968;70:213–220

37. Fleiss J, Cohen J, Everitt B. Large sample standard errors of kappa and weighted kappa. *Psychol Bull.* 1969;72:323–327

38. Dunn L, Dunn L. *Peabody Picture Vocabulary Test-Revised. Manual for Forms L and M.* Circle Pines, MN: American Guidance Service: 1981

39. Kendall M. *Rank Correlation Methods.* New York: Hafner; 1962

40. Leach C. *Introduction to Statistics: A Nonparametric Approach for the Social Sciences.* New York: John Wiley & Sons; 1979

41. Cicchetti D, Showalter D, Rourke B, Fuerst D. A computer program for analyzing ordinal trends with dichotomous outcomes: application to neuropsychological research. *Clin Neuropsychol.* 1992;6:458–463

42. SAS Institute Inc. *SAS/STAT User's Guide, Release 6.03 Edition.* Cary, NC: SAS Institute Inc; 1988

43. Cohen J. *Statistical Power Analysis for the Behavioral Sciences.* Englewood, NJ: L. Erlbaum Associates; 1988

19

Pharmacological Management of Pain in Children

Betty Pfefferbaum

University of Oklahoma College of Medicine, Norman

Carin A. Hagberg

University of Texas Southwestern Medical Center, Dallas

This article examines the use of analgesics and psychopharmacological adjuvants in children experiencing pain. Peripheral analgesics are effective for mild to moderate pain. Narcotics are effective but may produce dependence and tolerance as well as untoward side effects. Major tranquilizers, minor tranquilizers, tricyclic antidepressants, and stimulants have all been used as adjuvants in pain management. Major tranquilizers are now discouraged because of potential serious adverse effects. Benzodiazepines are relatively safe and decrease anxiety accompanying pain. Tricyclics may be used with caution. Stimulants have received little attention but may be useful in treating both pain and depression in the physically ill.

Only recently have clinicians and researchers begun to delineate effective strategies for pain management in children. Pediatricians often consult with mental health professionals, especially in the use of nonpharmacological interventions or when emotional and behavioral symptoms are present. Psychopharmacological agents are effective adjuvants especially when emotional distress accompanies pain. The child psychiatrist is likely to be consulted for children suffering from pain due to trauma, burns, cancer, and procedural and surgical treatments. Our experience suggests that child psychiatrists receive little exposure to pain management during training, unless by choice. Therefore, when called on for consultation in

Reprinted with permission from the *Journal of the American Academy of Child and Adolescent Psychiatry*, 1993, Vol. 32(2), 235–242. Copyright © 1993 by the American Academy of Child and Adolescent Psychiatry.

such cases, they lack information and confidence. Few systematic reviews of the use of analgesics in pediatric populations are available, and we found none in the child psychiatry literature. We review general principles of pain management, peripheral and central analgesics, and psychopharmacological adjuvants.

GENERAL MANAGEMENT PRINCIPLES

Assessment of pain requires a careful history, physical examination, and evaluation of concurrent emotional and behavioral problems. It is important to establish a trusting relationship with the child. This process begins with believing the complaint of pain (Foley, 1985) and encouraging the child to help define goals and assess the effectiveness of its management. When working with children it is important to provide age-appropriate information about all aspects of treatment. Nonpharmacological management of pain may be adequate alone or in combination with pharmacological intervention.

Treatment should focus on the underlying cause of pain, the pain itself, and any associated symptoms. The use of pharmacological agents in pain management should be guided by the same general principles applied to the pharmacological treatment of any symptom or disorder. These include identifying and monitoring target symptoms and adverse effects, using the lowest effective dose, and establishing a schedule for drug administration that takes into consideration the child's size and conditions that affect drug metabolism. Because children dislike injections, oral administration is the preferred route of administration for most situations unless an intravenous or subcutaneous line is in place. The child's age and size, disease state, and previous analgesic requirements guide treatment choices. Knowledge of the drug, including its side effects, interactions with other drugs, and propensity to cause dependence and tolerance, is critical because specific prescribing information for use in children is often unavailable. The use of adjuvant psychopharmacological agents is based largely on clinical experience and studies in adults. Periodic reassessment of drug effectiveness is critical.

Gastrointestinal absorption is influenced by pH-dependent diffusion and gastric emptying time. Absorption of psychotrophic drugs appears to be more rapid in children than in adults. Numerous factors influence drug distribution including the relative proportion of total body and extracellular water and the proportion of body fat, both of which change significantly during development (Riddle, 1991). Evidence suggesting more rapid disposition of drugs in children is usually explained by their more rapid hepatic metabolism (Jatlow, 1987). For many drugs, the metabolic rate reaches a high for patients between 1 and 5 years old, gradually declining to an adult rate by about age 15 (Riddle, 1991). The process of biotransformation explains the relatively low bioavailability of oral forms of some drugs as compared with parenteral forms. Dosing need simply be adjusted to allow for this effect. The kidneys are the primary organs for drug excretion and achieve adult level function during infancy (Riddle, 1991).

Riddle (1991) summarized what little is known about the pharmacokinetics of psychoactive drugs in children. Comparable doses of chlorpromazine and haloperidol produce lower plasma concentrations in children than in adults. Disposition is more rapid in children, and the drugs undergo extensive biotransformation (Jatlow, 1987). Pharmacokinetic studies of diazepam indicate a shorter half-life in children probably because of developmental factors related to hepatic microsomal enzymes. Developmental differences may not exist for benzodiazepines such as lorazepam and oxazepam that undergo conjugation without first being metabolized by hepatic microsomal enzymes (Riddle, 1991). Biotransformation of tricyclics is extensive in physically healthy children (Ryan, 1990) but may be less so in children with hepatic dysfunction, thereby necessitating a decreased dose or increased dosing interval. The half-life of nortriptyline is significantly shorter in children than in adolescents, and the oral clearance of the drug is significantly greater (Geller et al., 1987). A divided dose schedule is therefore recommended for children. Methylphenidate usually is prescribed at long dosing intervals relative to its half-life. Therefore, steady state concentrations are low by bedtime and at the usual next morning administration (Jatlow, 1987). Disease states, especially those affecting hepatic and renal functioning, must be considered when prescribing drugs for physically ill children.

PERIPHERAL ANALGESICS

Peripheral analgesics are effective for relief of mild or moderate pain such as the low intensity pain of headache, myalgias, arthralgias, and other integumental structures. They also may be used in the management of chronic pain. However, peripheral agents generally do not work well for severe pain or pain of visceral origin. The most commonly used peripheral agents are aspirin and acetaminophen, which have both analgesic and antipyretic effects. Peripheral agents are available in combination with other agents such as buffers, caffeine, antihistamines, and antispasmodics. These combinations are usually more expensive and produce more side effects than do aspirin or acetaminophen alone. Each drug has a "ceiling dose" at which further increases offer no improvement in analgesia. Although dependence and tolerance are not problems associated with these agents, serious side effects may occur, especially with prolonged use (Lacouture et al., 1984). Their side effects are usually the limiting factor in the length of time the agents may be used.

Recommended doses of aspirin are 10 mg/kg per dose or 65 mg/kg per day. When given orally, aspirin is absorbed within 30 minutes and reaches its peak level in 1 to 1½ hours (Schechter, 1985, 1987). Side effects include gastrointestinal irritation, ulcer formation, bleeding, and interference with platelet aggregation. Administration with food, milk, or water often is recommended to decrease gastric symptoms. Aspirin should be avoided for children who have compromised hematopoetic functioning; the use of nonacetylated salicylates such as choline magnesium salicylate is preferable in these patients. Because of its association with Reye's syndrome, aspirin should be avoided in children with viral illnesses. Fatal metabolic acidosis may occur with overdose. Although aspirin is safely and easily used, it is not harmless.

Acetaminophen is comparable with aspirin in dosage but differs from it in several respects. Acetaminophen achieves its peak effect faster, does not exert anti-inflammatory properties or cause gastrointestinal or hematological problems, and is not associated with Reye's syndrome (Schechter, 1985, 1987). Overdose is potentially fatal causing hepatic toxicity 24 to 36 hours after ingestion. If an overdose is recognized within 24 hours, treatment with acetylcysteine is effective and well tolerated. An initial loading dose of 140 mg/kg should be given, followed by 70 mg/kg every 4 hours until the serum acetaminophen level is zero.

Other peripheral agents, including nonsteroidal anti-inflammatory agents, are available. They tend to be more expensive than aspirin and acetaminophen and have not been approved for use in children. They should be considered for those who cannot tolerate aspirin or acetaminophen or for those with particular diseases.

CENTRAL ANALGESICS

The potent narcotic analgesics, morphine and related compounds, are the mainstays of treatment for severe pain, yet many persons remain hesitant to use them. Narcotics should be used when peripheral agents are not tolerated or are inadequate for pain relief. They play a major role in the management of acute and severe pain especially that arising from surgery, bone fracture, or visceral disorders such as biliary and ureteric colic. They are useful in management of chronic intractable pain such as that accompanying terminal cancer. Their major advantage over peripheral agents is their analgesic effectiveness. The major disadvantages are respiratory depression, dependence, and tolerance. Narcotics should be avoided in patients with head injury or craniotomy, seizures, undiagnosed acute abdominal conditions, and intoxication (Clark et al., 1988). Caution should also be exercised when narcotics are given with CNS depressants.

Unlike peripheral analgesics, narcotics do not have therapeutic ceiling doses because pain is a natural antagonist to opiates (Hill, 1988). The primary effect of narcotics on the CNS is analgesia, but untoward effects can occur. Sedation may mean the dose is too high. Concern about euphoria as a side effect is exaggerated, and its occurrence does not necessarily lead to addiction. Dysphoria associated with confusion about symptoms or a feeling of loss of control is a more common reaction, especially in children (Lacouture et al., 1984; Stimmel, 1983). Nausea and vomiting are common. Constipation, which does not diminish over time, can be treated with mild laxatives or stool softeners. Respiratory depression is the most serious side effect of opioids, but preliminary studies suggest that by 3 to 6 months of age, healthy infants have no greater respiratory depression from opioids than do adults (Berde, 1989). Respiratory depression can occur even at typical doses and may present a problem in patients in whom carbon dioxide retention is likely (Fields, 1987). Pain is an antagonist to central respiratory depression (Twycross and Lack, 1990) and patients whose pain is unrelieved will not develop respiratory depression. Concern about respiratory depression therefore should not preclude use of these drugs at doses adequate for pain relief, especially with the advent of current monitoring devices. Hypoxemia can be easily detected with pulse oximetry, a noninvasive means of estimating arterial oxygen saturation by measuring absorption of infrared light projected through a fingertip (Zeltzer et al., 1989). other effects including hypotension, miosis, cough suppression, and urinary retention are transitory (Clark et al., 1988; Way and Way, 1987).

Morphine is an excellent pain medication and is the standard by which to measure dosage and treatment effects of other narcotics. It is inexpensive, readily available, and has been studied extensively in pediatrics. The opioids are absorbed from the gastrointestinal tract and reach peak concentrations within 30 to 60 minutes after oral administration. They are metabolized primarily in the liver, and because of extensive biotransformation, oral doses may be greater than parenteral doses. The pediatric dose is 0.2 to 0.4 mg/kg orally every 4 hours. The intravenous dose is 0.08 to 0.1 mg/kg every 2 hours (Berde, 1989) or 0.025 to 2.6 mg/kg per hour by continuous intravenous drip (Miser et al., 1980; Schechter, 1985). Studies of continuous intravenous infusion in children have concluded that this route is safe and effective, but variable, and should be initiated after a trial of standard intravenous administration (Bray, 1983; Miser et al., 1980). The subcutaneous dose is 0.025 to 1.79 mg/kg per hour (Miser et al., 1983; Schechter, 1985).

Codeine is similar in structure to morphine. It is the most commonly prescribed opioid for moderate pain. It provides more effective analgesia than do the peripheral agents and has a low incidence of serious side effects compared with the more potent narcotics. It is well absorbed orally and has a low first pass effect. Peak effects occur in 1 to 1½ hours. The pediatric dose is 0.5 to 1 mg/kg orally every 4 hours or 3 mg/kg per day (Schechter, 1987). Codeine is available in pure preparations and in combinations with aspirin and acetaminophen. The use of combination agents is controversial. Some contend that the dose of codeine in these preparations is small and ineffective; others maintain that because the combination products contain both peripherally and centrally active components, more analgesia is possible than with either agent alone (Ross and Ross, 1988; Schechter, 1985).

Meperidine is a popular synthetic narcotic that is biochemically different than morphine and has a shorter duration of action. However, its metabolite, nor-meperidine, can produce CNS excitation with tremors, muscle twitching, hyper-active reflexes and seizures (Inturrise and Umans, 1986; Ross and Ross, 1988). Normeperidine has a longer half-life (15 to 30 hours) than meperidine and accu-mulates when used for long periods of time (Crockett, 1989). Renal failure results in higher concentrations of normeperidine and increased toxicity (Inturrise and Umans, 1986). Severe reactions and death have been documented when meperi-dine is administered to patients receiving monoamine oxidase inhibitors, an effect that has not been observed with morphine (Lacouture et al., 1984). Given these potentially serious and sometimes fatal reactions, the use of meperidine in chil-dren is not recommended.

Methadone, a synthetic opioid is well absorbed and long acting. The elimination half-life in children averages roughly 19 hours (Berde, 1989). Methadone is released slowly into the blood resulting in relatively constant plasma levels with continuous analgesia (Stimmel, 1983). Because of efficient oral/parenteral bioavailability, typical starting doses are 0.1 to 0.15 mg/kg every 4 hours regard-less of route initially (two to four doses) followed by either smaller doses every 4 hours (0.05 to 0.08 mg/kg) or the original dose at longer intervals (6 to 12 hours) (Berde, 1989). Because of its long duration of action, some prefer methadone, especially if given orally, over continuous opioid infusion. Plasma levels peak in 4 to 6 hours though analgesia is strongest in 1 to 2 hours (Ross and Ross, 1988). The half-life may increase in 2 to 3 days when given regularly (Ross and Ross, 1988), and the dosing interval can be lengthened. Withdrawal symptoms are less severe and more prolonged than those associated with morphine (Clark et al., 1988).

Fentanyl and its analogues (sufentanil, alfentanil) differ from morphine in their potency and duration of action. The short duration of effect makes these agents especially useful for painful procedures such as bone marrow aspirations and burn dressing changes. The recommended dose for fentanyl is 1 to 2 μ/kg intravenously per dose, or if given by continuous infusion, 2 to 4 μ/kg/hour (Shannon and Berde, 1989). These agents are highly lipophilic and show less rostral spread when administered spinally or epidurally. Fentanyl is most conveniently adminis-tered via a continuous epidural infusion although it can be administered mucosally (nose drops or in sweetened oral form) or transdermally (Shannon and Berde, 1989). When compared with fentanyl, sufentanil is five to ten times as potent whereas alfentanil is one-fifth to one-tenth as potent.

Dose and Schedule

Pain is more effectively managed if treatment occurs before it becomes severe. Insufficient dose or prolonged dosing intervals of an analgesic may cause inadequate relief resulting in frustration, anxiety, or depression. In such situations, the child loses confidence in the physician and even higher doses of the analgesic may be necessary to achieve pain control. It is common practice to dose by bolus on demand, which exposes patients to the toxicities of opioids, provides only intermittent benefit, and generates behaviors characteristic of addiction. If the analgesic is given at scheduled intervals based on the drug's duration of action, a maintenance dose that usually is lower than a demand dose can be established, thus preventing wide variation in analgesia (Farr, 1978).

Portenoy (1988) offers suggestions about doses of opioids in cancer patients that have general applicability. The physician should begin with the lowest effective dose and titrate against beneficial and adverse effects. The dose can be doubled if no analgesia results after the first dose; if partial analgesia results, the drug should be given on a scheduled basis every 4 hours with a rescue dose available every 2 hours until the total daily dose requirement is determined. The rescue dose can be estimated as one-eighth of the scheduled dose. The rescue drug can be the same drug used in the scheduled regimen unless methadone is being used, in which case, morphine is a better rescue drug because of its shorter half-life. Use of demand administration is discouraged except with rescue doses or when the need is uncertain as when first titrating methadone (Portenoy, 1988).

Narcotics with short half-lives (such as morphine) must be given at least every 4 hours; those with long half-lives (such as methadone) may be given every 6 hours. Steady state plasma levels are reached in four to five half-lives. Opioids with long half-lives may accumulate and cause toxic effects if not monitored closely. Methadone can be given as needed initially, and the scheduled dose can be determined in approximately one week when the drug's cumulative effects are evident (Portenoy, 1988).

Routes of Administration

Oral administration is preferred unless an intravenous line is already in place for other reasons. Parenteral administration appears to provide a greater effective narcotic dose because the drug does not undergo biotransformation, but if an oral dose equianalgesic to the parenteral one is administered, pain relief will be comparable. The intravenous route offers complete bioavailability, immediate effect, and comfortable administration if a line is in place. Rapid pain relief can be achieved initially with an intravenous bolus dose and maintained with follow-up doses either orally or parenterally. Continuous intravenous infusion provides a more constant effect than does repeated bolus dosing (Berde, 1989). Continuous subcutaneous infusion avoids the need for constant access to an intravenous port (Miser et al., 1983). Children usually are aware of the different effects of intravenous and oral narcotics, and a preference for the rapid effects associated with the intravenous route does not mean the child is addicted. These alternate routes are unnecessary if adequate oral doses are used. The oral to parenteral ratios are 3-6 to 1 for morphine, 1.5 to 1 for codeine, and 2 to 1 for methadone (Berde et al., 1990; Hill, 1988). A direct conversion from intravenous to oral routes often is unsuccessful, and use of both routes or a rescue dose for an interim may facilitate the transition.

Patient-controlled analgesia (PCA) employs a computer controlled infusion pump with a selected lockout interval and maximum cumulative dose that allows the patient to administer a small bolus of drug by pressing a button. Extensive studies demonstrate patient satisfaction with this method (Berde, 1989). At Children's Medical Center of Dallas, PCA has been used routinely in children older than 8 years. Patients often benefit from the sense of control accompanying this approach and generally titrate the dose to provide a moderate degree of comfort with minimal side effects. Further studies have shown that the effectiveness of PCA is improved with a continuous basal infusion of opioids (Sinatra et al., 1989). Meperidine has been restricted from use in continuous infusion or PCA with basal infusion because, as stated earlier, an accumulation of its metabolite, normeperidine, has potential CNS toxicity (Berde, 1989).

Regional blockade has become popular in recent years (Berde, 1989). It consists of the application of medications locally to modulate or block transmission of afferent nociceptive impulses. It is particularly important when systemic opioids are contraindicated, such as in children at high risk of developing apnea. Comparisons of systemic and regional analgesia have shown superior analgesia and fewer side effects with neural blockade (Berde, 1989). Epidural analgesia is probably the most versatile regional analgesic technique and at Children's Medical Center of Dallas is administered to children as young as 5 months of age. Medications can be administered by a single injection or repeatedly via catheter. Local anesthetics and opioids are used most often in regional blockade, and low-dose infusions of a combination of the two appear more effective than either alone.

Dependence, Tolerance, and Addiction

Extensive drug abuse in the youth of this country heightens concern about the use of analgesics. For the most part, these concerns are unfounded and can be attributed to a misunderstanding of terms such as "dependence," "tolerance," and "addiction." Physical dependence is an altered physiological state produced by the repeated administration of a drug, which necessitates its continued use to sustain its effects or prevent withdrawal symptoms. Psychological dependence produces a similar response, but it is accompanied by subjective rather than objective symptoms if the drug is discontinued (Stimmel, 1983). Tolerance refers to the diminished effect of a drug at the same dose and the need to increase the dose to achieve similar results. The need for higher doses, however, does not necessarily represent tolerance; it may mean advancing disease and indicates a need to reevaluate the medical condition (Portenoy, 1988). Tolerance is managed by increasing the dose or giving the analgesic more frequently. Dependence and tolerance occur with many drugs.

Addiction refers to a social and behavioral phenomenon characterized by compulsive drug use, intense desire for a drug, concern about its acquisition, and a high tendency to relapse after withdrawal (Jaffe, 1985). Although the dosage of pain medication may need to be increased to maintain analgesic effects or tapered gradually to control the effects of dependence, addiction in patient populations (except psychiatric patients) is rare (Newburger and Sallan, 1981). Dependence and tolerance often accompany addiction, but addiction does not necessarily occur with dependence and tolerance.

Withdrawal symptoms usually occur in patients who have taken narcotics for more than 2 weeks and then cease abruptly. Mild withdrawal symptoms may go undetected. The onset, intensity, and duration of withdrawal effects depend on the drug used. For morphine, symptoms begin 6 to 8 hours after the last dose and peak at 36 to 48 hours (Way and Way, 1987). Withdrawal effects include irritability, sleep disturbance, hypothermia, hyperventilation, tremor, mydriasis, lacrimation, rhinorrhea, anorexia, vomiting, diarrhea, and pain (Miser et al., 1986; Way and Way, 1987). Patients should be withdrawn from narcotics slowly by decreasing the drug by one-fourth of the total daily dose every 2 to 3 days. Supportive measures such as treatment with sedatives or long-acting narcotics during this period may be useful (Miser et al., 1986).

Toxicity

Overdose or toxicity with narcotics is rare in clinical settings when the drugs are properly used and the patient is closely monitored. Physical findings associated with toxicity include respiratory depression, coma, miosis, and reduced urinary output. Assuring ventilation is of primary concern and may require acute measures such as tracheal intubation or tracheotomy. Naloxone, a pure narcotic antagonist, can be administered intravenously to counter toxic effects, but it is not an innocuous drug. Intravenous bolus injections have resulted in pulmonary edema, hypertension, cardiac dysrhythmias, and cardiac arrest making it essential that the diagnosis of toxicity be clinically well established before using this intervention (Stoelting,

1987). For this reason, nalbuphine, an agonist antagonist, has been suggested instead of naloxone because it causes fewer hemodynamic changes (Kaplan, 1987). A prompt response to these agents indicates narcotic toxicity; failure to respond indicates another cause for the symptoms. If the patient does suffer from narcotic overdose or toxicity, repeated or continuous intravenous doses or depot intramuscular doses may be necessary (Yaster and Deshpande, 1988). The pediatric dose of naloxone is 0.01 mg/kg intravenously or intramuscularly; if necessary doses may be repeated every 2 to 3 minutes (Schechter, 1987).

PSYCHOPHARMACOLOGICAL ADJUVANTS

Children verbalize their distress in terms they understand. Pain is often used to identify other symptoms including anxiety and depression. Therefore, it is important to carefully evaluate the child's distress. Psychotherapeutic interventions and adjuvant psychopharmacological drugs may be beneficial. Drugs to consider include major tranquilizers, minor tranquilizers, antidepressants, and stimulants. The choice of drug should be tailored to the specific needs of the child and the goal should be to identify the simplest regimen with the most effective combination of drugs.

Major Tranquilizers

The role of phenothiazines in the management of pain is controversial (Fields, 1987). Narcotics may cause nausea and vomiting, symptoms for which phenothiazines are often administered. Phenothiazines have been used in adults for postoperative and chronic pain (Fields, 1987). Major tranquilizers can be used when sedation is desired or for severe anxiety or agitation. However, adverse effects can be serious and limit the usefulness of these agents. Side effects include sedation and anticholinergic symptoms. These drugs cause respiratory distress and orthostatic hypotension, of concern with narcotic administration. They may lower the seizure threshold and produce EEG changes. Neuroleptic malignant syndrome, laryngeal dystonia, and agranulocytosis are rare but potentially life-threatening complications, and tardive dyskinesia can be irreversible. Cardiac conduction disturbances, pigmentary retinopathy, and hepatic dysfunction can also occur (Teicher and Glod, 1990).

Because of concern about tardive dyskinesia, standard care now dictates obtaining informed consent from the parent and child and careful examination for abnormal movements before and during treatment. It is wise to begin treatment with the smallest possible dose and advance slowly as needed and tolerated. Schechter (1985) recommends 2 mg/kg per day of chlorpromazine, or 0.05 to 0.075 mg/kg per day of haloperidol. Complete blood cell count profiles, urinalysis, blood urea nitrogen, blood chemistries, and liver function tests should be obtained at baseline and regular intervals. The following case illustrates the usefulness of these agents for pain complicated by severe agitation.

Case study. A 10-year-old awoke from surgery in an agitated state with pressured speech and hyperactive behavior. His parents were concerned that he might have suffered an adverse reaction to the narcotic used postoperatively and requested that it be discontinued. The child, however, complained of severe pain and became self-destructive with head banging. Haloperidol 2 mg was given intravenously with excellent results. The child slept for several hours but on awakening, resumed his pressured speech, hyperactive behavior, and complaints of pain. Additional doses of haloperidol 0.5 mg intravenously were administered as needed for agitated behavior and proved effective in the management of behavioral symptoms and pain.

Minor Tranquilizers

Benzodiazepines are excellent for severe anxiety episodes in the course of an illness and for anticipatory and situational anxiety accompanying invasive procedures common in the management of many illnesses (Jay et al., 1987; Pfefferbaum et al., 1987b; van Hoff and Olszewski, 1988). Benzodiazepines commonly are administered orally or intravenously for children undergoing painful frightening medical procedures because they act rapidly and have amnestic properties. Jay et al. (1987) compared low doses of diazepam to cognitive behavioral interventions in children undergoing invasive treatment procedures. The authors concluded that diazepam reduced anticipatory anxiety but not behavioral distress. The findings do not conclusively demonstrate lack of efficacy as the doses were low and administered orally. Pfefferbaum et al. (1987b) found alprazolam to be beneficial when given orally three times a day for 3 days before invasive procedures. Midazolam, another short-acting benzodiazepine, is two to three times as potent as diazepam. At Children's Medical Center of Dallas, 0.3 mg/kg to 0.5 mg/kg (20 mg maximum) of midazolam, mixed with a sweet liquid, is given preoperatively for anxiety in children 9 months old or older. Because children often describe their anxiety in terms of pain and because these symptoms often coexist, it may be difficult to determine which symptom is being treated. The following case illustrates this point.

Case study. A 13-year-old girl was severely anxious and uncooperative after hemipelvectomy for osteogenic sarcoma. On hearing about discharge plans, she became agitated, and began banging her head, pulling her hair, and screaming that she was in pain. She responded to lorazepam 2 mg by mouth, which was eventually given on a scheduled basis every 6 hours when her anxiety, usually verbalized in complaints of pain, did not abate.

Benzodiazepines have anxiolytic, muscle relaxant, and anticonvulsant effects.

Side effects include sedation, ataxia, slurred speech, diplopia, and tremor that generally are not serious. Some persons experience depressed mood (Schechter, 1985), behavioral disinhibition, and psychosis (Petti et al., 1982; Pfefferbaum et al., 1987a). The following case is illustrative.

Case study. A 14-year-old amputee in treatment for osteogenic sarcoma also had a history of attention deficit disorder, hyperactivity, and conduct disorder for which he was receiving pemoline 37.5 mg P.O. in the morning and 18.75 mg P.O. in the afternoon. A trial of amitriptyline in low doses was initiated for sleep disturbance and was continued after discharge. A community physician discontinued the tricyclic in favor of triazolam. The first dose of triazolam 0.25 mg P.O. resulted in sleep of 4 hours duration, but after the second dose the next night, the patient experienced visual hallucinations and insomnia. Triazolam was discontinued and the symptoms were eventually managed with low doses of chlorpromazine 50 mg P.O. at bedtime and 10 mg P.O. in the afternoon.

Benzodiazepines are most appropriate in acute situations. Tolerance may occur with prolonged use. Physical dependence is a well-known problem, and abrupt withdrawal is not recommended after prolonged use. Withdrawal symptoms include sleep disturbance, irritability, anxiety, concentration difficulties, sweating, nausea, weight loss, palpitations, muscle pains, tremor, seizures, and psychosis (Salzman, 1989).

Antidepressants

Tricyclic antidepressants are well-established adjuvants for pain management in adults and are thought to exert primary analgesia separate from antidepressant effects (Massie and Lesko, 1989). They are used in adults with postherpetic neuralgia, diabetic neuropathy, tension and migraine headache, rheumatoid arthritis, chronic low back pain, and cancer (Fields, 1987). Imipramine is the standard agent in children. Amitriptyline, a more sedating drug, is also useful. These agents are particularly useful in children with sleep disturbance. According to Shannon and Berde (1989), benzodiazepines and barbiturates have little place in the management of sleep disturbances in children with severe pain. They advocate nightly administration of small doses of tricyclics for normalization of sleep.

Case study A 15-year-old experienced severe pain, anxiety, and depression following surgical removal of an undifferentiated sarcoma. He was treated initially with narcotics and lorazepam. When he developed sleep disturbance, his anxiety increased and amitriptyline 25 mg P.O. was added at bedtime. He responded well and soon realized that his pain increased when he was anxious or sad. He continued to experience pain, anxiety, and depression, but these symptoms became more tolerable when his sleep improved.

Treatment with tricyclics usually begins with a low dose at bedtime advancing with a divided dose schedule. Single starting doses as low as 0.1 mg/kg may be given in the evening (Shannon and Berde, 1989). Although the usual dose recommended for the treatment of depression in physically healthy children is 2 to 5 mg/kg per day, benefit for pain and associated symptoms may be achieved at lower doses of 1 to 2 mg/kg per day (Pfefferbaum-Levine et al., 1983).

Side effects of tricyclics include sedation, which may be desirable, and anticholinergic effects, which adolescents may not tolerate. These drugs may cause cardiac dysrhythmias, and increased respiratory distress when used with narcotics. Orthostatic hypotension can be quite disconcerting if the patient and family are not informed of the possibility of its occurrence.

Tricyclic toxicity is serious and can result in respiratory depression, hypotension, cardiac dysrhythmias and conduction deficits, congestive heart failure, confusion, coma, hyperactivity, hyperpyrexia, and muscular rigidity (Stimmel, 1983). Monitoring of chemistry profile, especially liver function, and cardiac status should accompany treatment with these drugs. Daily doses greater than 3.5 mg/kg per day in physically healthy children warrant electrocardiograph monitoring (McDermott et al., 1989). Schroeder et al. (1989) found increased heart rate and increased QT interval in children treated with desipramine, but no dysrhythmias or clinically significant changes in blood pressure.

The recent sudden deaths of several children on tricyclics have aroused renewed concern about the cardiotoxicity of these drugs (Riddle et al., 1991). Tingelstad (1991) recommends taking a careful medical history including history of cardiac arrhythmia, heart disease, syncope, hearing loss, or family history of heart disease or sudden cardiac death before initiating treatment with tricyclics. In addition he recommends a baseline 12-lead ECG, and if a significant dysrhythmia is found, a 2-minute rhythm strip, and similar ECG tracings and plasma drug levels during the loading phase and at steady state. When considering a tricyclic for the child in pain, a cardiology consult is indicated for any positive cardiac history, family history, or abnormal ECG findings.

The decision to monitor tricyclic blood levels should be made on an individual basis; however, monitoring is warranted when: (1) the patient fails to respond to the expected dose or duration of treatment, (2) using a tricyclic for which therapeutic levels are established, (3) drug toxicity or drug interaction is suspected, (4) the clinical condition changes unexpectedly, (5) the dose exceeds the recommended limit, and (6) the patient is very young or has cardiac, hepatic, or renal dysfunction (Orsulak, 1986).

Withdrawal symptoms may occur if tricyclics are discontinued abruptly. These include mood changes, agitation, sleep disturbance, appetite changes, gastrointestinal symptoms, and somatic complaints. Tapering the drug will help distinguish between rebound effects, withdrawal effects, and symptoms indicating that the drug should be continued.

Stimulants

Forrest et al. (1977) demonstrated the advantages of using stimulants with narcotics. The combination may allow the use of lower doses of narcotics, thereby decreasing the potential for adverse CNS and respiratory effects. Stimulants are effective in countering the sedative effects of narcotics. They have little if any analgesic effect when used alone (Tesar, 1982). Their use in the treatment of chronic pain has not been investigated, and there are no known studies of their use in pediatric pain management, but Schechter (1987) recommends doses of 2 to 10 mg per day of dextroamphetamine in addition to a narcotic for pain management in children. They may be given twice a day, but the last dose should be given by early afternoon to prevent insomnia.

Case reports support the use of stimulants to treat depression in physically ill adolescents who cannot tolerate tricyclics or in whom a rapid response is critical (Kaufmann and Murray, 1982; Walling and Pfefferbaum, 1990). The child psychiatrist's familiarity with these drugs makes their use appealing and they are reasonable adjuvants to consider.

There are several advantages to the use of stimulants. Efficacy can be determined within days inasmuch as their onset of action is rapid. Side effects are minor, usually occur early in treatment, are usually transient, and are reversible. They include anorexia, insomnia, agitation, anxiety, aggressive behavior, confusion, tachycardia, dysrhythmias, and blood pressure changes. Although tolerance and abuse can occur, they have not been considered of serious concern in physically ill adults (Satel and Nelson, 1989).

CONCLUSION

Pain is a complicated subjective experience that may require pharmacological intervention. Treatment should be initiated after careful assessment and monitored frequently because there may be great individual variation in response. Peripheral analgesics are effective for mild to moderate pain, but when they are inadequate, narcotics can be used safely. Knowledge of drug profiles allows for selection of an appropriate agent, dose, and route for essentially any pain situation. Dependence and tolerance but not addiction develop with many agents and should not pose undue alarm. When associated emotional or behavioral symptoms complicate the picture, adjuvant pharmacological and nonpharmacological treatment methods may be necessary. Major tranquilizers, minor tranquilizers, antidepressants, and stimulants are effective.

REFERENCES

Berde, C. B. (1989), Pediatric postoperative pain management. *Pediatr. Clin. North Am.,* 36(4):921–940.

Berde, C., Ablin, A., Glazer, J., et al. (1990), Report of the subcommittee on disease-related pain in childhood cancer. *Pediatrics,* 86(5):818–825.

Bray, R. J. (1983), Postoperative analgesia provided by morphine infusion in children. *Anaesthesia,* 30:1075–1078.

Clark, W. G., Brater, D. C. & Johnson, A. R. (1988), Narcotic (opioid) analgesic drugs. In: *Goth's Medical Pharmacology,* ed. W. G. Clark, D. C. Brater, & A. R. Johnson, St. Louis: C. V. Mosby, pp. 319–336.

Crockett, R. K. (1989), Pain management in the pediatric emergency department. *Int. Pediatr.,* 4(1):14–18.

Farr, W. C. (1978), Oral morphine for control of pain in terminal cancer. *Arizona Medicine,* 35(3):167–170.

Fields, H. L. (1987), *Pain,* New York: McGraw-Hill.

Foley, K. M. (1985), The treatment of cancer pain. *New Engl. J. Med.,* 313(2):84–94.

Forrest, W. H., Brown, B. W., Brown, C. R., et al. (1977), Dextroamphetamine with morphine for the treatment of postoperative pain. *New Engl. J. Med.,* 296:712–715.

Geller, B., Cooper, T. B., Schluchter, M. D., Warham, J. E. & Carr, L. G. (1987), Child and adolescent nortriptyline single dose pharmacokinetic parameters: Final report. *J. Clin. Psychopharmacol.,* 7(5):321–323.

Hill, C. S. (1988), Narcotics and cancer pain control. *Oncology,* 33(3):1–18.

Inturrisi, C. E. & Umans, J. G. (1986), Merperidine biotransformation and central nervous system toxicity in animals and humans. In: *Advances in Pain Research and Therapy,* Vol. 8, eds. K. M. Foley & C. E. Inturrisi. New York: Raven Press, pp. 143–153.

Jaffe, J. H. (1985), Drug addiction and drug abuse. In: *Goodman and Gilman's The Pharmacological Basis of Therapeutics,* eds. A. G. Gilman, L. S. Goodman, T. W. Rall & F. Murad. New York: MacMillan, pp. 532–581.

Jatlow, P. I. (1987), Psychoatrophic drug disposition during development. In: *Psychiatric Pharmacosciences of Children and Adolescents.* Washington, DC: American Psychiatric Press, pp. 29–44.

Jay, S. M., Elliott, C. H., Katz, E. & Siegel, S. E. (1987), Cognitive-behavioral and pharmacologic interventions for children's distress during painful medical procedures. *J. Consult. Clin. Psychol.,* 55(6):860–865.

Kaplan, J. A. (1987), *Cardiac Anesthesia,* Vol. 1. Philadelphia: W. B. Saunders, p. 74.

Kaufmann, M. W. & Murray, G. B. (1982), The use of D-amphetamine in medically ill depressed patients. *J. Clin. Psychiatry,* 43(11):463–464.

Lacouture, P. G., Gaudreault, P. & Lovejoy, F. H. (1984), Chronic pain of childhood: a pharmacologic approach. *Pediatric Clin. North Am.,* 31(5):1133–1151.

Massie, M. J. & Lesko, L. M. (1989), Psychopharmacological management. In: *Handbook of Psychooncology Psychological Care of the Patient with Cancer.* New York: Oxford University Press, pp. 470–491.

McDermott, J. F., Werry, J., Petti, T., Combrinck-Graham, L. & Char, W. F. (1989), Anxiety disorders of children or adolescents. In: *Treatments of Psychiatric Disorders. A Task Force Report of the American Psychiatric Association.* Washington, DC: American Psychiatric Association, pp. 401–446.

Miser, A. W., Miser, J. S. & Clark, B. S. (1980), Continuous intravenous infusion of morphine sulfate for control of severe pain in children with terminal malignancy. *J. Pediatr.,* 96:930–932.

Miser, A. W., Chayt, K. J., Sandlund, J. T., Cohen, P. S., Dothage, J. A. & Miser, J. S. (1986), Narcotic withdrawal syndrome in young adults after therapeutic use of opiates. *Am. J. Dis. Child.,* 140:603–605.

Miser, A. W., Davis, D. M., Hughes, C. S., Mulne, A. F. & Miser, J. S. (1983), Continuous subcutaneous infusion of morphine in children with cancer. *Am. J. Dis. Childh.,* 137:383–385.

Newburger, P. E. & Sallan, S. E. (1981), Chronic pain: principles of management. *J. Pediatr.,* 98(2):180–189.

Orsulak, P. J. (1986), Therapeutic monitoring of antidepressant drugs: current methodology and applications. *J. Clin. Psychiatry,* 47:39–50.

Petti, T. A., Fish, B., Shapiro, T., Cohen, I. L. & Campbell, M. (1982), Effects of chlordiazepoxide in disturbed children. *J. Clin. Psychopharmacol.,* 2(4):270–273.

Pfefferbaum, B., Butler, P. M., Mullins, D. & Copeland, D. (1987a), Two cases of benzodiazepine toxicity in children. *J. Clin. Psychiatry,* 48(11):450–452.

Pfefferbaum, B., Overall, J. E., Boren, H. A., Frankel, L. S., Sullivan, M. P. & Johnson, K. (1987b), Alprazolam in the treatment of anticipatory and acute situational anxiety in children with cancer. *J. Am. Acad. Child Adolesc. Psychiatry,* 26(4):532–535.

Pfefferbaum-Levine, B., Kumor, K., Cangir, A., Choroszy, M. & Roseberry, E. A. (1983), Tricyclic antidepressants for children with cancer. *Am. J. Psychiatry,* 140:1974–1976.

Portenoy, R. K. (1988), Practical aspects of pain control in the patient with cancer. Atlanta, GA: American Cancer Society, pp. 7–32.

Riddle, M. A. (1991), Pharmacokinetics in children and adolescents. In: *Child and Adolescent Psychiatry,* ed. Lewis, M. Baltimore, MD: Williams & Wilkins, pp. 767–770.

Riddle, M. A., Nelson, J. C., Kleinman, C. S., et al. (1991), Sudden death in children receiving Norpramin: a review of three reported cases and commentary, *J. Am. Acad. Child Adolesc. Psychiatry,* 30:104–108.

Ross, D. M. & Ross, S. A. (1988), *Childhood Pain Current Issues, Research, and Management.* Baltimore, MD: Urban & Schwarzenberg.

Ryan, N. D. (1990), Heterocyclic antidepressants in children and adolescents. *J. Child Adolesc. Psychopharmacol.,* 1(1):21–31.

Salzman, C. (1989), Treatment with antianxiety agents. In: *Treatments of Psychiatric Disorders. A Task Force Report of the American Psychiatric Association.* Washington, DC: American Psychiatric Association Press, pp. 2036–2052.

Satel, S. L. & Nelson, J. C. (1989), Stimulants in the treatment of depression. *J. Clin. Psychiatry,* 50:241–249.

Schechter, N. L. (1985), Pain and pain control in children. *Curr. Problems Pediatr.,* 15(5):6–67.

Schechter, N. L. (1987), Pain: acknowledging it, assessing it, treating it. *Contemp. Pediatr.,* 4:16–46.

Schroeder, J. S., Mullin, A. V., Elliott, G. R., et al. (1989), Cardiovascular effects of desipramine in children. *J. Am. Acad. Child Adolesc. Psychiatry,* 28(3):376–379.

Shannon, M. & Berde, C. B. (1989), Pharmacologic management of pain in children and adolescents. *Pediatr. Clin. North Am.,* 36(4):855–871.

Sinatra, R., Chung, K.S., Silverman, D. G., et al. (1989), An evaluation of morphine and oxymorphone administered via patient-controlled analgesia (PCA) or PCA plus basal infusion in postcesarean-delivery patients. *Anesthesiology,* 71:502–507.

Stimmel, B. (1983), *Pain, Analgesia, and Addiction: The Pharmacologic Treatment of Pain.* New York: Raven Press.

Stoelting, R. K. (1987), *Pharmacology and Physiology in Anesthetic Practice.* Philadelphia, PA: J. B. Lippincott, p. 94.

Tesar, G. E. (1982), The role of stimulants in general medicine. *Drug Therapy,* 12:186–195.

Teicher, M. H. & Glod, C. A. (1990), Neuroleptic drugs: indications and guidelines of their rational use in children and adolescents. *J. Child Adolesc. Psychopharmacol.,* 1(1):33–56.

Tingelstad, J. B. (1991), The cardiotoxicity of the tricyclics. *J. Am. Acad. Child Adolesc. Psychiatry,* 30(5):845–846.

Twycross, R. G. & Lack, S. A. (1990), *Therapeutics in Terminal Cancer.* New York: Churchill Livingstone.

van Hoff, J. & Olszewski, D. (1988), Lorazepam for the control of chemotherapy-related nausea and vomiting in children. *J. Pediatr.,* 113(1):146–149.

Walling, V. R. & Pfefferbaum, B. (1990), The use of methylphenidate in a depressed adolescent with AIDS. *J. Dev. Behav. Pediatr.,* 11(4):195–197.

Way, W. L. & Way, E. L. (1987), Opioid analgesics and antagonists. In: *Basic and Clinical Pharmacology,* ed. B. G. Katzung. Norwalk, CT: Appleton Lange, pp. 336–349.

Yaster, M. & Deshpande, J. K. (1988), Management of pediatric pain with opioid analgesics. *J. Pediatr.,* 113(3):421–429.

Zeltzer, L. K., Jay, S. M. & Fisher, D. M. (1989), The management of pain associated with pediatric procedures. *Pediatric Clin. North Am.,* 36(4):941–964.

20

Nine-Year Outcome of the Vermont Intervention Program for Low Birth Weight Infants

Thomas M. Achenbach, Catherine T. Howell, Melanie F. Aoki
University of Vermont, Burlington
Virginia A. Rauh
Columbia University, New York City

Twenty-four low birth weight children who had received an experimental intervention (LBWE) during the neonatal period, 31 control children who had received no treatment (LBWC), and 36 normal birth weight children were compared. The intervention involved seven hospital sessions and four home sessions in which a nurse helped mothers adapt to their LBW babies. At age 9, LBWE children scored significantly higher than LBWC children on the Kaufman Mental Processing Composite, Sequential, Simultaneous, Achievement, Arithmetic, and Riddles scales, after statistical adjustments for socioeconomic status. The LBWE children had also advanced more rapidly in school than had LBWC children. Parent (Child Behavior Checklist) and teacher (Teacher's Report Form) ratings of school functioning were more favorable for LBWE than LBWC children, with especially strong effects on Teacher's Report Form scores for academic performance and the attention problems syndrome. At age 9, LBWE children were not significantly inferior to normal birth weight children on any measure. These results bear out a progressive divergence between the LBWE and LBWC children that first became statistically significant in cognitive scores at age 3. The findings suggest that the intervention prevented cognitive lags among LBW children and that this eventually had a

Reprinted with permission from *Pediatrics*, 1993, Vol. 91(1), 45–55. Copyright © 1993 by the American Academy of Pediatrics.

favorable effect on academic achievement, behavior, and advancement in school. The progression from no significant differences between LBWE and LBWC children on early cognitive and achievement scores to significant and pervasive differences in later functioning argues for long-term follow-up periods to evaluate properly the power of behavioral interventions to compensate for biological risks.

Low birth weight (LBW) is a common risk factor that may have a variety of developmental sequelae.[1,2] The number of LBW children is likely to remain high owing both to the substantial incidence of LBW and to medical technology that enables LBW infants to survive. The developmental risks for many LBW children may stem more from mismatches between the level of their biobehavioral functioning and the world they confront than from specific organic abnormalities.

Various interventions for LBW children have been reported. Some have provided extra stimulation to compensate for sensory deprivation assumed to result from isolation during neonatal intensive care.[3-5] Other interventions have been designed to change parental attitudes and behavior[6-9] or to provide individualized treatment for LBW infants whose postnatal development was found to be delayed.[10] Several have been designed to improve the child-rearing practices of low socioeconomic status (SES) mothers.[11-13] Probably the most ambitious intervention has been a massive 3-year educational and family support program directed toward improving the environments of LBW children from predominately low-SES minority backgrounds.[14,15]

Beneficial effects have been demonstrated shortly after the termination of several of the foregoing interventions.[3,8,11-14] The longest outcome study that we found for these interventions included a 3-year follow-up.[16] In this study, observers rated the home environments of intervention children more favorably than those of control children, but cognitive tests and parents' reports yielded no significant differences between the groups. On some measures, statistical interactions indicated that control children weighing less than 1500 g at birth were doing more poorly than comparable intervention children. However, these findings are limited by the small number of subjects weighing less than 1500 g—only three in the control group, four in one intervention group, and two in the other intervention group.

To shed light on the possible effects of early interventions for LBW children over a much longer period than previously reported, the present paper reports the 9-year outcome of an intervention that took place during the first few postnatal months. The intervention differed from most others in that it was not designed specifically to overcome handicaps associated with sensory deprivation or low SES. Instead, it was designed to optimize mother-infant interactions for LBW children whether or not they experienced the added risks of sensory deprivation or low SES.

Because every study has idiosyncratic aspects, no single study of such an important issue can be conclusive. Our intervention was based on the knowledge and technology available at the end of the 1970s, when the intervention was designed. However, considering the current lack of other long-term tests of interventions for LBW children, our outcome data for ages 4,[17] 7,[18] and now 9 years provide a baseline for comparison with any studies that do eventually report long-term outcomes.

MOTHER-INFANT TRANSACTION PROGRAM

To facilitate the long-term development of LBW children, the Mother-Infant Transaction Program (MITP)[17,19,20] was designed to optimize caretaking interactions by enhancing mothers' adjustment to their LBW infants. Emphasizing the transactional nature of development,[21] the MITP had the following aims: (1) to enable the mother to appreciate her baby's specific behavioral and temperamental characteristics; (2) to sensitize her to the baby's cues, especially those that signal stimulus overload, distress, and readiness for interaction; and (3) to teach her to respond appropriately to those cues in order to facilitate mutually satisfying interactions.

The MITP was implemented by a neonatal intensive care nurse who worked with the mother and baby in seven daily sessions during the week prior to the baby's discharge from the hospital, plus four home sessions at 3, 14, 30, and 90 days after discharge, as described previously.[17,19,20] The nurse adjusted the pace and emphasis of the sessions to each mother's needs. Techniques included modeling, demonstration, verbal instruction, and practical experience handling the baby. Throughout the intervention sessions, the nurse encouraged the mother to feel confident and comfortable with her baby.

Each in-hospital session dealt with a different aspect of the baby's functioning, such as self-regulation and interaction, behavioral signs of distress, predominant states, and techniques for bringing about the quiet alert state most responsive to social interaction. In the last two hospital sessions, the nurse helped the mother achieve sensitivity and responsivity in daily caretaking routines and prepare for life at home.

In the first home visit, the nurse explored the mother's adjustment to care at home, identifying her strengths and supporting her self-confidence. At the 2-week home visit, the nurse helped the mother build a repertoire of interactive play with the child. At the 1-month visit, the nurse and mother explored the child's emerging behavioral style and ways to enhance the "fit" between mother and child by taking account of the child's rhythms and capacities. The final visit reviewed all the recent changes the mother had noticed in her child. The mother was then presented with a logbook of the baby's development.

There was no intervention after the 90-day home visit. The children's subsequent educational experiences were extremely varied, as they attended many different schools. The 91 children tested at age 9 attended 63 different schools, with no more than 3 attending any one school. Only 1 child in the MITP group and 2 children in the LBW control group had been in Head Start.

It was hypothesized that the program would improve mothers' knowledge, skill, confidence, and satisfaction in caring for their LBW infants. The effects on the mothers were expected to improve mother-infant transactions, which, in turn, would reduce the risk of developmental lags.

The hypothesized effects on mothers were confirmed by significantly more favorable scores for maternal self-confidence, satisfaction with the mothering role, and maternal perceptions of infant temperament among mothers in a group randomly assigned to receive the experimental MITP intervention (LBWE) than in a group randomly assigned to a no-intervention control condition (LBWC).[17,19] Within the LBWE group, the nurse's ratings of quality of mothering and receptivity to the program were significantly correlated with subsequent cognitive test scores from 6 to 48 months.[17] Long-term effects on the LBWE children were expected to include better developmental and academic progress than would be found for the LBWC children.

The senior author of the present paper was not involved in designing or implementing the MITP. He became involved as the principal investigator of the follow-up studies at ages 2 through 9, but was neutral with respect to the hypothesized benefits of the MITP.

PREVIOUS FINDINGS ON CHILDREN'S DEVELOPMENT

We have previously reported comparisons between LBWE, LBWC, and normal birth weight (NBW) peers on developmental measures at ages 6, 12, 24, 36, 48, and 84 months.[17,18] In brief, no significant differences were found between the LBWE and LBWC groups at 6 or 12 months, when both groups lagged significantly behind the NBW group. At 2 years, the LBWE group scored higher than the LBWC group on the Bayley Mental Developmental Index (MDI),[21] but the difference reached only the $P < .10$ level of significance. Thereafter, the divergence between the LBWE and LBWC groups increased, with the LBWE group scoring significantly higher on the McCarthy General Cognitive Index[23] at age 3 years ($P < .05$) and 4 years ($P < .01$). The divergence continued to increase at age 7 years, when the LBWE group obtained a mean score of 107.4 on the Mental Processing Composite (MPC) of the Kaufman Assessment Battery for Children,[24] compared with 96.6 for the LBWC, a difference that was significant at $P < .001$. (The Kaufman scores are equivalent to IQs.) Not only did the LBWE children move steadily ahead of the LBWC children, but they also caught up to the NBW children. From age 3 years to 7 years, the mean test scores of the LBWE children were very similar to those of the NBW children.

The superiority of the LBWE group was highly significant not only in terms of being $P < .001$, but also in terms of the *magnitude* of the difference, which was large enough to be of considerable practical importance for the children's academic adaptation and progress. The difference of 10.8 points on the Kaufman MPC at age 7 was equivalent to 0.96 of a standard deviation, which is a large effect according to Cohen's[25] criteria for effect sizes. Furthermore, a significantly greater proportion of LBWC than LBWE children scored below the Kaufman's standardization mean of 100, and more LBWC than LBWE children scored below 100 at every SES level where any child scored less than 100 (Hollingshead[26] SES levels 2 through 5).

The progression from no significant differences between the LBWE and LBWC groups to increasingly significant and large differences in later years suggests a "sleeper effect" that has important implications for preventing adverse cognitive and behavioral outcomes. Because important cognitive and behavioral outcomes may not be measurable until later and/or because the effects on transactional patterns may be cumulative over long periods, proper evaluation of interventions like the MITP may have to continue into developmental periods well beyond those in which the intervention occurs.

In the case of the MITP, our earlier findings of major differences in developmental test scores were not accompanied by findings of significant differences in academic achievement. At age 7, when a standardized measure of academic achievement was first administered, the LBWE children did outscore the LBWC children, but the difference reached only $P = .11$. Poor academic achievement may be an important sequela of LBW, but not until the ages when important variations in achievement become measurable. Because most of the children tested at age 7 were at first grade or lower levels of schooling, there may have been a "floor effect" on our measurement of academic achievement. In other words, the level of achievement was too low to permit detection of differences associated with the MITP. We hypothesized that by age 9, however, the children's achievement levels would be advanced enough to provide a more sensitive test of effects associated with the MITP.

PURPOSES OF THE PRESENT STUDY

The purposes of the present study were (1) to determine whether the LBWE children would continue to outperform the LBWC children on measures of cognitive development 9 years after the intervention; (2) to test the hypothesis that the LBWE children would now surpass the LBWC children on standardized measures of school achievement at age 9, when important variations in achievement would be more measurable than at earlier ages; and (3) to determine whether differences in school functioning would be manifest in standardized ratings by parents and teachers.

METHODS

Subjects

The characteristics of the subjects at birth, the intervention program, early assessment procedures, and outcomes through age 4 were described by Rauh et al.[17] Outcomes through age 7 were reported by Achenbach et al.[18] To summarize, the subjects were born in the Medical Center Hospital of Vermont between April 1980 and December 1981. With parental consent, infants who weighed less than 2250 g and were free of congenital anomalies and severe neurological defects were assigned to an experimental (LBWE) or control (LBWC) group by the toss of a coin. Prematching of subjects on important variables before assignment to treatment according to a randomized blocks design was precluded by the need to recruit and assign subjects as they were born. An NBW comparison group ($>$ 2800 g, $>$ 37 weeks' gestation) was recruited from babies born after each LBWC baby. The target sample sizes of 40 per group were based on the statistical power needed to detect medium effects of 8% of variance via analysis of variance[15] with probability .84 and on the N that could be expected to be available within the funding period. Follow-up studies beyond 2 years were not initially anticipated but were made possible by a series of small 2-year grants from the March of Dimes Birth Defects Foundation.

We administered 9-year tests to 24 LBWE, 31 LBWC, and 36 NBW children. The disparity in sample sizes reflects differences that existed from the intervention period, plus attrition caused by the deaths of 2 LBWE children; 1 LBWC who moved abroad; 2 LBWE, 3 LBWC, and 1 NBW who moved without forwarding addresses; 2 LBWE and 2 LBWC who were eliminated when they manifested cerebral palsy; 5 LBWE, 2 LBWC, and 4 NBW families who declined further participation; and 1 LBWE and 1 LBWC who were too busy for the most recent testing but continued participating in other ways. Subjects were tested if they lived in the United States, including one as far away as California and two in Colorado. Not counting the two children who died and the four who were excluded because they manifested cerebral palsy, we thus obtained age 9 tests on 86.7% of the 111 subjects. Table 1 summarizes the initial demographic and biomedical characteristics of the 91 subjects who were tested at age 9.

TABLE 1
Demographic and Biomedical Characteristics of Children With Age 9 Test Scores*

Characteristics	LBWE (n = 24)	LBWC (n = 31)	NBW (n = 36)
Biomedical			
Birth weight, g	1652.2 ± 402.1	1534.4 ± 389.8	3457.4 ± 420.5
Gestational age, wk†	32.3 ± 2.2	32.0 ± 2.8	39.9 ± 1.2
Apgar (5 min)	8.1 ± 1.2	7.8 ± 1.0	9.4 ± 0.6
Days hospitalized	38.9 ± 27.4	37.0 ± 26.1	3.4 ± 2.1
Medical complications‡	8.2 ± 3.1	9.6 ± 3.7	2.1 ± 1.9
Demographic			
Maternal age, y	28.1# ± 4.6	25.1 ± 4.7	26.6 ± 4.6
Maternal education, y	14.0** ± 2.5	12.4 ± 1.7	14.2 ± 2.8
Social class§	3.0** ± 1.1	3.9 ± 0.8	2.9 ± 1.1
Brazelton scores‖ (interactive)	4.5 ± 0.9	4.8 ± 0.5	2.8 ± 1.2
Female	63	36	47
Firstborn	67	61	56
Small for gestational age¶	17	26	0
Cesarean delivery	29	29	17
Very low birth weight (<1500 g)	42	45	0

* Quantitative data represent mean ± SD, and categorical data are given as percentages. LBWE, low birth weight experimental; LBWC, low birth weight control; NBW, normal birth weight.
† Determined by Dubowitz assessment.[27]
‡ Total number of antenatal, perinatal, and postnatal problems.[28]
§ Hollingshead Two-Factor Index of Social Position.[26]
‖ Interactive score from *A Priori Profiles for the Brazelton Neonatal Assessment Scale*[29] administered by a nurse trained to reliability.
¶ Less than 10th percentile on Colorado Intrauterine Growth Charts.[30]
# $P < .05$, LBWE > LBWC; if the number of tests were corrected for chance expectations, none would be considered significant.[35]
** $P < .01$, LBWE > LBWC; if the number of tests were corrected for chance expectations, none would be considered significant.[35]

Assessment Procedures

We will focus on assessment of cognitive development, academic achievement, and school behavior, although other forms of assessment have also been used, such as home observations during the first year, a nurse's ratings of mothers' responses to the program, mothers' self-reports, and ratings of preschool behavioral/emotional problems.[17,31]

Previously reported cognitive developmental measures have included the Bayley Scales of Infant Development[22] at ages 6, 12, and 24 months; the McCarthy Scales[23] at ages 3 and 4 years; and the Kaufman Assessment Battery for Children[24] at 7 years. To equalize length of development since conception, the infant and preschool tests were administered at ages adjusted for length of gestation. Thus, for example, when NBW children were tested 48 months after birth, children born 2 months early were tested 50 months after birth.

At ages 7 and 9 years, we geared testing to the school calendar rather than to gestation-adjusted age. We did this because the effects of school experience might outweigh the now relatively small gestational age differences. Since the children's birthdays were spread over 2 years, we tested them in the summer of the year of their ninth birthday. Because birthdays were distributed throughout the year and some children started school late, repeated grades, or were placed in transitional classes between kindergarten and first grade, they were not all at exactly the same point in their school careers. However, we analyzed the tests' age-based standard scores that are designed to correct for variations in the actual age of testing. We computed the standard scores on the basis of chronological age since birth. The mean postbirth age at testing was 9.0 years, SD = 0.3

The choice of measures was based on the quality of their standardization, reliability, evidence for validity, and continuity of subtests within the mental ages to be spanned. Achenbach et al[18] have detailed the reasons for using the Kaufman at ages 7 and 9. For testing the hypothesized differences between LBWE and LBWC children, the Kaufman has the advantage of providing achievement and cognitive measures standardized on the same national sample. The achievement subtests appropriate for 9-year-olds are designated as *Arithmetic; Faces & Places* (child names the fictional character, famous person, or well-known place shown pictorially); *Reading/Decoding* (child identifies letters and reads and pronounces words); *Reading/Understanding* (child acts out commands that are given in printed sentences); and *Riddles* (child infers a concept when given several of its characteristics). Age-based standard scores are computed for each of the five achievement subtests. A total Achievement score is computed from the mean of these standard scores.

The Kaufman assesses the child's overall cognitive level in terms of the MPC, which is similar to a Full-Scale IQ. The MPC is scored from scales designated as *Sequential Processing* (child solves problems by arranging input in sequential or serial order, eg, by repeating numbers spoken by the examiner) and *Simultaneous Processing* (child solves problems by integrating input simultaneously, eg, by analogic reasoning).

To provide a measure of receptive vocabulary, we also administered the Peabody Picture Vocabulary Test-Revised, Form L (PPVT-R),[32] which merely requests the child to point to a picture corresponding to a word spoken by the examiner. As with our earlier assessments, the tests were administered in the families' homes by a master's-level examiner who was not informed of the subjects' group membership. The same examiner performed all the 9-year tests except one in Colorado and one in Maryland, for which local examiners were hired.

To assess parents' and teachers' perceptions of the children, the parents completed the Child Behavior Checklist for Ages 4–18 (CBCL),[33] while teachers completed the analogous Teacher's Report Form (TRF).[34] Both forms include 118 items for scoring particular behavioral/emotional problems, plus two open-ended problem items and items for assessing competencies manifested by the child. The CBCL and TRF items differ somewhat according to the home vs school context in which the child is seen, but the 1991 scoring profiles enable both instruments to be scored in terms of a common set of eight syndromes.[33,34]

RESULTS

SES Differences

Despite randomized assignment, the LBWE group had a higher mean Hollingshead[26] social class score than the LBWC group. This difference did not result from differential attrition but occurred by chance in the initial assignment to treatment vs control conditions.[17] Among the 111 subjects having complete initial data, the mean Hollingshead scores were as follows: LBWE = 3.2, LBWC = 3.9, NBW = 3.0, with SD ranging from 0.9 to 1.2. For the 91 tested at age 9, the mean LBWC score was still 3.9, while the LBWE was 3.0 and the NBW was 2.9, with SD ranging from 0.8 to 1.1, as shown in Table 1. The LBWC SES was significantly lower than that of the other groups at both points ($P < .01$).

If we correct the 14 comparisons in Table 1 for the number expected to reach $P < .05$ by chance,[35] all three nominally significant differences on maternal age, SES, and education could be considered chance.[35] Nevertheless, we controlled for SES differences by covarying initial Hollingshead scores in the group comparisons. To control for a more current index of SES that might be associated with the children's test performance, we also covaried the number of years of maternal education at the age 9 testing in separate analyses of covariance (ANCOVAs) of the age 9 test scores. (ANCOVAs are analyses of variance in which a potentially confounding variable such as SES is statistically equalized ["covaried"] among groups in order to prevent it from affecting group differences in the dependent variable, such as test scores. The statistical package was SAS/STAT.[36])

Biomedical Vulnerability

There were no significant differences between the LBWE and LBWC groups in any of the initial biomedical variables listed in Table 1. Nevertheless, because the LBWC group had slightly less favorable scores than the LBWE group on several of these variables, we constructed a composite biomedical vulnerability index. We did this by performing a principal factor analysis of birth weight, 5-minute Apgar score, medical complications score, and classification as small for gestational age (ie, < 10th percentile on charts by Lubchenco et al.[30]) as described by Achenbach et al.[18] A 1 × 2 ANCOVA comparing the LBWE and LBWC subjects with initial SES as covariate showed no significant difference between the LBW groups on factor scores for biomedical vulnerability (F < 1). (In all ANCOVAs using one covariate, we first tested differences between the slopes of the dependent variable on the covariate. If slopes differed enough to reach $P = .20$, we used the separate slopes to adjust the dependent variable for the covariate.)

Even though the groups did not differ in biomedical vulnerability scores, we took the precaution of performing 1×2 ANCOVAs of test scores using the biomedical vulnerability score as a covariate. However, its inclusion as a covariate did not reduce the significance level of the differences between LBWE and LBWC groups on any age 9 test scores from the level obtained using only SES as a covariate. To keep the analyses as straightforward and as comparable as possible with our previous reports, we therefore present the ANCOVAs of test scores in which initial SES and maternal education at the age 9 testing served as the only covariates.

ANCOVAs of Test Scores

We first tested the regression slopes of each test score on the covariate of initial SES for the LBWE, LBWC, and NBW groups. The only analyses in which the slopes differed enough to reach even the $P = .20$ level were the Kaufman Arithmetic, Faces & Places, and Reading/Decoding subtests. As a precaution, we used ANCOVAs with separate slopes for each group in these three analyses.

Table 2 summarizes the 9-year test scores and F tests from 2 (sex) $\times$ 3 (group) ANCOVAs with Hollingshead SES score as the covariate. The only significant sex differences were higher scores by boys than girls on the Kaufman Arithmetic ($P = .026$), Riddles ($P = .046$), and Simultaneous ($P = .029$) scores. There were no significant interactions between sex and group. We present the mean scores for each group in tabular form for comparison with the results of similar analyses of earlier scores presented by Rauh et al[17] and Achenbach et al,[18] who also used initial Hollingshead SES as the covariate.

After adjustment for SES, the mean scores of the LBWE group were higher than those of the LBWC group on all 10 achievement and cognitive measures. A priori contrasts with 1,87 degrees of freedom showed that the superiority of the LBWE over the LBWC group was significant on the Kaufman Achievement, Arithmetic, Riddles, MPC, Sequential, and Simultaneous scales. If we correct for the 2 of 10 comparisons expected to reach $P < .05$ by chance, the Riddles and Sequential subtests were the most likely to reflect chance differences, because they yielded the smallest F values that reached $P < .05$.[35] The difference reached $P = .088$ on the PPVT-R. The LBWE group did not differ significantly from the NBW group on any measure (all $P \geq .168$).

The ANCOVAs using maternal education at the age 9 testing as the covariate yielded still larger differences favoring the LBWE over the LBWC group on all test scores. The following differences were now significant that had not been sig-

TABLE 2

Mean 9-Year Test Scores Adjusted by Analysis of Covariance for Socioeconomic Status*

Test Scores	LBWE (n = 24), Mean ± SD	LBWC (n = 31), Mean ± SD	NBW (n = 36), Mean ± SD	F(1,87)†	P
Kaufman Assessment Battery for Children					
Total Achievement	110.1 ± 14.8	99.7 ± 17.3	107.7 ± 16.1	5.46	.022
Arithmetic	105.5 ± 18.1	94.5 ± 12.8	111.2 ± 18.5	5.93	.018
Faces & Places	107.9 ± 15.0	104.2 ± 17.6	107.6 ± 13.5	<1.00	.405
Reading/Decoding	107.2 ± 14.5	103.8 ± 18.9	105.0 ± 15.2	1.37	.497
Reading/Understanding	105.2 ± 13.6	98.5 ± 18.2	102.3 ± 15.5	2.13	.148
Riddles	111.3 ± 13.8	103.4 ± 14.2	110.9 ± 14.6	4.39‡	.039
Mental Processing Composite	110.5 ± 11.7	97.2 ± 13.7	110.3 ± 13.7	11.87	<.001
Sequential	105.6 ± 11.5	96.6 ± 15.9	105.6 ± 12.6	5.01‡	.028
Simultaneous	109.8 ± 12.8	97.9 ± 12.6	111.8 ± 13.0	11.05	.001
Peabody Picture Vocabulary Test	108.5 ± 12.9	101.1 ± 17.1	105.9 ± 15.3	2.97	.088

* LBWE, low birth weight experimental; LBWC, low birth weight control; NBW, normal birth weight.

† A priori contrasts between LBWE and LBWC.

‡ These two tests were the most likely to be significant by chance, because their F values were the smallest that reached $P < .05$.[35]

nificant when initial SES was the covariate; PPVT, $P = .029$; Faces & Places, $P = .049$; and, at $P = .056$, Reading/Understanding. In addition, the F values increased and the P values decreased in all other comparisons, bringing the only remaining nonsignificant difference to $P = .105$ for Reading/Decoding. Thus, whether the covariate was the original SES measure computed from parental occupation and education at the child's birth or mother's concurrent educational level, the results clearly showed that the LBWE group performed significantly better on both the ability and achievement measures, after controlling for SES.

Long-term Developmental Course

Cognitive test scores. To depict the long-term developmental course of the children's cognitive performance, Fig 1 displays the mean cognitive test scores for the LBWE, LBWC, and NBW groups at each testing from 6 months to 9 years. The scores were obtained from the Bayley MDI at ages 6, 12, and 24 months; the McCarthy General Cognitive Index at ages 3 and 4 years; and the Kaufman MPC at ages 7 and 9 years.

To provide a common metric across the different tests, we converted the tests' standard scores to z scores at each testing, with the effects of SES differences controlled by ANCOVA. For example, the 6-month Bayley scores for all subjects shown in Fig 1 were converted to z scores with mean $= 0.0$ and SD $= 1.0$. To control for the initial SES differences, a 1×3 (LBWE vs LBWC vs NBW) ANCOVA was performed on the 6-month z scores, with initial SES as the covariate. Corrected for the covariate of SES, the z scores were then averaged within each group to obtain the mean 6-month score displayed for that group in Fig 1. Thus, whereas 0.0 was the z transformed mean of the 6-month Bayley scores for all the subjects, Fig 1 shows that the mean of the LBWC group was about 0.33 SD below the overall mean; the mean of the LBWE group was 0.07 below the overall mean; and the mean of the NBW group was 0.35 above the overall mean.

The sample included all 81 children who had the 6-month and 9-year tests and who missed no more than one test at ages 12 months through 7 years. For the 7 children who missed one test over this period, the mean of the z scores obtained on the tests preceding and following the missed test was used in place of the missing score. As Fig 1 shows, the small differences between the LBWE and LBWC groups at ages 6, 12, and 24 months were followed by a progressive divergence of their scores thereafter. Even from age 7 to 9 years, the scores of the LBWC group continued to drop in relation to those of the LBWE and NBW groups. By age 9, the LBWC mean was 0.51 SD below the overall mean, while the mean of the LBWE was 0.24 SD above the overall mean and the mean of the NBW was 0.29 SD above the overall mean.

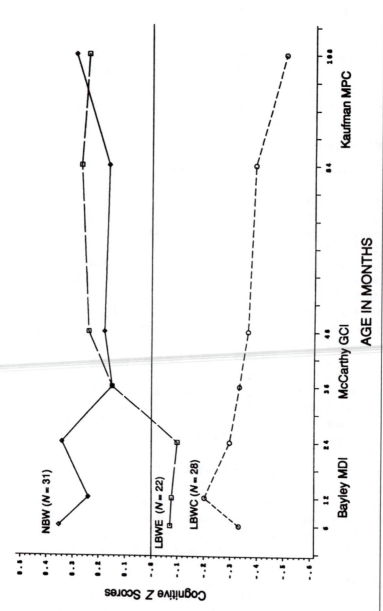

Figure 1 Cognitive scores converted to z scores at each testing for children who were tested at 6 months and 108 months and who missed no more than one test from age 6 to 108 months (z scores adjusted for initial socioeconomic status[26] by analysis of covariance). If a child missed a test, the mean of the child's z scores from the immediately preceding and following tests was used. NBW, normal birth weight; LBWE, low birth weight experimental; LBWC, low birth weight control; MDI, Mental Developmental Index; GCI, General Cognitive Index; MPC, Mental Processing Composite.

Achievement test scores. In addition to supporting the hypothesis that LBWE children would outperform LBWC children on cognitive measures at age 9, the results also supported the hypothesis that LBWE children would now score significantly higher than LBWC children on a standardized measure of academic achievement. To depict the developmental course of achievement, Fig 2 shows the mean Kaufman Achievement scores at ages 7 and 9, the only ages at which academic achievement was tested. Because the same test was used at both ages, there was no need to create a common metric by converting to *z* scores. Instead, the mean of the standard scores actually obtained on the Kaufman is displayed for all children in each group who were tested at both ages 7 and 9. Like most cognitive test scores, the Kaufman Achievement scores have a standardization mean = 100 and SD = 15. As was done for the cognitive test scores, the achievement scores in Fig 2 have been adjusted for differences in SES by ANCOVAs in which initial SES was the covariate.

As Fig 2 shows, there was a divergence between the LBWE and LBWC achievement scores from age 7 to 9. This was analogous to the divergence shown

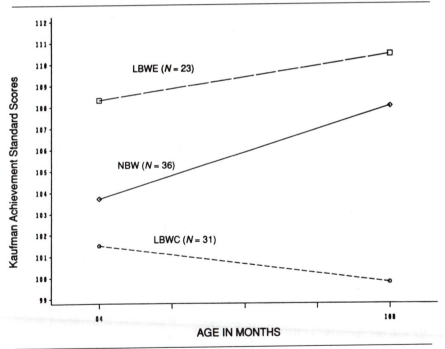

Figure 2 Kaufman Achievement test scores at ages 84 and 108 months, adjusted for initial socioeconomic status[26] by analysis of covariance. LBWE, low birth weight experimental; NBW, normal birth weight; LBWC, low birth weight control.

in Fig 1 for cognitive scores from age 3 to 9. At age 7, the LBWE children were already obtaining achievement scores about 7 points higher than the LBWC children (after adjustment for SES), although this difference did not reach the $P = .05$ level of significance. When tested in a 3 (LBWE vs LBWC vs NBW) $\times$ 2 (age 7 vs 9) repeated-measures ANCOVA, the age 7 mean of 108.3 obtained by the LBWE children differed at $P = .093$ from the age 7 mean of 101.5 obtained by the LBWC children. By age 9, the LBWE mean had risen to 110.4, while the LBWC mean had dropped to 99.8, a difference of 10.6 points that was now significant at $P = .009$. (The mean scores and P value differ slightly from those in Table 2, because Table 2 includes all 91 subjects who were tested at age 9, whereas the repeated-measures ANCOVA and Fig 2 include only the 90 subjects who were tested at both ages 7 and 9.)

Not only did the achievement scores of the LBWE children exceed those of the LBWC children, but, as Fig 2 shows, the LBWE scores also exceeded those of the NBW, albeit not significantly so. Although the divergence of z scores on the cognitive measures shown in Fig 1 reflects divergence relative to the mean of the subjects in our sample, the divergence of the achievement scores in Fig 2 is relative to the Kaufman's national standardization sample. Thus, the improvement in LBWE scores and the decline in LBWC scores from age 7 to 9 reflect not only the children's performance relative to that of our sample, but also relative to American schoolchildren in general.

The fact that the NBW children improved from an age 7 mean of 103.7 to an age 9 mean of 108.0 suggests that the divergence may be due at least partly to the more effective measurement of group differences in achievement at age 9 than at age 7. Because expectations for academic achievement are quite minimal at age 7, "floor effects" may limit the power of achievement tests to detect group differences. By age 9, however, the typical levels of achievement had advanced enough to permit better detection of group differences. The divergence in scores may therefore partly reflect the advancing precision of measurement from a point where each group was close to the mean of all the individual scores to a point where group divergences from the overall mean could be more accurately captured.

The same phenomenon may have contributed to the divergence between LBWE and LBWC cognitive scores. That is, although both groups were well below the NBW children during the first 2 years, differences between the LBWE and LBWC children increased as the possibilities for measuring higher order cognitive functions increased with developmental level. It should be remembered, however, that the declines in LBWC scores shown in Figs 1 and 2 do not reflect actual decrements in performance. The LBWC children were also continuing to advance on both the cognitive and achievement measures, but the divergence shows that their *rate* of advance lagged increasingly behind that of the LBWE children.

Effects Associated With MITP vs SES

In all the foregoing comparisons, we used ANCOVA to adjust test scores for differences in SES. After adjustment for SES, all comparisons showed better performance by LBWE than LBWC children, and most of the differences were statistically significant. The evidence for the effect of the MITP on the performance of LBW children does not necessarily mean that SES had no effect, however. Other research has shown that the general quality of the environment associated with SES can have significant effects on long-term outcomes for children who have biomedical risk factors such as LBW.[37]

To quantify the relative effects of the MITP and SES on the test scores of the LBW children, we performed multiple regressions of each age 9 cognitive and achievement test score on the two predictor variables of MITP experimental vs control condition and concurrent maternal education in terms of years of schooling, which is apt to be the SES measure most closely related to age 9 test performance. Because 5 LBWE mothers but only 1 LBWC mother had more than 16 years of education, these 6 cases were omitted so that the regression slopes would be based on the same portion of the education distribution in both groups. We computed the percent of variance in each test score that was independently accounted for by MITP condition and by maternal education, with the effects of the other predictor variable partialled out. Because the NBW group was not relevant to these analyses, we included only the 19 LBWE and 30 LBWC children tested at age 9 whose mothers had 16 years of education or less.

Among the Kaufman scores that showed significant effects of the MITP in Table 2, the experimental vs control condition accounted for much more variance in cognitive scores than did maternal education differences. In the Kaufman MPC scores, MITP condition accounted for 19% of the variance, which is considered to be a medium effect according to Cohen's[25] criteria, while SES accounted for only 2% of the variance. (According to Cohen's criteria for multiple regression, effects that account for 2% to 13% of variance are small, 13% to 26% are medium, and $\geq$ 26% are large.) In the Kaufman Sequential and Simultaneous scores, MITP condition accounted for 11% and 16% of the variance, respectively, both much larger than the effects of SES, which accounted for 1% and 8% of the variance, respectively.

In the achievement scores, on the other hand, the MITP accounted for less variance than maternal education. For the Total Achievement and Arithmetic scores, the MITP accounted for 7% of the variance, compared with 17% and 11%, respectively, for maternal education. On Riddles, the other achievement subtest that showed a significant effect in Table 2, the MITP accounted for 5% of the variance in the multiple regression, compared with 14% accounted for by maternal education. Thus, even though the MITP appeared to have a much greater impact than SES differences on the cognitive performance of LBW children at age 9, SES still appeared to have relatively large effects on the specific knowledge tapped by the achievement tests.

Parent and Teacher Ratings

Behavioral/emotional problems and competencies are likely to be affected by stresses in a child's life, as well as by factors such as SES. In our analyses of the CBCL and TRF scores, we therefore controlled for the marital status of the parents (married or widowed vs separated or divorced), and for family problems reported by parents on the 12-item Family Assessment Device,[38] as well as for SES. These three variables were entered as covariates in ANCOVAs of CBCL and TRF competence and problem scale scores for the 79 LBW and NBW children who had complete data on all the parent ratings and the 75 who also had complete data on the teacher ratings. The importance of family problems was indicated by significant associations of the Family Assessment covariate with 11 of the 15 CBCL scales and 11 of the 17 TRF scales.

Socioeconomic status was significantly associated with only the CBCL Social and Total Competence scales and the TRF Academic Performance scale. Parental marital status was significantly associated with the CBCL Activities, Social, and Total Competence scales, but not with any TRF scales after the effects of SES and family problems were covaried out. The number of significant associations of SES and marital status with the rating scales did not exceed chance expectations.[35]

On both the CBCL and TRF scales that directly tap academic performance in school, LBWE children obtained significantly better scores than LBWC children ($P = .002$ on the CBCL School scale; $P = .006$ on the TRF Academic Performance scale). The differences found on the Kaufman scores (which were not known to the parents or teachers) were thus manifested in school performance that was evident to both parents and teachers. Although SES was also associated with the TRF Academic Performance scale, it represented a small effect (5% of variance), compared with the medium effect (8%) represented by the LBWE vs LBWC condition, according to Cohen's[25] criteria for effect sizes in ANCOVA. Furthermore, the LBWE children obtained significantly higher scores than the LBWC children on TRF ratings of how much the child was learning ($P = .010$) and on the total adaptive score computed by summing ratings on four adaptive characteristics ($P = .051$). Teachers also reported significantly fewer problems for LBWE than LBWC children on the TRF attention problems syndrome ($P = .002$) and on the Total Problems scale ($P = .043$). On all the remaining TRF adaptive and problem scores, LBWE children received more favorable ratings from teachers than did LBWC children. Although these specific differences were not significant, a binomial test was significant at $P < .001$ for the consistent superiority of the LBWE over the LBWC children on all 17 TRF comparisons (academic performance, four adaptive characteristics, sum of these four, eight syndromes, Internalizing, Externalizing, and total problems). Other than the School scale, the remaining CBCL scales did not show significant or consistent differences between groups.

As another index of school functioning, we compared LBW children who were in the grade expected for their age with those who were behind because they started school late (0 LBWE, 3 LBWC), repeated grades (5 LBWE, 12 LBWC), or were placed in transitional classes between kindergarten and first grade (2 LBWE, 2 LBWC). After making the SES distributions more similar by excluding children whose mothers had more than 16 years of education, the percentage of LBWC children who were below the expected grade was nearly twice as great as for LBWE children (53.6% vs 27.3%; $\chi^2 = 3.50$, $P = .061$). The significance level improved to $P = .057$ when mothers with more than 16 years of education were included. Nine of the LBWE vs 21 of the LBWC children had received any kind of special educational services (eg, early essential education, Head Start, tutoring, special class placement; $\chi^2 = 4.99$, $P < .05$). At the age 9 assessment, the grades completed were as follows: LBWE, 7 had completed grade 1, 17 grade 3, mean grade $= 2.71$; LBWC, 1 grade 1, 15 grade 2, 15 grade 3, mean grade $= 2.45$; NBW, 1 grade 1, 10 grade 2, 25 grade 3, mean grade $= 2.67$.

Comparisons Between Birth Weights ≤ 1,500 and > 1,500 Grams

Because pediatricians may be especially interested in children weighing 1500 g or less at birth, we compared outcomes for LBWE and LBWC children weighing 1500 g or less at birth vs those weighing more than 1500 g. We did this by performing 2 (LBWE vs LWBC) × 2 (≤ 1500 vs > 1500 g) × 2 (sex) ANCOVAs on the Kaufman MPC and Achievement scales and all CBCL and TRF scales.

The mean scores tended to be more favorable for children weighing more than 1500 g than for those weighing 1500 g or less on most scales within both the LBWE and LBWC groups. However, the main effect of birth weight was not significant in any analysis. Furthermore, only four interactions between birth weight and other variables were significant at $P < .005$. As this was fewer than the nine expected by chance in the 105 tests of interactions, they were likely to be chance findings. Although larger samples might yield significant differences between children weighing 1500 g or less vs more than 1500 g, the significant differences that we obtained between LBWE and LBWC children were not likely to have been affected by interactions with these ranges of birth weights.

DISCUSSION

The results demonstrated a significant divergence between the achievement test scores of 9-year-old LBWE and LBWC children that was analogous to the divergence between their cognitive test scores that first became significant at age 3. As depicted in Figs 1 and 2, both types of scores initially showed no significant differences between LBWE and LBWC children. Thereafter, however, the scores of the LBWE children rose while those of the LBWC children declined. The decline in the cognitive and achievement scores of the LBWC children does not mean that they lost ground or regressed, but that their *rate* of development fell behind that of the LBWE children. Figure 1 also shows that the LBWE children's cognitive development caught up to that of the NBW children at age 3 and did not differ significantly from that of the NBW children thereafter. Figure 2 shows that the total academic achievement scores obtained by the LBWE children were slightly ahead of those obtained by the NBW children at ages 7 and 9 and that the scores of both groups became significantly higher than those of the LBWC children at age 9. Furthermore, by age 9, the proportion of LBWE children who had advanced at the expected rate in school was greater than the proportion of LBWC children ($P = .061$). By all these measures, then, the LBWE group was progressing more rapidly than the LBWC group 9 years after the MITP neonatal intervention.

Although the LBW children had been randomly assigned to the experimental and control conditions, the mean SES of the LBWE children was higher than that of the LBWC children. This difference occurred by chance in the initial randomization and has persisted throughout the longitudinal reassessments. To take account of this difference, all our analyses, as well as Figs 1 and 2, have compared LBWE and LBWC children after controlling for SES. However, we also presented findings on the magnitude of effects attributable to SES relative to those attributable to the intervention. For the age 9 cognitive test scores, the effects attributable to the intervention ranged from 11% to 19% of the variance, compared with 2% to 7% attributable to SES differences, measured in terms of concurrent maternal education. For the age 9 achievement scores, however, the effects attributable to SES differences ranged from 11% to 17% of the variance, compared with 5% to 7% attributable to the MITP. Thus, at age 9, the intervention's effect on the specific kinds of knowledge tapped by achievement tests, though significant, was less than the effect of SES differences.

As academic achievement becomes increasingly dependent on the child's own cognitive prowess, it is possible that effects associated with SES will decline relative to effects associated with the intervention. This possibility is suggested by the finding that SES differences and the MITP both accounted for very similar percentages of variance in the age 4 cognitive scores (8.1% for SES, 9.8% for the intervention) but that these percentages were 2% and 19%, respectively, in the age 9 Kaufman MPC. The effect associated with the MITP thus appeared to increasingly outweigh the effect associated with SES as the LBW children advanced to higher levels of development.

By age 9, the cognitive advantage of the LBWE over the LBWC children was 13.3 points on the Kaufman (110.5 vs 97.2; Table 2). This difference amounted to 1.05 SD, based on the mean of the standard deviations for the two groups. According to Cohen's[25] criteria, this is a very large effect. The difference between the total Kaufman Achievement scores was 10.4 points (110.1 vs 99.7; Table 2), a difference equal to 0.65 SD. Although smaller than the cognitive difference, the difference between achievement scores also constituted a large effect according to Cohen's criteria. Furthermore, parent CBCL and teacher TRF ratings also showed significantly better school functioning for the LBWE and LBWC children in terms of academic performance and behavior problems. The highly significant difference on the TRF attention problems syndrome is especially important, because attention problems so often instigate referral for treatment or special education.

Comparisons with Other Studies

We know of no other published outcome studies of experimental interventions for LBW children that have continued so long after the intervention ended. There is thus no basis for determining whether other interventions were followed by such long-term differences between experimental and control groups. Unlike several interventions with low-SES, predominately minority children,[11-13] ours did not show significant effects on test scores obtained shortly after the intervention ended. Although the mean Bayley MDI scores of our LBWE children were higher than those of the LBWC children at 6, 12, and 24 months, the largest difference reached only $P < .10$ at 24 months.

The effects of other interventions on the Bayley scores of very-low-SES children demonstrate that it is feasible to improve the infant test scores of such children. It is possible, however, that our failure to find significant effects on Bayley scores was due to the more favorable perinatal conditions and home environments of our subjects than of the low-SES, minority children in the other studies. In contrast to the high proportion of very-low-SES, teenage, unmarried mothers in the other studies, the mothers in our study were from all five of Hollingshead's SES levels, only three were in their teens, and all mothers of children tested at age 9 were married when their child was born. Because most of the children in our study were thus likely to have better home environments than the control children in the studies reporting significant effects on the Bayley, the aspects of functioning measured by the Bayley may not have been as susceptible to influence by an intervention. In other words, the other interventions may have improved Bayley scores by compensating for very poor environments.

A study of mainly lower-middle-SES families with few unmarried or teenage mothers demonstrated significant increases in Bayley scores with age for LBW babies receiving one of two experimental interventions.[8] However, this study did not demonstrate significant superiority of Bayley scores in either intervention group over the LBW control group at termination. At a 1-year follow-up of 59% of the children, one of the LBW intervention groups obtained significantly higher Bayley motor scores than the LBW control group.[39] Significant effects on age 3 IQ were found immediately following the massive 3-year intervention provided by the Infant Health and Development Program,[14,15] which was aimed at overcoming serious environmental deprivation. This intervention was also followed by significantly more favorable ratings on the Child Behavior Checklist for Ages 2–3.[31,40]

Adding our findings to those of the previous studies suggests the following picture: Among LBW children whose home environments were quite substandard, Bayley tests administered shortly after interventions yielded significantly higher scores for experimental than for control groups. In our study and another one[8] that included many children living in more standard environments, however, interventions did not immediately produce significantly better Bayley scores in the experimental than the control groups. The Infant Health and Development Program[14,15] demonstrated that 3-year IQs and behavior problem scores can be improved among low-SES LBW children, at least immediately following the intervention. Our findings suggest that IQ, achievement, and behavior problem scores could be improved over a much longer period after an intervention for LBW children living in more standard environments. It is to be hoped that additional long-term outcome studies will be done to test interventions both for children who suffer the dual risks of LBW and substandard environments and for children who suffer only one of these risks.

Mechanisms of the MITP Effects

The MITP aimed to facilitate the development of LBW children by changing mothers' attitudes, sensitivity, and behavior toward their children. Such effects on mothers were expected, in turn, to establish more favorable transactional patterns that would facilitate the children's subsequent development. The hypothesized effects on mothers' attitudes were evidenced by significantly more favorable scores for maternal self-confidence, satisfaction with the mothering role, and maternal perceptions of infant temperament among LBWE than LBWC mothers.[17] Associations between early maternal behavior and later LBWE outcomes were indicated by significant correlations between both the quality of mothering and mothers' receptivity to the MITP, as rated by the nurse who worked with the mothers, and subsequent test scores from 6 to 48 months.[17]

It is difficult to prove precisely how the long-term development of the LBWE children may have been facilitated by the MITP. However, the MITP appears to have facilitated development by establishing more favorable mother-child transaction patterns than would otherwise emerge for LBW children. The "sleeper effect," whereby test scores showed increasing differences after age 3, suggests that any earlier improvements in the children's behavior were not detectable in the types of functions measured by the Bayley scales. The increasing LBWE-LBWC differences on cognitive tests and then on achievement tests implies that (a) more advanced test items were more sensitive to the affected functions; or (b) there was a cumulative effect on development, such that initial differences in functioning led to progressively greater disparities in cognitive skills and the acquisition of information; or (c) both (a) and (b) could have contributed. Whether (a), (b), or both explain the sleeper effect, large long-term effects on cognitive development are especially valuable, whether or not early functions are also measurably affected.

CONCLUSIONS AND IMPLICATIONS

Nine years after a relatively inexpensive intervention to improve mother-infant transactions, LBWE children obtained significantly more favorable scores than LBWC children on cognitive and achievement tests, as well as on standardized parent and teacher ratings of school functioning. The strongest differences in ratings were on scales tapping academic performance and the attention problems syndrome, after controlling for SES, family problems, and parental marital status. The intervention group had also been promoted more rapidly than the control group in school ($P = .061$) and had fewer special services.

Although SES effects were partialled out of the analyses of the other variables, SES also contributed to differences in performance, especially on achievement tests. The effects associated with the intervention were much larger than the effects associated with SES on the cognitive scores, but the achievement tests showed the opposite pattern. As higher levels of achievement are likely to depend more on the children's own cognitive prowess, it is possible that achievement scores will show increasing effects associated with the intervention relative to the effects associated with SES. In parent CBCL and teacher TRF ratings that showed significant differences between LBWE and LBWC children, SES was significantly associated only with teacher ratings of Academic Performance, and this effect of SES was smaller than the effect of the intervention condition.

The progression from no significant LBWE vs LBWC differences in early cognitive and achievement scores to significant differences in diverse measures of school-related functioning indicates the need for long-term follow-up to evaluate properly the power of behavioral interventions to compensate for biological risks. The findings also indicate that important long-term effects may be produced by a low-cost intervention that can be provided by personnel already employed by neonatal intensive care units. It should be feasible to apply the MITP to LBW infants in many hospitals, as well as to infants having other potentially handicapping conditions. Additional long-term outcome studies are needed to test the robustness of our findings under varying conditions.

ACKNOWLEDGMENTS

This research was supported by March of Dimes Birth Defects Foundation grants 12-88 and 12-186, National Institute of Mental Health grant MH-32924, and a biomedical research support grant from the University of Vermont College of Medicine.

We are grateful to Drs David C. Howell, Stephanie H. McConaughy, and Catherine Stanger for their help.

REFERENCES

1. Davie R, Butler N, Goldstein H. *From Birth to Seven: The Second Report of the National Child Development Study.* London, England: Longman; 1972
2. Zachau-Christiansen B, Mednick BR. Twelve-year follow-up status of low birthweight infants. In: Schulsinger F, Mednick SA, Knop J, eds. *Longitudinal Research: Methods and Uses in Behavioral Science.* Boston, MA: Martinus Nijhoff; 1981
3. Leib SA, Benfield G, Guidubaldi J. Effects of early intervention and stimulation on the preterm infant. *Pediatrics.* 1980;66:83–90
4. Scarr-Salapatek S, Williams ML. The effects of early stimulation on low birthweight infants. *Child Dev.* 1983;44:94–101
5. Solkoff N, Weintraub D, Yaffe S, Blase B. Effects of handling on the subsequent development of premature infants. *Dev Psychol.* 1969;1:765–768
6. Leifer AD, Leiderman PN, Barnett CR, Williams JA. Effects of mother-infant separation on maternal attachment behavior. *Child Dev.* 1972;43:1203–1218
7. Minde K, Shosenberg N, Marton P, Thompson J, Ripley J. Self help groups in a premature nursery: a controlled evaluation. *J. Pediatr.* 1980;96:933–940
8. Barrera ME, Rosenbaum PL, Cunningham CE. Early home intervention with low-birth-weight infants and their parents. *Child Dev.* 1986;57:20–23
9. Barrera M, Cunningham C, Rosenbaum P. Low birthweight and home intervention strategies: preterm infants. *J Dev Behav Pediatr.* 1986;7:361–366
10. Bormwich RM, Parmelee AH. An intervention program for pre-term infants. In: Field TM, Sostek AM, Goldberg S, Shuman HH, eds. *Infants Born at Risk: Behavior and Development.* New York, NY: SP Medical & Scientific Books; 1979
11. Field TM, Widmayer SM, Stringer S, Ignatoff E. Teenage lower-class black mothers

and their preterm infants: an intervention and developmental follow-up. *Child Dev.* 1980;51:426–436

12. Resnick MB, Eyler FD, Nelson RM, Eitzman DV, Bucciarelli RL. Developmental intervention for low birthweight infants: improved early developmental outcome. *Pediatrics.* 1987;80:68–74

13. Ross GS. Home intervention for premature infants of low-income families. *Am J Orthopsychiatry.* 1984;54:263–270

14. Infant Health and Development Program. Enhancing the outcomes of low-birthweight, premature infants. *JAMA.* 1990;263:3035–3042

15. Ramey CT, Bryant DM, Wasik BH, Sparling JJ, Fendt KH, LaVange LM. Infant Health and Development Program for low birth weight, premature infants: program elements, family participation, and child intelligence. *Pediatrics.* 1991;89:454–465

16. Barrera ME, Kitching KJ, Cunningham CC, Doucet D, Rosenbaum PL. A 3-year early home intervention follow-up study with low birthweight infants and their parents. *Top Early Child Special Educ.* 1990;10:14–28

17. Rauh VA, Achenbach TM, Nurcombe B, Howell CT, Teti DM. Minimizing adverse effects of low birthweight: four-year results of an intervention program. *Child Dev.* 1988;59:544–553

18. Achenbach TM, Phares V, Howell CT, Rauh VA, Nurcombe B. Seven-year outcome of the Vermont intervention program for low-birthweight infants. *Child Dev.* 1990;61:1672–1681

19. Nurcombe B, Howell DC, Rauh VA, Teti DM, Ruoff P, Brennan J. An intervention program for mothers of low-birthweight infants: preliminary results. *J Am Acad Child Psychiatry.* 1984;23:319–325

20. Rauh VA, Nurcombe B, Achenbach T, Howell C. The Mother-Infant Transaction Program: the content and implications of an intervention for the mothers of low-birthweight infants. *Clin Perinatol.* 1990;17:31–45

21. Sameroff AJ, Chandler MJ. Reproductive risk and the continuum of caretaking casualty. In: Horowitz FD, Hetherington M, Scarr-Salapatek S, Siegel G, eds. *Review of Child Development Research.* Chicago, IL: University of Chicago Press; 1975;4

22. Bayley N. *Bayley Scales of Infant Development.* New York, NY: Psychological Corporation, 1969

23. McCarthy D. *McCarthy Scales of Children's Abilities.* New York, NY: Psychological Corporation; 1972

24. Kaufman AS, Kaufman NL. *Kaufman Assessment Battery for Children.* Circle Pines, MN: American Guidance Service; 1983

25. Cohen J. *Statistical Power Analysis for the Behavioral Sciences.* 2nd ed. New York, NY: Academic Press; 1988

26. Hollingshead AB. *Two-Factor Index of Social Position.* New Haven, CT: Yale University, Dept of Sociology; 1957

27. Dubowitz LM, Dubowitz V, Goldberg C. Clinical assessment of gestational age in the newborn. *J. Pediatr.* 1970;77:1–10

28. Zax M, Sameroff AJ, Babigian HM. Birth outcome in the offspring of mentally disturbed women. *Am. J Psychiatry.* 1977;47:218–230

29. Adamson L, Als H, Tronick E, Brazelton TB. *A Priori Profiles for the Brazelton Neonatal Assessment Scale.* Boston, MA: Child Development Unit, Boston Children's Hospital; 1975

30. Lubchenco LO, Hansman C, Boyd E. Intrauterine growth in length and head circumference as estimated from live births at gestational ages from 26–42 weeks. *J Pediatr.* 1966;37:403–422

31. Achenbach TM, Edelbrock C, Howell CT. Empirically based assessment of the behavioral/emotional problems of 2–3-year-old children. *J Abnorm Child Psychol* 1987;15:629–650

32. Dunn LM, Dunn LM. *Peabody Picture Vocabulary Test-Revised.* Circle Pines, MN: American Guidance Service; 1981

33. Achenbach TM. *Manual for the Child Behavior Checklist/4–18 and 1991 Profile.* Burlington, VT: University of Vermont, Dept of Psychiatry; 1991

34. Achenbach TM, *Manual for the Teacher's Report Form and 1991 Profile.* Burlington, VT: University of Vermont, Dept of Psychiatry; 1991

35. Sakoda JM, Cohen BH, Beall G. Test of significance for a series of statistical tests. *Psychol Bull.* 1954;51:172–175

36. SAS Institute. *SAS/STAT User's Guide.* Release 6.03 edition. Cary, NC: SAS Institute; 1988

37. Werner E, Smith RS. *Kauai's Children Come of Age.* Honolulu, HI: University of Hawaii Press; 1977

38. Byles JA, Byrne C, Boyle MH, Offord DA. Ontario child health study: reliability and validity of the general functioning subscale of the McMaster Family Assessment Device. *Fam Process.* 1988;27:97–104

39. Barrera ME. Stability of early home intervention effects with preterm infants: one-year follow-up. *Early Child Dev Care.* 1987;27:635–649

40. Achenbach TM. *Manual for the Child Behavior Checklist/2–3 and 1992 Profile.* Burlington, VT: University of Vermont, Dept of Psychiatry; 1992